AF834639

Taite R. Anderson, DDS

THE ART OF ORAL SURGERY

edra
PUBLISHING

This edition first published 2024

©2024 Edra Publishing US LLC – All rights reserved

ISBN 9781962679251
eISBN 9781962679442

Editor: Paola Sammaritano, Edra S.p.A.

The rights of translation, electronic storage, reproduction, or total or partial adaptation by any means (including microfilms and photostatic copies), are reserved for all countries. No part of this publication may be reproduced, stored in a retrieval system, or transmitted in any form or by any means, electronic, mechanical, photocopying, recording, or otherwise, without permission in writing from the publisher.

Knowledge and best practice in this field are constantly changing: As new research and experience broaden our knowledge, changes in practice, treatment, and drug therapy may become necessary or appropriate. Readers are advised to check the most current information provided (i) or procedures featured (ii) by the manufacturer of each product to be administered, to verify the recommended dose or formula, the method and duration of administration, and contraindications. It is the responsibility of the practitioners, relying on their own experience and knowledge of the patient, to make diagnoses, to determine dosages and the best treatment for each individual patient, and to take all appropriate safety precautions. To the fullest extent of the law, neither the publisher nor the editors assume any liability for any injury and/or damage to persons or property arising out of or related to any use of the material contained in this book.

This publication contains the author's opinions and is intended to provide precise and accurate information. The processing of the texts, even if taken care of with scrupulous attention, cannot entail specific responsibilities for the author and/or the publisher for any errors or inaccuracies.

Readers should be aware that websites listed in this work may have changed or disappeared between when this work was written and when it is read.

The publisher has made every effort to obtain and cite the exact sources of the illustrations. If in some cases he has not been able to find the right holders, he is available to remedy any inadvertent omissions or errors in the references cited.

Product or corporate names may be trademarks or registered trademarks and are used only for identification and explanation without intent to infringe. All registered trademarks mentioned belong to their legitimate owners.

edra
PUBLISHING

Edra Publishing US LLC
3309 Northlake Boulevard,
Suite 203,
Palm Beach Gardens,
FL 33403
EIN: 844113980

info@edrapublishing.com
www.edrapublishing.com

Printed in May 2024 by "Erregiemme printing" S.r.l.

TAITE R ANDERSON

To my Lindsey, Ellyana, Silas, and Micah.

You are my compass, my anchor, and the wind that fills my sails through this journey of life. So much life has happened between the covers of this book. Thank you for supporting me and believing in me.

All my love,

Taite (Dad)

TABLE OF CONTENTS

INTRODUCTION

The Art of Oral Surgery is a curated gallery of images and text, each piece chosen to represent something different. I personally created each piece of visual art to enrich the ideas in the text. While writing this book was mostly enjoyable, I found the greatest joy in drawing, painting, photographing, editing and illustrating thoughts and concepts in ways that resonate with the reader. A curator doesn't try to capture *all* art in a single gallery. He chooses different pieces for different reasons. Likewise, I have chosen to write and illustrate chapters in different ways. In the first part of the book, I used my creative perspective to frame complex topics in pictures. I am a visual learner and needed to work through these big concepts visually to teach them better. The rest of the book is more scientific and technique oriented. With our background and training, I thought trying to apply an artistic perspective to the technical aspects would lose the nature of the information and wouldn't be helpful. The later chapters have more annotated surgical photography and illustrations.

As you read through the book, I invite you to ask yourself these questions: Why did he put this picture here? What is it telling me? As a picture is worth a thousand words, I hope each picture communicates more to you than what I could write between the covers of this book.

Writing this book pushed me to explore and dive into what I do, what I was taught, what I have learned, and what I have been challenged to unlearn—and why. This book is a humble offering of my thoughts and practices, and what seems to work in my hands today.

I have been writing this book for a few years. My work is oral and maxillofacial surgery, and my passion is seeing people grow and experience life's greatest beauty. For nearly 20 years, I have studied and learned everything I can about oral surgery. While dental school and residency formed a strong foundation, much of what I do and how I do it has evolved and developed by paying attention to what works and what doesn't in my private practice. Some of my best teachers have been course instructors, authors, patients, team members, colleagues and, of course, failure. (Failure is one of the best teachers. Just be careful not to learn too much at a time.) My drive to learn everything I can, from anything or anyone, all the time, is fueled by an insatiable curiosity. How? Why? These are two of my favorite questions, and I ask them over and over, to the point I sometimes drive people crazy. But asking these questions forces me to look beyond the obvious and invites me to explore possibilities.

My wife and I love to walk the beach and pick rocks at our home on Lake Michigan. It gives us a sense of awe at the grandeur of our universe. It slows us down in our fast-paced lives. It's a good day when we find a Petoskey stone. They look dull and inconspicuous amidst the other rocks on the beach, but with a little effort, they come to life again in a new way. I like to polish and ponder these 350-million-year-old pieces of fossilized coral. I always keep one in the left pocket of my jeans. Its smooth, soft edges ground me in reality. It is comfortable and inspiring to me, so I keep coming back to it. I see each stone as a unique piece of art that has been in the process of being created for hundreds of millions of years. And when I find one, I do my part to bring out its beauty.

In my journey and study of Petoskey stones, I have found peace in knowing that some art is never quite finished. What you are about to read may resonate with you. Some may say "I get it." Others may say, like the stone, "It isn't quite finished. It needs more polishing." And that's OK with me. I welcome your comments, because I am on a journey to develop ideas that make surgery and art more accessible while also bringing out their beauty. I want to hear your thoughts and input, your inspiration and challenges. If you can, please send me an email once you've finished the book and let me know your thoughts. That tells me the art brought some joy to you or that the limitations of the book brought uncertainty. Either way, I want to know. You can reach me at theartoforalsurgery@gmail.com

This polished Petoskey stone comes with me almost everywhere I go.

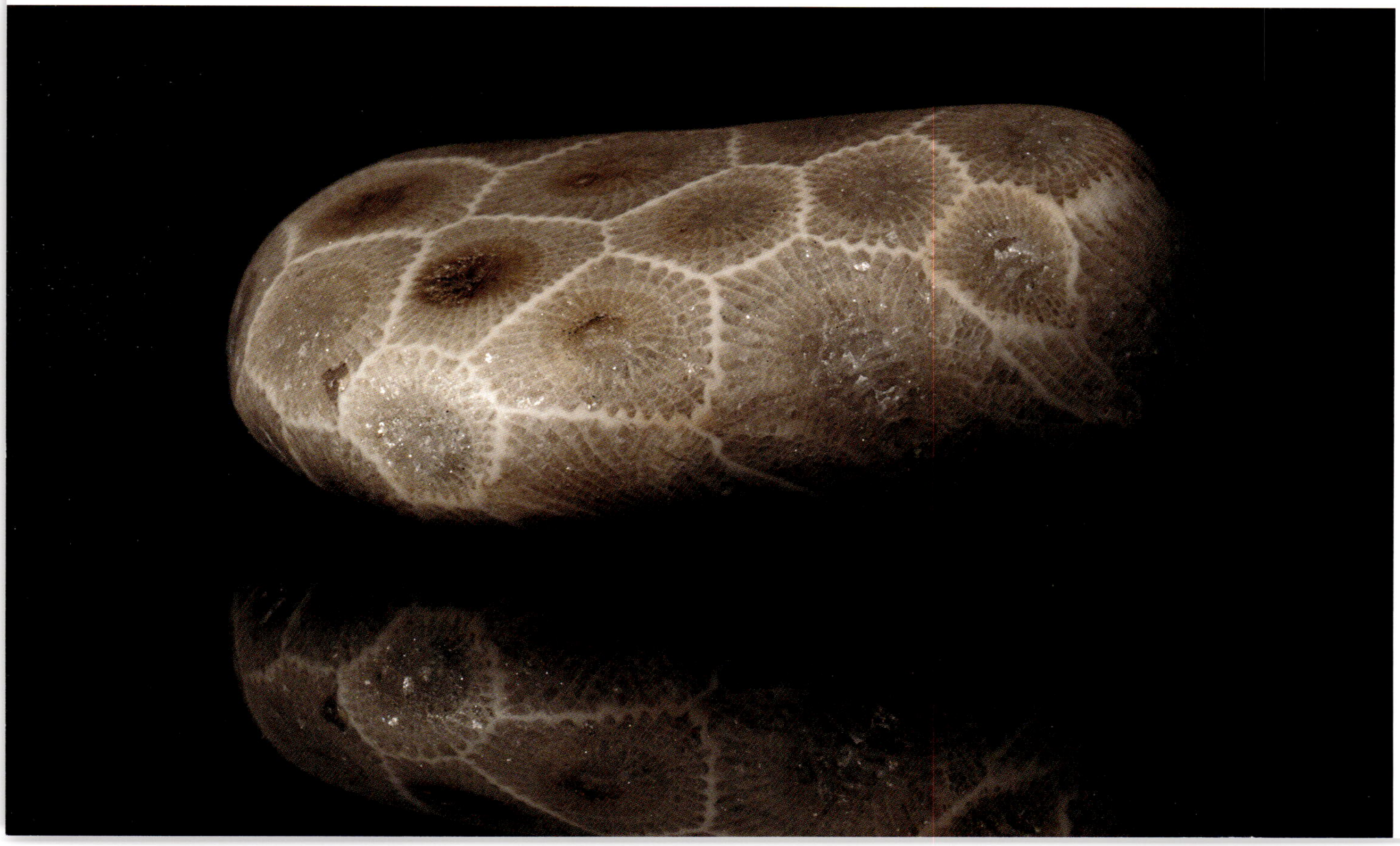

Pictures and illustrations

Bound by the limitations of ink on paper, I used annotations and markings to breathe life into the pictures. I hope the images offer you a helpful, dynamic and realistic perspective of surgery. The pictures in this book were picked from thousands of shots I took during routine surgeries in my solo private practice. I hope they portray an accessible and inspiring perspective. One thing I have come to love about modern art is how it calls out the beauty in the everyday moments of our everyday lives. That inspires me. I hope it inspires you too.

Anyone who has photographed their own work knows photography exposes flaws, and I am certainly not perfect. Some of the pictures show that. They are real pictures. I invite you to look for the messages in the pictures. Look for new insight on the art of oral surgery.

Citations

Before writing this book, I would rarely remember the source of what I learned. If the information seemed true and helpful, I would try to adopt it. The information in this book comes mainly from my experience, which was built on the shoulders of giants, so many brilliant minds and countless hours of research and thought. I wish I could cite the sources of all the information. Most of it seems like common knowledge to me now. There are many references throughout, but I am unable to comprehensively cite the sources of all the information in this text.

I hope you enjoy *The Art of Oral Surgery*.

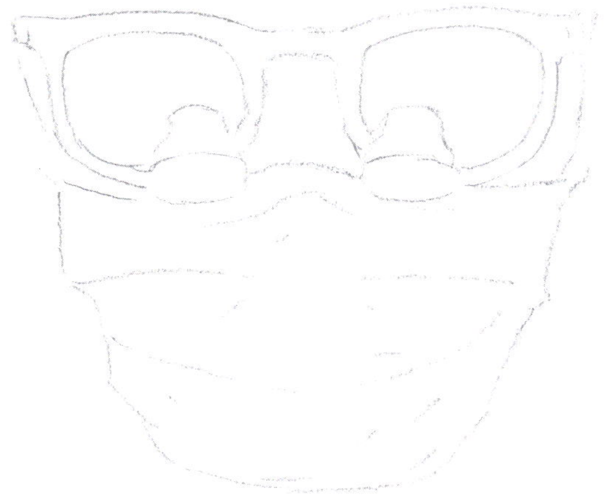

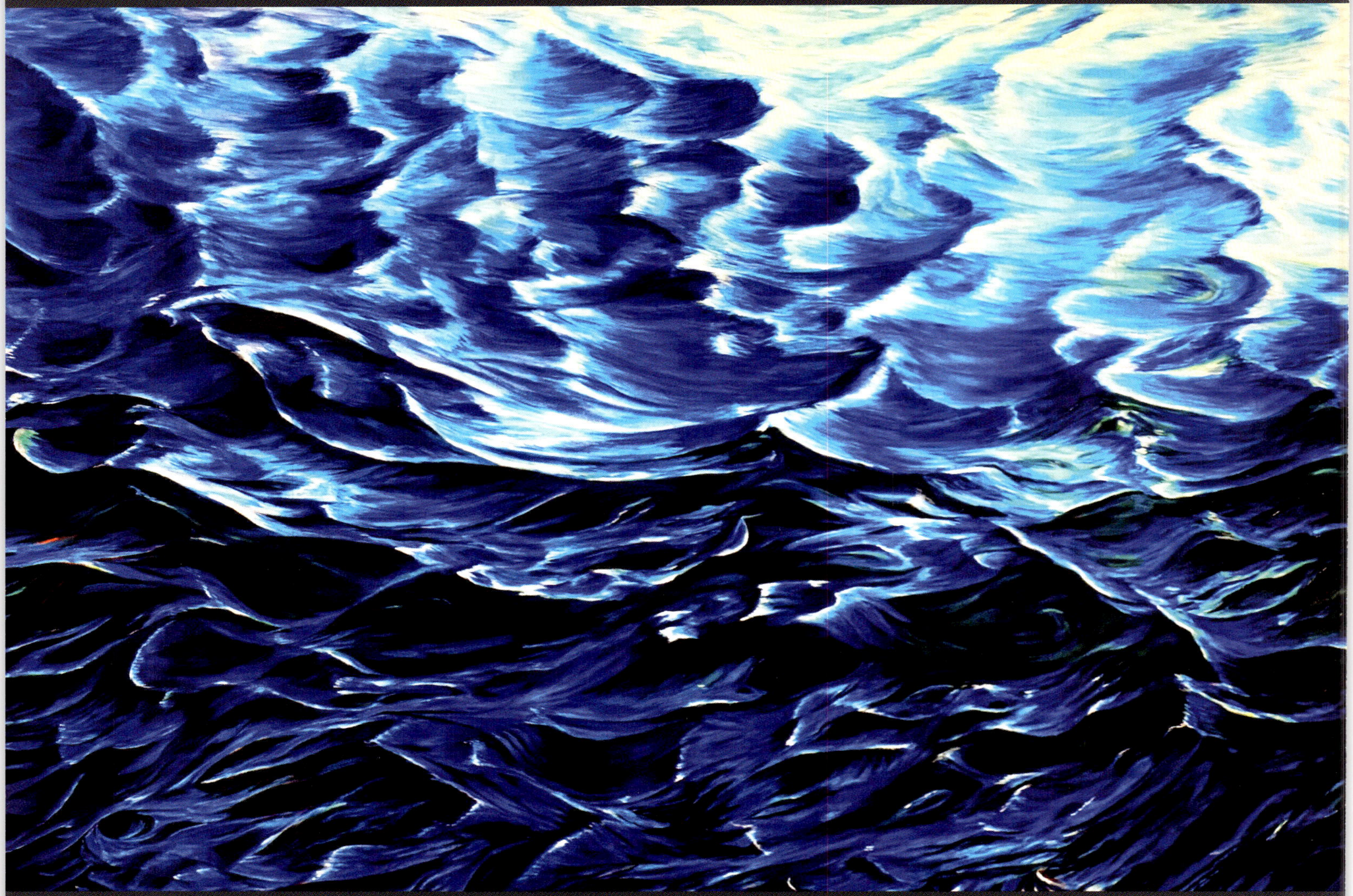

Healing Water. (40x60 inch acrylic on canvas.)

CHAPTER 1

THE ART OF HEALING

Why the Body Heals

Healing is as old as life itself. Every living thing must be able to heal to survive. As surgeons, it is not our touch that heals, as much as we may like to think it is. That may feel like a blow to the ego, but it is an invitation into a relationship with each patient. It is the body that heals. The cells and the tissue. It is designed to heal. As we study healing and master our craft, we are indeed participating in a much greater thing: life.

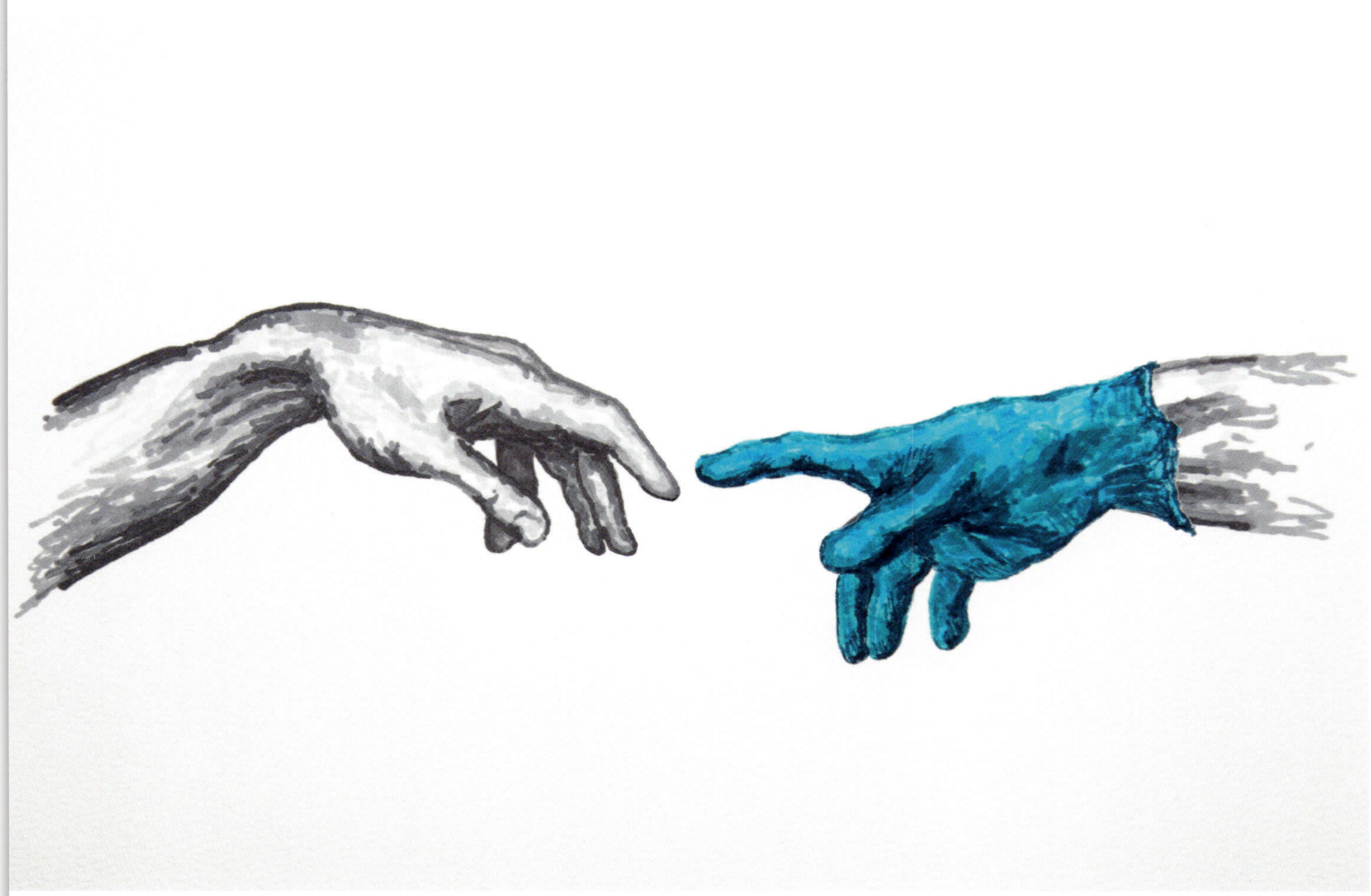

Figure 1-1 (Artwork inspired by Michelangelo.)

In oral surgery residency, we are brought up believing we have to know everything. That we are the end of the line and we just have to figure it out. The fear of being wrong and failure has been instilled in us. I'm not sure if it is our personality or our training that makes us that way, but I am pretty sure it makes surgeons a bit difficult to deal with at times. We like taking the simple and making it complicated. I do the opposite. I work to make the complicated simple and the simple even simpler. I have always been more interested in the questions, curious to learn and discover. Often, the beauty I find is in the depth and complexity, and yet the profound simplicity of life.

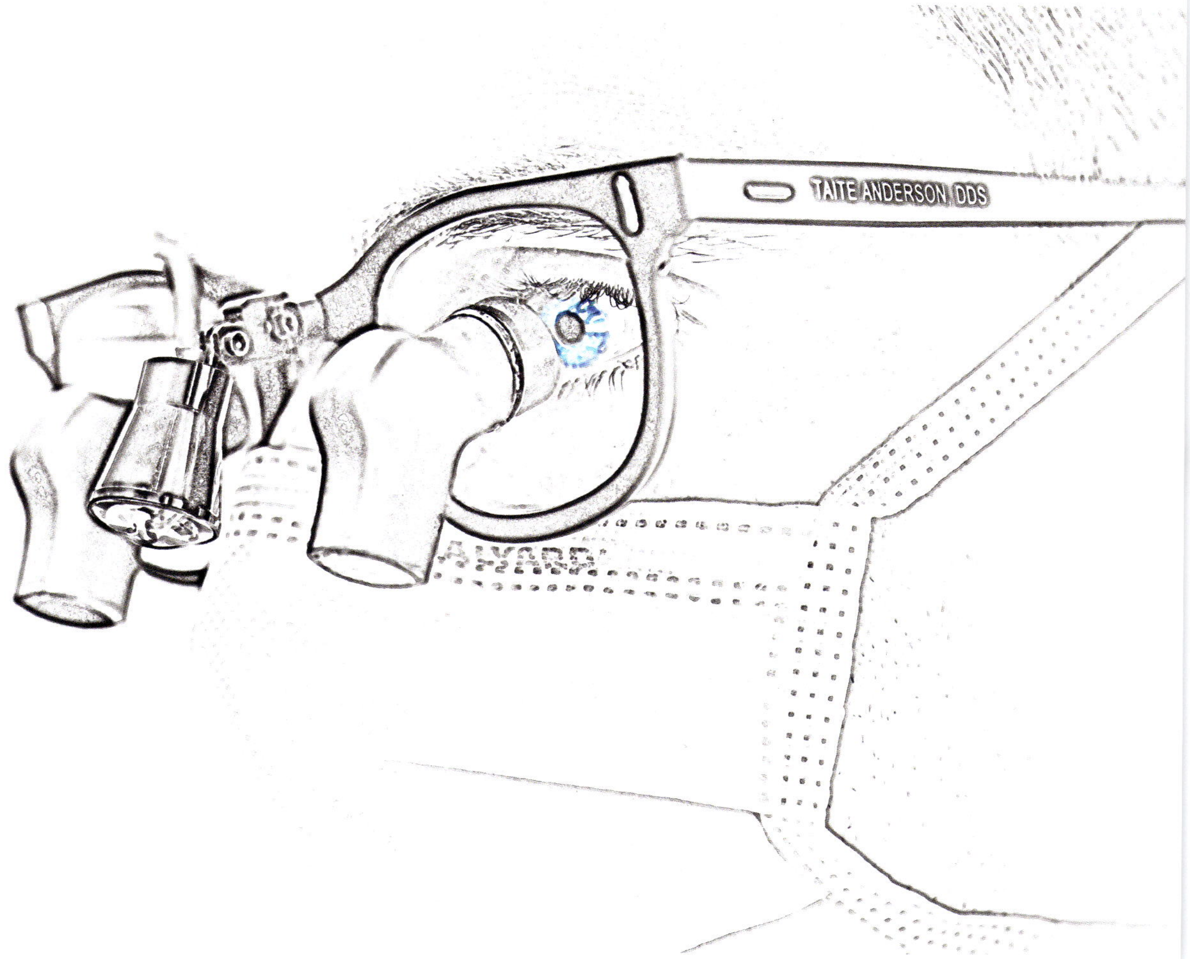

Figure 1-2 Self portrait. I want to share what I look for and what I see in surgery.

In my world as a surgeon, healing always begins with an injury. **We injure to heal**. We cut tissue and remove things that are causing problems—things the body is incapable of fixing on its own.

What makes the body heal? The cells, you may say. But the cells also cause an uproar, inflaming the tissue and destroying the body in the case of autoimmune disease. So, there must be something more. The cells are somehow guided along on their journey of healing.

Surgery is like Graffiti: Vandalism to some, and art to others. Cells see it as vandalism. They only see trauma. They respond to surgery the same way they respond to any injury. They need to heal. But **I see surgery as art**. It is the beginning of the healing that takes place after the patient leaves the surgery. The body already knows how to heal. It has been doing that since its beginning.

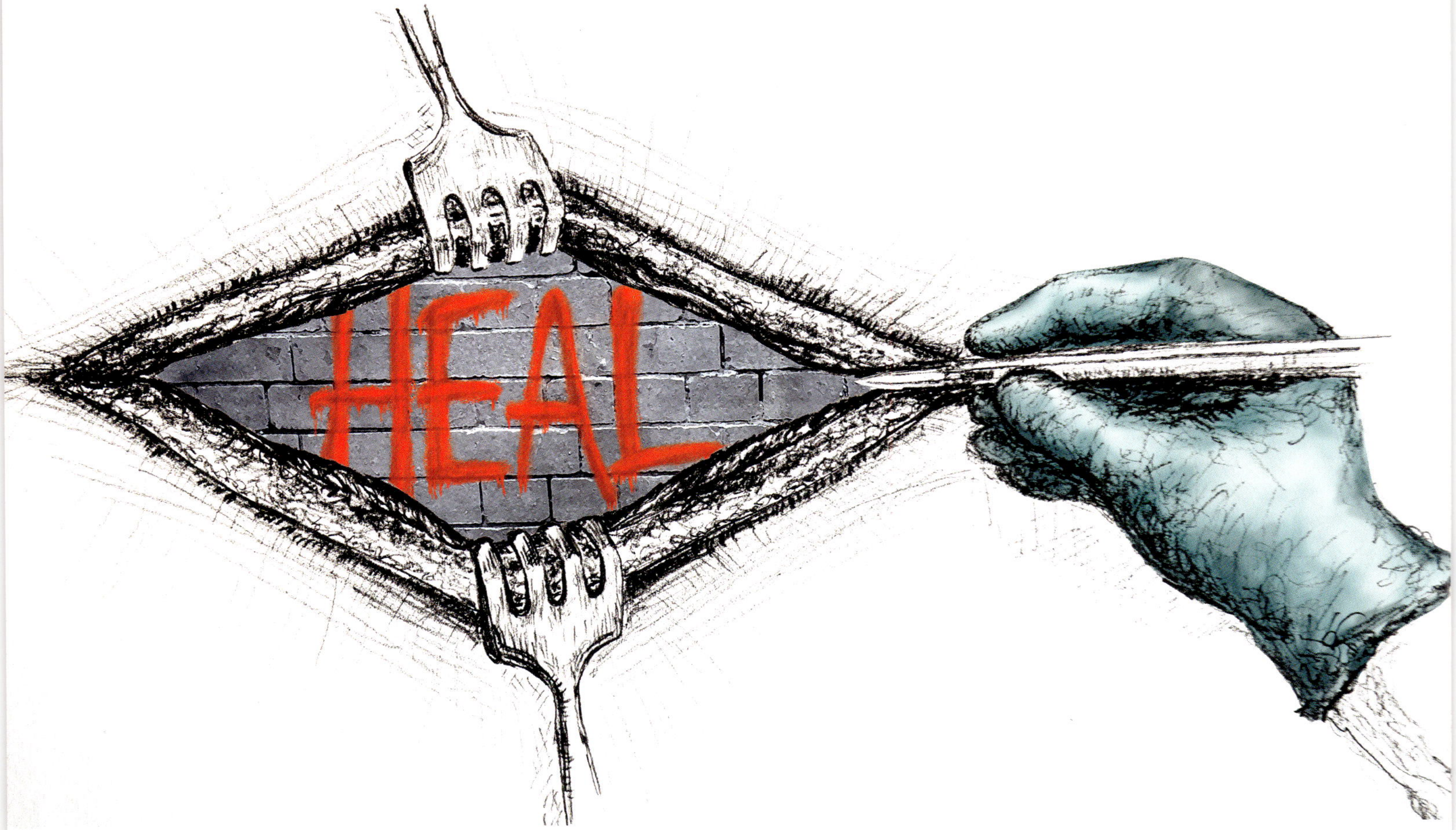

Figure 1-3 (Artwork inspired by Banksy).

The Body Heals: Basic Biology

Let's look at how we can leverage the art of healing in surgery. The most common surgical procedure on the planet is the extraction. Therefore, edentulism must be the most common surgical related defect. It is a problem.

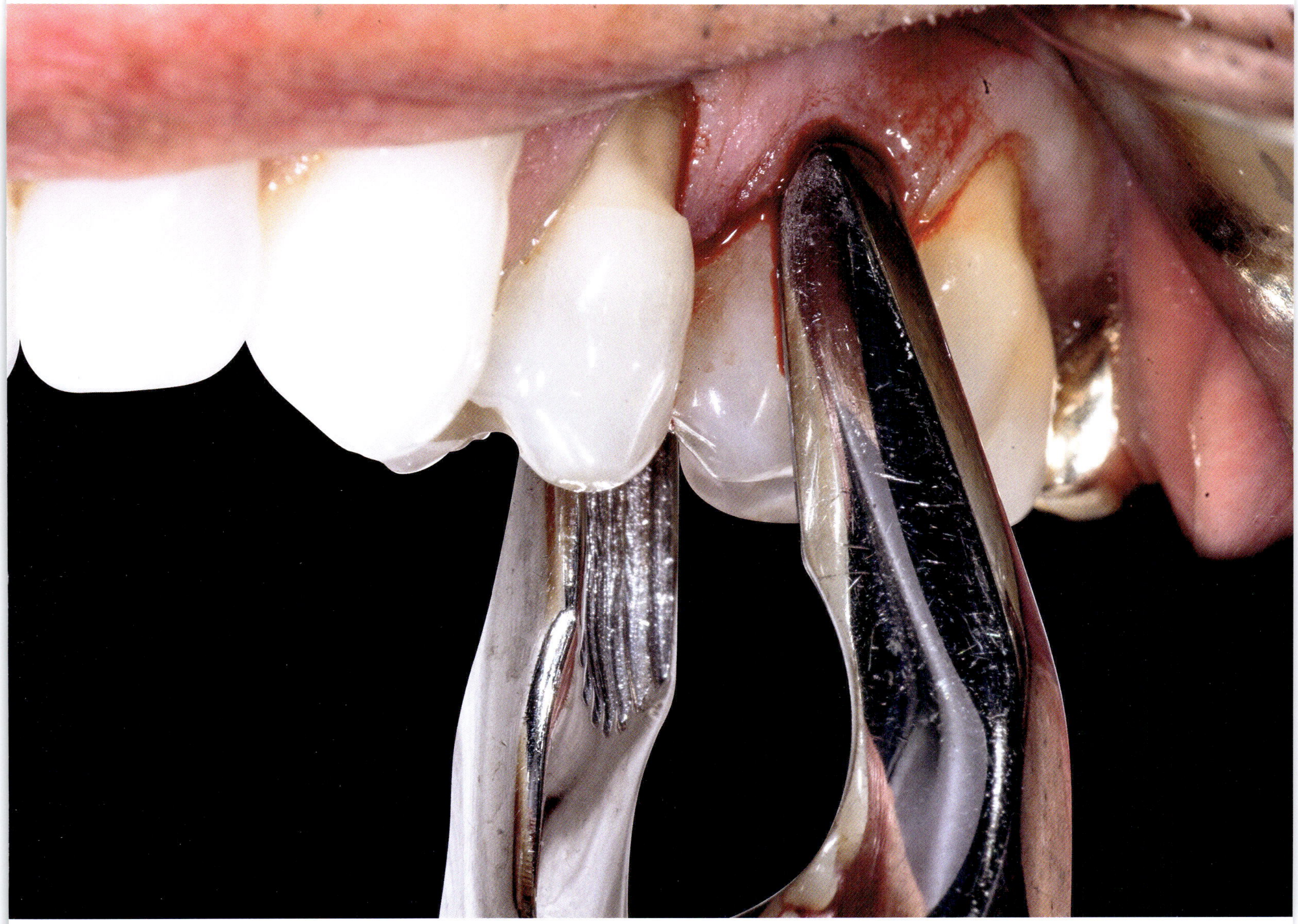

Figure 1-4

Placing an implant after an extraction is our attempt to recreate nature, using our understanding of science to restore beauty and function. We want to make the patient whole again. Implants are the solution to the problem, and they only work when healing is successful.

The goal is not simply getting the tooth out or screwing an implant in place. Holding a tooth in the forceps is not the objective. We want to be kind to the tissue, causing as little trauma as possible, for the cells' sake! If we want to be successful with our implants, we need to pay attention to the details of healing. If we just yank a tooth and jam in a screw, it will fail a lot more often. Failure is really easy. Success is the prize worth pursuing.

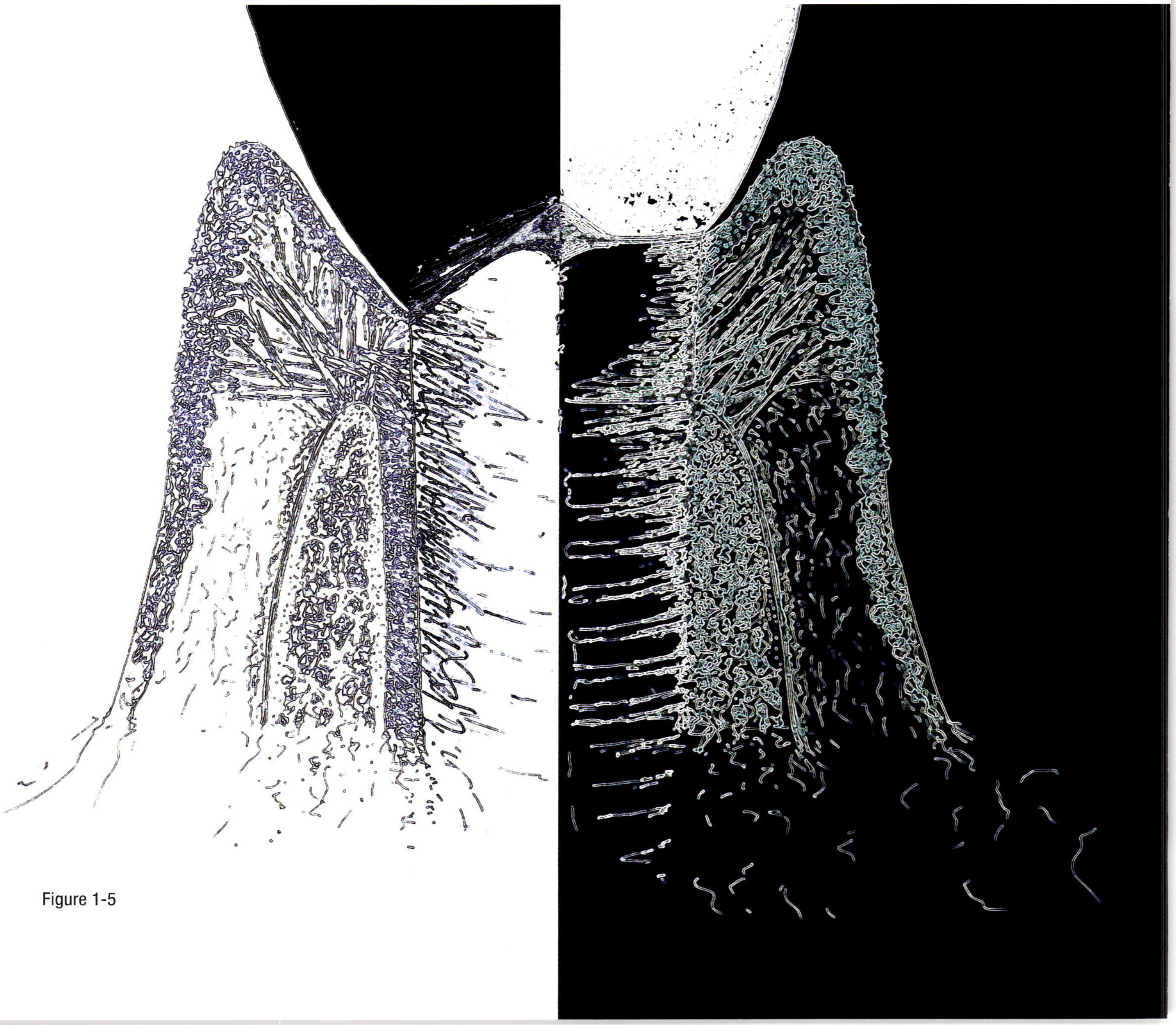

Figure 1-5

Let's look closer at what needs to happen in an immediate implant site for the screw to stay put, to integrate, and, ultimately, to succeed. Here's an extraction site with the hole prepped for an immediate implant. We can see the remnants of the periodontal ligament. If we look closer, we can see individual cells, like platelets.

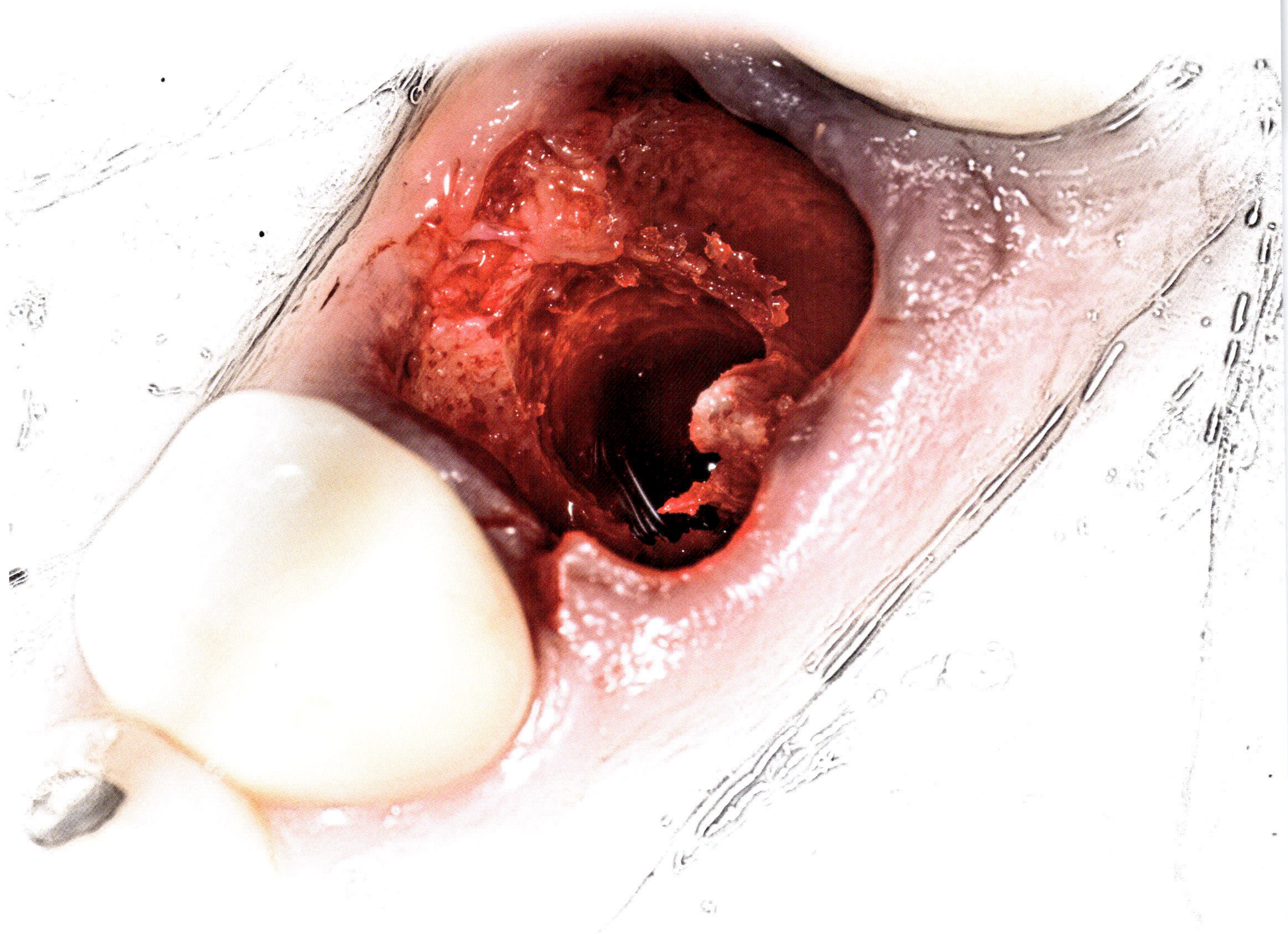

Figure 1-6

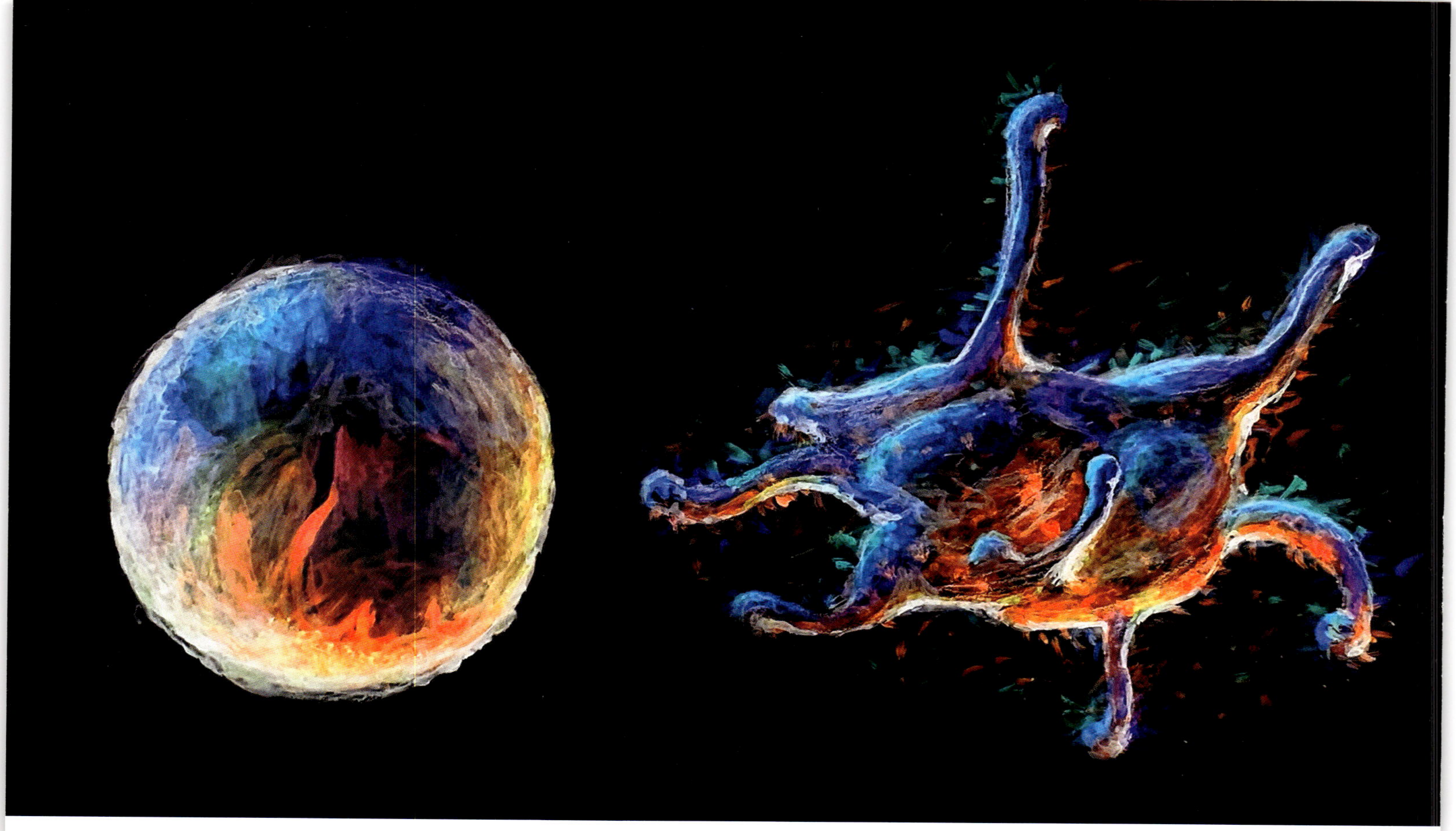

Figure 1-7 (Artwork inspired by Paul Cézanne.)

This is how I envision platelets. They usually hang out as simple, round, anucleate cytoplasmic cell bodies, but they are a powerhouse for healing. When activated, platelets grow sticky tentacles and release signaling proteins to stop bleeding and orchestrate healing.

Platelets play a big role in hemostasis, which is why we call them thrombocytes, thrombo for clotting and cyte for cell. But they are so much more than just a clotting cell. They participate in all phases of wound healing: hemostasis, inflammation, proliferation, maturation. Platelets also have a role in immunity. They are a powerhouse for healing. Filled with sacs of signaling proteins, they are always ready to stimulate cell growth, differentiation, inflammation and repair. When released, the proteins biochemically attach to receptors on nearby cells, telling them precisely what to do. It is almost like they pull biological levers on the cells to make things happen.

THROMBO	CLOTTING
CYTE	CELL

Figure 1-8

Some of the proteins they release are called growth factors. These regulate and maintain cellular growth. We label them according to their primary roles. For instance, Vascular Endothelial Growth Factor (VEGF) triggers the formation of new blood vessels.

As dentists, we tend to see these acronyms and gloss over. All these growth factors seem too complex and like they don't really matter. But they do. They all work together to heal. They are part of the everyday life of our bodies. They are a part of us. Like Andy Warhol transformed everyday objects into works of art, I want to call attention to how important and beautiful these things are. Appreciate them.

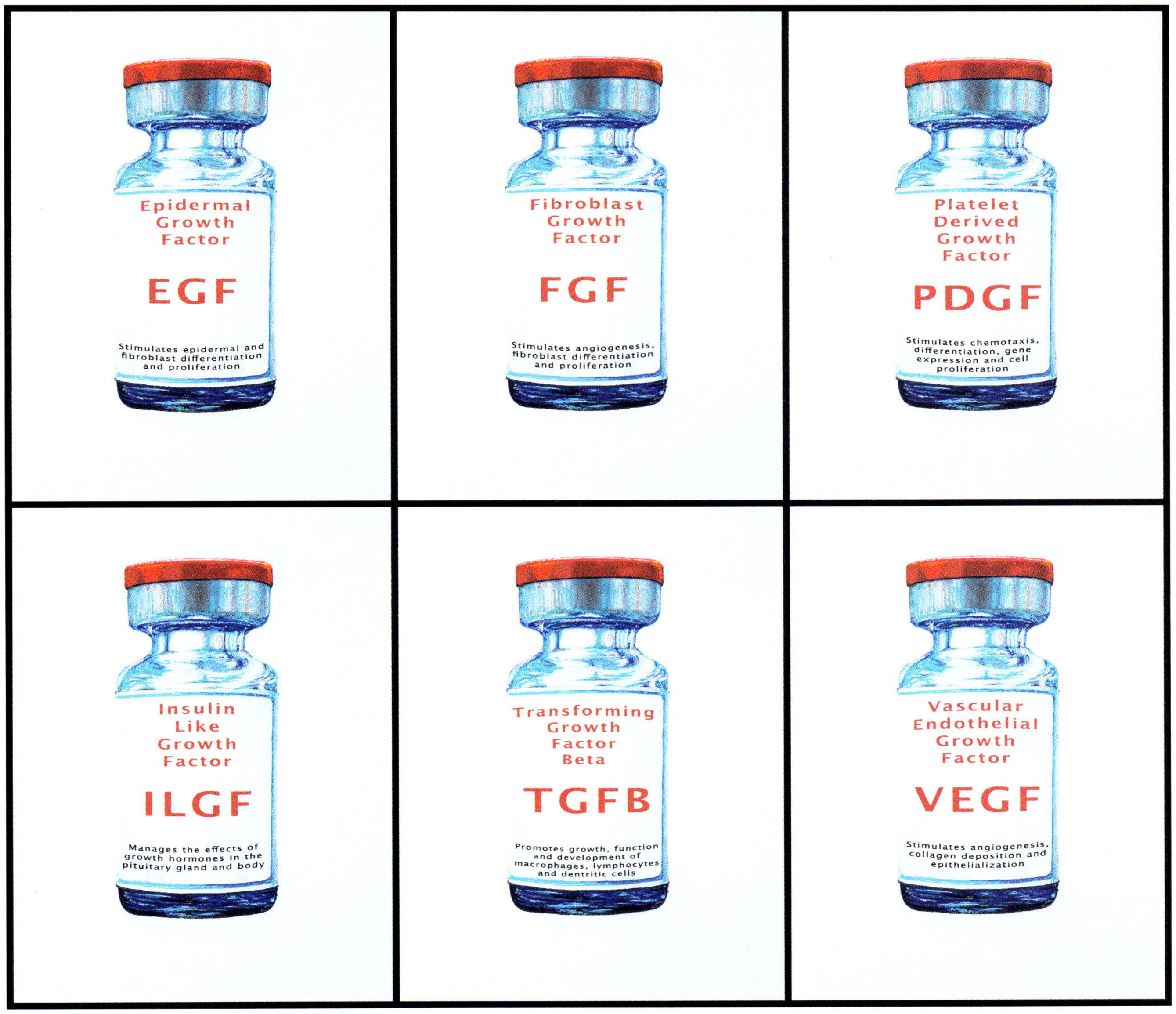

Figure 1-9 (Artwork inspired by Andy Warhol.)

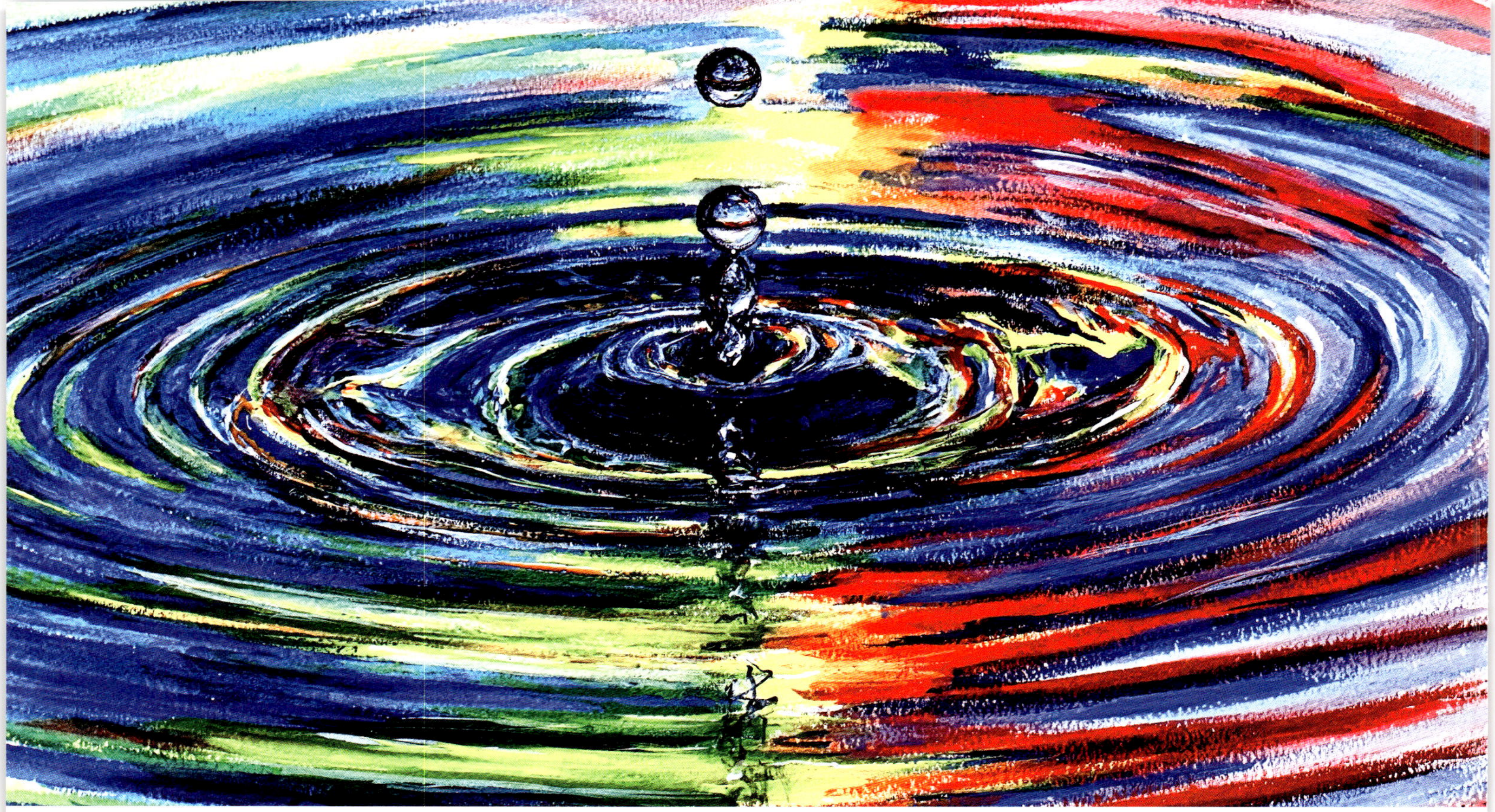

Figure 1-10 When growth factors are released, their signal ripples outward in all directions. Like ripples, growth factors themselves don't physically change much of anything. But they are directly responsible for so very much. The signal is amplified the closer you get to the droplet. Each small droplet impacts everything around it.

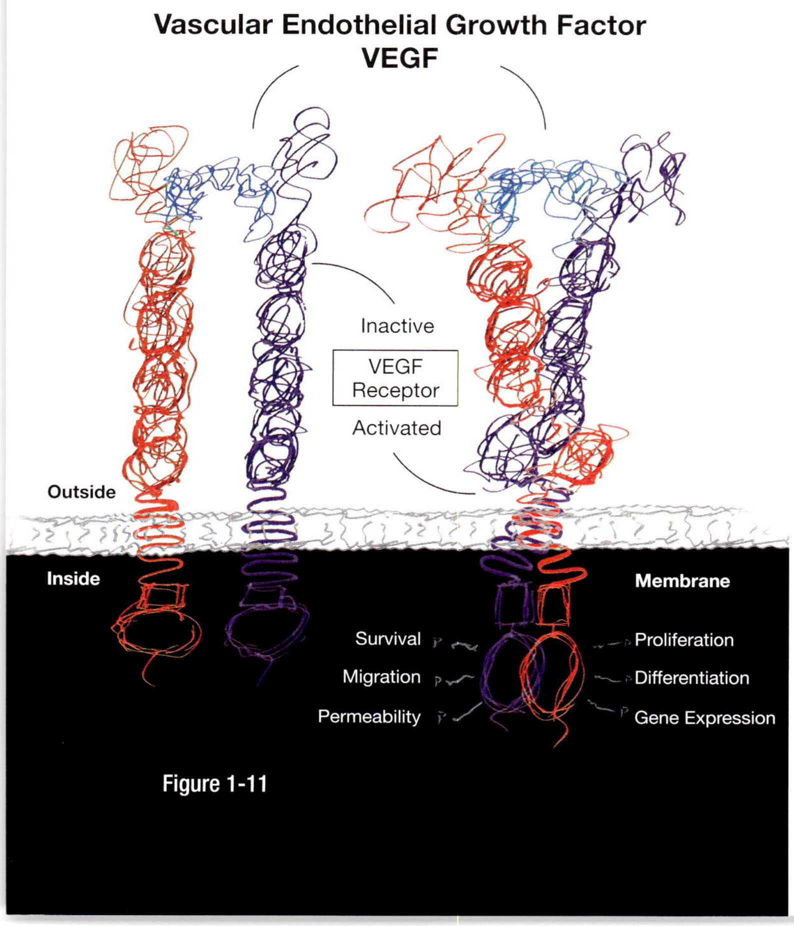

Figure 1-11

When VEGF is released from platelets (and other various sources) it spreads out through the extracellular space. It floats around for a while until it is grabbed by a perfectly matched dimeric protein structure sticking out from cell walls called a VEGF receptor. When this happens, the five outer dimers join and sort of warp around each other. As they contort and snap together, the whole complex twists into a new, more stable shape. This changes the shape inside the cell membrane, exposing an ATP binding site. Thus, a cascade of intracellular events is triggered, impacting gene expression and cell cycle regulation. And this is just one tiny step in the elaborate biochemical chain of events triggered by VEGF. It goes on and on.

Check this out. If you have a blood vessel next to an extraction site with an immediate implant, the platelets in the site release VEGF proteins. This signal causes some of the normal endothelial cells to transform themselves into highly specific tip and stalk cells. They completely change. The transformed tip cells lead the charge and grow antennae that follow the homing beacon toward the VEGF signal. This cell was just like the other endothelial cells before. Right behind it, another endothelial cell transforms into a stalk cell. It becomes a factory producing a new 3D vessel sprouting toward the site. If we want healing next to our implant, we want to crank up the VEGF signal to form new vessels. And angiogenesis is just one of VEGF's many valuable healing effects. It also triggers fibroblasts and keratinocytes to promote collagen formation and healing.

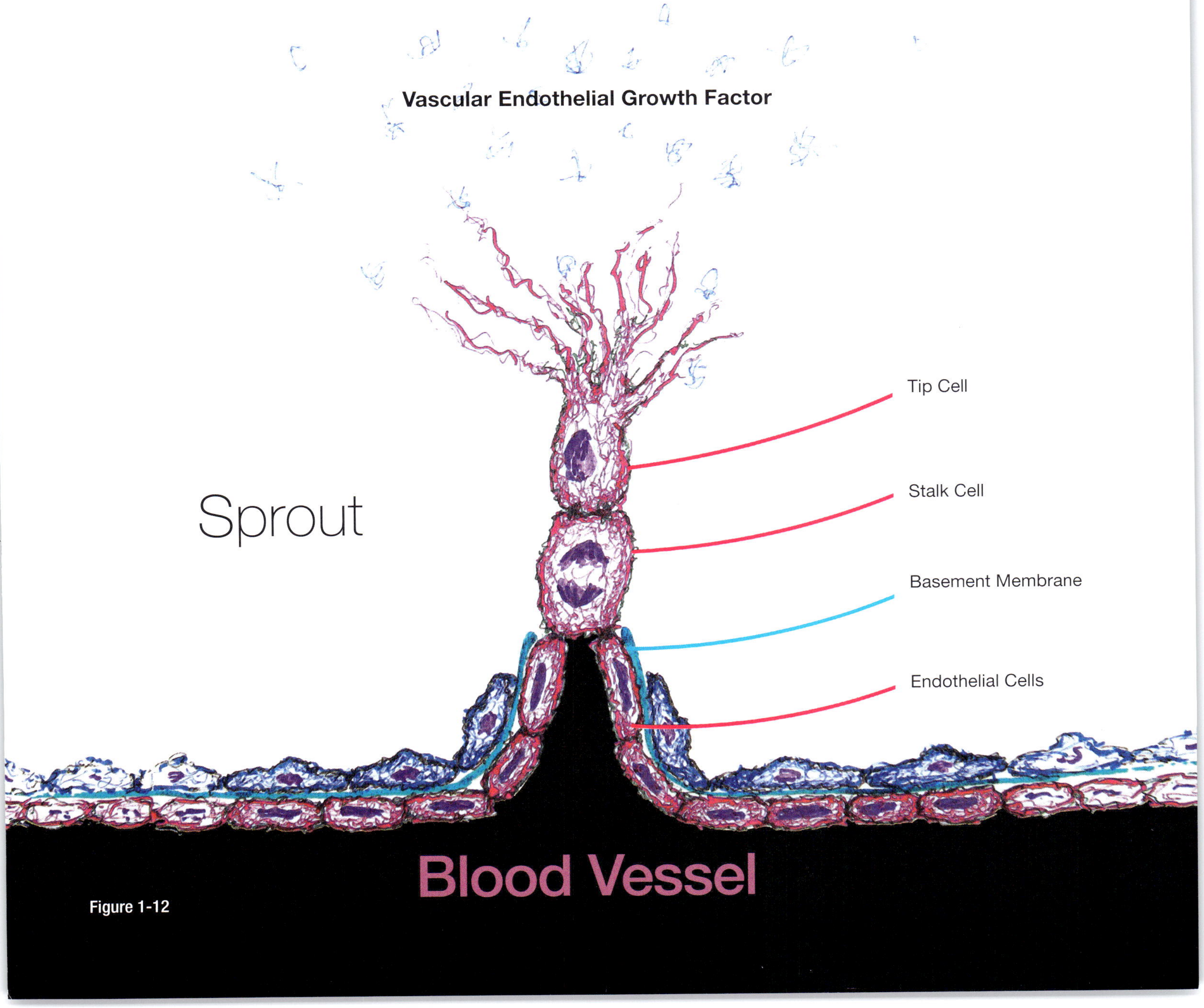

Figure 1-12

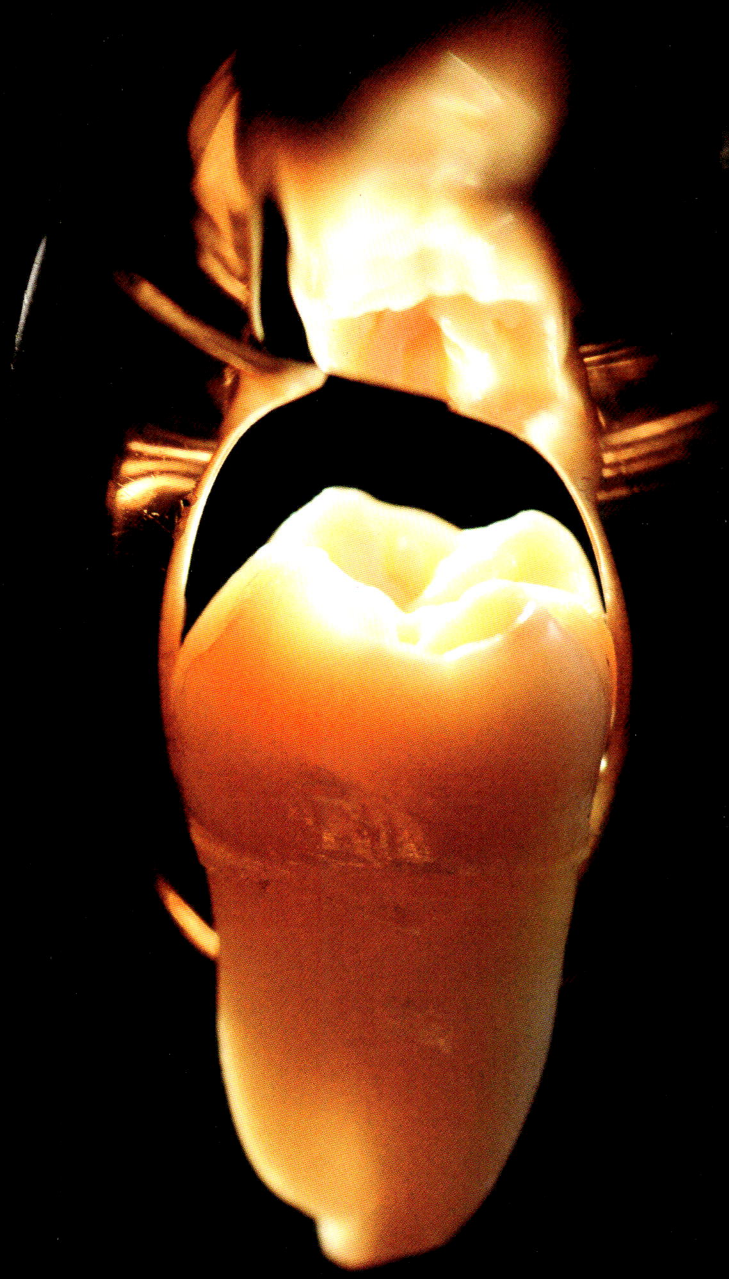

Figure 1-13

How do we heal through surgery? We start by viewing healing as the goal. An extracted tooth is not the goal. If getting the tooth out is the goal, we will inherently miss the boat on setting up for healing. During surgery, minimize trauma as much as possible with precise, calculated moves, and then let the body do its thing. It knows what to do. We study it. We learn from it. And we adapt what we do to accommodate it. We don't pound it into how we want it to be. (I wish we could. Wouldn't that be nice? "Pound to fit. Paint to match," my father-in-law used to say.)

But that doesn't work in healing. We want to get in, get the job done, and get out. We want to make the body think it was its own idea to heal in a way that meets our needs.

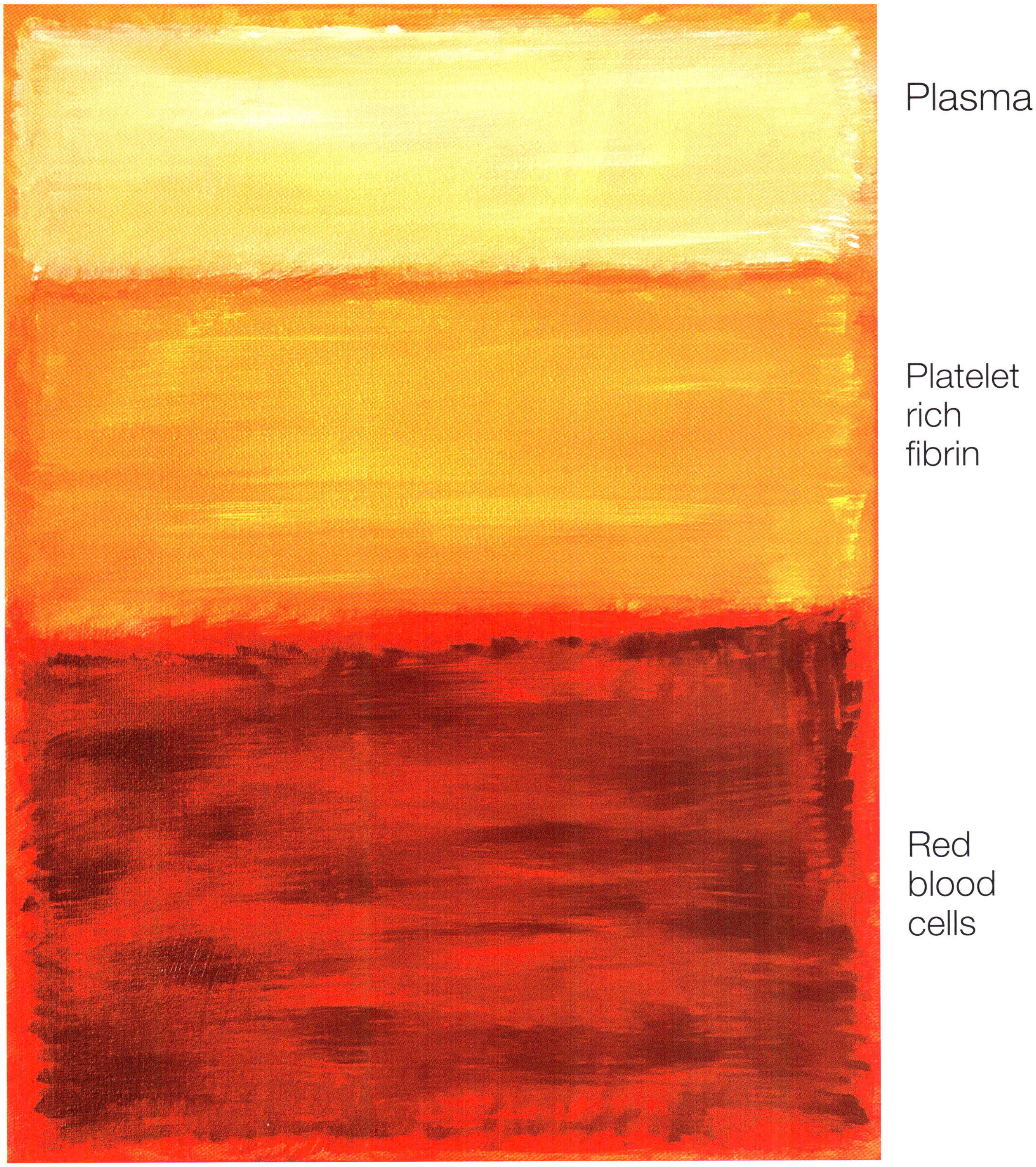

Figure 1-14 (Artwork inspired by Mark Rothko.)

How can we crank up healing right where we want it? In this case, right at the implant-bone interface? One way is by using Platelet Rich Fibrin (PRF). PRF is the concentrated portion of a patient's own blood, turbocharged for healing. It is basically whole blood spun down, which separates the components by density. The red blood cells are the densest and they fall to the bottom. Plasma stays at the top as it is mainly water and electrolytes. And in the middle is the gold. Concentrated platelets, growth factors, white blood cells and fibrin. This is the PRF.

Placing the PRF in the extraction site feeds it a healthy diet of:

- Platelets to stop the bleeding and coordinate the healing process.
- Growth factors slowly released over several weeks.
- White blood cells to defend against bacterial invasion.
- A hearty fibrin mesh to support the tissue in growth.

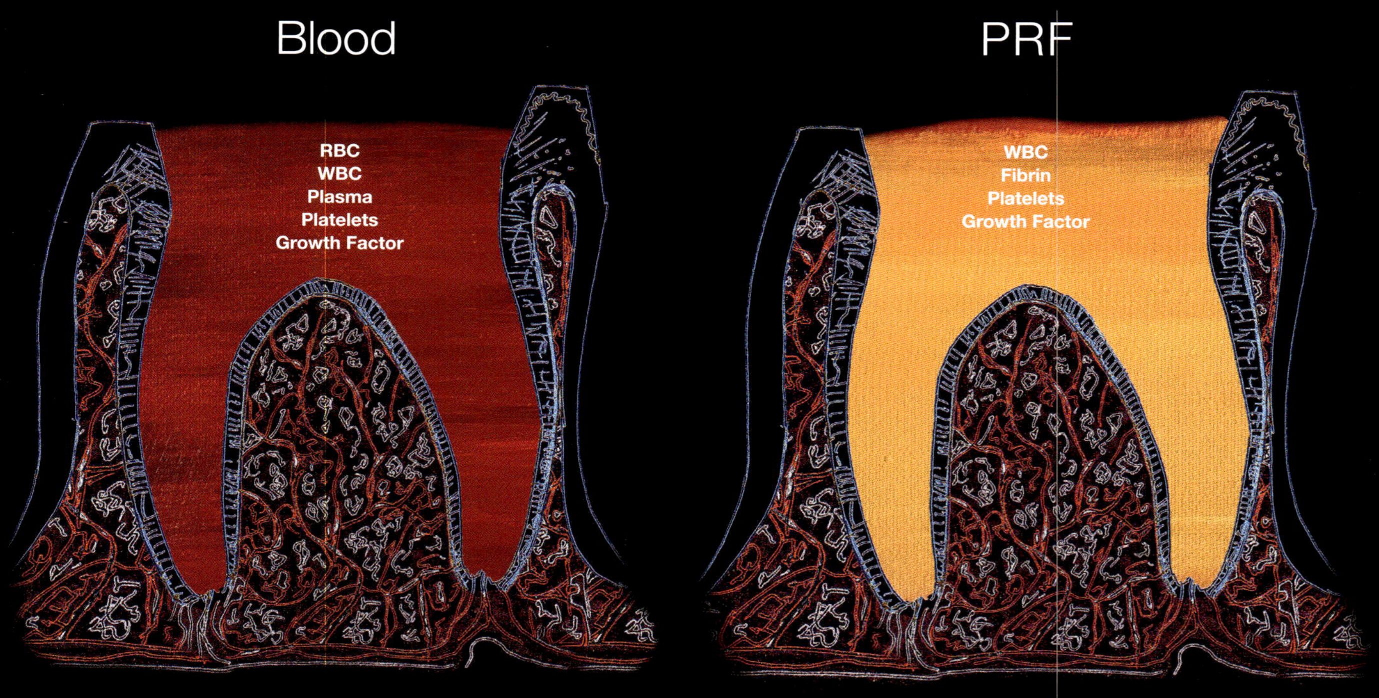

Figure 1-15

The extraction site doesn't need a regular blood clot. The red blood cells and plasma just dilute the healing potential. But it desperately needs platelets, leukocytes, and growth factors. It needs to lay down a framework for rebuilding, a fibrin mesh of protection. Instead of relying on whole blood, which also contains a bunch of non-healing related components, we spin down the blood and pluck out the good stuff. The gold.

We want the gold next to our implants.

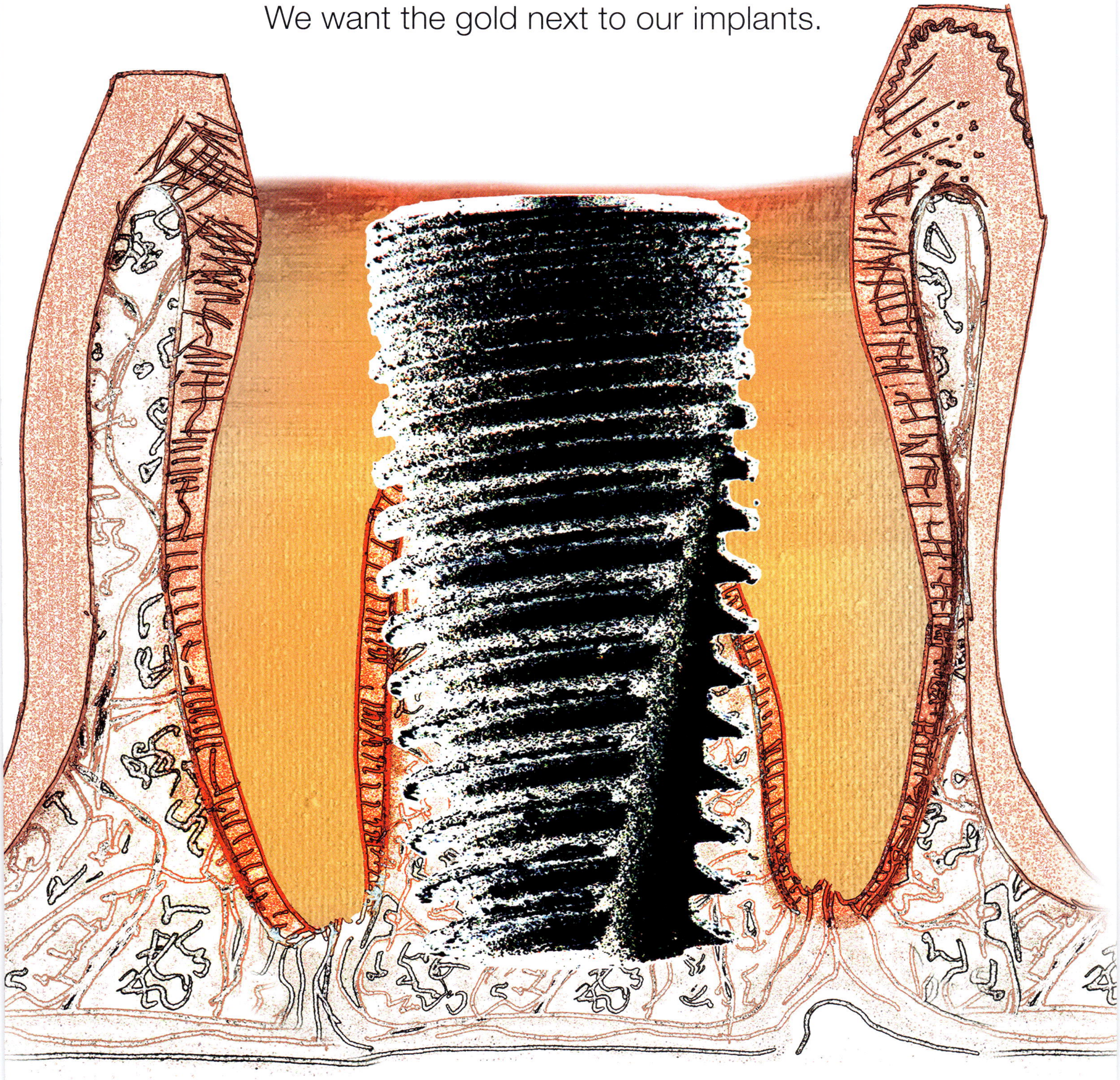

Figure 1-16

What does this actually look like in my practice? Let's look at an immediate molar implant case.

I routinely mix PRF with allograft to make a sticky bone graft that I place around the implant. I find it efficient to pack the bone when the Ostell peg is in place because it covers the implant and gives me space to work.

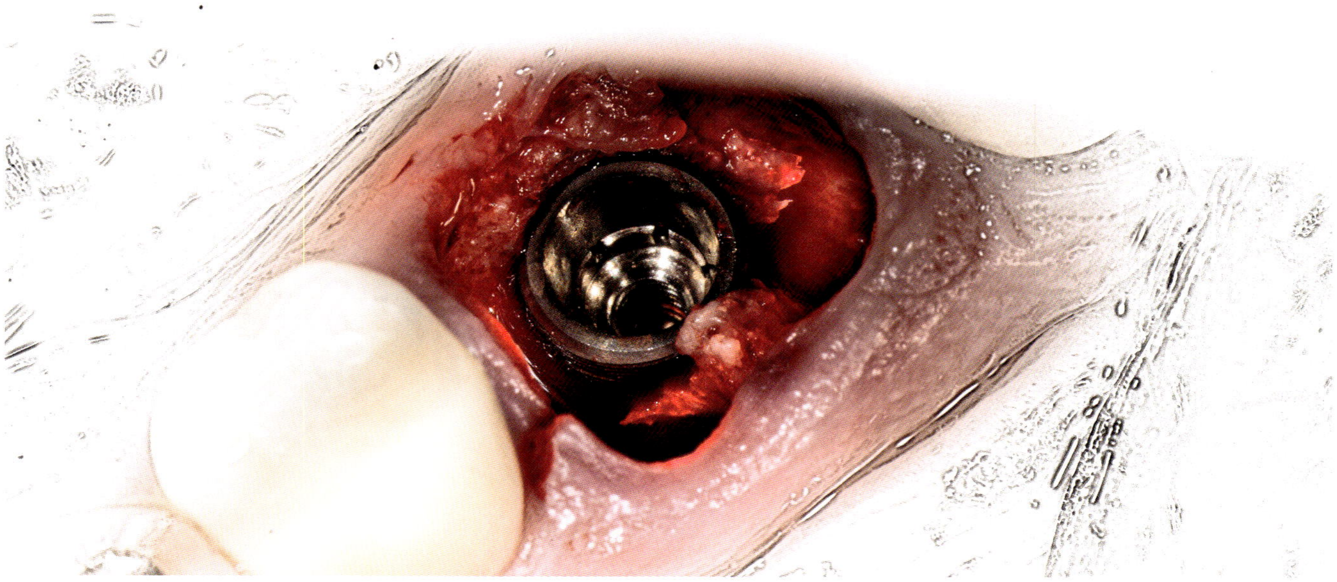

Figure 1-17

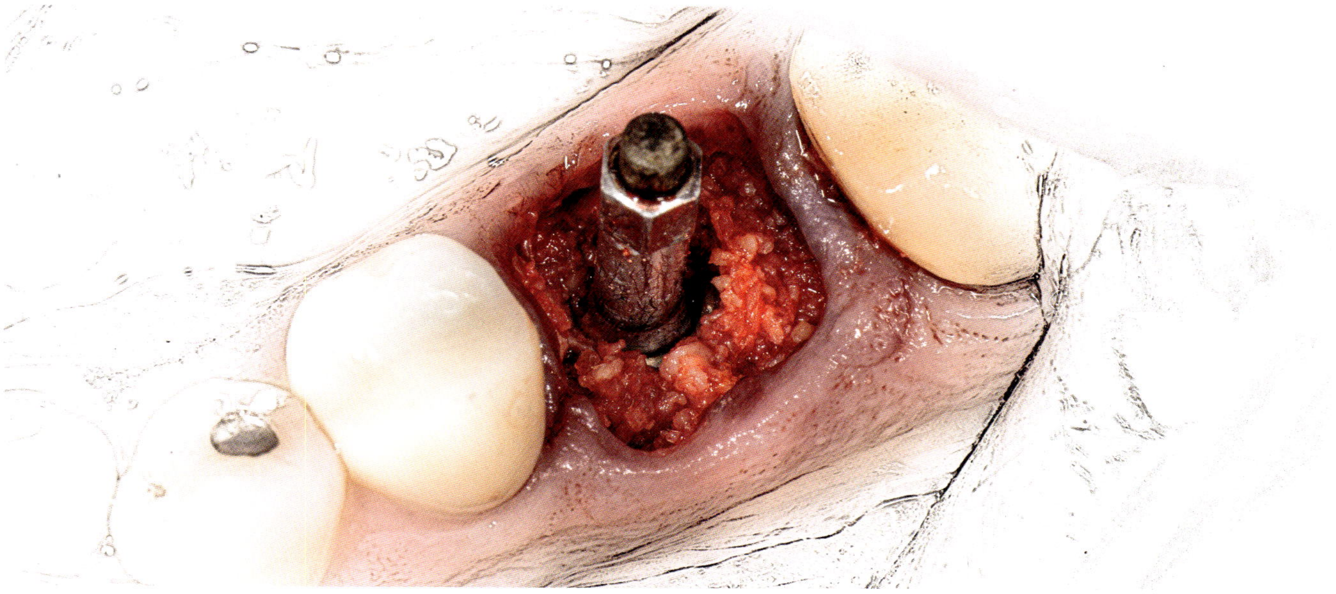

Figure 1-18

Then I place a flared healing abutment.

Before suturing, I tuck a PRF membrane around the abutment. Each of these steps is aimed directly at the healing process. At osseointegration. At making the patient whole.

Implant companies know the key to osseointegration is in the implant's outermost atomic layer. It needs to play well with the bone. It needs to adapt to the process of healing at the cellular and even atomic level. The surface must respect VEGF and promote angiogenesis, among other things. Many unique surface treatments have been studied and applied to implants, all claiming some benefit in short or long-term stability.

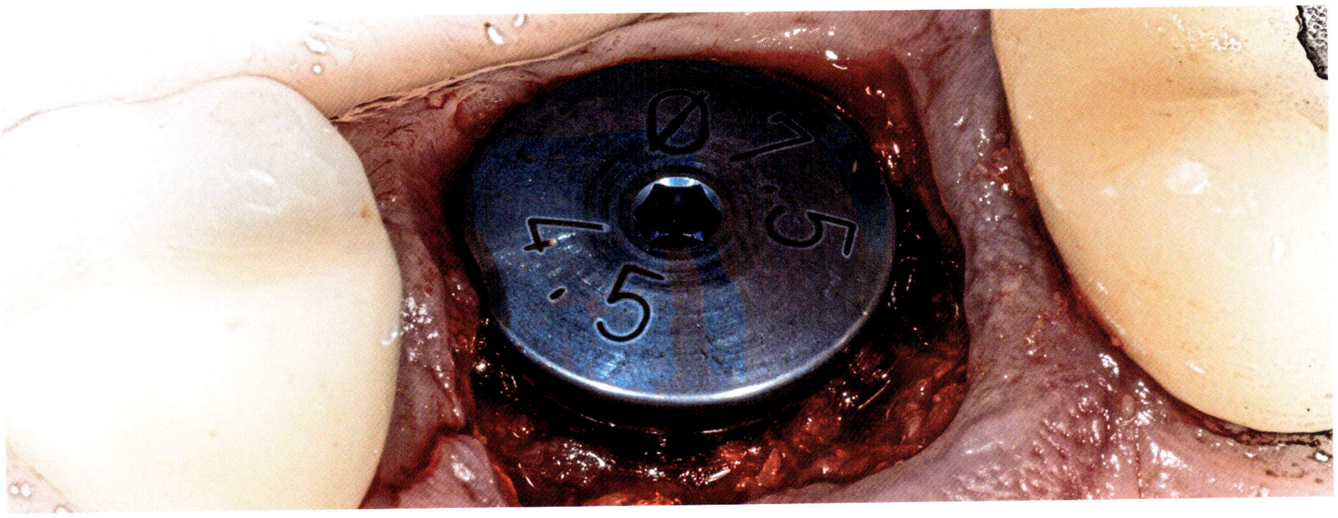

Figure 1-19

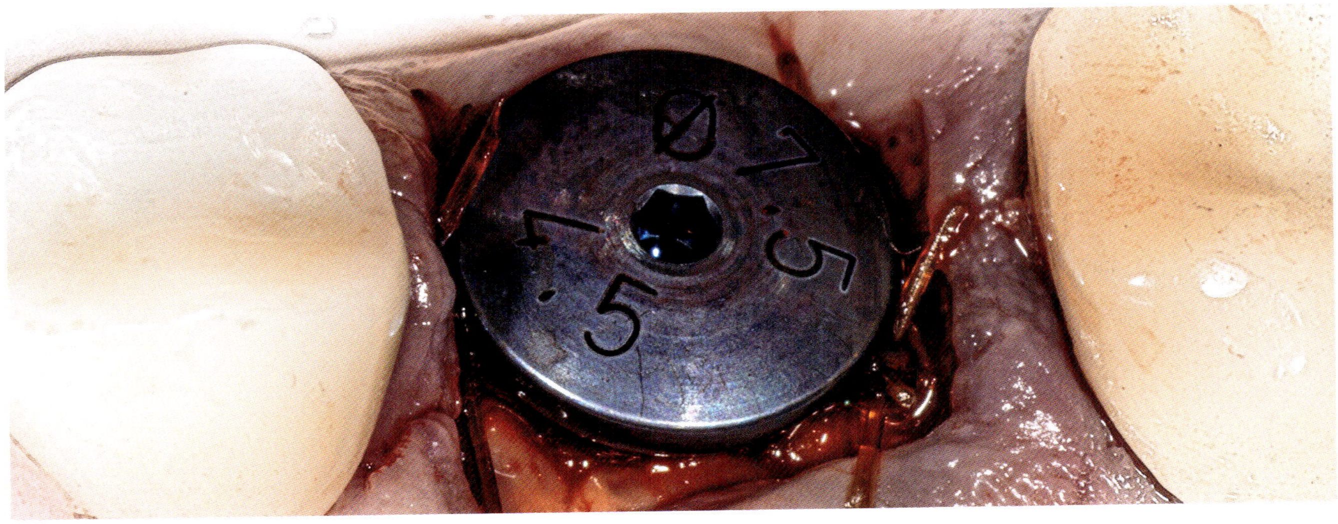

Figure 1-20

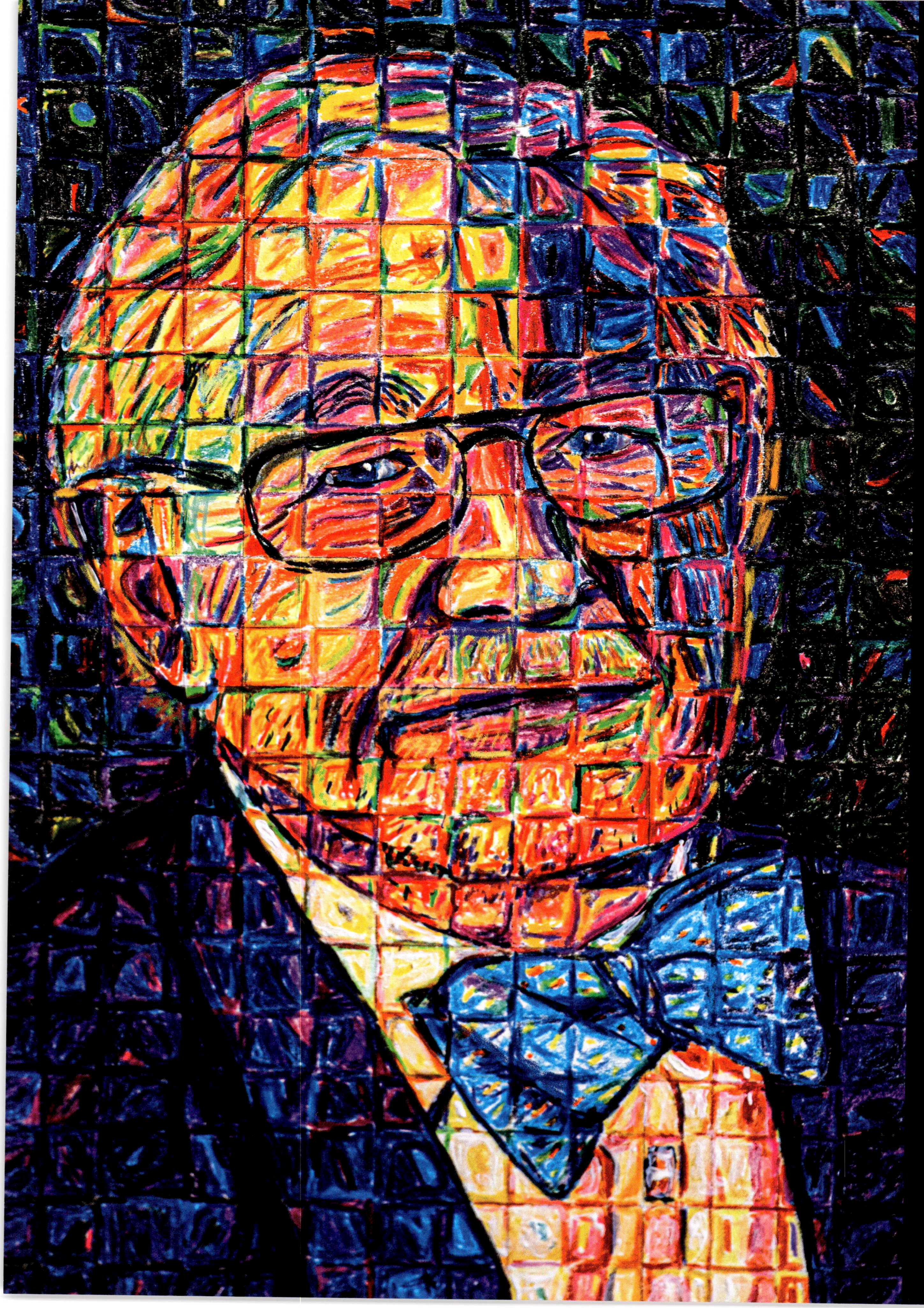

We owe many thanks to the pioneer in osseointegration. Per-Ingvar (P-I) Brånemark has left quite a legacy. He looked closely at the world around him, asking questions, looking for understanding. He discovered and developed many of the foundational pieces, the bedrock of implant dentistry. I think he too found beauty in the details, and in putting the pieces together.

◂
Figure 1-21 Portrait of the late Per-Ingvar (P-I) Brånemark, a visionary who explored details and brilliantly wove them together to create the art of implantology. (Artwork inspired by Chuck Close.)

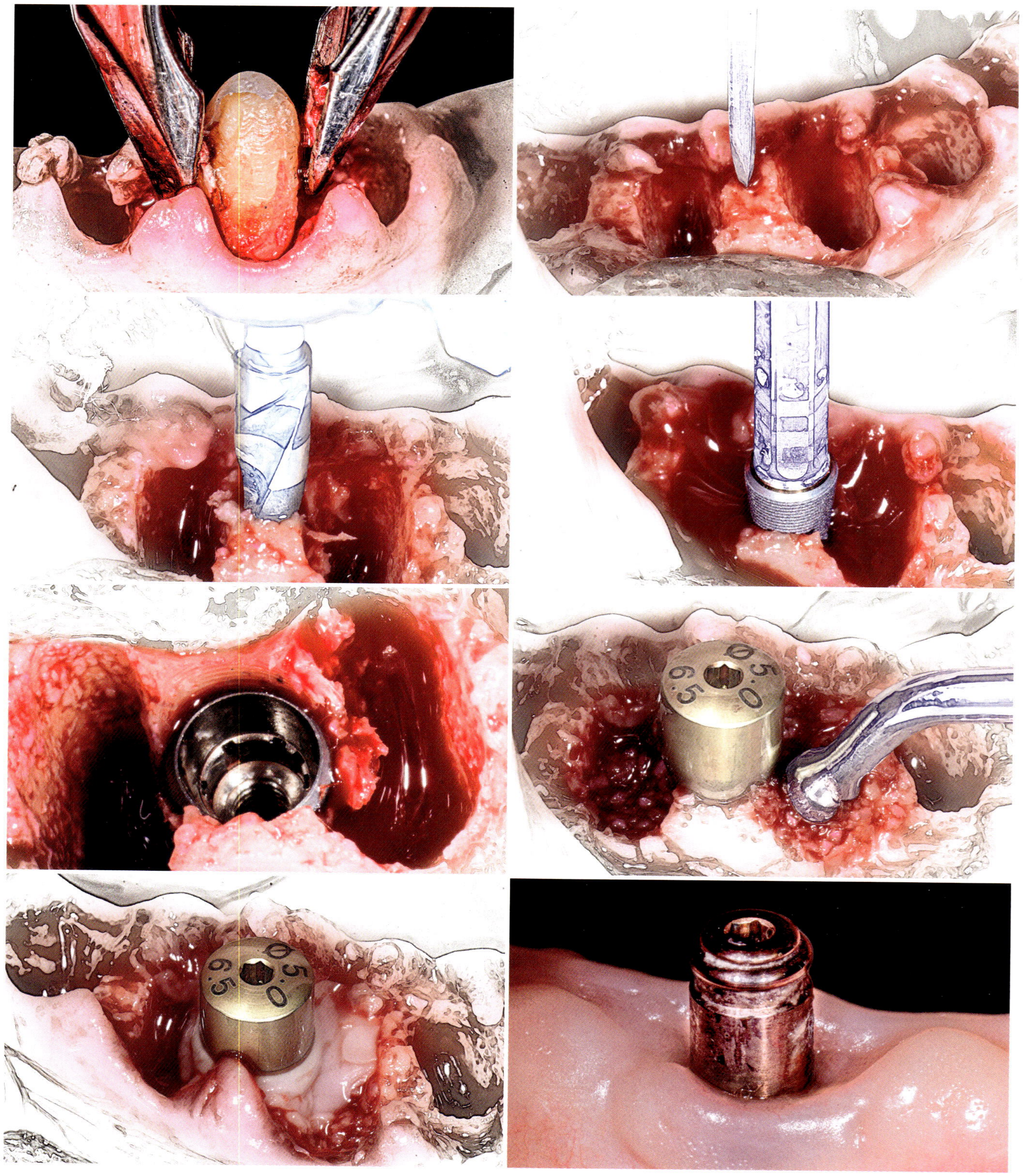

Figure 1-22

And these are just a few small components of the larger healing masterpiece.

When you are figuring out when, where and how to place an implant, it is not just about the screw, the angle or position. It's really not about you… It is very much about the age-old healing process at the most microscopic level of the patient's mouth.

When you think about the art of oral surgery, remember healing is the most fragile and important element. It is the essence of what we do. It's not the screw. It's not the integrated treatment plan. It is in the healing. Break it down even more. Pay keen attention to the details and leverage them and you are certain to have greater success. I want you, and really your patients, to succeed.

Minimize Trauma, Maximize Perfusion

The body is physiologically programmed to succeed at sustaining life. Think about all the different ways it protects and restores itself. The more we understand about this, the better we can serve our patients and achieve the surgical outcomes we all desire.

The brain is the first line of defense, long before the immune system. Be smart.

"If you're gonna be stupid, you gotta be tough."
Grandpa Bill

Let's think for a moment about what it takes for soft tissue to heal. When tissue is incised, cells are disrupted and destroyed. The blood supply replenishing life in the cells is compromised. It is almost like a microscopic battle scene. The recovery process afterward is dependent on three things: the extent of the damage, the return of the blood supply, and the stamina of the surviving cells.

At its most basic level, all vital tissue requires perfusion. Severe lack of perfusion, more precisely lack of oxygen, is not compatible with tissue repair. This is impacted by macroscopic mechanical injury as well as the post injury inflammatory response.

Maintaining oxygenation is a primary mechanism to optimize tissue healing. We can see how our surgery will affect recovery by observing tissue integrity and color. When blunt injury causes a change in color to blue or white, there is a major disruption in blood supply. (This is different from blanching the tissue under pressure, in which the color immediately returns as the intact vessels refill with blood.) A lack of perfusion pushes the tissue to a hypoxic state, increasing and amplifying tissue necrosis[1].

The power of healing flows through our blood. Through it, the basic elements of healing are transported throughout our body. Some of the resources and signaling pathways are present locally where cells are damaged or being repaired, but the majority of healing is dependent on blood supply. Reperfusion of the injured tissue is therefore a critical step in healing. Where there is ischemia, the capillary network needs to be reestablished. At the direction of angiogenic cytokines, like VEGF, access holes are bored into the existing blood vessels. The sprouting capillaries migrate into the ischemic tissue and organize a new capillary network, restoring oxygenation, and replenishing nutrients to the tissue.

Thankfully, the tissue in most oral surgery procedures already has adequate blood supply before surgery, with the exception of some less common pathologies like medication or radiation induced osteonecrosis. If we protect the tissue, we optimize healing potential.

Surgery is a continuum of reversible and irreversible cellular injury. Remember, the moment a scalpel touches the tissue, there is injury. Set the injury up for healing.

The Continuum of Healing

The immensely complex process of wound healing is frequently divided into three or four overlapping and successive phases: hemostasis, inflammation, proliferation, maturation. I encourage you to think about how each of these steps is impacted during surgery. This awareness can help guide and improve your surgical technique and, ultimately, the patient's outcome.

Optimize hemostasis

With the commencement of the clotting cascade at the first injury to blood vessels, an elaborate series of events takes place.

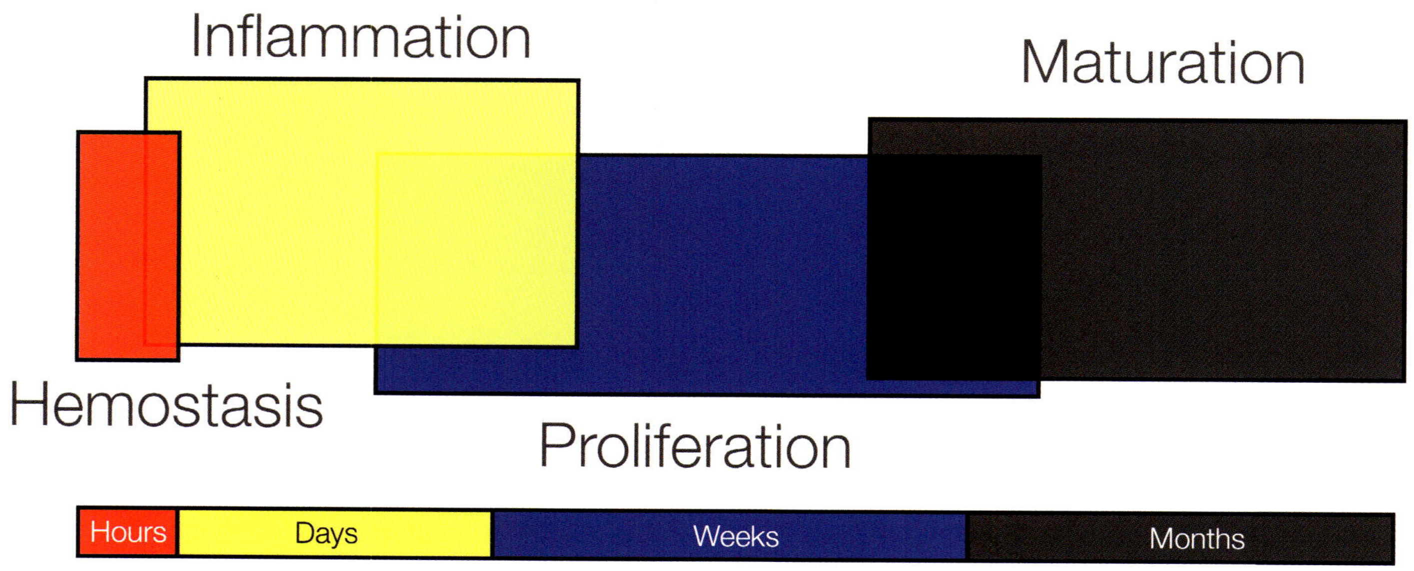

Figure 1-23 Successive phases of healing overlap and interact to keep the process moving.

Think about how to help the body achieve hemostasis from the moment you pick up an instrument.

- Minimize tissue trauma. Sometimes you can see larger blood vessels in the surgical field. If you are able, try to protect them. Minimizing scope of dissection can also reduce bleeding and promote hemostasis. Clean incisions and dissection will optimize the site for hemostasis, especially compared to a site with torn and jagged tissue.
- Patient derived biomaterials, such as platelet rich fibrin, have tremendous potential to promote hemostasis. They provide an incredible fibrin network and supply increased concentrations of cells and factors to the injury site, stacking the deck in the patient's favor.

Reduce inflammation

Less trauma = less inflammation = better healing. Inflammation is a two-edged sword. It is an asset in directing cellular activity and we need it to heal. If we tried to bypass this step completely, we would significantly impair healing. We need to respect inflammation, but we can also reduce its liability.

- Minimize tissue trauma.
- Inflammation is part of the body's response to protect and heal itself in the face of an invasion or injury. Minimize the injury and potential for invasion and you minimize the inflammation.
- Oxidative stresses of anoxic tissue. When tissue is starved of oxygen, even temporarily, this stresses the tissue and increases inflammation. Protect perfusion during and after surgery.
- Consider the patient as a whole. There may be a role in considering dietary and environmental inflammatory exposures. A systemically inflamed patient will likely have more localized inflammation.

Leverage proliferation

There is a direct relationship between tissue trauma and the need for proliferation. More trauma requires more proliferation.

- Minimize the need for proliferation.
  - Macerated tissue and traumatized bone require much more proliferation from the adjacent cells to restore the site to its previous condition. Careful techniques in soft tissue and hard tissue management will decrease the resources needed to heal.
- Maximize opportunities for proliferation.
  - The osteoprogenitor cells in the periodontal ligament have tremendous potential to promote proliferation of bone. Any time we are able to preserve the periodontal ligament in the socket during an extraction, we maximize the tissue's assets.
  - Maintain scaffold and structure for bone formation in a socket. A two walled defect is set up for a different recovery than a five walled defect. When the buccal plate, in particular, is protected and maintained, the opportunity for proliferation in the site is optimized.

Orchestrate maturation

Influence the maturing tissue's properties. The final wound healing phase is maturation. This is the real goal of what we do. If we keep this in mind each step of the way, we will impact the outcome much more profoundly. What type of mature tissue do we want? What will best serve the patient?

- Quantity of tissue: Consider what adequate volume of soft or hard tissue looks like. A simple example is a single tooth extraction. If the restorative plan consists of a three-unit fixed bridge restoration, it may not seem very important to preserve the hard and soft tissue. We know resorption will occur anyway. But the contours of the remaining tissue will influence food impaction around the bridge and the amount of bone support around the abutment teeth. If the plan is implant replacement, it is easy to see the importance of adequate ridge width and height. And not just adequate bone for a titanium screw, but sufficient tissue contours to optimize the emergence profile and implant loading. But if the plan is just to leave the space empty, then does it matter much how the tissue matures? Surely a broader, more stable ridge will serve the patient better even if there is no replacement. It is indeed an asset, especially when compared to a narrow, short ridge.

- Quality of tissue. Not only is volume of mature tissue important, but the quality and characteristics are also a key part of the equation. This is tremendously important for both soft and hard tissue. If given the choice to place an implant into type four soft bone or type one dense bone, the dense bone will win every time. We want the most stable outcome. Stable keratinized gingiva versus mobile non-keratinized mucosa? Pick gingiva every time. When considering the art of healing, we need to think about short- and long-term aspects. Maximize the long-term assets and think about setting up the best tissue quality.
- When closing an extraction site, if we coronally advance a flap and obtain primary closure, the best-case scenario for our keratinized gingiva is the final position of the advanced flap. This immediately reduces the potential amount by the width of the socket. Compare that to a repositioned flap with an entire socket site that can heal over with keratinized gingiva. This simple change increases the amount of keratinized gingiva by at least five or more millimeters.
- Consider the esthetics of tissue architecture. Especially in the esthetic zone, the volume of tissue is only the beginning. If there is thick, boggy, non-keratinized gingiva showing at high smile, there's significant room for improvement. If the same volume of tissue is pink and symmetric, it may be wildly successful. Managing not only the quantity but also the potential quality of the tissue is a high calling in the art of oral surgery.

Stress and Healing

We must consider the patient as a whole when we discuss healing. The patients who want to heal and believe they are healing will most certainly heal better than those who are anxious and stressed about it. Stress directly impacts healing. The cortisol release related to stress has a profound impact on healing. While this hasn't been studied at great length yet that I know of, I believe this may be a critical, and often overlooked, aspect of healing.

There was an interesting study that hit home for me. During dental school finals, the study subjects showed a 30% slower recovery from a palatal wound than during their summer break[2]. Dental school finals are no joke, as we all know. But compare that level of stress with the stress some patients are carrying: ill family members, domestic instability, job loss. There are many things in life more stressful than dental school finals. An awareness of how stress impacts healing doesn't decrease the stress, but it could impact and guide how you discuss things with patients or how quickly you proceed to the next stages of their planned treatment.

The Continuum of Healing Simplified

There is a distinct start to healing. It begins the moment of injury. At some point, the tissue is done healing. The transition between phases of healing is not so clearly demarcated. It flows from one to the next. To keep it simple during surgery, I like to think of the immediate, early and late phases of healing. How can I have a positive impact in each of these phases? Similarly, I want to pay attention to what might have a negative impact on immediate, early and late healing.

Healing is truly incredible. It is complex and difficult to grasp. That's why I like to think about it in those three phases.

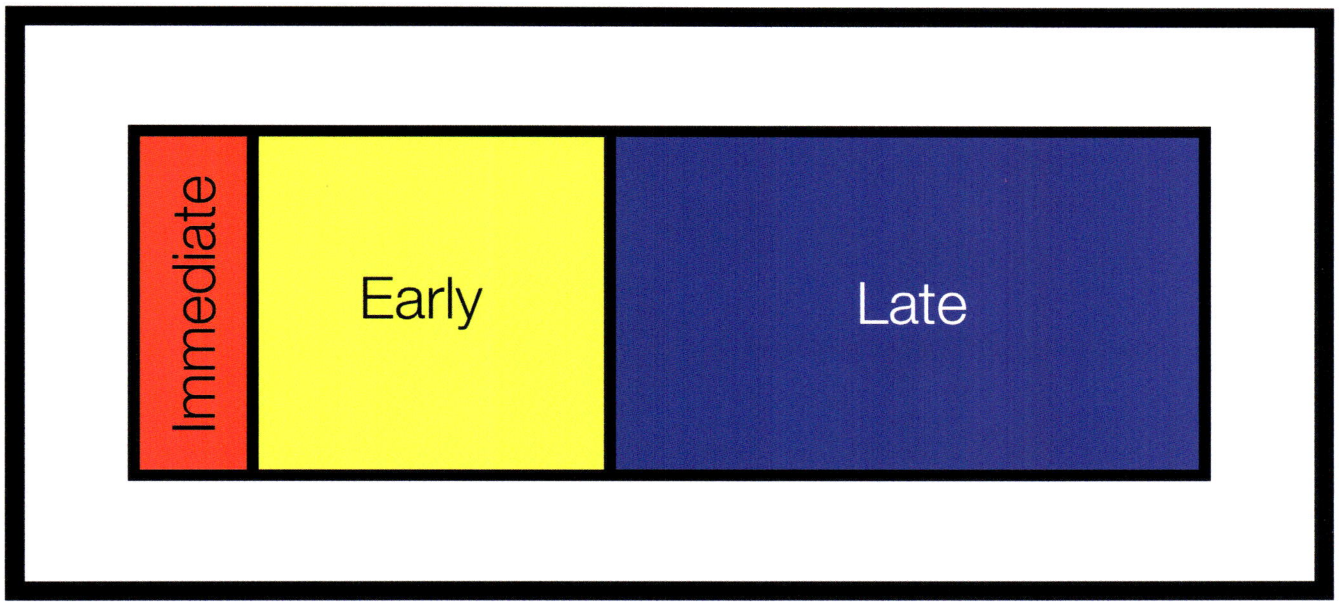

Figure 1-24 During surgery, I like to simplify my thoughts to the immediate, early and late healing phases. What can I do to help cells heal in these three phases?

References

1. Arias JI, Aller MA, Arias J. Surgical inflammation: a pathophysiological rainbow. J Transl Med. 2009 Mar 23;7:19.
2. Marucha PT, Kiecolt-Glaser JK, Favagehi M. Mucosal wound healing is impaired by examination stress. Psychosom Med. 1998;60(3):362-365.

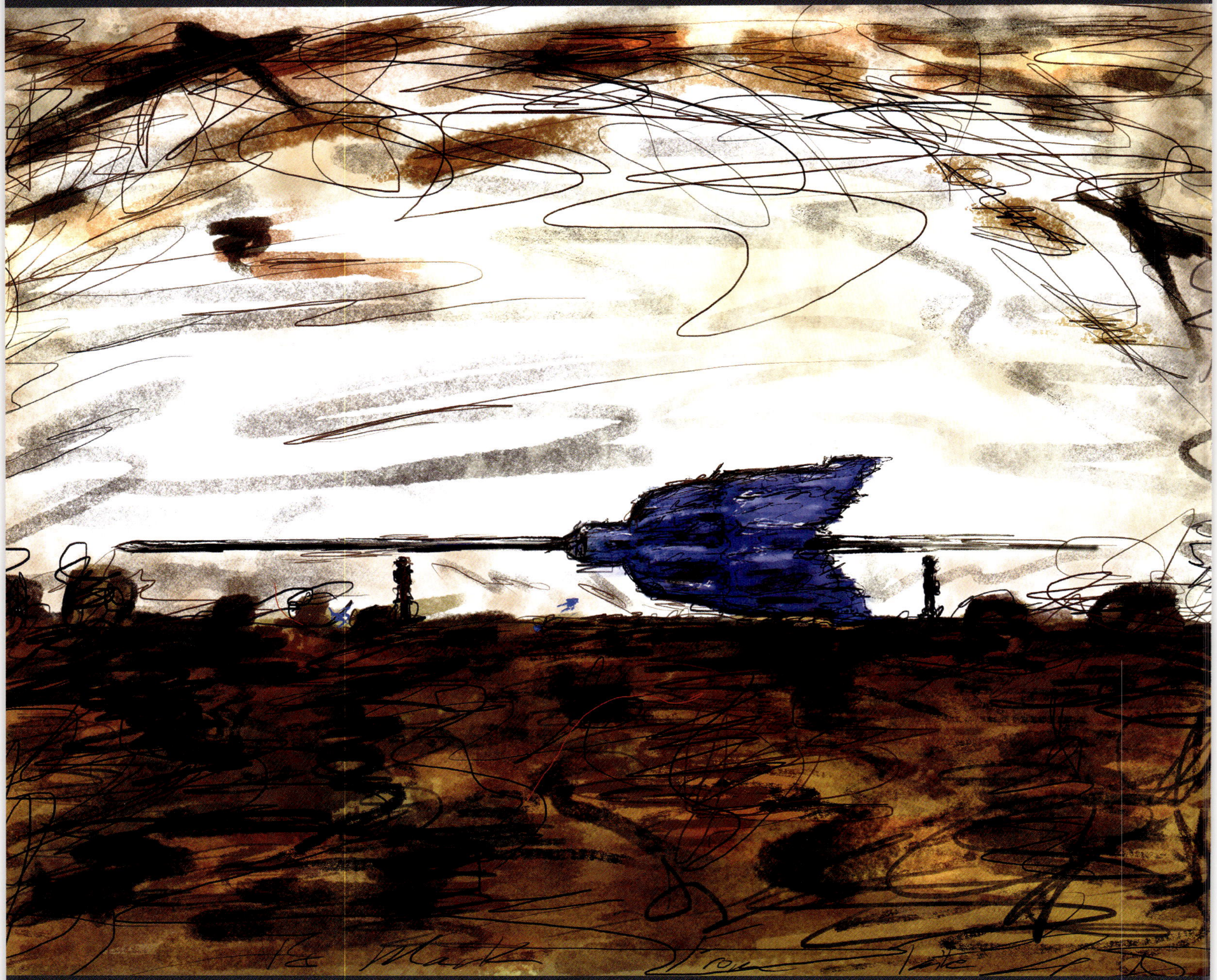

Patients often see local anesthetic needles as enormous, even ominous. To the cells, they are. Keep them in mind with everything you do. It all matters to them. (Artwork inspired by Claes Oldenburg.)

CHAPTER 2

THE ART OF TISSUE MANAGEMENT

SURGERY = INJURY

The outcome of any surgery depends on many variables, with tissue management one of the most prominent and influential. How well was the hard and soft tissue treated during surgery? That story is told by the tissue and the patient during recovery.

Attention to Detail

Tissue management should not be confused with surgical skill. They are related but distinct. Highly skilled surgeons with incredible abilities still must choose to be kind to the tissue. Every moment of surgery and every move of an instrument participates in surgical injury. The tissue is splayed open, unprotected and vulnerable. Internal flesh is exposed and helpless. In that moment, there is nothing the cells can do to protect themselves.

How do I honor the tissue and its role in healing? Afterall, the cells of the surgical site do most of the heavy lifting. Their job only begins when ours is finished. Even if the surgery goes on for hours, the healing goes on for days, weeks even months.

Protecting the vulnerable always begins with awareness. If we are not aware of the potential danger and harm, how can we defend against further, unnecessary injury?

There are several areas of vulnerability to respect during surgery:

Individual cell integrity

Each of your individual cells carries your entire DNA sequence. All your genetic information is housed inside every one of them. They each have their own protection (cell wall) and power plant (mitochondria). Consider the millions of individual cells involved in any given procedure. By themselves, they are incredibly fragile. As part of a living being, they could even be considered sacred. They deserve respect. When an individual cell is traumatized, it releases proinflammatory mediators such as prostaglandins and histamine. These increase tissue trauma and stimulate pain receptors. Think about maintaining and protecting individual cells.

Cell adhesion

Remember the "adherens junctions" from biology class? These are the intercellular junctions, the mechanical attachments, that hold epithelial cells together. Desmosomes are like a spot weld. They are circular adherens junctions that seem to be especially effective at resisting abrasion in the spinous layer of the epithelium.

Hard and soft tissue cell surfaces have specialized proteins that bind them to other cells and the extracellular matrix. These cell adhesion molecules, called linker proteins, are embedded in the cell wall. They are responsible for maintaining intercellular structural integrity. They hold the fabric of the tissue together. If you think about these attachments and respect them when manipulating the tissue, you likely will be more cautious and attentive to the details. This will serve you and your patients well.

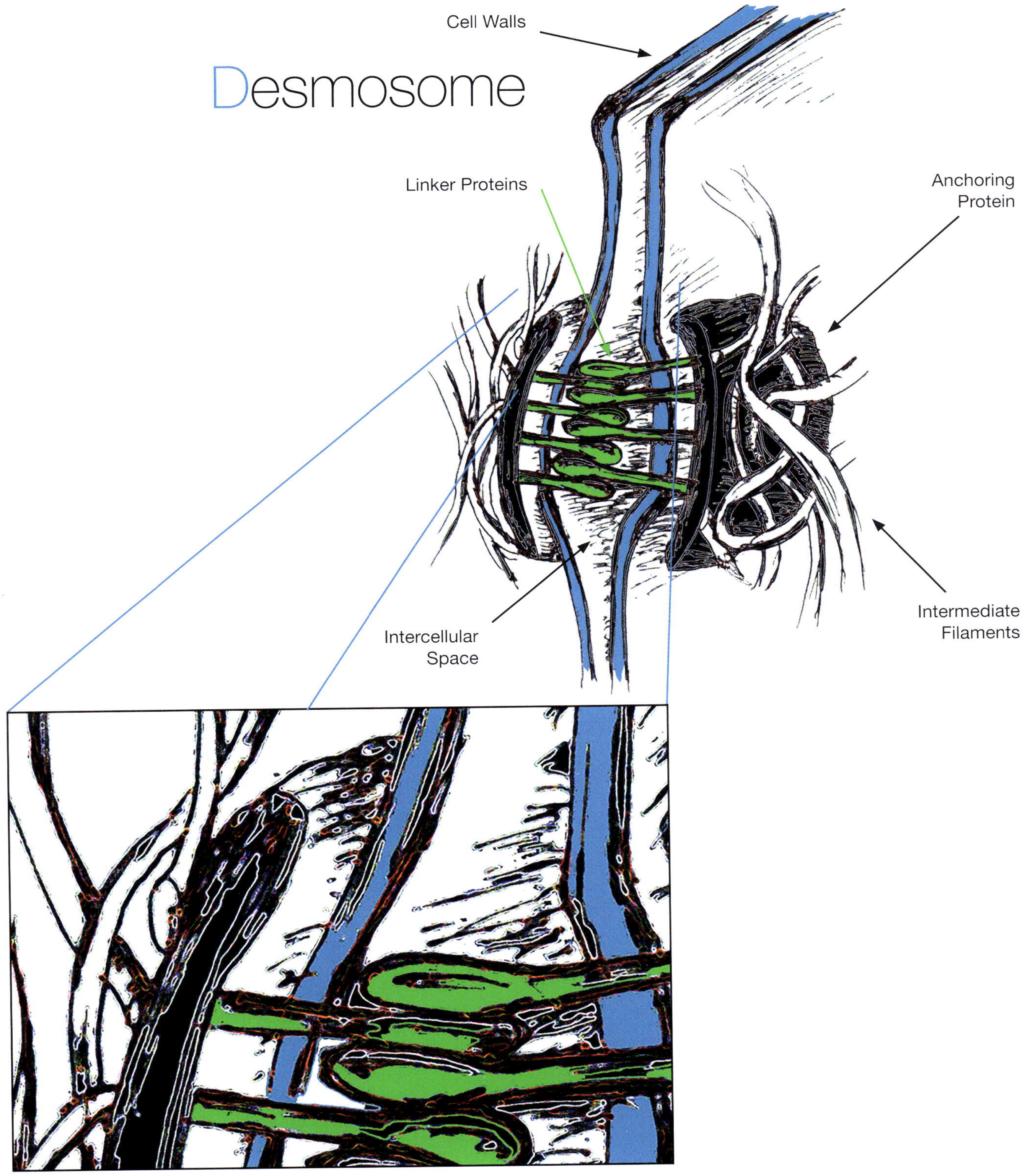

Figure 2-1 Linker proteins (*green*) are anchored within each cell. They extend through the cell wall (*blue*) where they link with the adjacent cell. These interdigitations form a network of spot welds holding the tissue together.

Tissue layers

Tissue is generally stronger within a given layer than it is between layers. It is easy to separate between the layers unintentionally or inadvertently, which can be a problem. For instance, submucosal connective tissue has a tendency to peel off the periosteum when reflecting a full thickness flap. But a clean subperiosteal dissection can easily release the periosteum off underlying bone. Awareness and attention to the middle layers helps protect this vulnerability. It is important to be able to visualize the tissue layers when performing surgery.

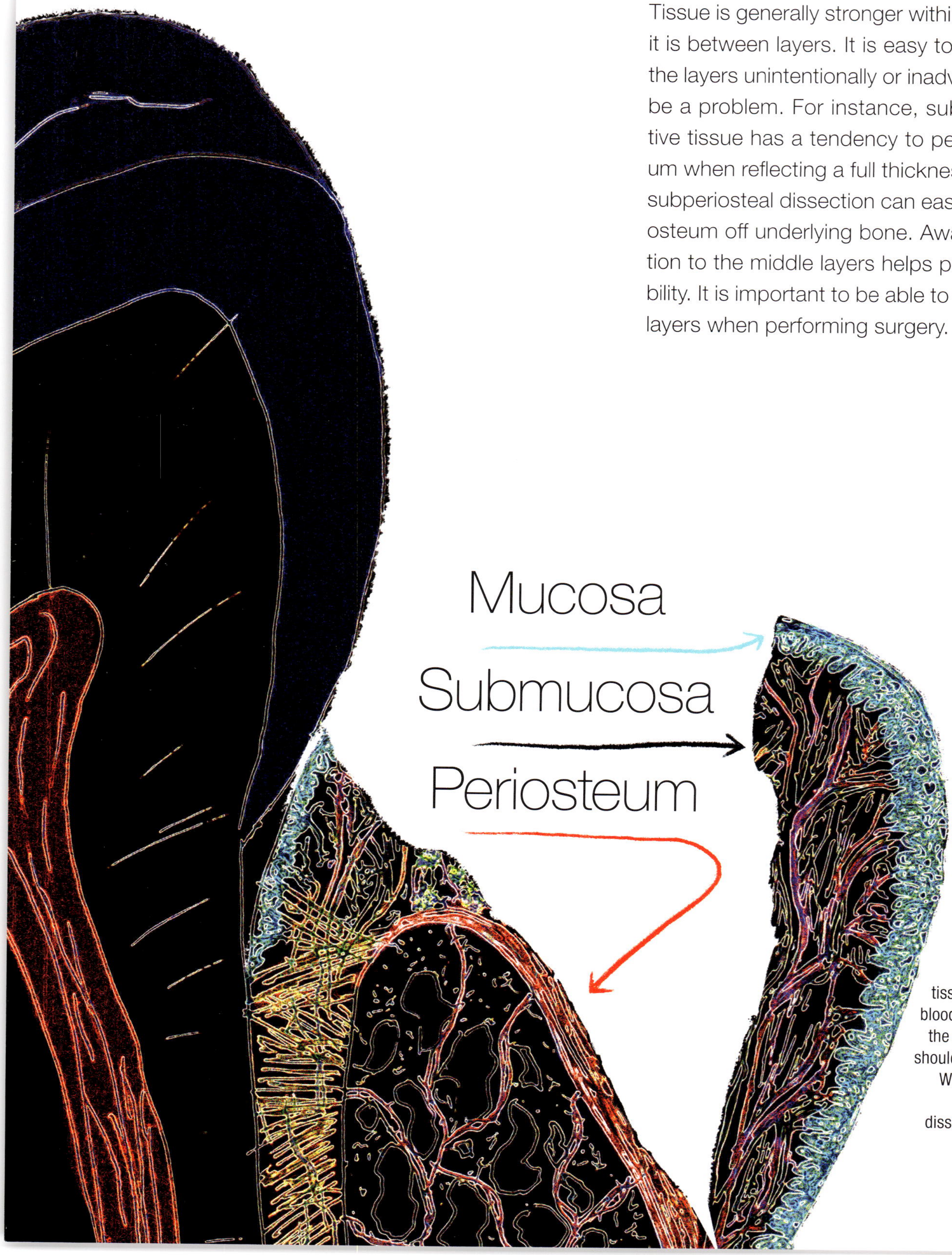

Figure 2-2 When reflecting a flap, it is easy to dissect a supraperiosteal layer. This strips the overlying tissue and compromises the blood supply. When accessing the underlying bone, the flap should include the periosteum. When a split thickness flap is needed, ensure the dissection is clean and in the correct plane.

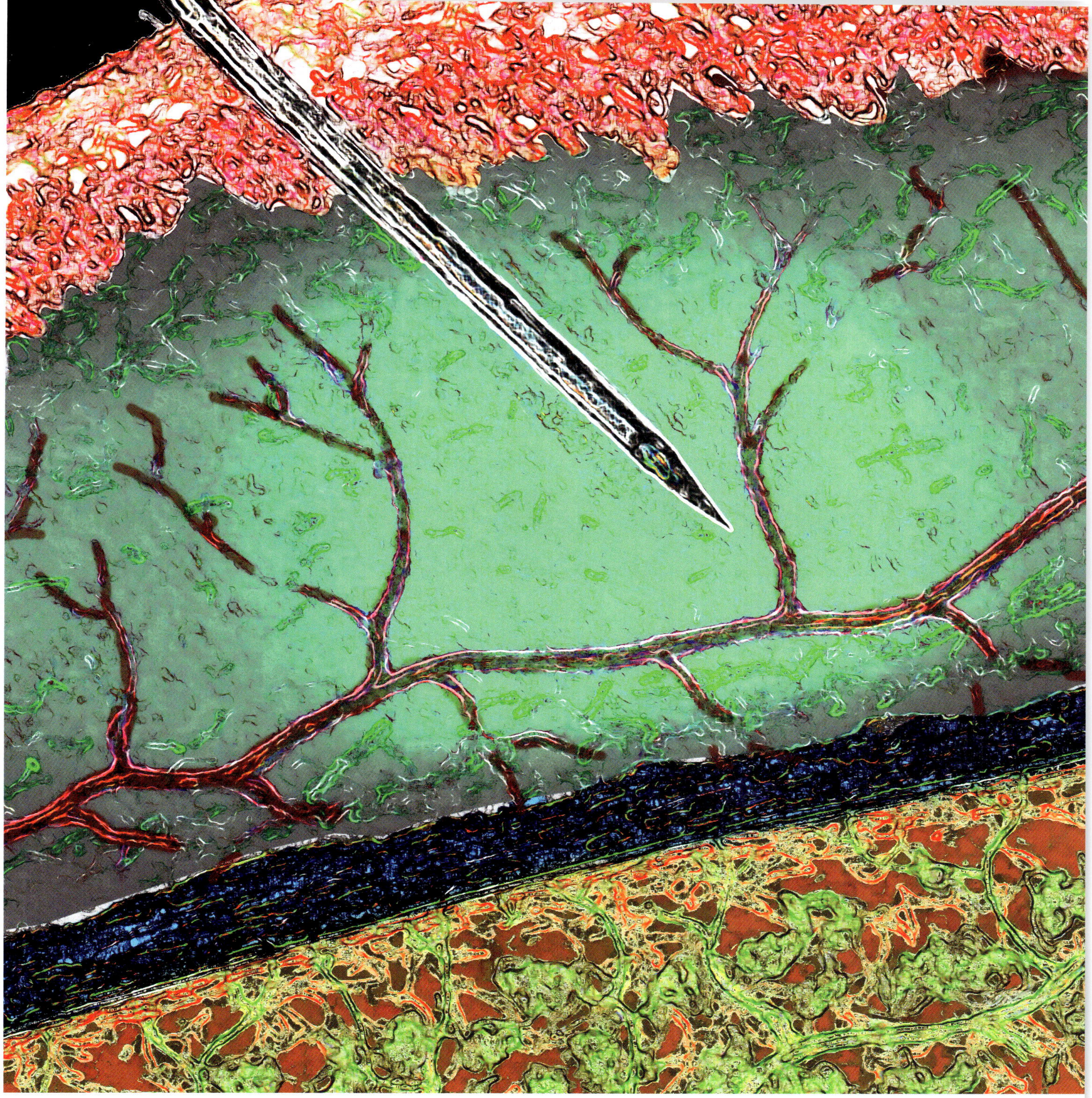

Figure 2-3 Needles injure tissue. The distension of the local anesthetic stretches intracellular attachments and can dissect between tissue planes. The local anesthetic itself can chemically injure the tissue, especially nerves. Being aware of the consequences of our actions is foundational to the art of oral surgery. (Artwork inspired by Vincent van Gogh.)

Trauma occurs even when administering local anesthetic. It fills the tissue with fluid, dissecting the layers. In addition to physical trauma, many patients experience psychological trauma from injections. People seem to think the 30-gauge needle is enormous. (Almost like a Claes Oldenburg sculpture. It is that big to the cells. (See figure page 26.) We do well when we empathize with patients who are scared of the needle.

Blood supply

Vessels are incredibly effective at delivering blood throughout the body. The large vessels feed smaller and smaller vessels down to capillaries and the cells themselves. The smaller the vessels, the more fragile and susceptible they are to injury during surgery. They are easily torn and crushed, especially the smallest capillaries. Larger vessels are more resilient, but they are responsible for much more tissue. The larger the vessel, the greater the impact when damaged. Handling tissue gently reduces the disruption of the blood supply that is imperative to healing. Preserve the blood supply to preserve life.

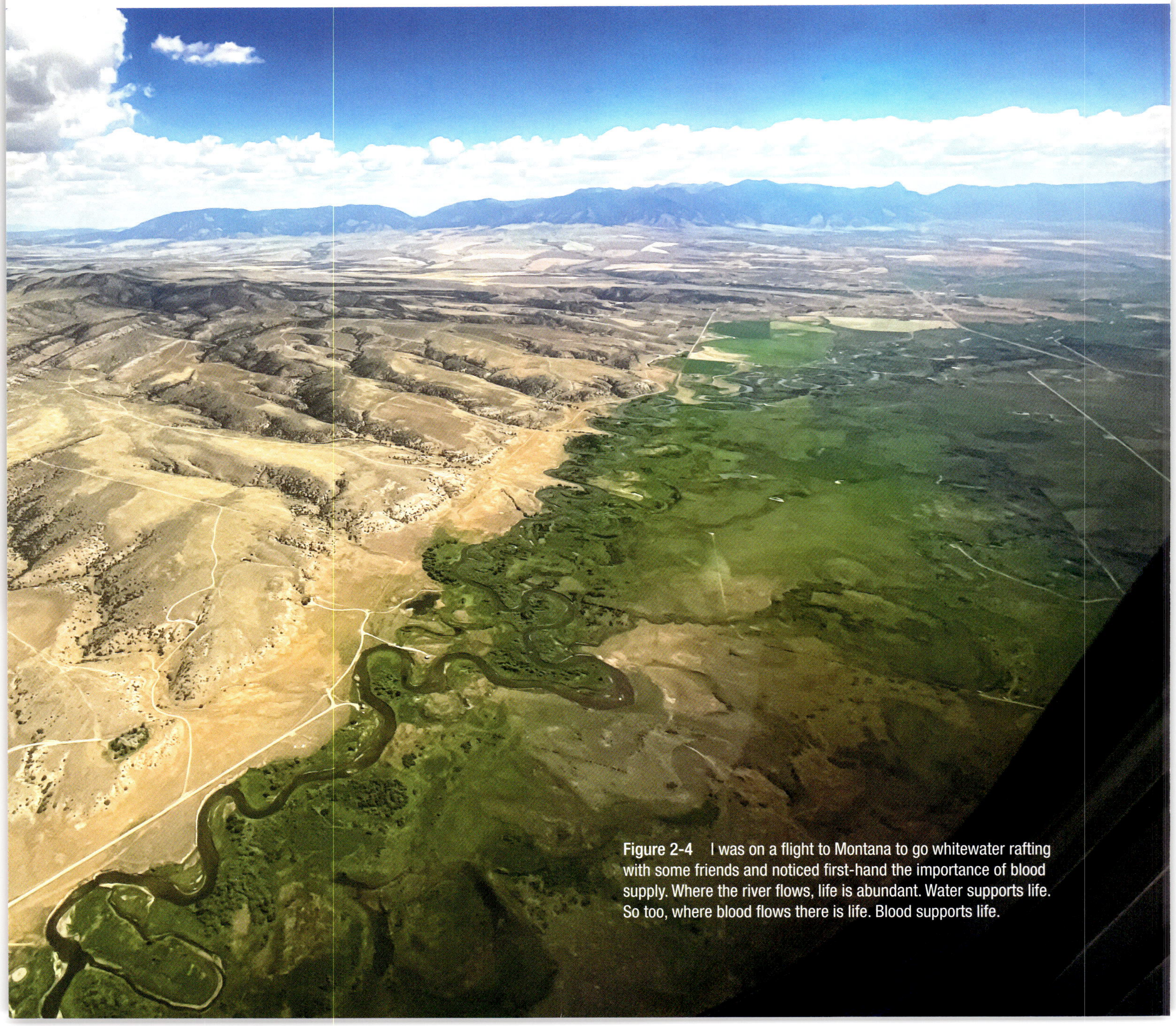

Figure 2-4 I was on a flight to Montana to go whitewater rafting with some friends and noticed first-hand the importance of blood supply. Where the river flows, life is abundant. Water supports life. So too, where blood flows there is life. Blood supports life.

Blood flow

A beautifully designed, perfectly elevated flap can easily be strangulated and suffer when it is not manipulated and handled with care. Retracting a flap can kink or occlude the vessels. Pay attention to the flap's position and color. During prolonged surgery, consider removing the retractor and giving it a break to allow blood to flow. Let the tissue breathe. Maybe you need a break for a moment too. Take a deep breath, all the way in and all the way out. Stretch your back and neck.

Some hypoxia is good. It actually promotes wound healing, but too much is deadly. When the tissue is starved for too long, it can trigger excessive inflammation and even trigger apoptosis and necrosis. Surgery always causes localized hypoxia. Excellent tissue management maximizes the benefits and minimizes harm.

Tissue hypoxia is a key factor in stimulating wound healing. The master regulator in tissue oxygen homeostasis is a fascinating little dimeric protein called Hypoxia-Inducible Factor-1 (HIF-1). When there is enough oxygen (normoxic conditions), the HIF-1 protein gets tagged for destruction by proteasomes (the enzymes responsible for destroying damaged or unneeded proteins in a cell). When there isn't enough oxygen (hypoxic conditions), HIF-1 is not tagged for destruction, and it survives. It regulates multiple gene expression pathways, including VEGF. It recruits cells to the site, promotes the production of extracellular matrix and cell division, and helps the cells survive hypoxic conditions[1]. This hypoxia paradox represents much of the art of oral surgery. We need some, but too much of a good thing can become harmful.

Cleanup

Early in the healing process, resident macrophages begin cleaning up the mess of cellular debris. These white blood cells increase in number by recruiting others and by signaling monocyte differentiation. In conjunction with various enzymes and lymphatic tissue, they have the enormous job of digesting the wreckage that remains. They clear out junk to make way for healing. They are tiny machines. At about 21 microns (0.000813 inches) in diameter, I am sure they appreciate all the help we can give them[2].

Tug of war

As a kid, did you ever line up on that huge rope at recess and look behind you to see a brute anchoring your team? With that kid on your side, you just knew you were going to win. You still had to pull, but you weren't so worried about the rope ripping your hands.

Soft tissue handling is kind of like a game of tug of war. If I were a betting man, I would put my money on stainless steel over mucosa. Periosteum over lamina propria. Thick retromolar tissue over thin buccal gingiva. When we play tug of war, someone is going to win.

A few things to consider:

- Good intentions can be misguiding. There are times when I intend to perform minimal flap elevation and I end up with a longer surgical time and tattered tissue. Intending to minimize soft tissue trauma can result in more trauma. Vigilance in soft tissue management pays high rewards and turns good intentions into reality. Think about how your flap design and development serve you and the patient. Then think about it again while retracting tissue during the procedure. Maintaining this awareness will not only guide the task at hand, but it can also be a teacher for future surgeries.

- If you ask more of a small flap than it can offer, something will give, often at the expense of tearing the gingiva or mucosa. Be careful and attentive to what you are asking of the tissue while developing, reflecting and retracting a flap.
- There is a cuff of more adherent, fibrous tissue surrounding teeth right at the alveolar crest. This should be cut before any tension is placed on the tissue.
- When you begin reflecting a full thickness flap, if there isn't a clean incision completely through the periosteum, the periosteum tends to stay put. The plane of dissection will often progress along the basement membrane. This significantly increases surgical trauma and creates space for edema, hematoma formation, and the spread of infection. The periosteum is much more stable than the overlying tissue. When it is adequately incised, the dissection progresses much more predictably.

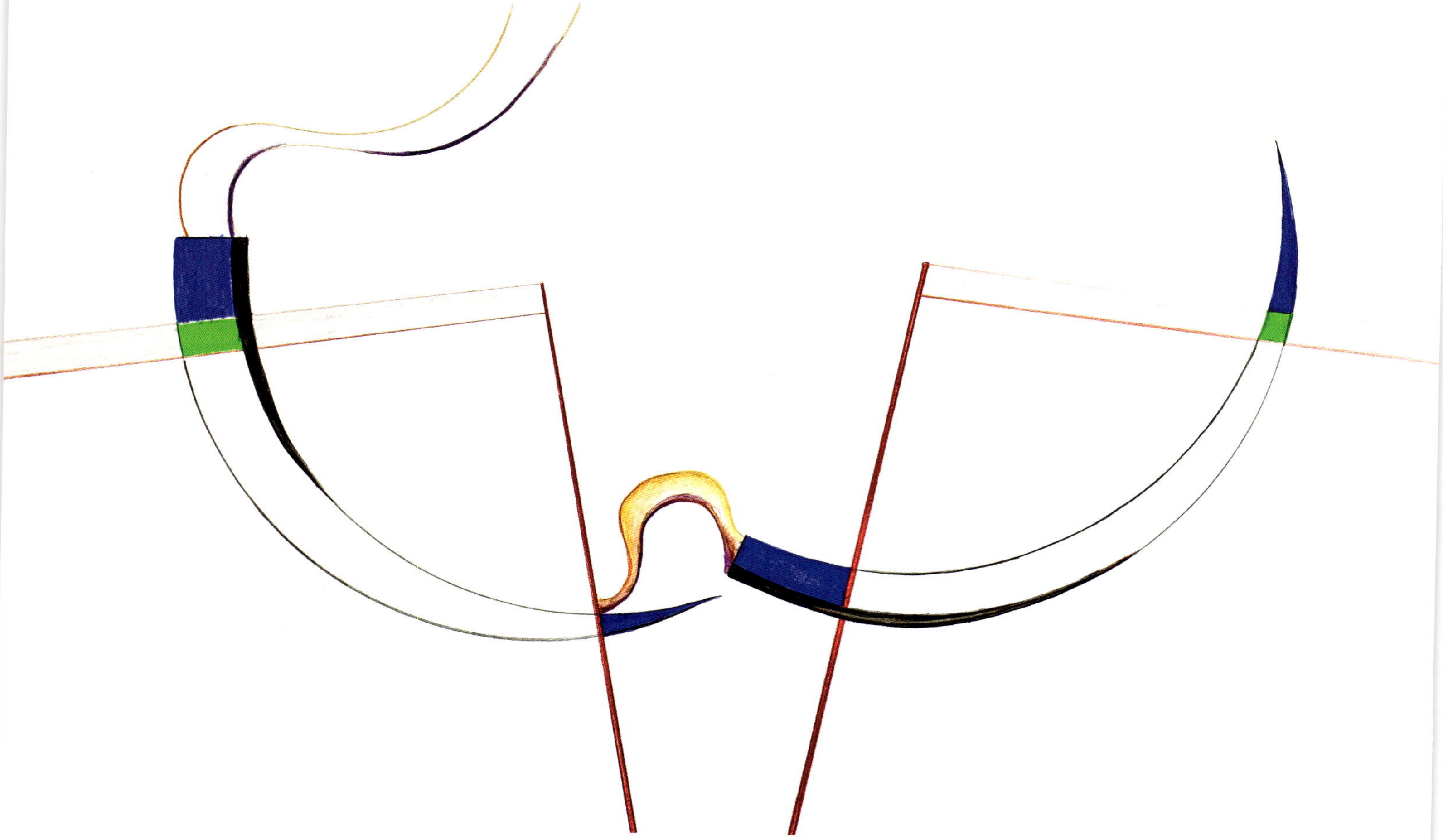

Figure 2-5 Envision the tissue edges coming together as you pass the needle through one side and then the other side of the incision. (Artwork inspired by Wassily Kandinsky.)

Suturing

Suturing is often the final step in surgery and is what the patient sees. Accurately and precisely reapproximating the edges looks good both to us and the cells involved. The cells heal best when realigned properly across the incision. The basement layer cells want to be next to other basement layer cells. When passing the needle, take equal bites of the tissue on both sides. This is one of the simplest elements of suturing. If it looks and feels like you have about the same amount on each side, you likely will be close enough.

The cross section of a needle can either be non-cutting (round) or cutting (triangular). The cutting needle is designed to penetrate with a sharp tip and then incise the tissue as it passes through. This makes passing through the tissue much easier than a non-cutting or round needle. It improves control over the needle path and protects the tissue from further trauma. But there is an increased risk of tearing the tissue if the needle does not passively move through it. Additionally, tension from the suture on the cut can pull the thread through the tissue more easily.

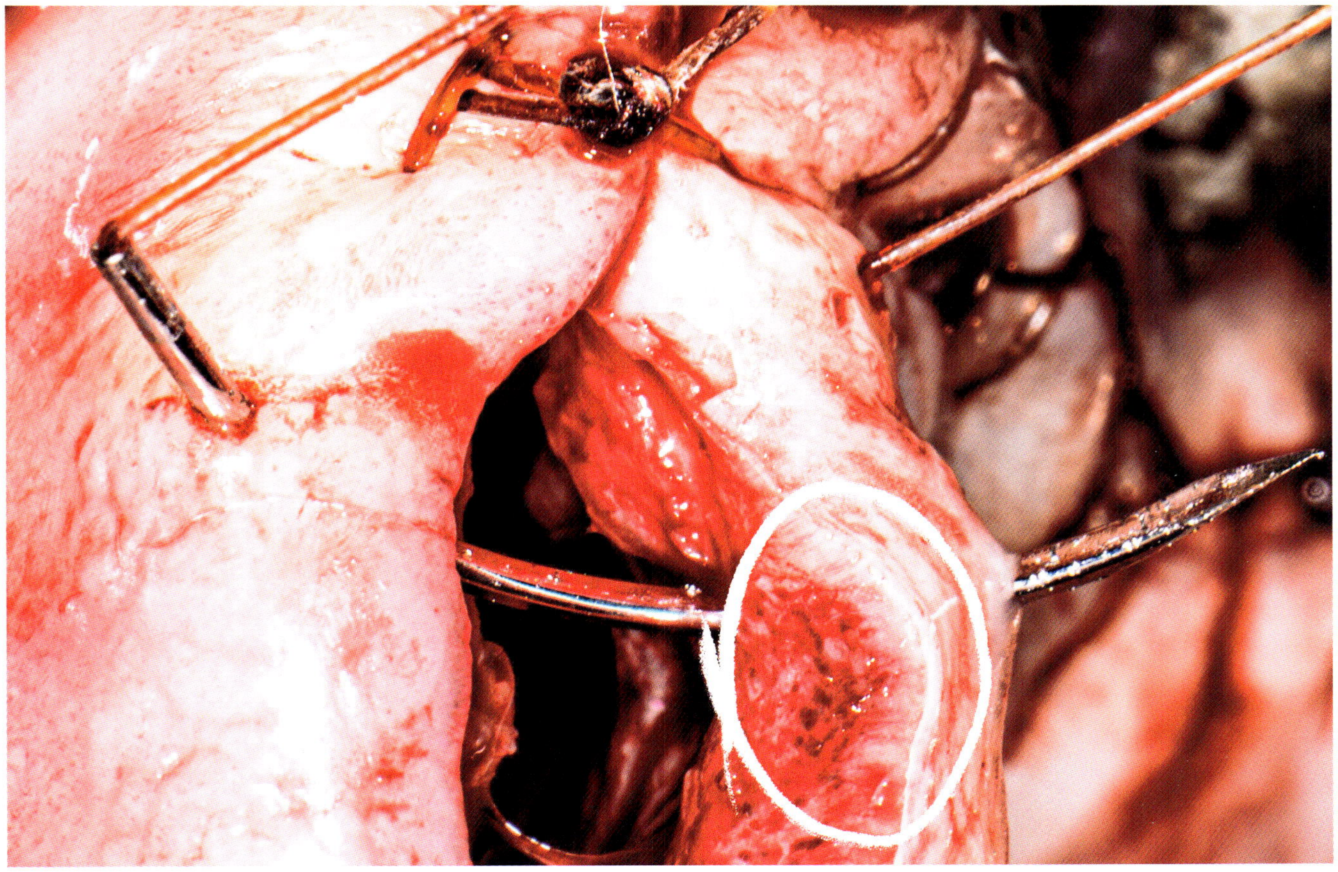

Figure 2-6 Note the layers of the palatal tissue. You can see the superficial epithelium and underlying connective tissue. We want the suture to be passed in a way that brings them together across the incision like they were before surgery.

Because of the complicated angles and positions, passing a needle through tissue often involves some tension and, of course, trauma. Many clinicians opt to use reverse cutting needles to help minimize both. While it has the same benefits as a cutting needle, the reverse cutting needle leads with the non-cutting edge instead of the cutting edge. This makes it more forgiving to the tissue during the healing process.

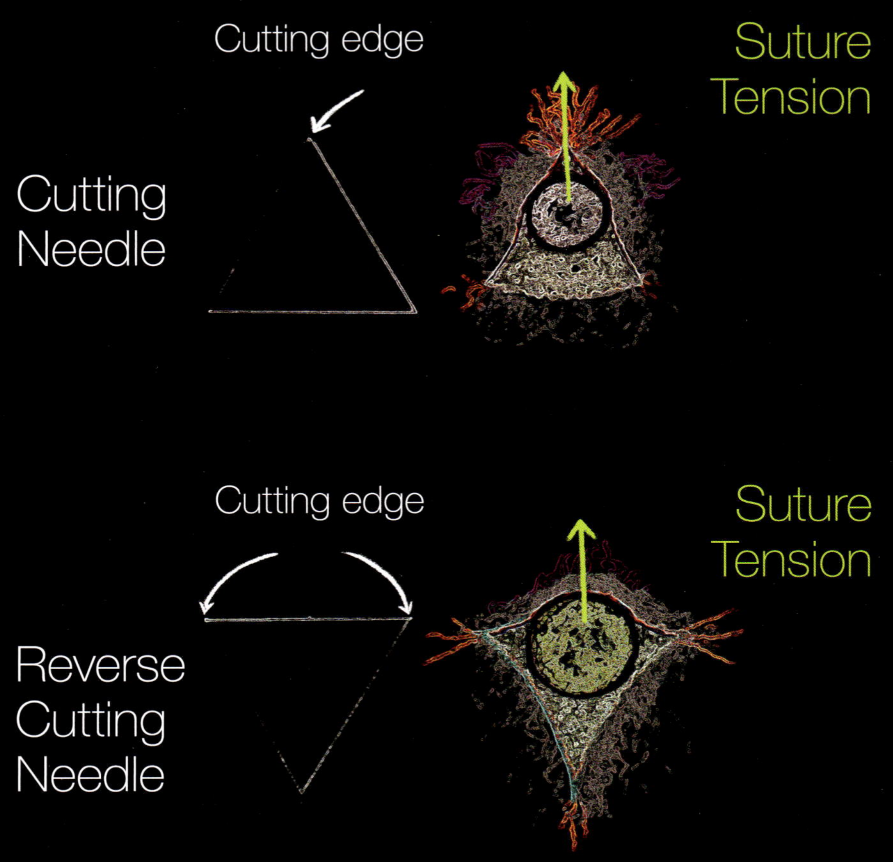

Figure 2-7 Tension from the suture can tear the tissue. A cutting needle results in more stress on the tissue than a reverse cutting needle.

Knot tying

If you can't tie a knot, tie a lot.
Friction holds a knot together. The two pieces of line or suture are wrapped in a pattern that allows the friction between them to hold them in position under tension. Their pattern and the amount of friction is dictated by the type of knot. If they are not wrapped or tied properly, they won't create the favorable friction necessary to hold the knot together.

A suture only holds as well as the knot that ties it. It should be snug enough to hold, but not so tight that it causes harm. The final tie can be pulled much tighter than the initial throw. Make sure the knot is tight enough just before cutting the ends.

There are many more topics to discuss regarding suturing, but we simply cannot cover it all in this book. Just remember the type of suture material you use will impact the tissue's response. Resorbable sutures cause increased tissue inflammation as enzymes break them down. The instruments used to handle the tissue can protect it or harm it. Grasp the tissue with adequate force to control it, but not so much to cause damage. Properly using tissue pickups with teeth is protective, but the teeth can lacerate tissue if they slip, or they can macerate tissue if they are squeezed too tightly.

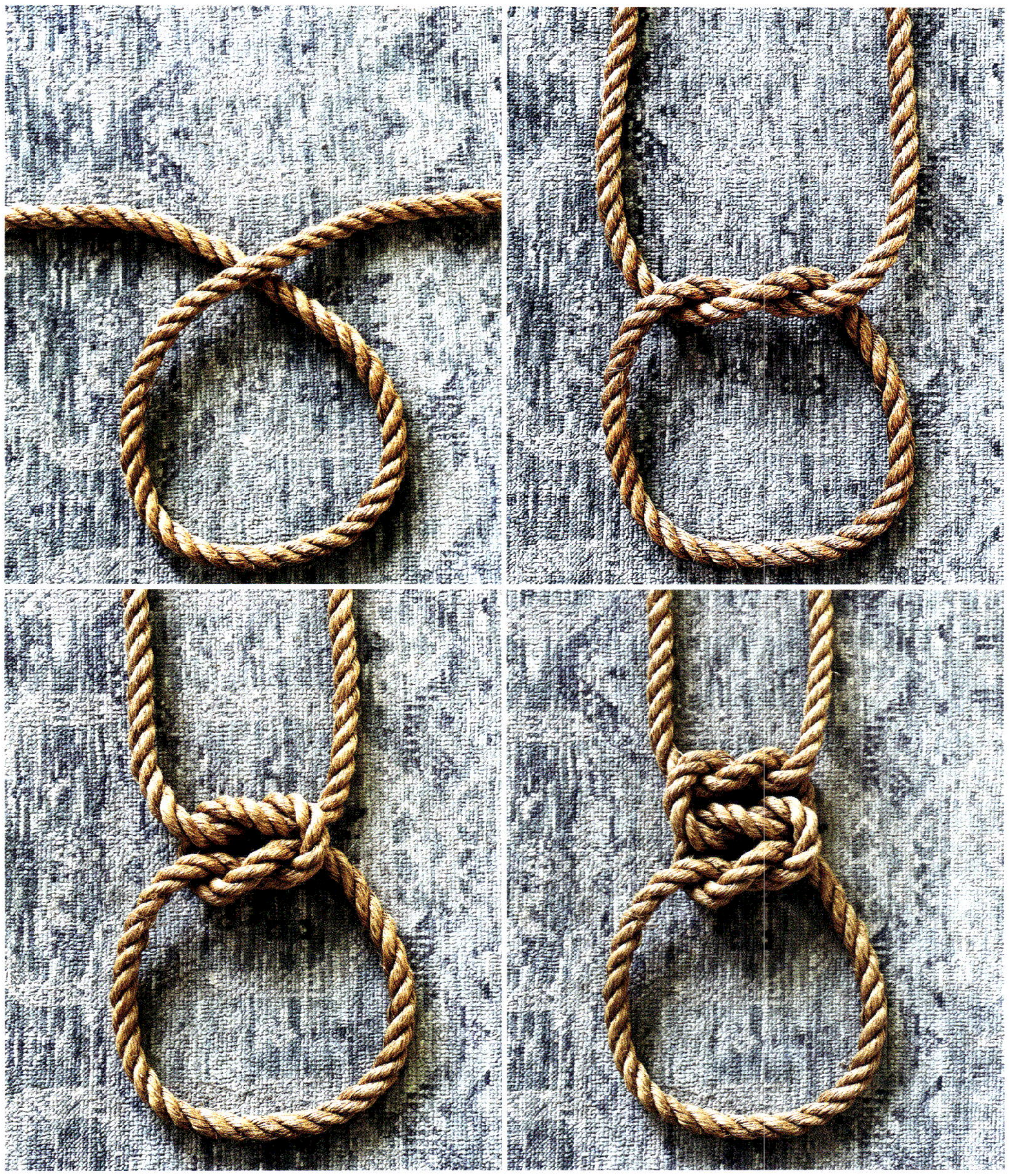

Figure 2-8 Each step in tying a knot increases friction between the two lines. Notice how these surgeon's knots stack neatly on each other. If they are not squared properly, they will not hold well. (This hemp line, courtesy of Bill Carnes, was salvaged from the Mississippi River, where it bound barges together.)

References

1. Hong WX, Hu MS, Esquivel M, et al. The Role of Hypoxia-Inducible Factor in Wound Healing. Adv Wound Care (New Rochelle). 2014 May 1;3(5):390-399.
2. Koh TJ, DiPietro LA. Inflammation and wound healing: the role of the macrophage. Expert Rev Mol Med. 2011 Jul 11;13:e23.

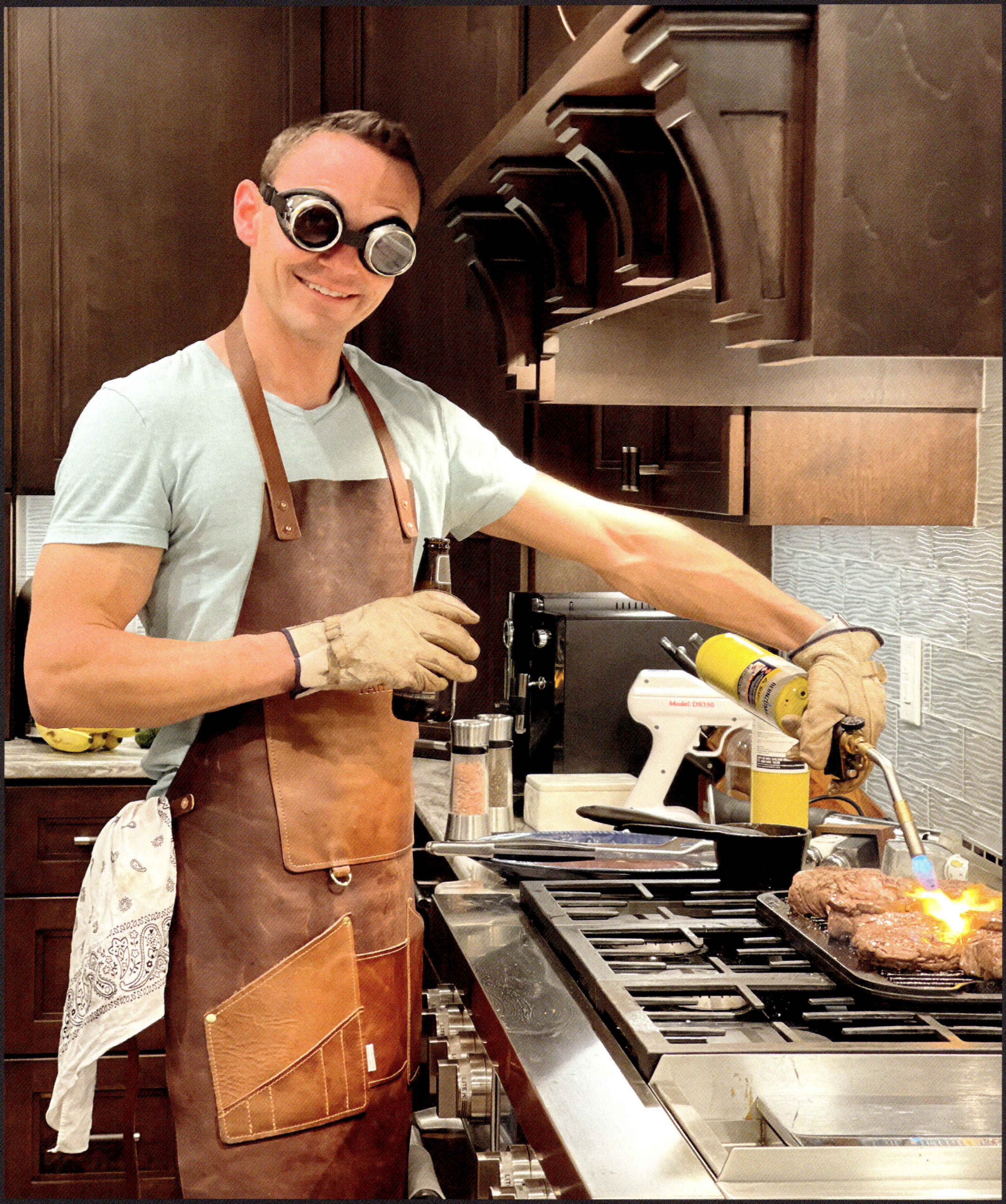

Fun with Maillard; my favorite way to prepare steak.

CHAPTER 3

THE ART OF PREPARATION

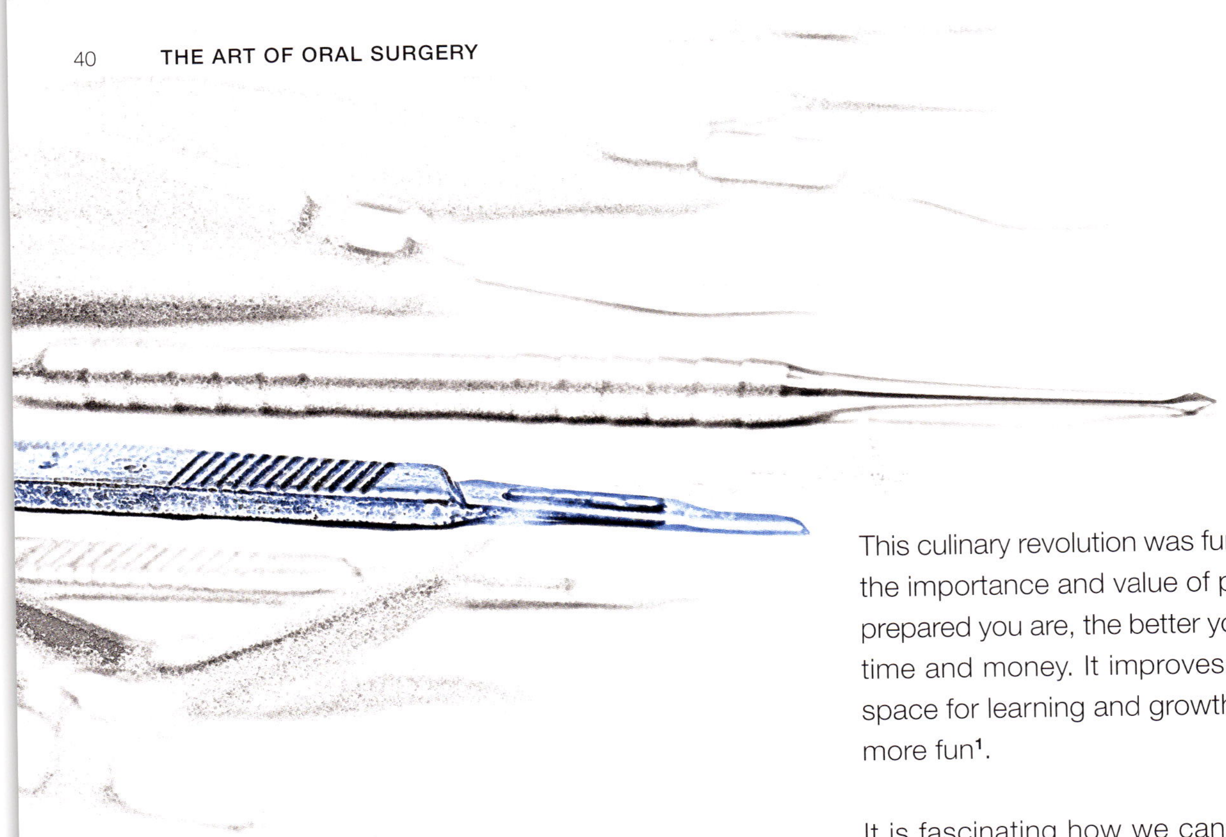

Mise en place. Everything in its place

Efficiency. Predictability. Consistency.

The modern restaurant was born when Georges Auguste Escoffier combined his military experience with his culinary passion and entrepreneurial spirit. Under growing pressure to serve more patrons with haute cuisine (high cooking), this French chef created a concept around the turn of the 20th century that now governs every respectable kitchen in the world: mise en place (pronounced "me-zohn plahs"), which means everything in its place. Predictable results with uncompromising quality could only be achieved through a system focused on preparation. He knew culinary art and developed a system to reproduce its beauty. In fact, the system provided much better quality and predictable results while making space to explore and create within culinary art. When everything is prepared and ready, it allows you to pay closer attention to the work at hand.

This culinary revolution was fundamentally based on the importance and value of preparation. The more prepared you are, the better you perform. This saves time and money. It improves outcomes. It creates space for learning and growth. And it makes it a lot more fun[1].

It is fascinating how we can learn from other disciplines and apply different principles to our own work. (See Atul Gawande's work on applying aviation checklists in "Checklist Manifesto.") The mise en place concept applies directly to the art of oral surgery. Escoffiere's title and role as a chef who happened to be an entrepreneur and teacher is very similar to ours as dentists, entrepreneurs and teachers.

Steps of mise en place: Be as efficient as possible

- **Prepare the chef/surgeon**. *Know the recipe*. How well do I know my procedure? Can I anticipate each step? Can my team anticipate each step?
- **Prepare the ingredients/supplies**. *Gather, measure, mince and chop*. Do I have everything I need at hand? Biologics, hardware, medications, emergency medications?
- **Prepare the space**. *Gather and organize tools and arrange everything according to their use*.

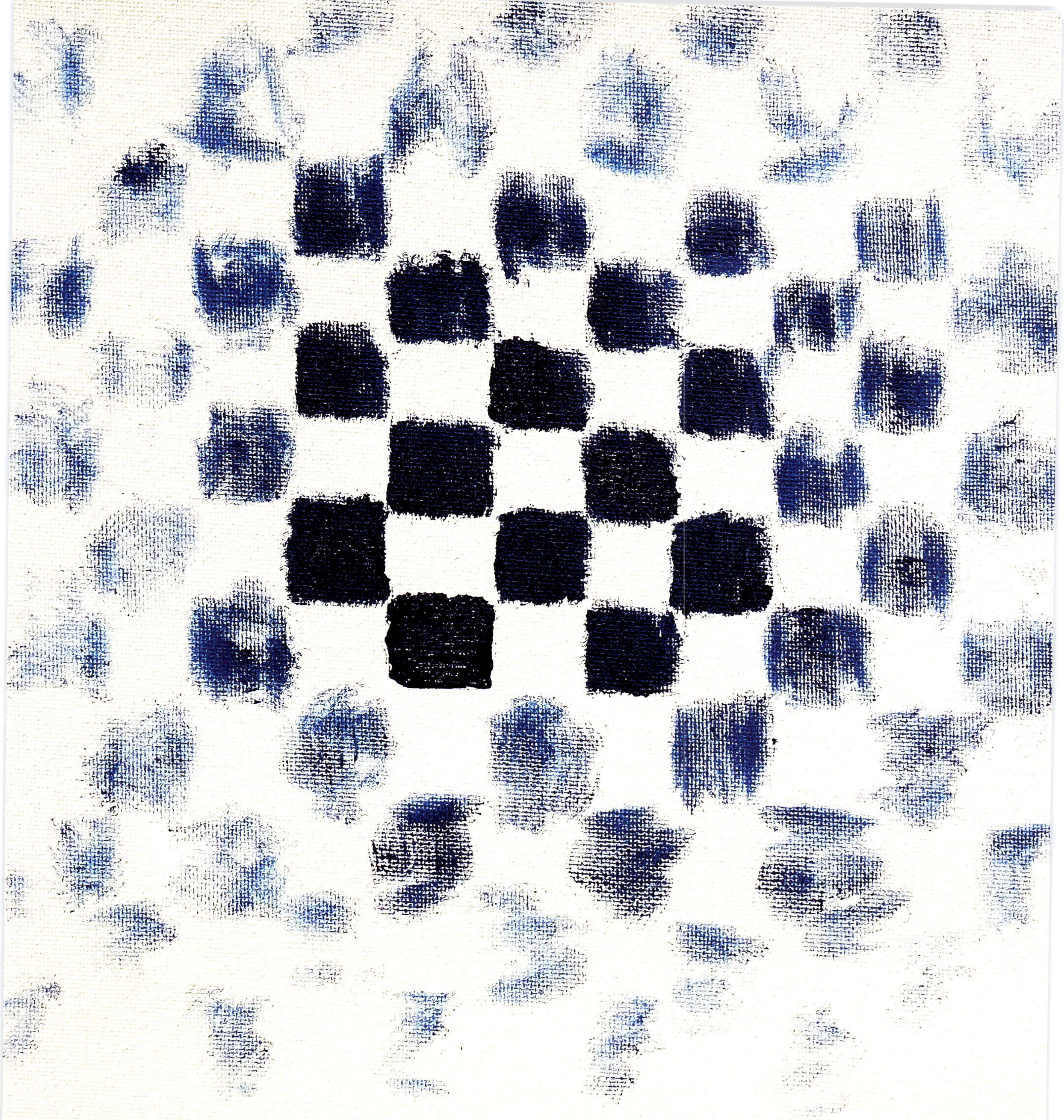

Figure 3-1 Our closest moves are always the clearest, but we must be prepared for what may happen at the periphery. The farther out we can anticipate, the better we can prepare for what is to come. (Artwork inspired by Virginia Chamlee.)

Visualize every aspect of the procedure's flow from the surgeon's perspective and, equally important, from the assistant's. Even look at the patient's perspective. The organized and prepared workspace is the face of mise en place, or as my incredible assistant Kailey always says, "Everything has a place. Everything in its place."

- **Clean as you go**. *Messy station = messy mind.* Maintaining order during surgery helps maintain a clear mind. My hand should know where to go without me looking. In my practice, I call this "resetting the tray."

You're only as good as your mise.
Save time. Stay organized.

Know the procedure

Preparation begins with knowing the procedure. What is the patient scheduled for? Does that match what will really happen? Mise en place starts with everyone on the team knowing the plan, understanding the process and being able to adapt to the potential changes inherent in surgery. Things change. Being ready and able to adjust for changes develops from a broader understanding of the procedure. We don't plan on a sinus perforation, but we all know what we need to do if it occurs—and we are ready for it as a team.

Gaining experience takes time. An experienced team knows what to expect. Educating your team and standardizing processes with your team accelerates their knowledge, confidence and preparedness exponentially. It gives them the potential to function like long-time veterans in a very short amount of time. This type of intentional preparation is well worth the effort. Engaged teams want to know. They want to understand. They want to participate at that higher level. Equip their brains to keep up with you and you will find they propel you and your practice to new heights.

Know your instruments

Any well-equipped kitchen must have a proper knife block. Each knife is designed with very specific intent and engineering. You cannot easily slice tomatoes with a bread knife or cut a watermelon with a paring knife. And while we typically use a knife for its sharp edge, sometimes it is the back of the blade, known as the spine, that is used when bruising lemongrass or milking an ear of corn. Similarly, the cutting edge of a scalpel is typically used to incise. It also can be used in a sweeping motion for stripping or scraping tissue, a technique Dr. Istvan Urban describes as similar to strumming a guitar. The back of the blade also can be used to score tissue so it can be realigned easily. Even the handle can be used for blunt dissection.

A clever person could probably sift through a block of knives and find a useful blade for preparing a fine dish. But true chefs know their knives like the back of their hand. Afterall, they become an extension of their hand. They know all the various tools, techniques, ingredients and principles of how it all works together to create a nourishing work of art.

Set up your workspace

My mise en place in my clinic is built on the most common instruments for my most common procedures. They make up the basic tray I have in every surgery. Each specific procedure has its own instruments added to the setup. This is all outlined in our Standard Operating Procedures (SOP) with photos and an explanation. Additional instruments that I anticipate needing are opened on the surgical table. Other instruments I may need are also readily available, placed unopened in the room on the back counter. Ideally, we have everything we would reasonably expect to use for the procedure in the room. This includes biologics for grafting and medications for sedation. Visualizing the flow of the procedure when setting up helps identify which instruments to open and which to have available.

The eight basic trays in my practice are all identical. The instruments are positioned in their order of use, mine on the right and my assistant's on the left. I work my way from right to left, from incision, to tissue reflection, luxation, elevation, curettage, and then closure. Forceps are up top as they vary depending on the procedure. The cleaner and more organized my setup, the more efficient and better I can perform my surgery. When I am done with an instrument, I try to place it back where it belongs. (This is a constant work in progress for me...) Resetting the tray keeps it neat and efficient. I even find it makes a difference in how I feel about the surgery. My basic tray setup has changed many times over the past decade and will continue to evolve as I hone my skills and develop new ones.

In the operating room, my setup looks totally different, but the concept is the same. The instruments are planned and prepared. My assistant knows each instrument and its use. And everything is in order.

Figure 3-2 Fiber-handle chisels lined up and ready for mandibular bilateral sagittal split ramus osteotomy.

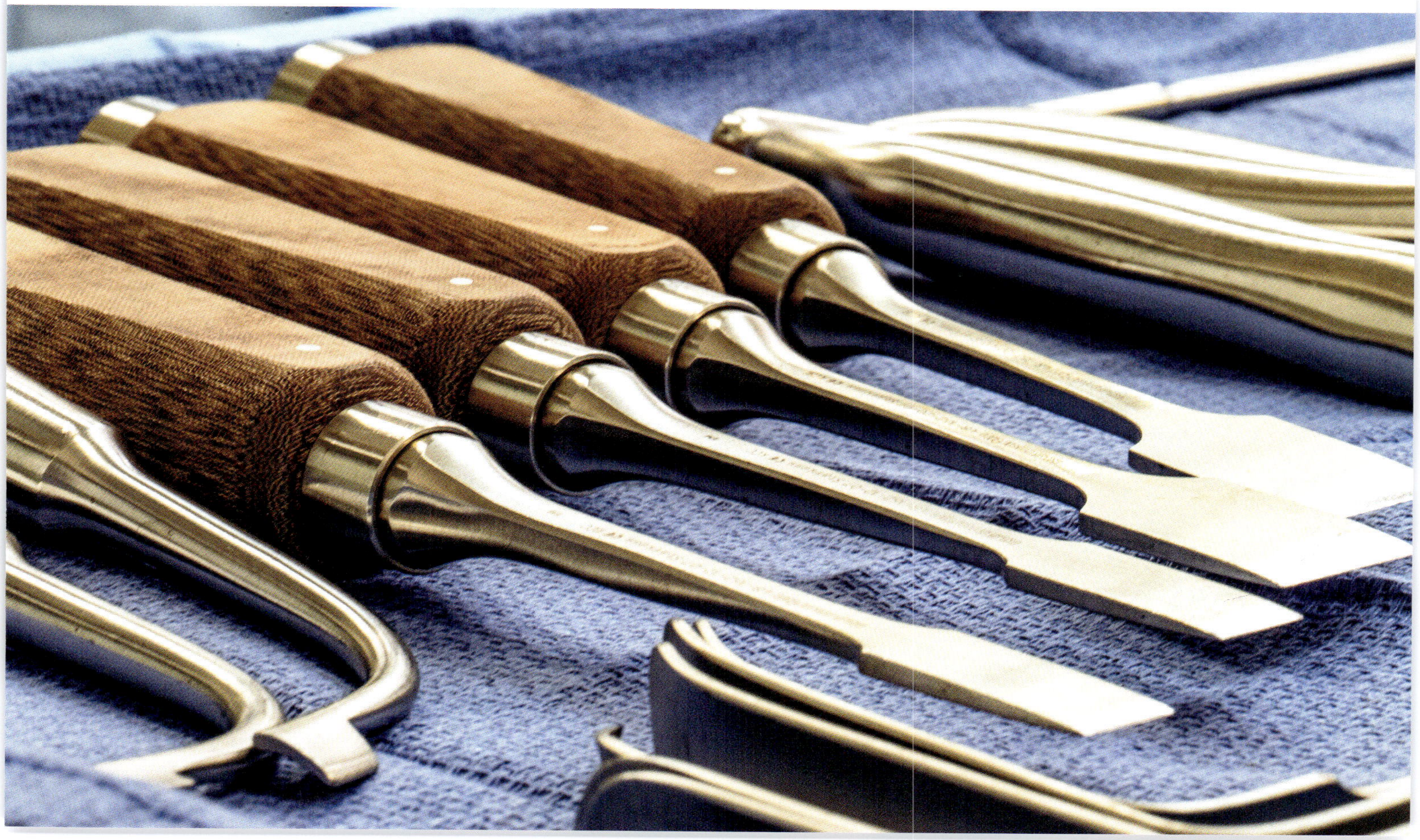

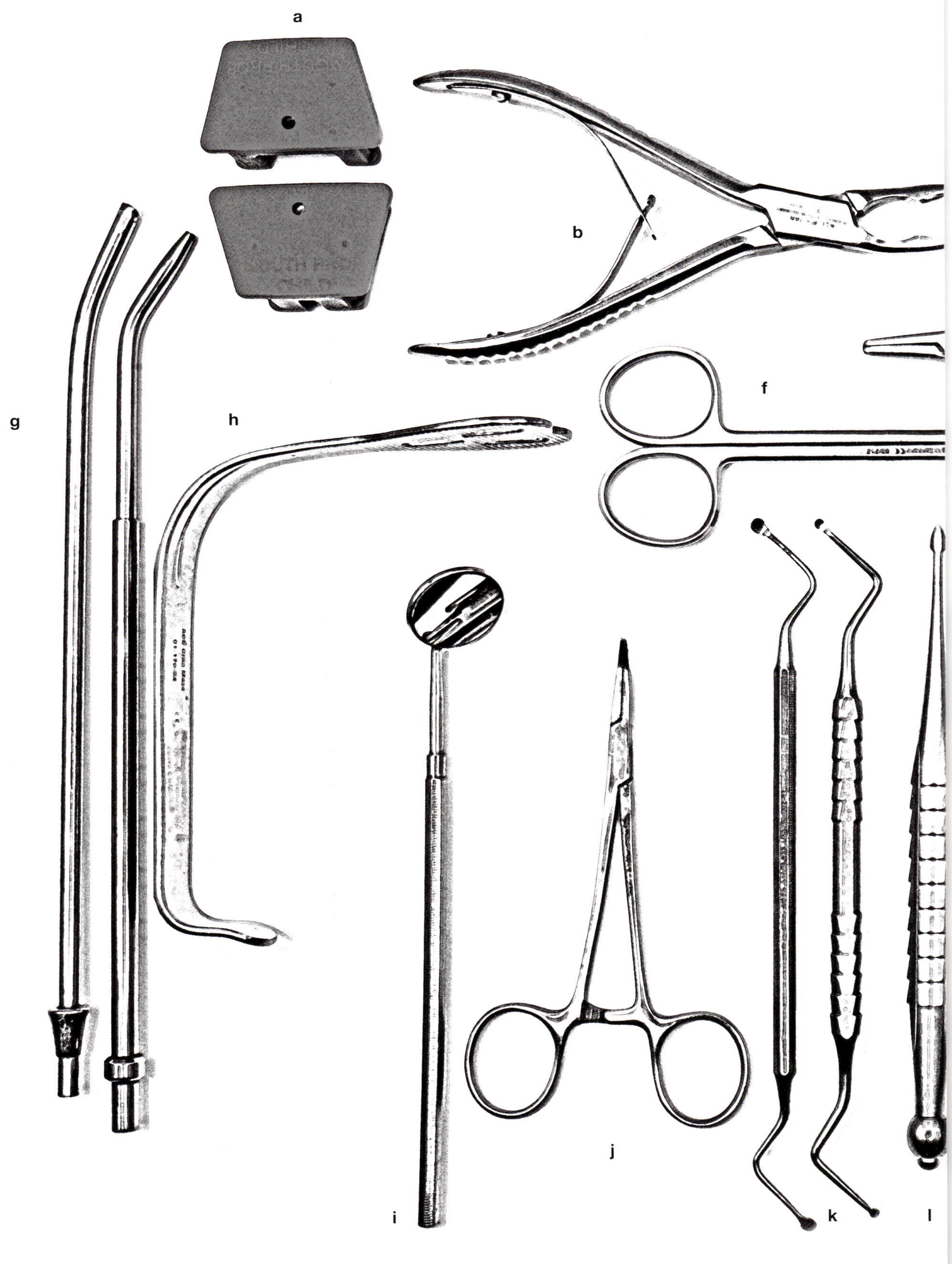
a
b
f
g
h
i
j
k
l

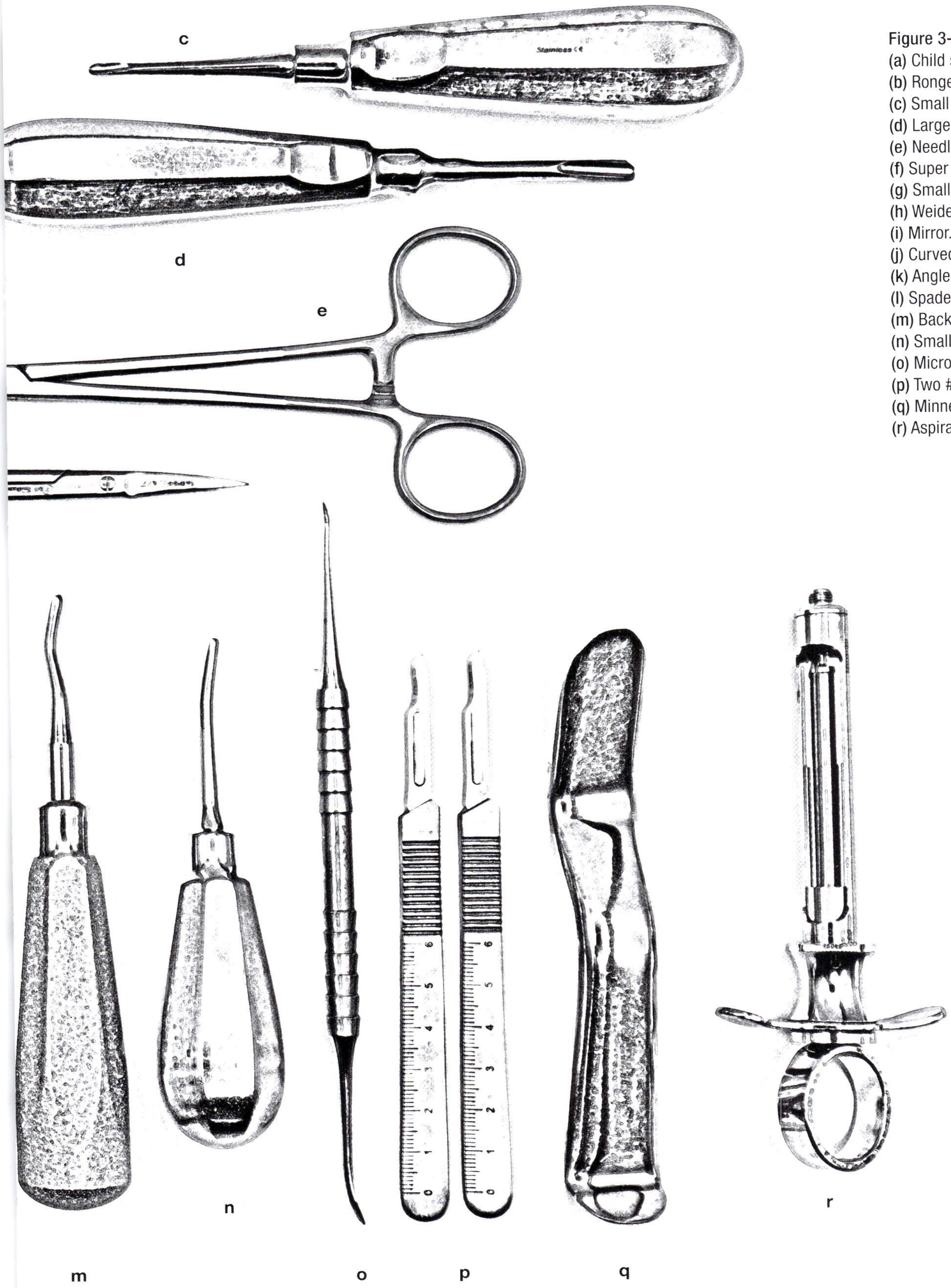

Figure 3-3 Basic tray.
(a) Child sized bite blocks.
(b) Rongeurs.
(c) Small straight elevator.
(d) Large straight luxator.
(e) Needle drivers.
(f) Super cut scissors.
(g) Small and medium suction.
(h) Weider tongue retractor.
(i) Mirror.
(j) Curved hemostats.
(k) Angled curettes.
(l) Spade elevator.
(m) Back action elevator.
(n) Small Bein luxator.
(o) Micro Buser.
(p) Two #15 blades.
(q) Minnesota retractor.
(r) Aspirating syringe.

To be efficient with tray setup, consider asking yourself a few questions:

- Which instruments do I need every time? Most of the time?
- Is there something that would make this easier, quicker or less traumatic?
- Do I have what I need to get out of trouble?
- What instrument always feels like it is missing?

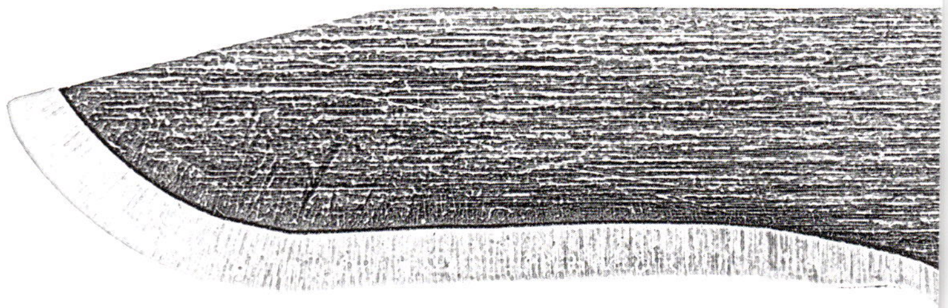

Figure 3-4 No. 15 blade.

Instruments

Surgical blades

No. 15 blade: The most common and versatile blade. (The Chef's knife, if you will.) The belly of the blade is the primary cutting surface. When incising a full thickness flap, the broad curved edge provides a long, sharp bevel capable of cutting through mucosa and periosteum. The moderately pointed tip can complete an incision in tighter areas, such as when approaching a tooth. The back of the tip can be used in spit thickness dissection to develop the supraperiosteal plane. The belly of the blade can scrape a surface clean, like when exposing the mentalis in a stepped genioplasty approach or when clearing the bone of all soft tissue in preparation for guided bone regeneration.

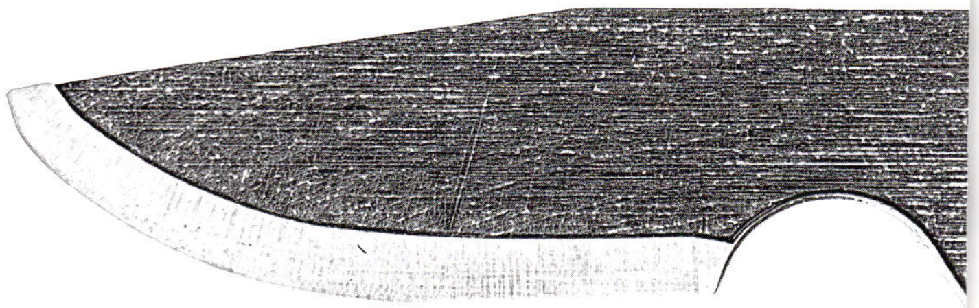

Figure 3-5 No. 15c blade.

No. 15c blade: A more nimble, little brother to the 15 blade. Its slender tip is well suited for a clean sulcular incision, following the anatomy of the teeth without scoring or tearing the fragile sulcular epithelium. It also can be quite useful when manipulating soft tissue around an implant, like in the Palacci technique or palatal roll.

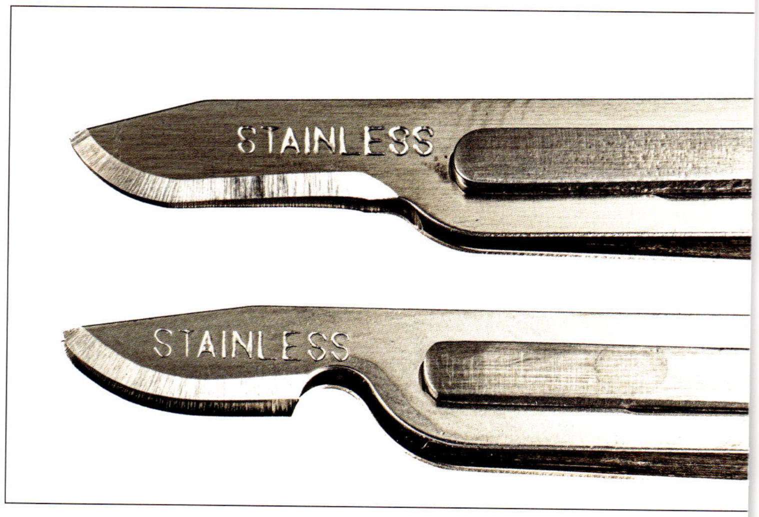

Figure 3-6 Comparison of 15 (*top*) and 15c (*bottom*) blades. The slender 15c can get into tighter spaces, like the sulcus. The 15 seems to provide better control when cutting thicker tissue, such as to expose impacted third molars.

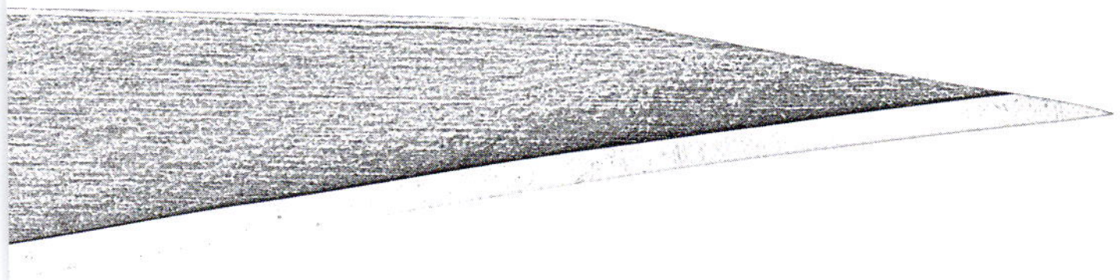

Figure 3-7 No. 11 blade.

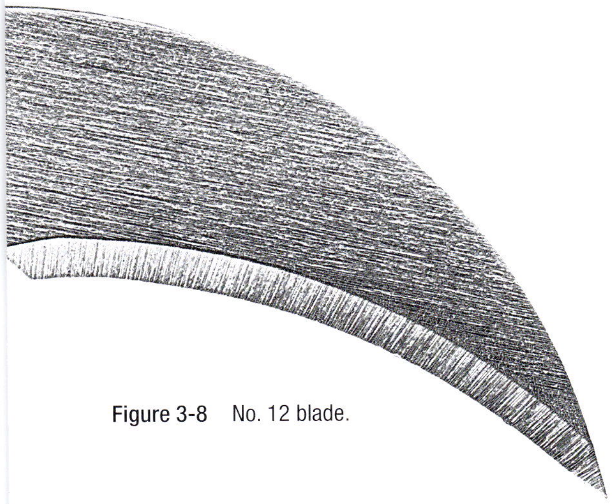

Figure 3-8 No. 12 blade.

No. 11 blade: This blade is sharp and pointed. It's great for a stab incision to access a loculation of pus in an acute abscess. The fine tip is also effective at scoring or releasing periosteum when mobilizing tissue for an advancement flap (similar to a No. 12 blade).

No. 12 blade: A reverse curved blade with a very acutely angled tip. This highly specialized blade assists in full thickness dissection on the distal of a posterior tooth. It helps prevent unfavorable blind tissue tearing. It also can be used to release the periosteum when advancing a flap for implant related surgery or for incising the periosteum to access the buccal fat pad when closing an oral-antral communication with a multilayered, pedicled flap closure. (Check out Chapter 6 for more information on buccal fat pad advancement).

Beaver blade: With an entirely convex, smooth cutting edge, this blade is ideal for split thickness soft tissue dissection. Its shape allows it to provide feedback to the operator when passing through the tissue, helping to maintain the correct plane of dissection.

My experience in oral surgery is there are two types of clinicians: big trays and little trays. Little trays don't have as many friends who are instrument reps.

Specialized micro blades: There is an entire array of various specialized micro blades for different soft tissue procedures. When learning new techniques, pay attention to the different instruments recommended. Try them. You may like them, or you may go back to your own knife block.

A proper knife, properly used, saves surgical time for the surgeon and healing time for the patient. It efficiently cuts the tissue and promotes an optimal healing site by minimizing trauma to the tissue. It may seem wasteful to use multiple blades for a single procedure, but a scalpel's razor-sharp blade dulls quickly, especially when cutting against bone or tooth. It even loses its edge from cutting through soft mucosal tissue. In my practice, the tray for a routine set of third molars gets two No. 15 blades. I always cut the lower first with a fresh blade. The distobuccal tissue on lower third molars can be quite tenacious. I want my sharpest edge to pass through that tissue. A clean cut there saves time and reduces inflammation. After the blade has dulled some from this initial cut, I find it can still easily incise the less dense tuberosity tissue overlying the upper third molars. If I unintentionally pick up a used blade for a lower third molar, I can immediately tell by how it cuts. That is why I set the blades in their proper place. The blade on the right is for the patient's right side, and the one on the left is for the left side. I don't want to think about which blade I already used. (When chefs reach for their knife block, their hand should know exactly where to go.)

Stewardship is important, but not at the expense of excellence. When in doubt, just get a fresh blade.

Scissors

The cutting edge of scissors should be respected like the scalpel blade. Tissue scissors can lose their edge when used to cut anything but soft tissue. Dull tissue scissors macerate as opposed to cutting cleanly. Protect them.

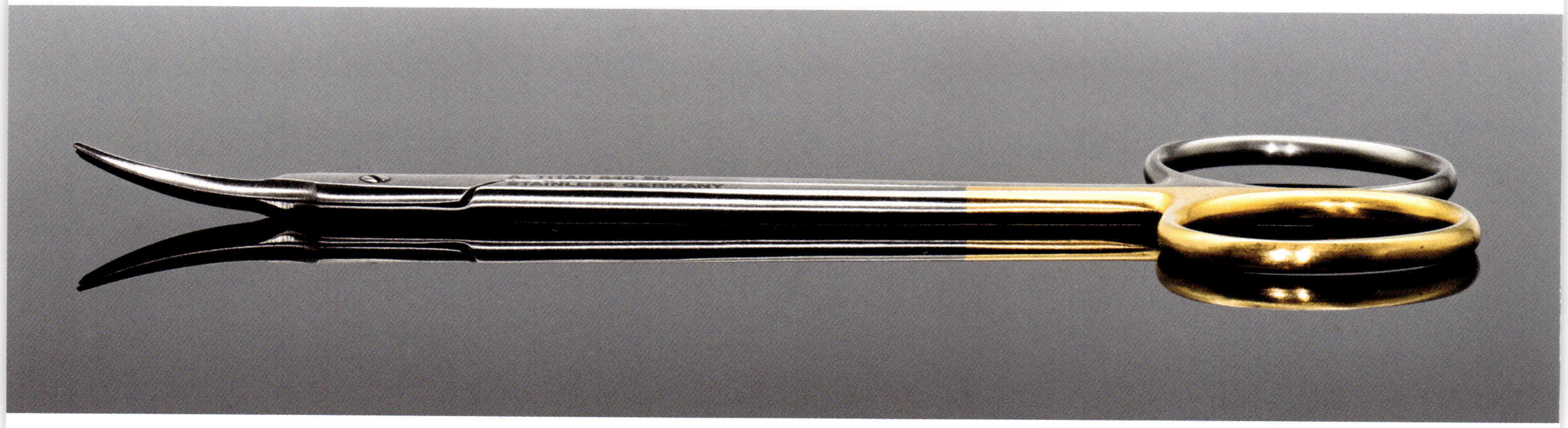

Figure 3-9 These delicate iris scissors are used for soft tissue dissection, such as biopsy or flap development. I often use larger Kelly scissors with a super-cut design, which combines a sharp upper blade with a finely serrated lower blade to keep tissue or sutures from slipping out when cutting.

Forceps

The Latin origin of the word forceps comes from formus (hot) and capere (take) and means "something with which to grasp hot things"[2]. But when I see the English word "forceps," it seems to accurately represent its purpose in dentistry. Forceps are used to apply a force. In our case, that force is applied to and through a tooth. Envision the force as a continuous flow of energy. It needs to go from your hand, through the instrument to the tooth, and then through the cementum to the periodontal ligament, where it ultimately performs its action.

The mission objective of forceps is to optimize engagement to remove the tooth with minimal collateral damage. You want an instrument that will get a good grip on the tooth without crushing it. The contours and design of the forceps beaks should maximize engagement of the accessible tooth structure to keep this flow of force continuous.

We can greatly increase our force and decrease pressure when we increase the contact surface area. The greater the contact between the forceps and the tooth, the lower the pressure. When forceps contact a tooth in a very small area, they apply much higher pressure with the same force. We want our forceps to hug the tooth with as much contact area as possible. This optimizes the force while minimizing the pressure.

In an effort to keep it simple, I've narrowed forceps down to a few categories:

- Universal (engage the crown)
- Straight beaked (engage root structure)
- Specialized (engage furcation or smaller root fragments)

The universal forceps are the standard 150, 151 and Ash. The contour of the beaks is versatile, allowing a good grip on the crown.

FORCE v PRESSURE

Force extracts teeth. Pressure breaks teeth.

Figure 3-10 (Artwork inspired by Ford v Ferrari.)

Figure 3-11 Universal, straight beaked, and specialized diamond tip forceps. Each engages the tooth structure differently.

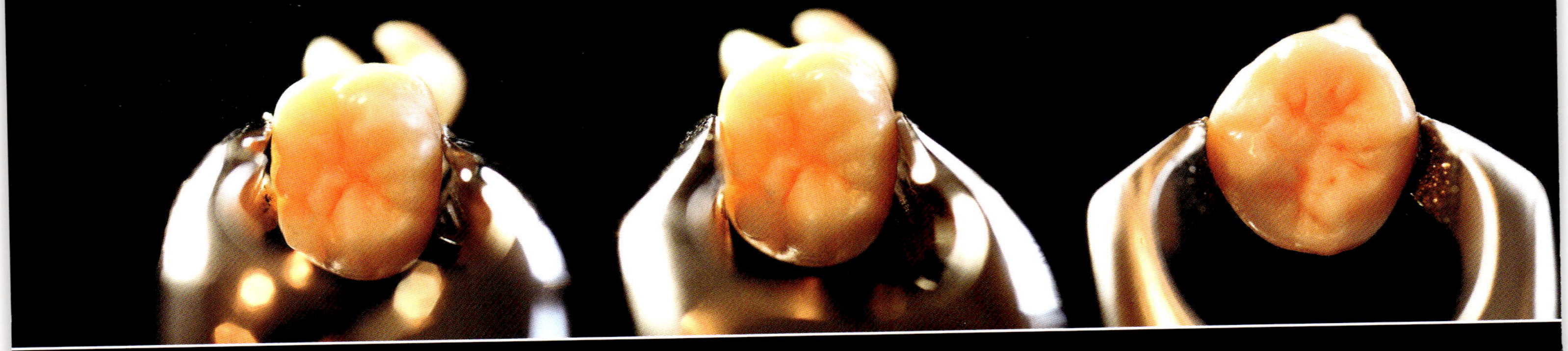

Figure 3-12 The beaks of Ash forceps contour around the crown and engage with a serrated edge.

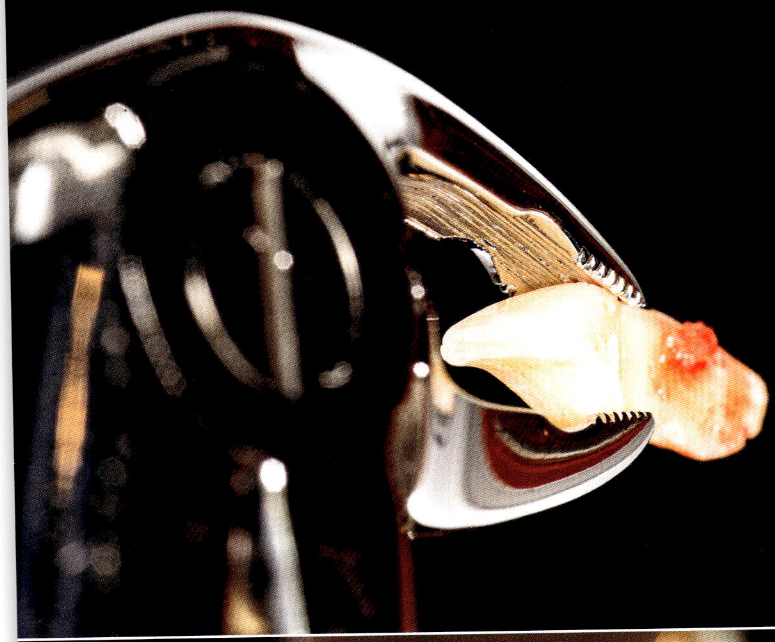

Figure 3-13 Notice how the contour of the straight beak engages the crown. It works best on teeth without a bulbous crown or to engage root structure.

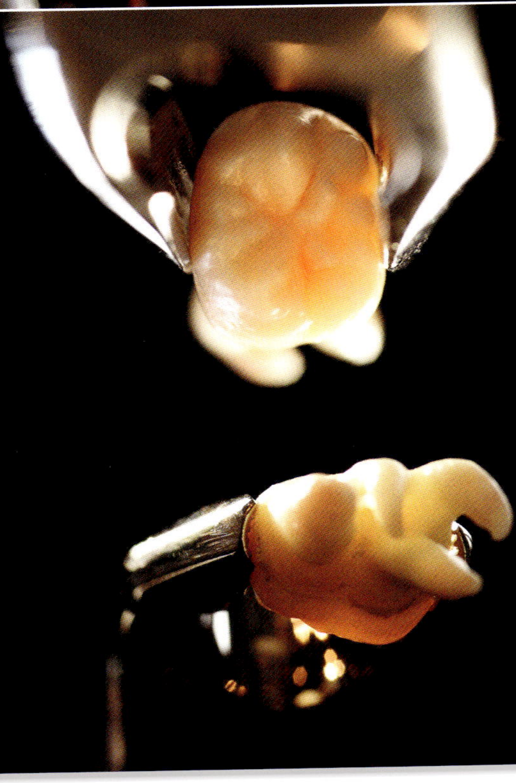

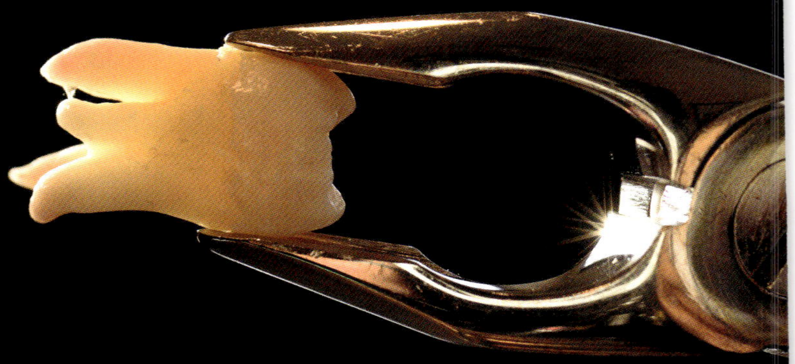

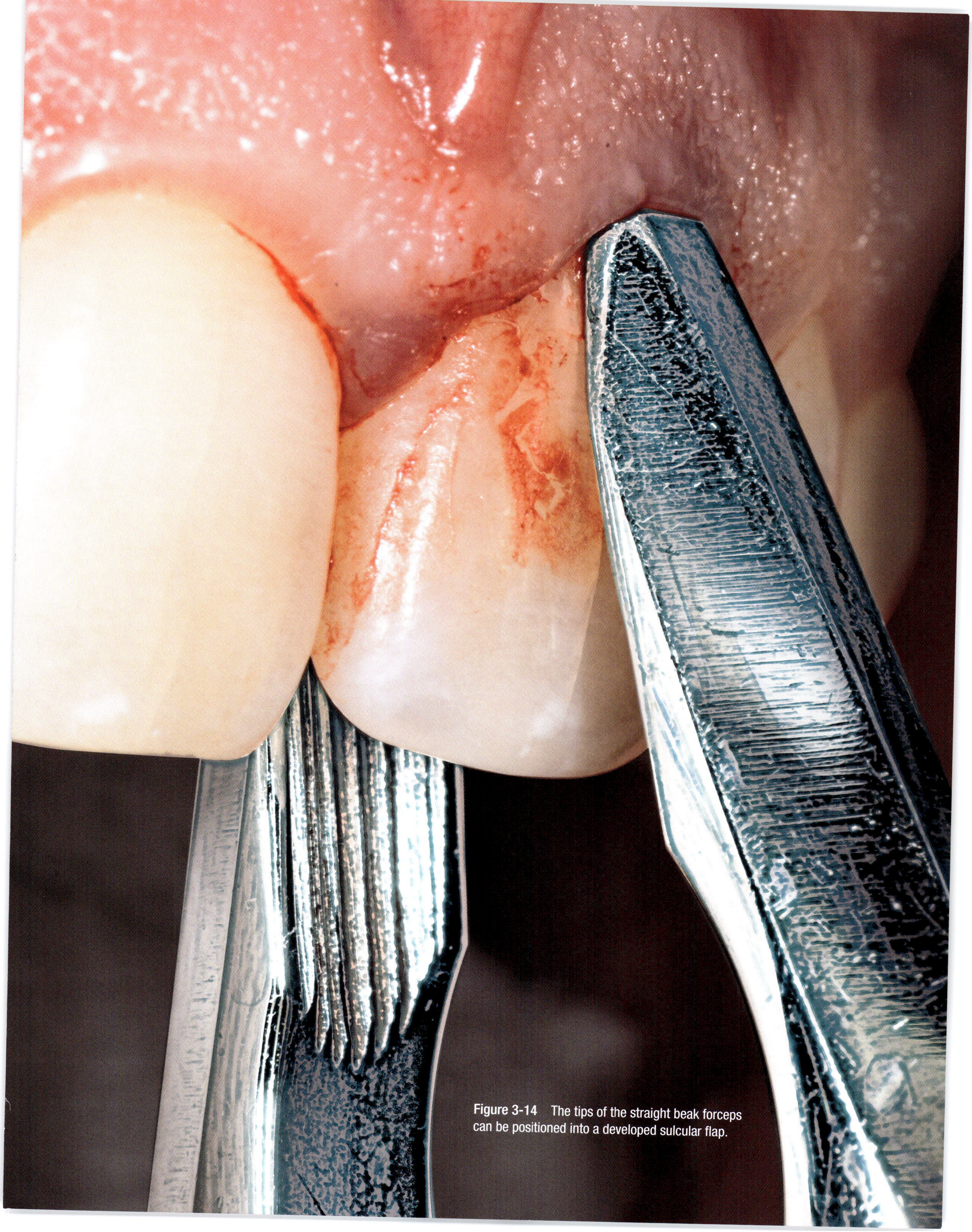

Figure 3-14 The tips of the straight beak forceps can be positioned into a developed sulcular flap.

Specialized forceps have different designs and features.

Cowhorn (#23). These are designed to engage the furcation of lower molars using an inclined plane on the tooth furcation to project the tooth out of the alveolus. As the beaks press into the furcation, they wedge the tooth off the interradicular bone with an up and down pumping action, further displacing the beaks apically with each pump. The functionality of the cowhorn is further explored in the exodontia chapter.

Root tip forceps (upper and lower). The narrow tips combine strength and access. They are small enough to access some tight spots, but strong enough to grip the tooth structure and hopefully deliver it. These forceps help preserve bone by getting into tighter spots, potentially limiting the amount of bone removal needed to grip the tooth.

There are some variations on these overall themes, including size, shape, angle and surface coating. One such improvement is a diamond coating. This serves to increase the friction between the tooth and the forceps, theoretically increasing its effectiveness. Countless brilliant ideas have blossomed into different forceps designs over the years. There are many specific and unique designs available. Try some of them to find out what works well for you. It is worth exploring.

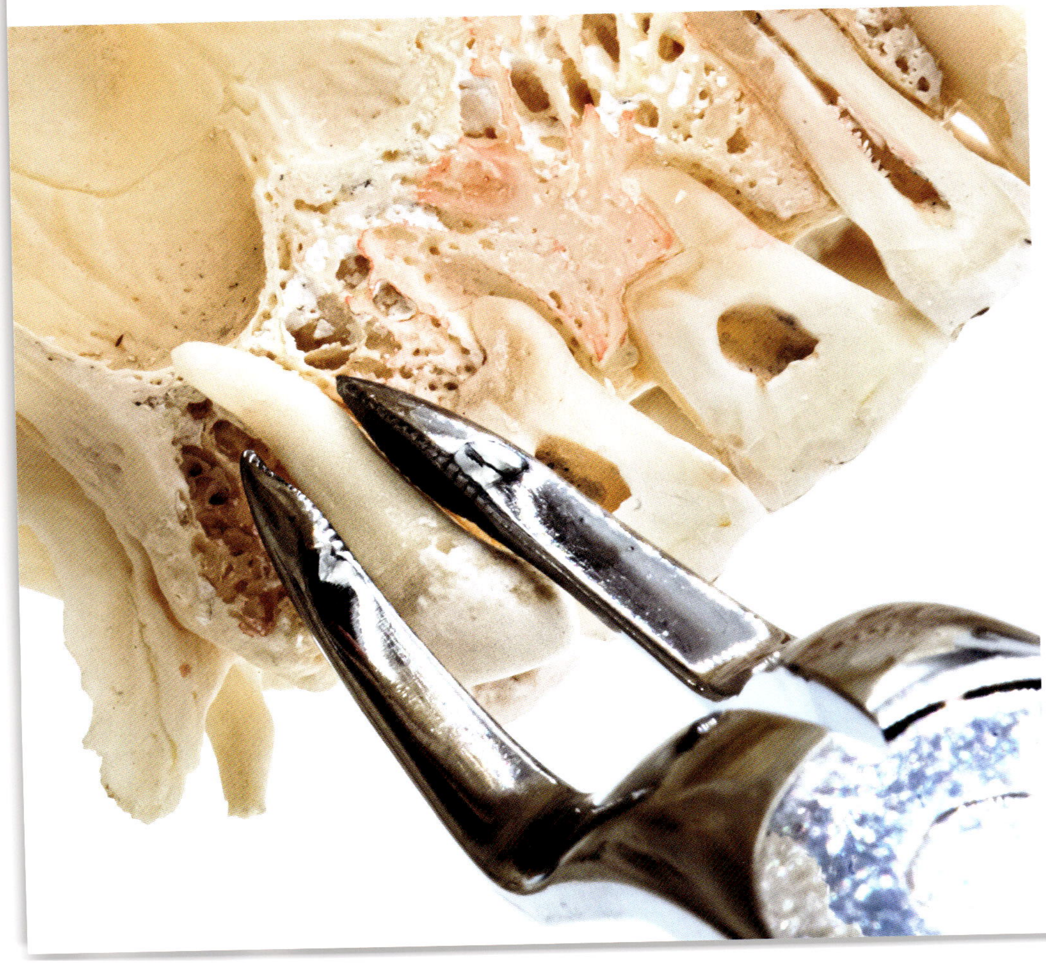

Figure 3-15 Root tip forceps have slender beaks, improving the ability to grasp a root tip. While they are smaller than other forceps, this image illustrates that they still take up some space. Depending on the situation, bone removal still may be necessary when using root tip forceps.

I'll never forget what a dentist named Bob told me while we were extracting teeth in a sweaty classroom in rural Honduras. After having gone on something like 100 short term dental mission trips, he advised me to **master a few instruments**. "The fewer instruments I needed, the more streamlined I would be," he said. The minimalist approach has served me well in my practice. The advantage is amplified on the mission field. It was on this mission trip during my second year of dental school that I got bit by the "oral surgery bug." From then on, I felt like oral surgery is what I was made to do.

Periotome. Luxator. Elevator.

These three types of instruments seem to overlap in form and function. They each release the periodontal ligament, freeing the tooth for extraction. There is a continuum between these instruments, with the periotome the most delicate and the elevator the largest.

The periotome is the slenderest of these instruments. It is designed to sever the periodontal ligament by applying vertical force between the tooth and bone. Proper use of a periotome facilitates the fabled "atraumatic extraction." It decreases the lateral or expansion forces often relied upon in routine simple exodontia. As such, it limits the amount of osseous damage and optimizes the healing site. With the thin nature of the instrument, very limited rotational or leveraging forces can be applied without bending or damaging it.

The Micro Buser is a cross-over between a periotome and a luxator. Its slender tip can sever the periodontal ligament, but its more robust shank can withstand the force of rotation and even elevation at times. It can be used to progress through the first steps of the extraction algorithm, severing and elevating soft tissue flaps, severing the ligament and even luxating or delivering the tooth. It may seem this instrument is mentioned ad nauseam throughout the book because of how useful and practical it can be.

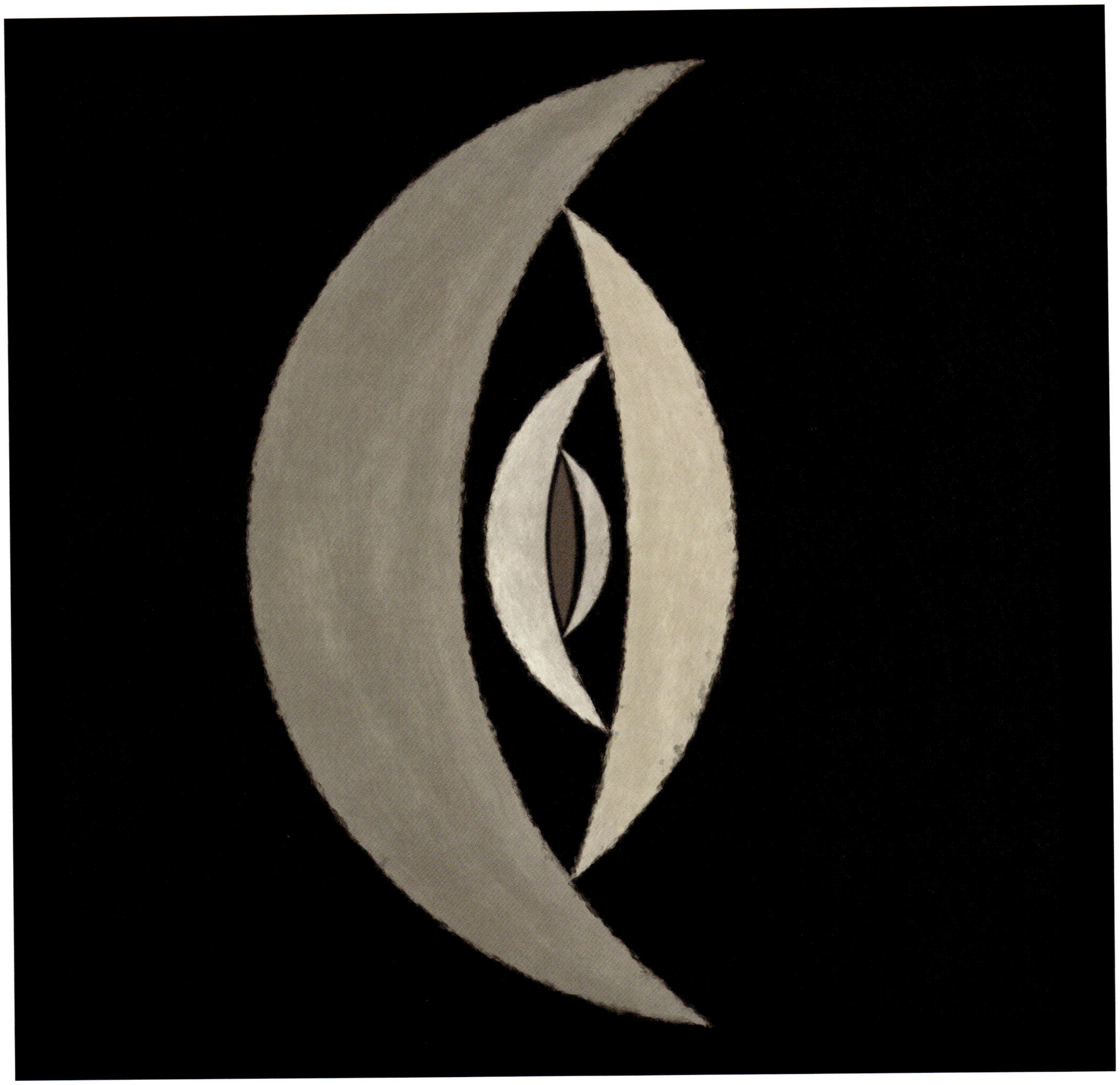

Figure 3-16 Sizing up. As you progress through an extraction, the instruments generally get larger. The smallest, the periotome, is biconvex, while the Micro Buser is crescent shaped. Then comes the small Bein luxator, followed by the spade elevator and lastly, the large elevator. This is not always a step-wise approach from one to the next. Use what seems to be working. If you are struggling, try thinking bigger or smaller. (Artwork inspired by Geraldo de Barros.)

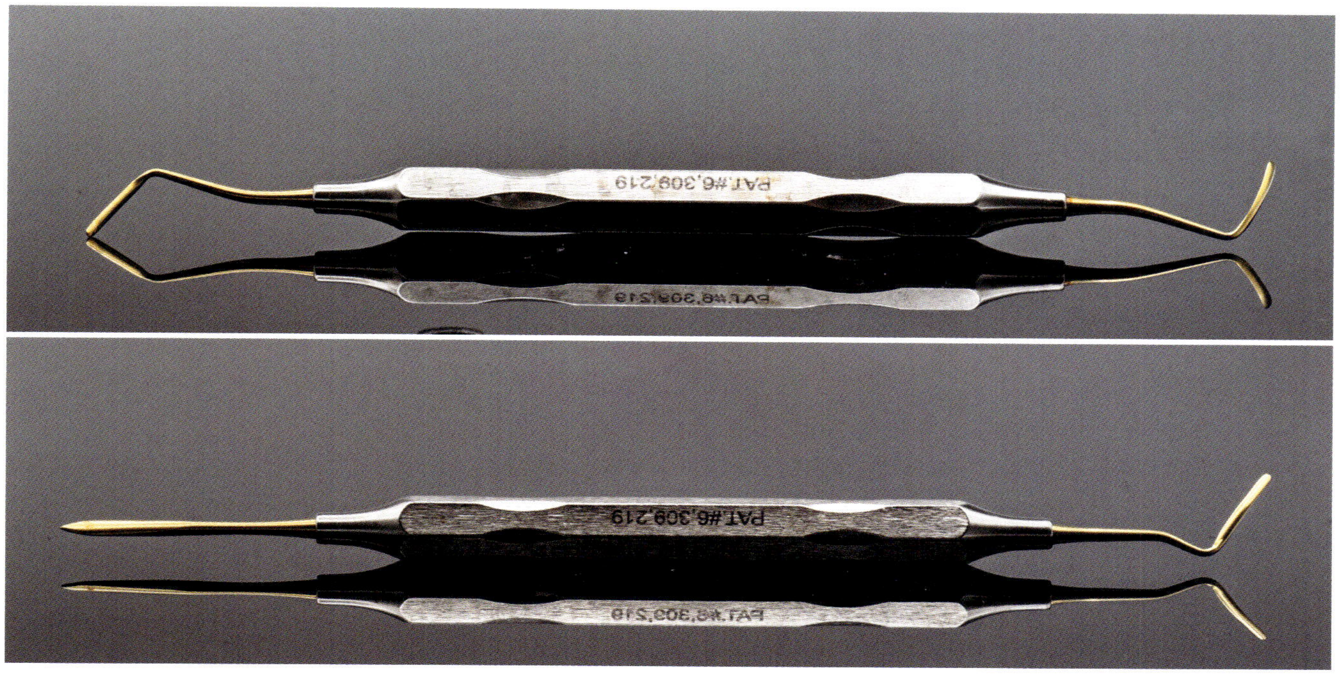

Figure 3-17 The periotome is designed to sever the periodontal ligament. Its slender nature limits its use to very light force.

Figure 3-18 The Micro Buser is much more versatile than its larger relatives because of its refined shape and delicate tip.

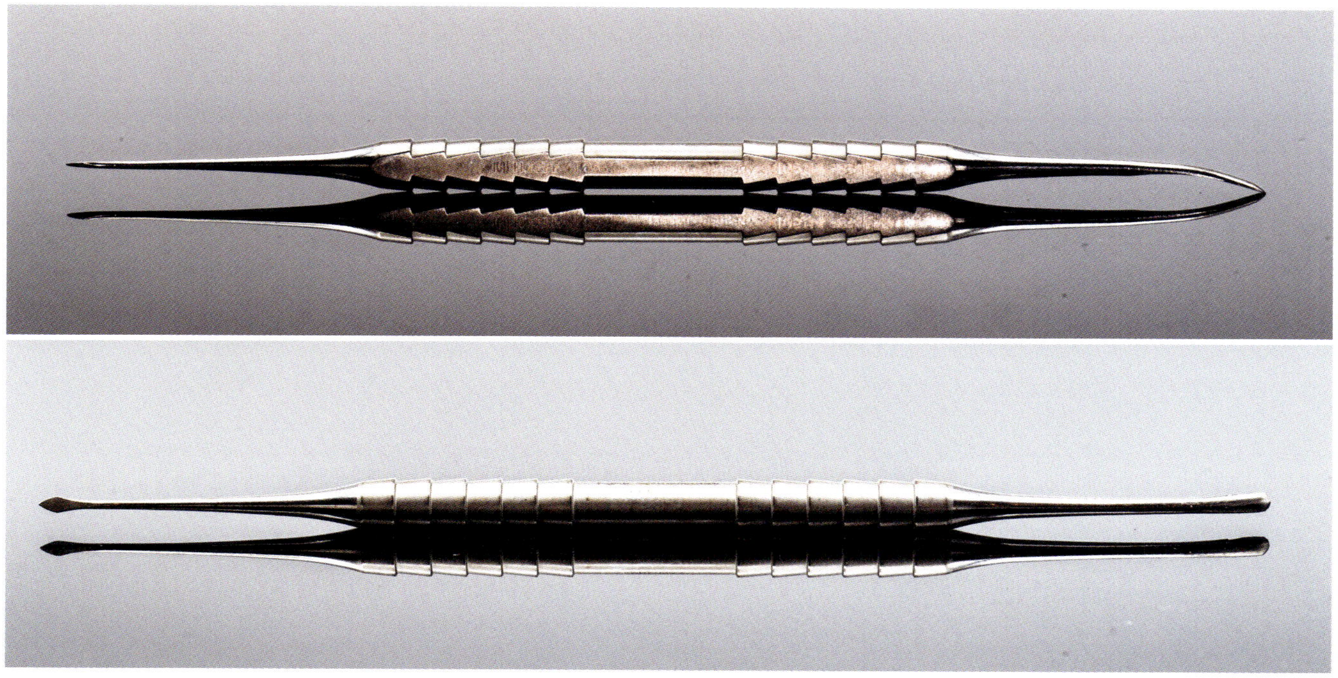

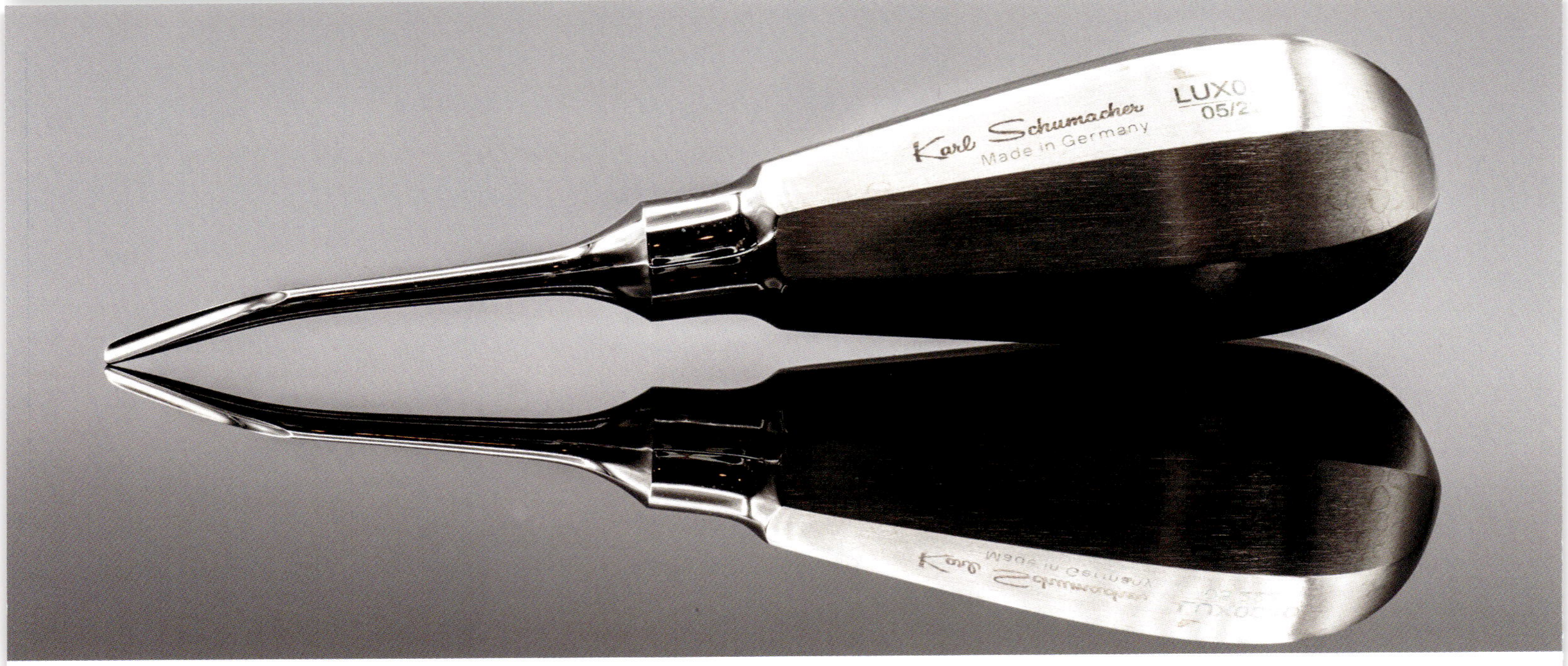

Figure 3-19 Bein luxating elevator 2.5 mm curved.

The small luxator is another versatile instrument. The sturdy shank and relatively nimble and slender tip allow it to engage limited tooth structure with relatively impressive results. It can be passed into very narrow interproximal spaces between lower anterior teeth or impacted third molars. It fits into the ligament space and often can be advanced quite a way down the root. The handle is relatively short to reduce the leveraging forces and fracture risk.

The spade elevator combines the diamond shaped tip of the Micro Buser with the strength of a luxator. The pointed tip can function like a periotome, and it can be manipulated like a luxator (with rotation) or elevator (with leverage). This is particularly useful when there is limited support for leverage, or if the purchase point is compromised. The sharp point also can be navigated into small ligament spaces or between tight roots. The broad back of the spade spreads out forces, serving to protect the surrounding bone, such as a thin buccal plate. Attention to the tip's condition optimizes the benefits of this instrument. If it is dull or chipped, it may become more of a liability than an asset.

Figure 3-20 Spade elevator.

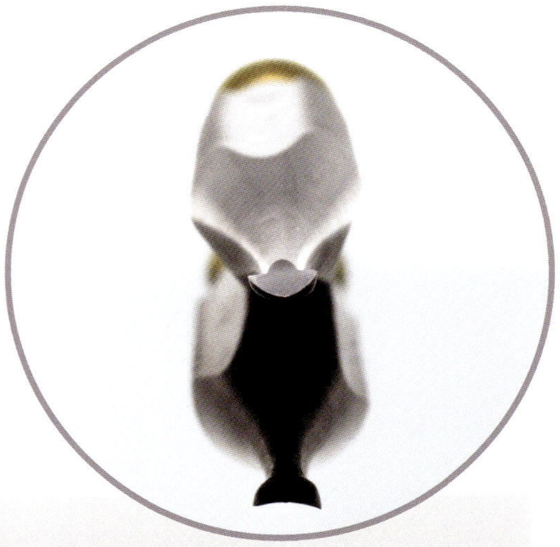

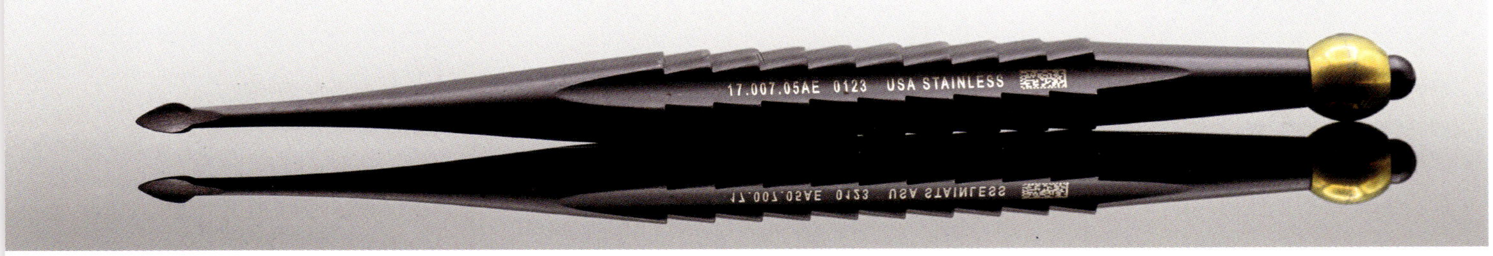

The elevator is the heftiest of these types of instruments, serving as a lever to loosen the tooth and expand the socket. Like a meat cleaver, it can generate significant force and must be respected. With its shape and design, the lever action uses the alveolar crest or the adjacent tooth as the fulcrum. The elevator's strength may give the operator a false sense of security, as significant forces can be applied to the surrounding structure, potentially unknowingly harming them. A crown or Class V restoration is a classic example. They can easily be dislodged or delaminated when elevating an adjacent tooth with minimal force.

The back action elevator is the workhorse elevator; it is slim lined, yet substantial in heft. It is not as agile as some of the smaller elevators or luxators, but if there is room for it, it will get the job done. The angled shank improves access over a straight elevator. Its backward angled curvature allows clean access to elevate on more posterior teeth. It can get around the corner better than any other I have found. As a true elevator, it is quite sturdy and won't back down when more force is applied.

The small and large straight elevators are the most elementary instruments on my tray. While they are less commonly used in my hands, I still want them available for every extraction. The small straight elevator seems most handy when elevating on the distal of a tooth if the angle of the back action is unfavorable. It can serve as an intermediary between the small luxator and the back action, splitting the

Figure 3-21 The back action elevator works well from the premolars and back. The curvature improves the angle of access, making it easier for us and kinder to the patient's lips and cheeks.

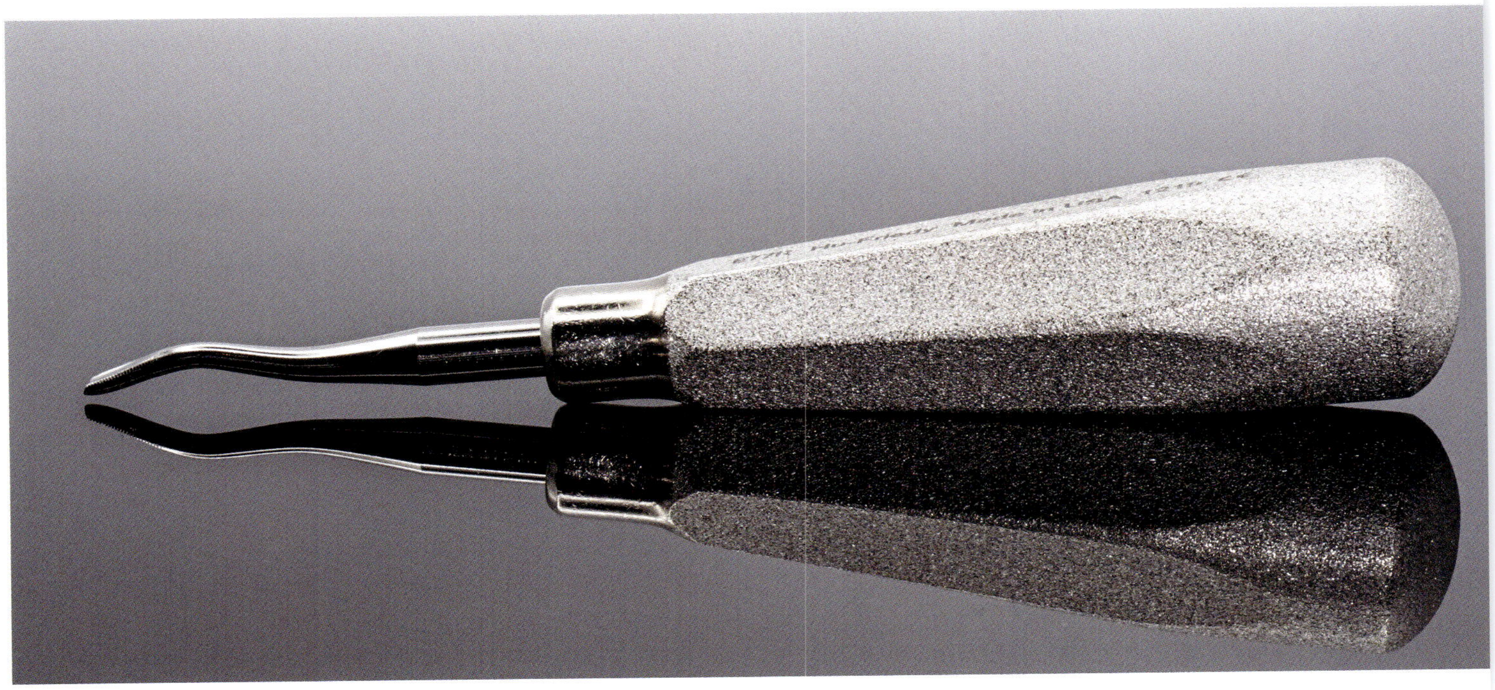

difference in size and brute strength. The large elevator's advantage is its lever action can cross a larger space, bridging a larger gap created by a surgical bur or luxation. It also can provide a little more horsepower with its larger lever arm when an intact root is stubbornly retained by dense bone. But with the increased leverage, it also can be a liability when the increased force leads to further fracturing of the root.

There is a constant ebb and flow between these instruments. My team is ready with the next instrument in the lineup, though at times I move backward in the algorithm, using an instrument again or skipping ahead to a different one.

There have been three different small luxators on my surgical tray over the past decade. The first generation I acquired when I purchased the practice felt uncomfortable in my hand. On the tradeshow floor at a meeting, I spent time handling multiple options from multiple manufacturers. I found a few I liked and bought them. Of these, I figured out which one I liked best and bought eight more (one for each tray and one spare). The luxator I chose had a warranty that I used too frequently as the instrument broke easily. It was nice they didn't charge me for the replacement, but it cost me a lot of surgery time retrieving broken tips. I tried several more options at another tradeshow. I now have a Bein 2.5 mm luxating elevator on each tray. It has a slender tip and a comfortable handle. The angle is very versatile and functional. And they rarely break.

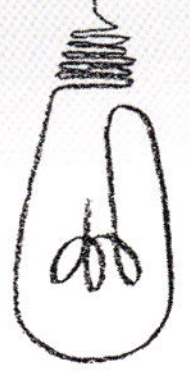

With the thin nature of these instruments, they have the potential to break, leaving behind a small portion of metal that must be removed. The noise and feel of a broken instrument is distinct from fracturing bone or tooth. It has a metallic ping. When the tip of a luxator or elevator breaks, the remaining piece is usually jammed in a tight spot. That's probably why it broke. It got pushed a little too hard, and now it is stuck.

Don't lose sight of it. Try to locate it immediately and come up with a plan for retrieval. Sometimes you can grab it with a hemostat or get it with the suction. It may be wedged between the tooth you are removing and the bone or adjacent tooth—and it can be very tightly lodged in there. Consider removing some tooth structure to access the piece or work to mobilize the tooth to free the fragment. That little piece can easily seem to disappear. Take it slow.

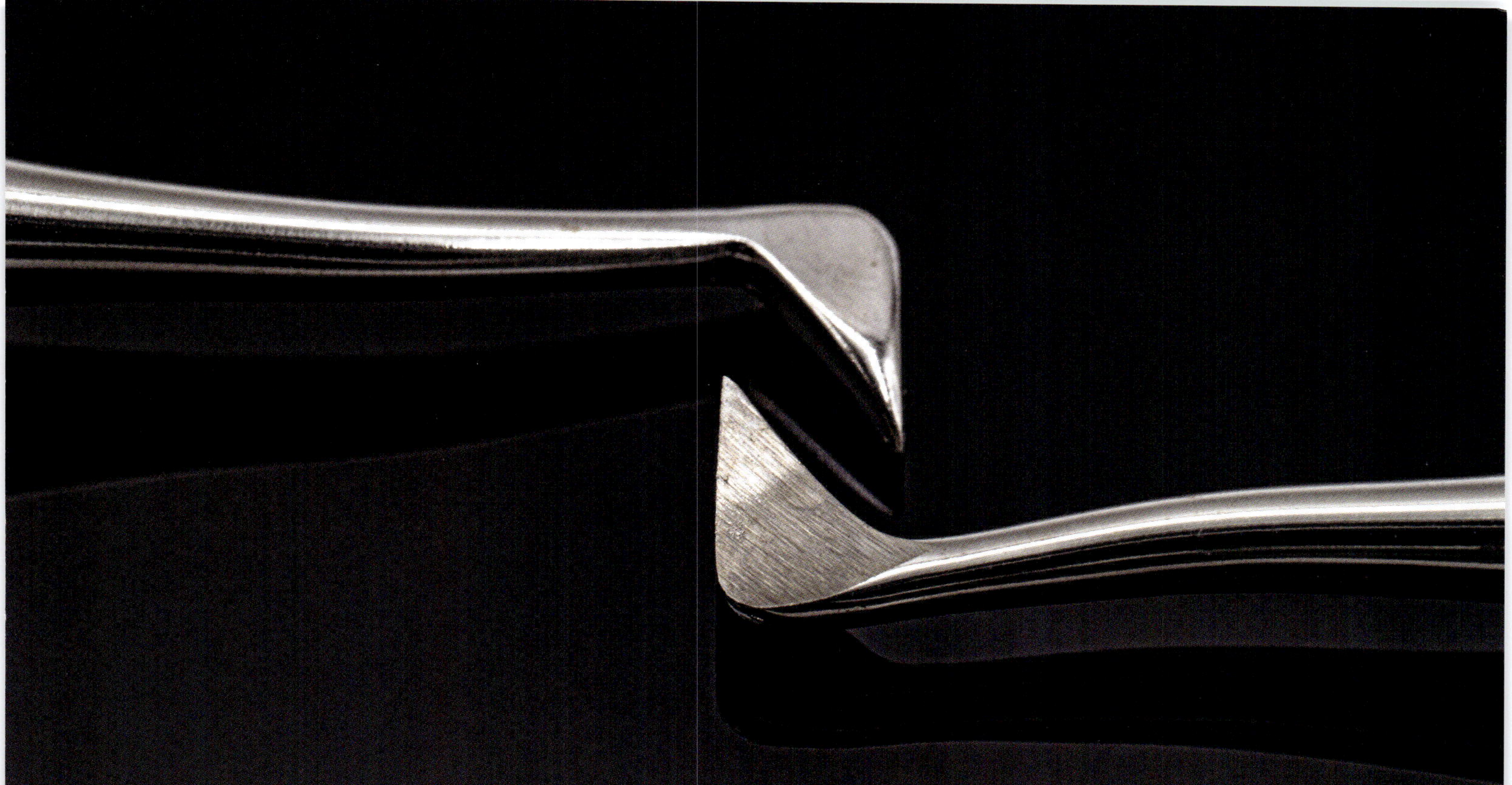

Figure 3-22 The yin and yang of the Cryer elevators. The sharp tip, curved head, and offset angle enables them to engage root structure in a unique way. They also have the potential to harm the interradicular bone as shown below.

Cryer elevator

This elevator comes in handy when one root of a lower molar is stuck. If one root is out, the sharp tip can engage the remaining root structure and generate a good bit of upward force. The interradicular bone can be removed with rotational movement. This can help remove the tooth, but it also can damage the remaining socket. All instruments have a yin and yang. They are used to injure so the patient can heal.

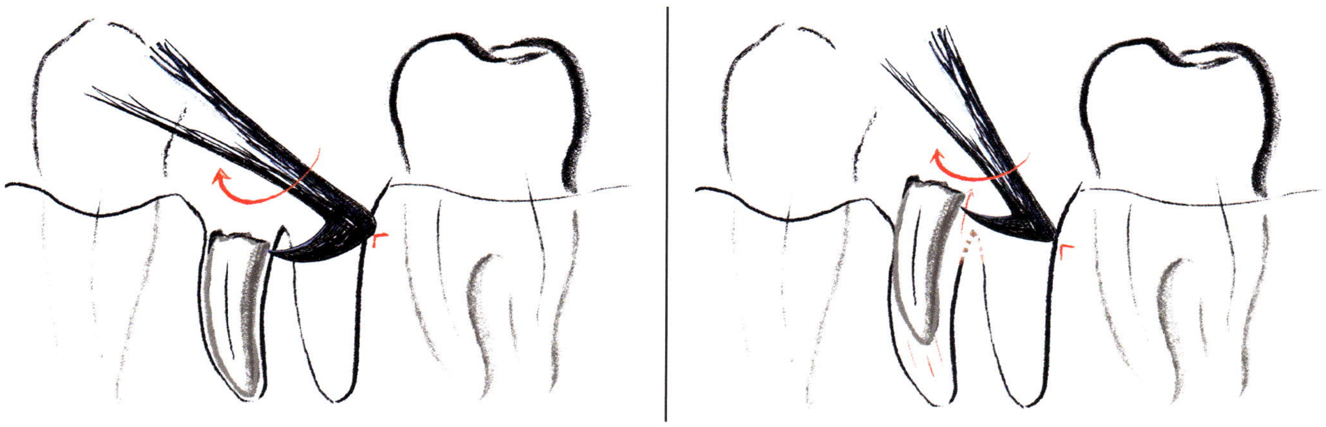

Figure 3-23 The sharp tip engages the root structure while the instrument is rotated, fulcruming off the socket wall. Use caution as this can damage the interradicular bone. Consider the entire socket and future plans when deciding if and how to use this instrument.

Retractors

The Minnesota retractor often feels like an extension of my left hand. In conjunction with the sweetheart tongue retractor, it seems most visualization problems can be eliminated by retracting the cheeks and tongue. These retractors are relatively blunt, but they can cause significant tissue trauma if too much pressure is applied. When using the Minnesota retractor to retract a full thickness flap, great care must be taken to ensure the instrument's tip remains in solid contact with the bone. If not, the reflected flap easily slides under the instrument and will be traumatized from pressure and movement from the retractor. The periosteum, in particular, must be cared for as it is responsible for a significant amount of blood supply to the surgical site, and it is highly innervated. Great care in this detail pays dividends in the patient's recovery.

The tongue retractor seems to have three main challenges. It can be difficult to get it to stay put with a large or highly mobile tongue. It can easily gag the patient and damage the mandible's thin lingual mucosa. The dense underlying bone does little to help the area heal. These injuries can be more painful for the patient and take more time to heal than the surgery. In light of these challenges, this instrument is valuable in creating a functional workspace and protecting the patient's airway.

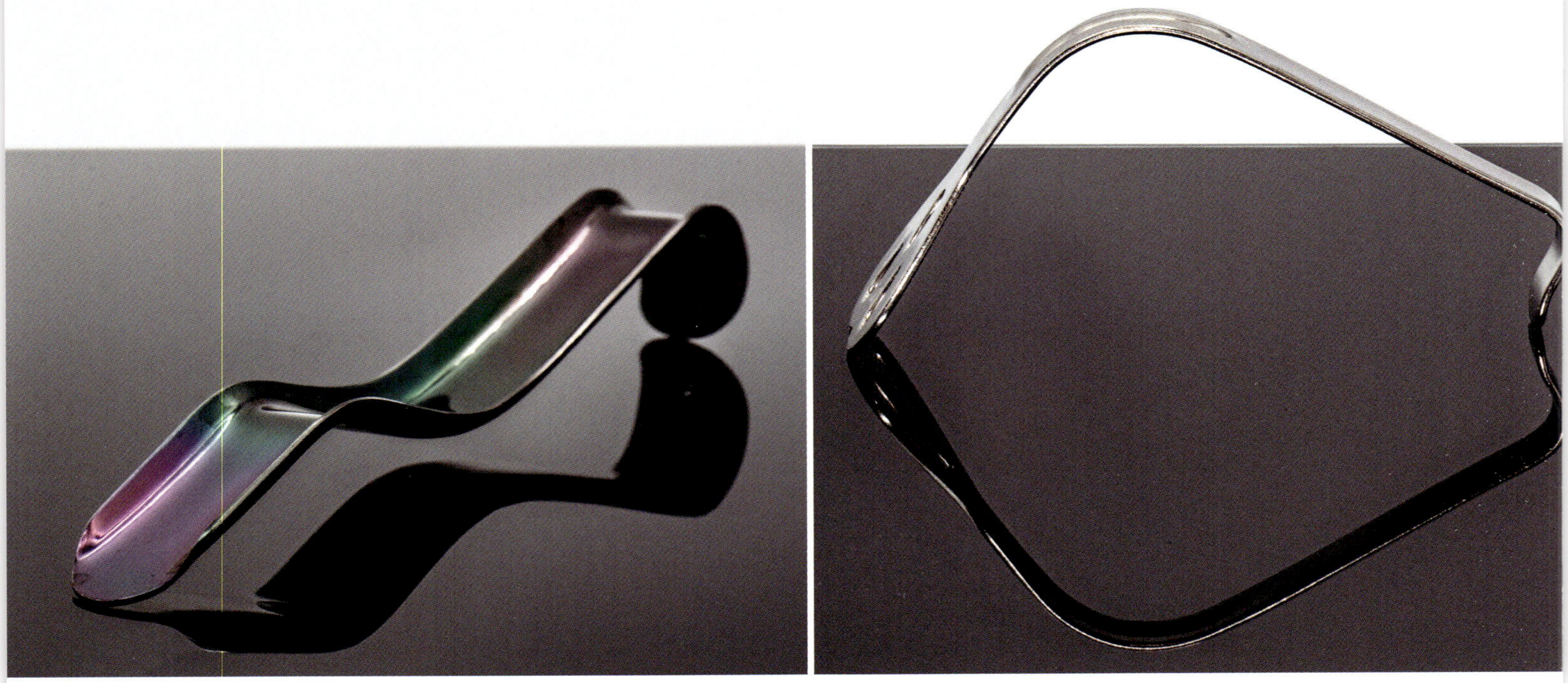

Figure 3-24 The Minnesota retractor feels like an appendage. It is almost always in my left hand during surgery (*left*). The Weider or "sweetheart" retractor protects the tongue and airway during surgery (*right*). It can be a mouth full for the patient. It also has potential to rub against the lingual mucosa and harm it. Use it with care.

Angled curettes

These multi-talented instruments are most frequently used to debride pathologic tissue at the apex of an extraction site. The concave surface allows clinicians to intuitively scoop out unwanted tissue. When inverted, the convex surface can debride the margins of an apical lesion, ensuring complete removal of pathologic tissue, which is quite necessary to achieve the best results for ridge preservation. But they can also come in quite handy when engaging a small portion of retained root tip in a difficult surgical extraction. They can sneak in and function as a small luxator in tough to reach areas. They can tease out a small upper molar root tip or retrieve a fractured segment of a lower molar when the lingual plate is compromised.

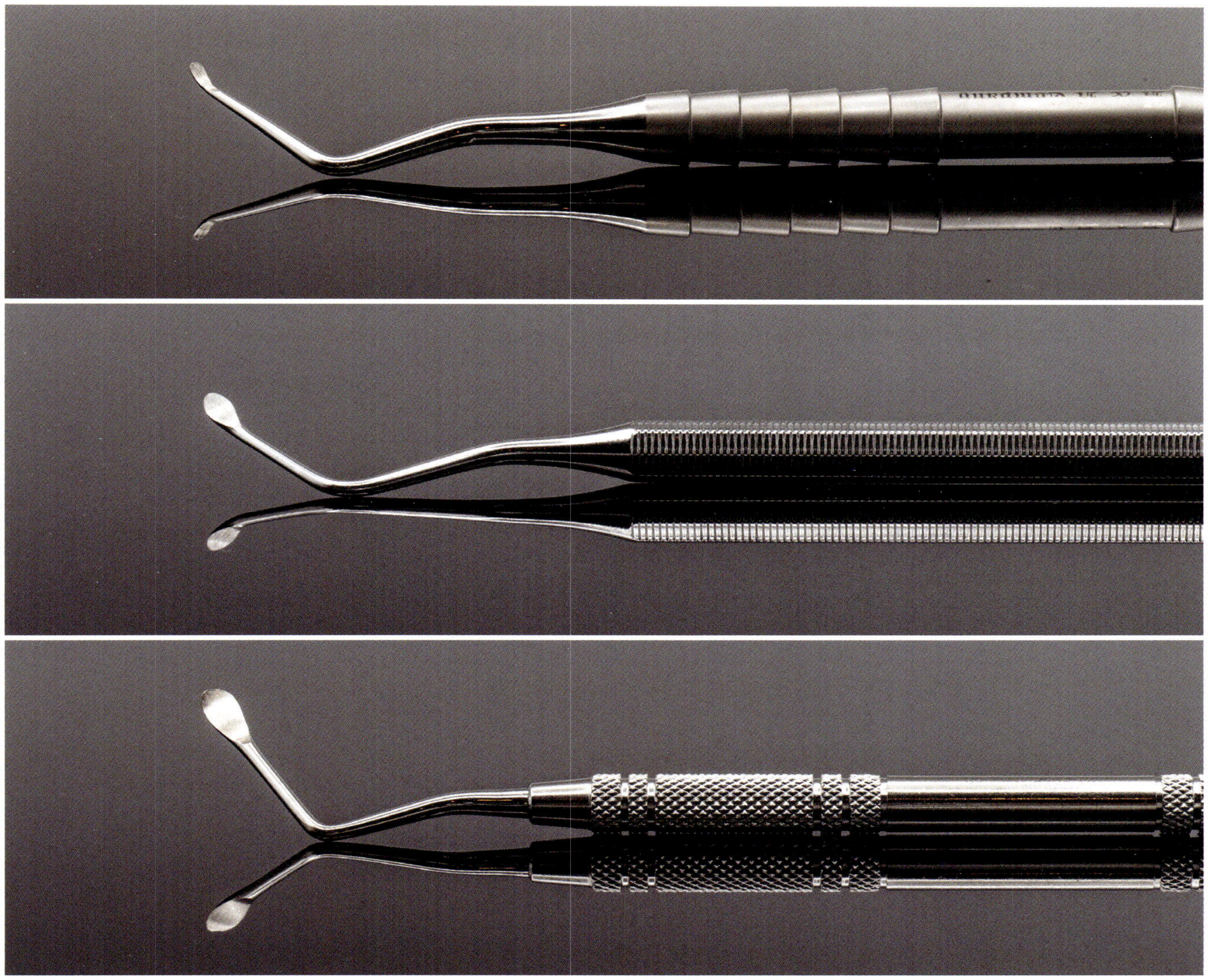

Figure 3-25 As their name suggests, angled curettes can be used to perform curettage of the tissue. Their shape and angles make them useful in other situations too. Think about the slender tip and offset angle when elevating intraosseous pathology, sinus membrane, or even a small root tip.

Curved hemostats

Hemostats can both squeeze and spread. They are effective at grasping small portions of tooth structure or tenacious soft tissue from an extraction site. They are also effective at spreading tissue in dissection when accessing the buccal fat pad or bluntly exploring a deep space odontogenic infection. Their slender design makes them well suited for retrieving small root fragments after the piece has been mobilized. The flat beaks do not engage curved tooth structure very well. If the root fragment is squeezed a little too tight, the piece can shoot out of the beaks of the hemostat. That is one reason to protect the patient's airway, and everyone's eyes.

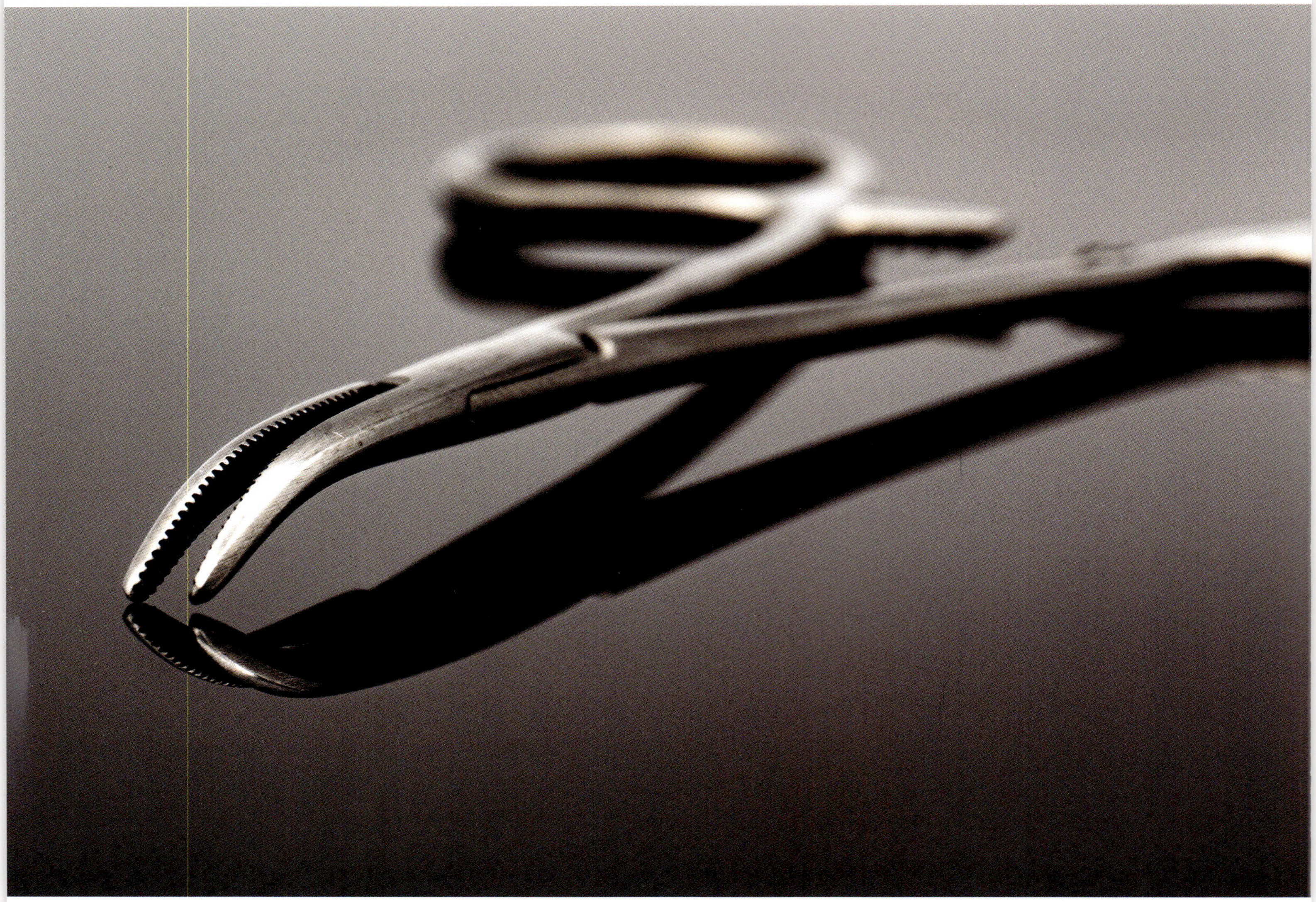

Figure 3-26 Curved hemostats.

Rongeur

This instrument is far more versatile than its name suggests. French for rodent or “gnawer,” the rongeur is designed to effectively gouge or remove bone. It can be quite useful for removing soft tissue and retrieving loose fragments of tooth. Rongeurs even can be used as forceps if there is a small space or relatively mobile segment of tooth that needs to be removed. The beaks articulate with a sharp edge that can grossly excise loose soft tissue, but will not give a clean cut. Be cautious when using them as forceps. The sharp occluding edges have a higher chance of fracturing tooth structure. Small straight beaked forceps or root tip forceps may be a better alternative in these situations.

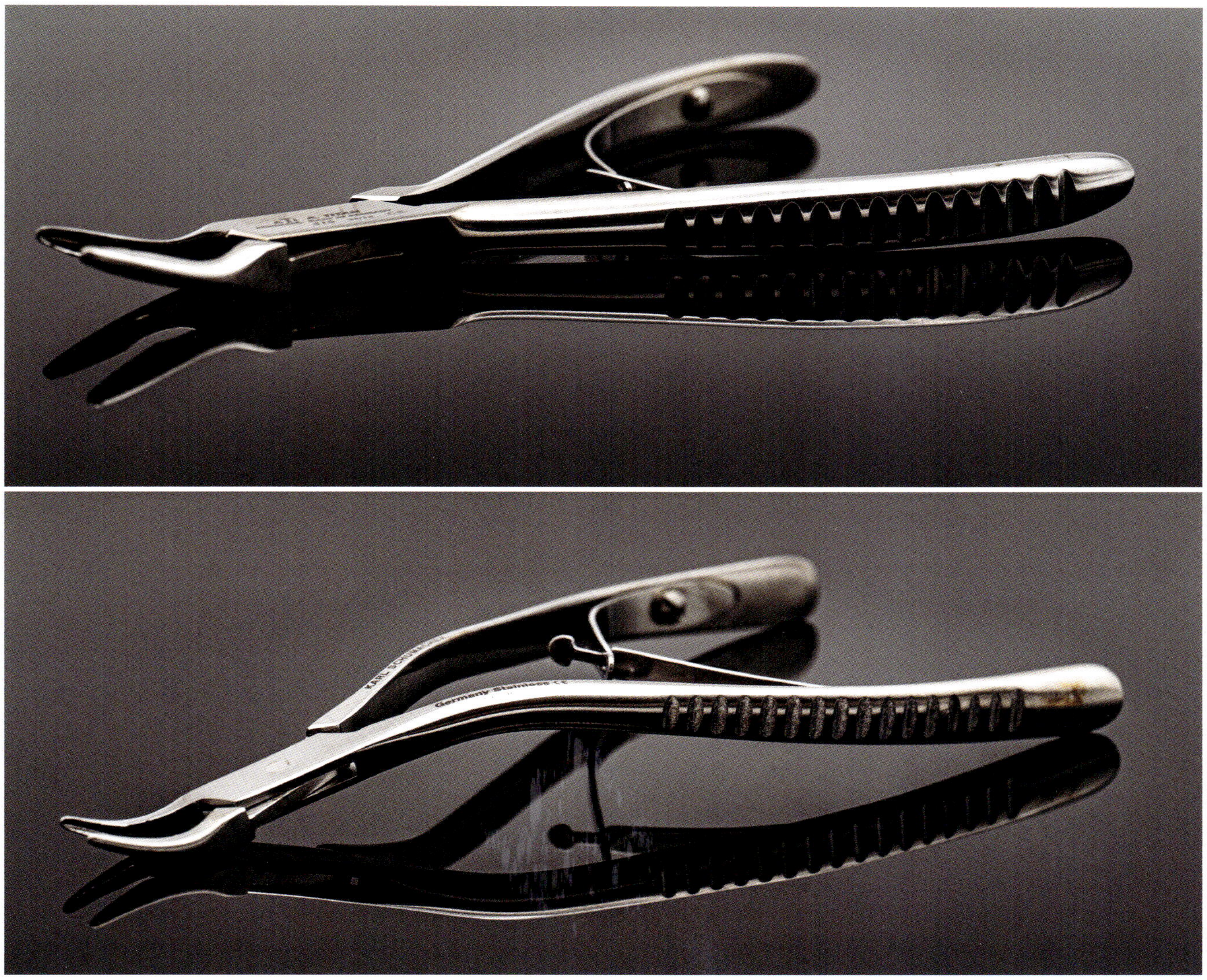

Figure 3-27 Straight and curved rongeurs are versatile instruments for retrieving root fragments, performing alveoloplasty and removing soft tissue.

Needle driver

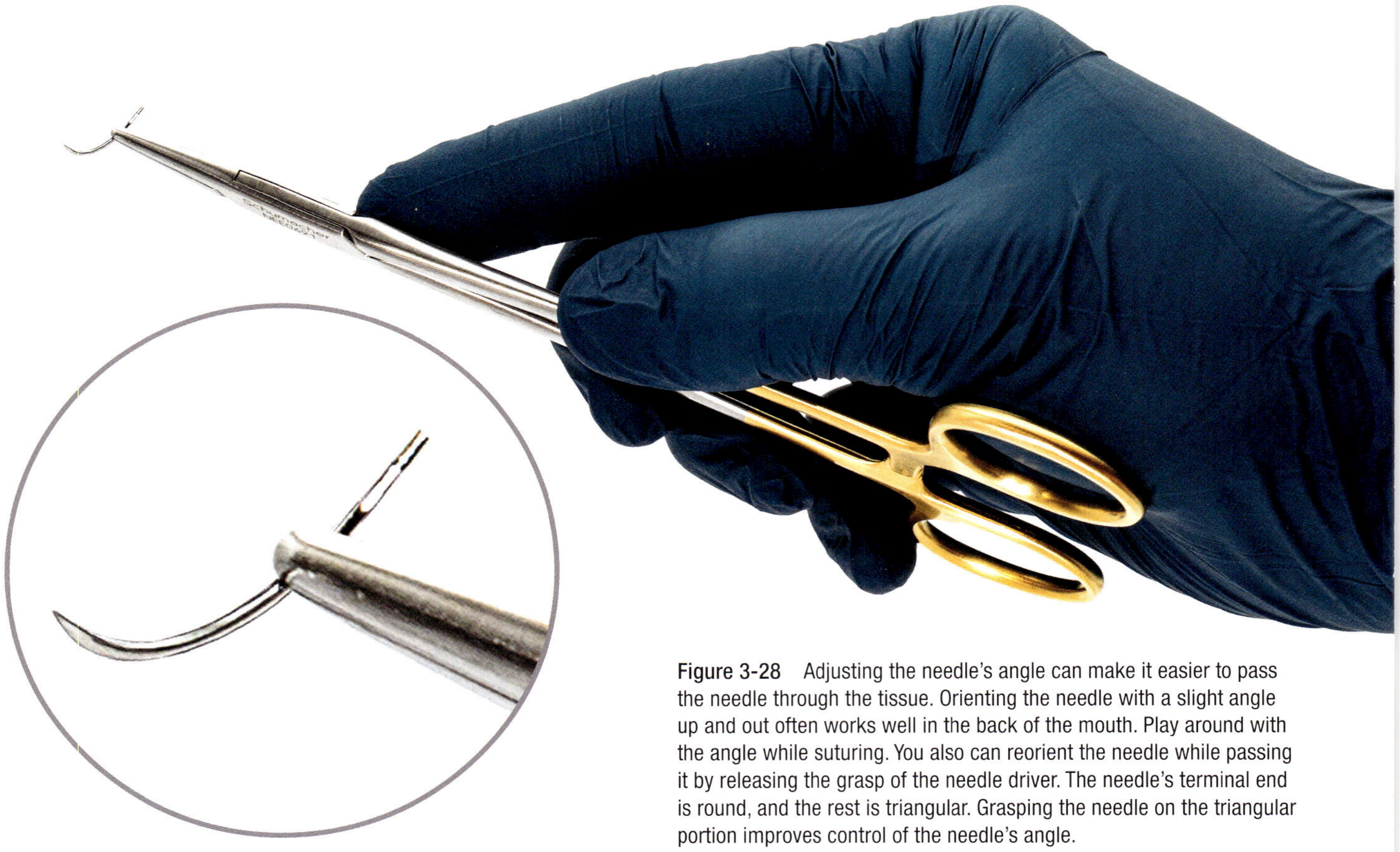

Figure 3-28 Adjusting the needle's angle can make it easier to pass the needle through the tissue. Orienting the needle with a slight angle up and out often works well in the back of the mouth. Play around with the angle while suturing. You also can reorient the needle while passing it by releasing the grasp of the needle driver. The needle's terminal end is round, and the rest is triangular. Grasping the needle on the triangular portion improves control of the needle's angle.

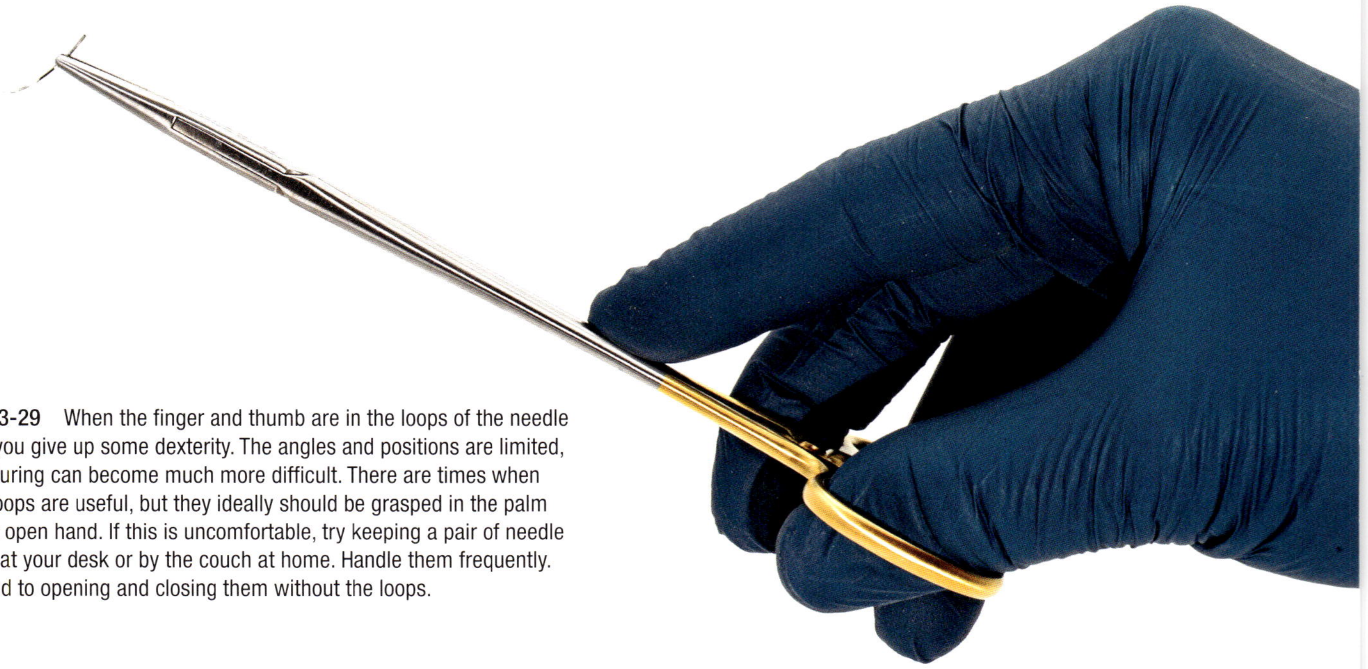

Figure 3-29 When the finger and thumb are in the loops of the needle driver, you give up some dexterity. The angles and positions are limited, and suturing can become much more difficult. There are times when these loops are useful, but they ideally should be grasped in the palm with an open hand. If this is uncomfortable, try keeping a pair of needle drivers at your desk or by the couch at home. Handle them frequently. Get used to opening and closing them without the loops.

Castroviejo needle driver

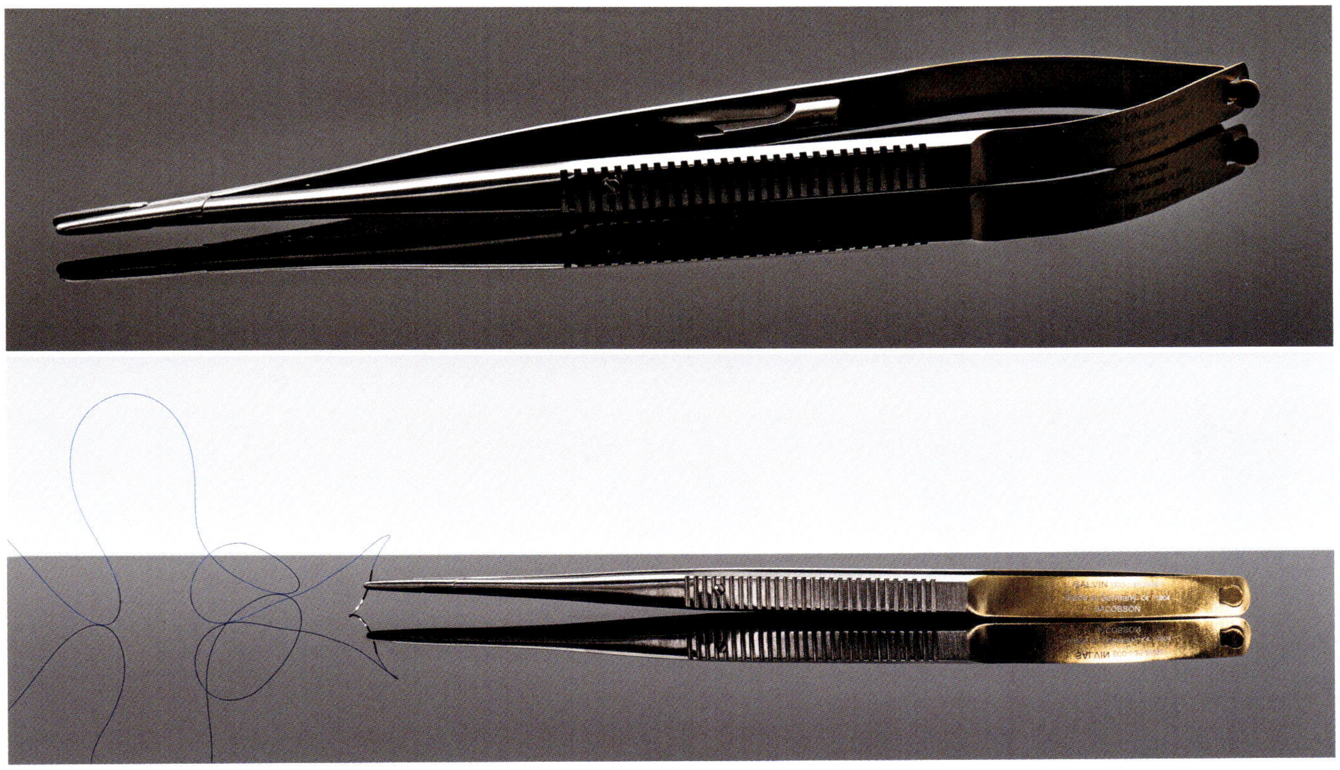

Figure 3-30 This is a nice little instrument when manipulating delicate soft tissue, especially with a 5-0 or smaller suture. The mechanics allow the clamp to be released while holding it in a pencil grip. This allows for different angles to pass suture through the tissue.

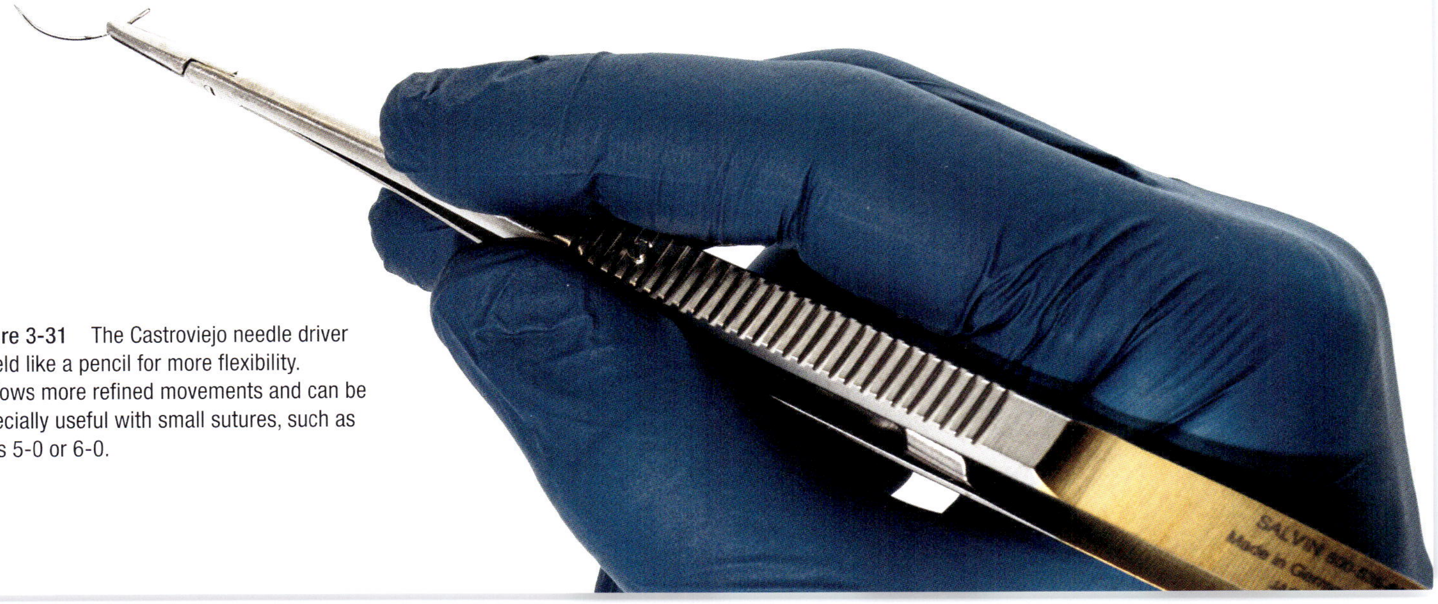

Figure 3-31 The Castroviejo needle driver is held like a pencil for more flexibility. It allows more refined movements and can be especially useful with small sutures, such as sizes 5-0 or 6-0.

Surgical handpiece

The type of surgical drill you use doesn't matter as much as how the drill is handled. Self-irrigation is tremendously helpful, but it can be ineffective if you are not careful. Watch where the irrigation goes. Make sure it clears the debris. If sludge builds up, you know it is not irrigating adequately and the tissue will suffer from thermal injury. In training, we used air powered units. In my private practice, I have been quite pleased with the high-speed electric straight drill from Bien-Air. The contrangled surgical drill can be very helpful when drilling in tight posterior areas. It seems to have less horsepower but has proven to be quite helpful at times, especially for fractured molar roots.

Burs

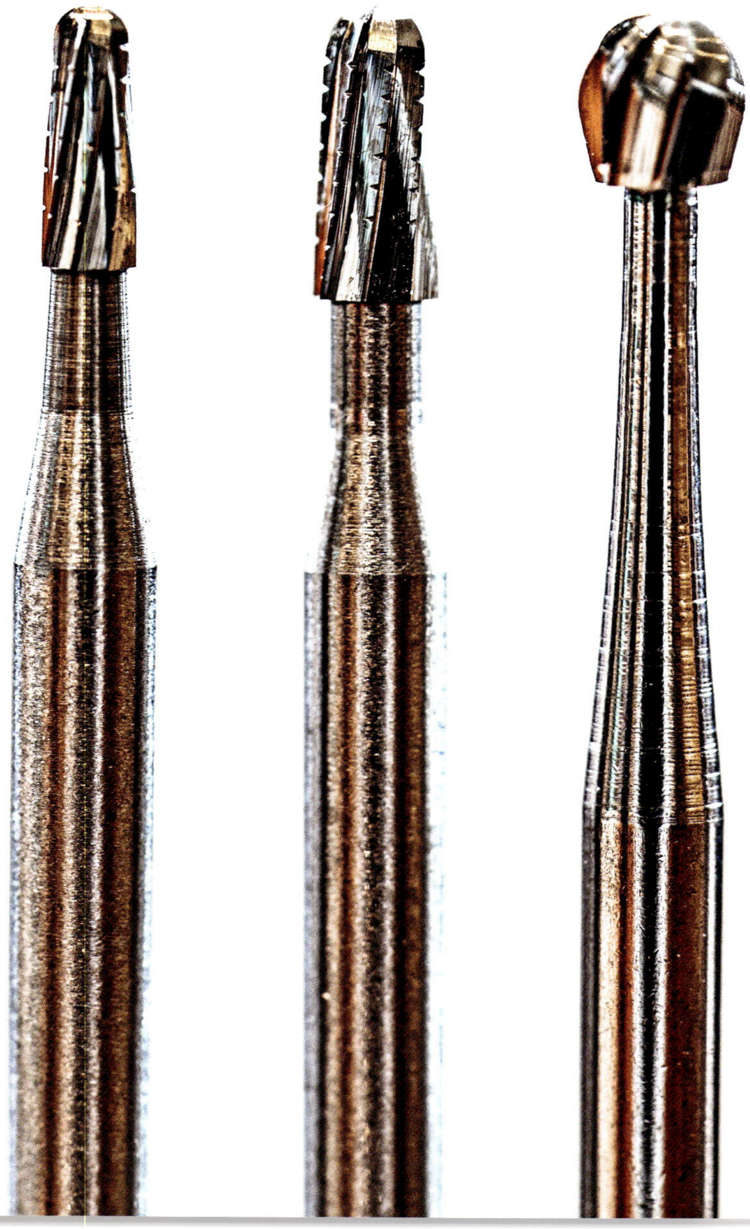

Figure 3-32 These are the most common burs I use. 1702 (*left*) is an end and side cutting cross-cut fissure bur mostly used when retrieving fractured roots. 1703 (*middle*) is a slightly larger end and side cutting cross-cut fissure bur and is the workhorse for removing bone and sectioning teeth. No. 10 round (*right*) is a round bur used for root reduction in coronectomy and bone removal in antrostomy for direct sinus augmentation. These three drills get me through most of my procedures (except implant preparation).

Dimensions

Know the dimensions of key instruments. You can create a quick reference to keep you and your patient safe during surgery. Here are some examples of helpful measurements and when it is beneficial to know them:

- Surgical bur diameter: space between roots and teeth
- Bur landmark lengths: safe drilling depth to protect nerve and sinus
- Bevel on scalpel: split thickness grafts
- Length of scalpel blade: split thickness grafts

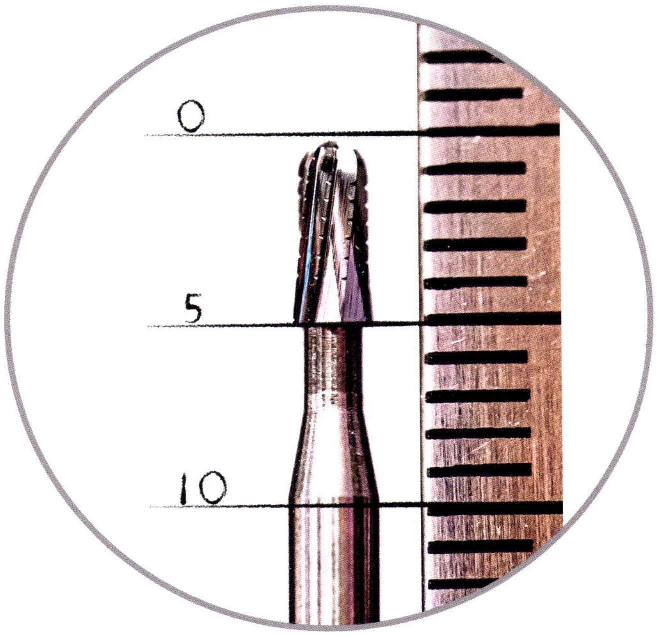

Figure 3-33 It is tremendously helpful to know the length of the different parts of the bur. It can help estimate what drilling depth will be most efficient with the cuts, so you stay out of trouble and don't have to worry about cutting too deep.

Beyond Instruments

The value of mise en place goes well beyond lining up instruments. It goes beyond properly loading the suture and surgical bur, setting up the room, preparing the team and patient. It even goes beyond the architectural design and flow of the room and office. It is an entire thought process, thinking through everything before you start. It is a way of life.

Evaluation

I am convinced anyone, and I mean anyone, can be trained to see the world as an artist. You just need to look for it. The more practice and attention you put into looking for the beauty that's all around us, the more aware you will become. If you don't look for it, you certainly won't see it.

You only see what you look for, whether it is in the visible spectrum or not. Our brains are hardwired to look for what we know. This is a tremendously valuable asset in human evolution and survival, but it must be understood and respected or it can blind us to the obvious. When performing an evaluation, it is helpful to have a system established to look beyond what the patient came in for, within reason of course. We must train ourselves to look for both the obvious and the not-so-obvious.

As James Clear says in "Atomic Habits," "We don't rise to the level of our goals, we fall to the level of our systems."

Like cones in the retina that can only perceive and transmit signals in the visible spectrum of red through purple, modern medicine can only see what it knows. The amount of the electromagnetic spectrum that cannot be seen by the human retina far exceeds the 380 to 750 nm that can be seen. A patient has the right to be off the visible medical spectrum. We continue to expand our understanding and broaden the spectrum, but if a patient has a condition in the ultraviolet wavelength, we may not be able to explain it with our current understanding. The associated cognitive dissonance can be torture for a patient who just doesn't fit into our current understanding. Think outside the box. There is a lot going on out there.

Figure 3-34 (Artwork inspired by Pink Floyd's album cover: The Dark Side of the Moon.)

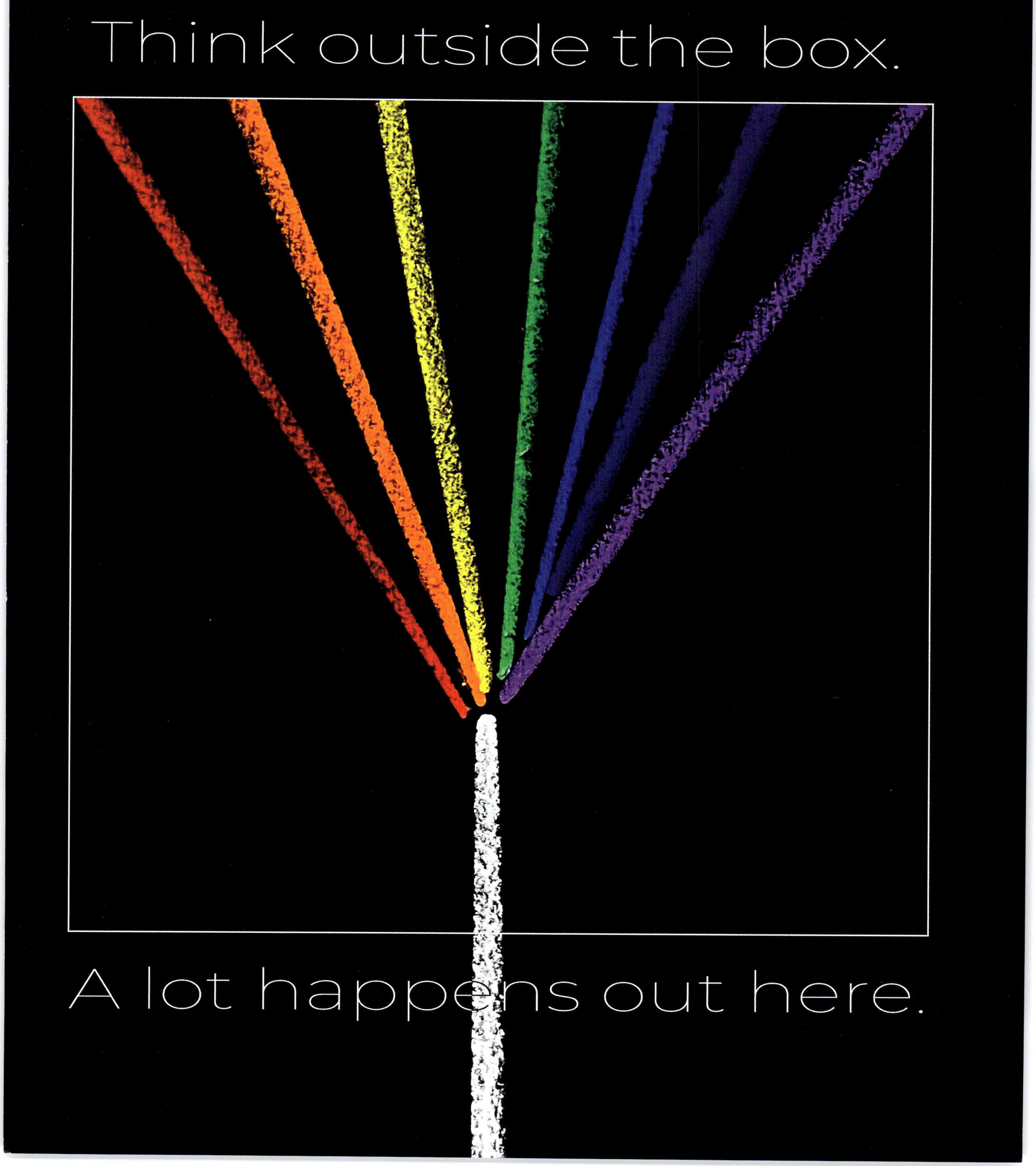
Think outside the box.
A lot happens out here.

Radiographic evaluation

Navigation is all about knowing where you are and where you are going. Nautical charts are to the sailor as radiographs are to the surgeon. They show both what is beneath the surface as well as what is above. As the sailor can be easily misled by passing waves and deceived by distances on the water, he needs a chart and compass to guide him. But these tools alone will not ensure safe navigation without skill in using them. So too the surgeon can be led into danger without the navigational direction of a radiograph. Even with the most sophisticated imagery, the mouth's unique anatomy and tight quarters can cause a state of near delusion at times. These few pages cannot contain everything you need to know about navigating safely through surgery, but I hope they shed light on practical principles that are applicable for the novice and experienced surgeon alike.

What you see on the surface provides some direction, but it can mask the hidden structures beneath. A navigational chart shows submerged rocks and shoals, providing relative distances and measurable bearings to guide vessels safely. Radiographs show relative angles and planes. They can be measured, either by estimation, as in a panoramic radiograph, or with precision, as in a CBCT. They don't show

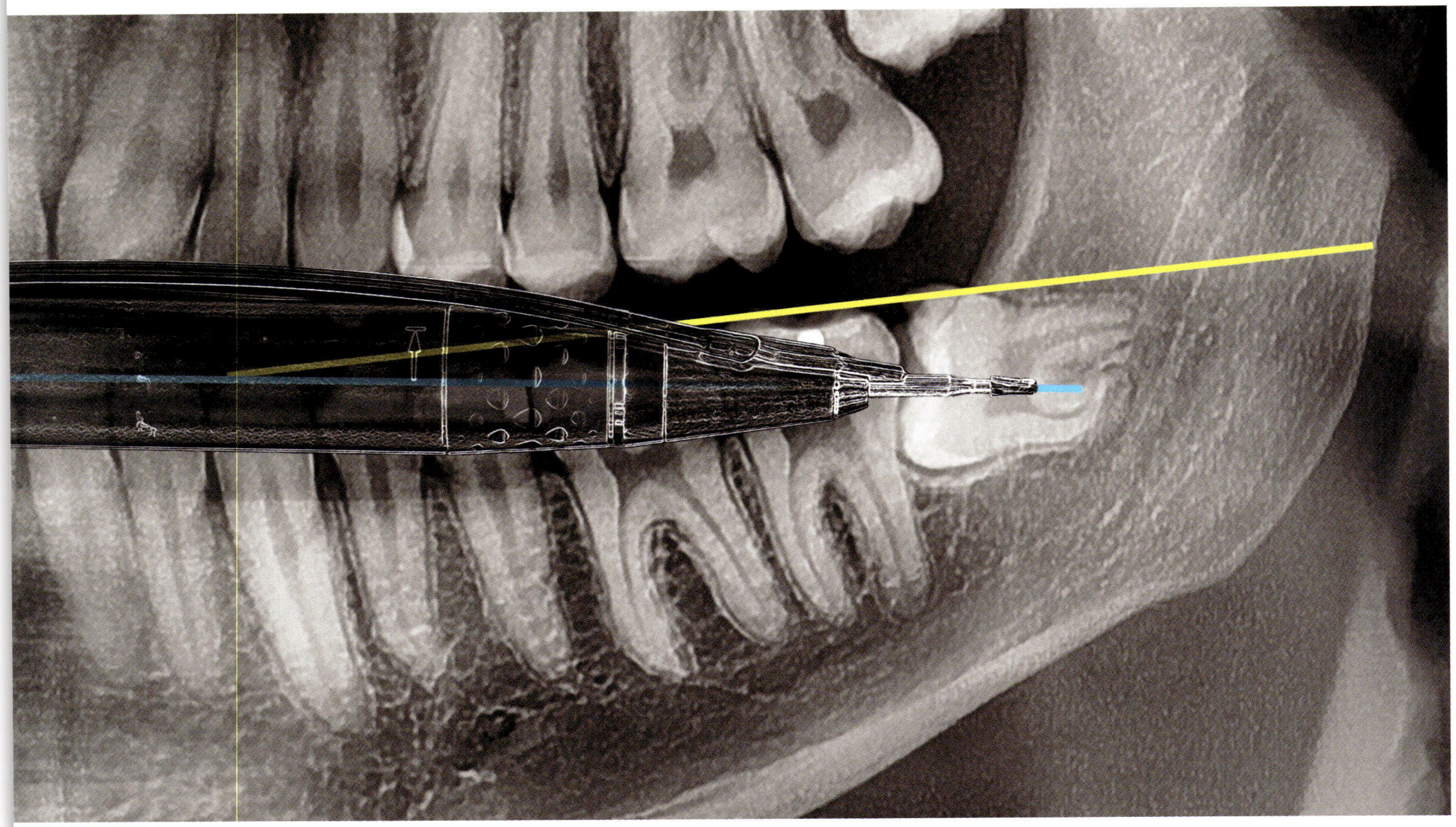

Figure 3-35 The occlusal plane (*yellow*) can be used to estimate the best angle for the drill (*blue*). The height of the second molar helps gauge vertical drilling position.

everything, but they usually show enough to safely guide the surgery.

A few key landmarks can help you get your bearing in surgery. The occlusal plane provides perspective in relation to the underlying anatomy. Running a line perpendicular to the occlusal plane on the radiograph and then envisioning it in the mouth can help you get your bearings before cutting tooth or bone. Relative distances and angles can be estimated by looking at the crowns of adjacent teeth on the radiograph and then translating that into the mouth.

The unknown is untreatable. We cannot fix something if we don't even know it is there. Failure to diagnose is one of the most common reasons for litigation. While it may not always result in legal action, missing a diagnosis most certainly can result in harm to the patient. Establishing good habits and systems is self-preserving and keeps things fun.

By default, our brains look for what they think should be there. We are hardwired to see what we are looking for. To prepare our brains to look for what is actually there, it can be helpful to routinely start at the periphery of an image and work toward the center. There are many systematic approaches to reviewing radiographs that can achieve the same goal of objectively seeing what is present. We need to be experts at the fundamentals. As we grow and develop, we must keep returning to the fundamentals of our art. We will discover and see things we would have missed otherwise. We are never too good to go back to the fundamentals, especially in evaluation.

The single periapical image seems fairly simple to evaluate, but you know how tricky it can be to identify apical pathology at times. If you aren't looking for apical lesions, they are very easy to miss.

A full field cone beam CT scan holds a tremendous amount of information that needs attention. This is not meant to be a comprehensive review of how to read a CBCT, but I would like to share some things I have found helpful when looking at images. It may help you see it in a slightly different way too.

CBCT viewing setup

A panoramic or curved view with very thin slicing can provide a quick and accurate initial assessment of the dentition and surrounding bone as a whole. Scrolling back and forth through the viewing trough makes it easy to identify periapical pathology.

Is there any pathology in the teeth or periodontium? Any asymmetry, apical lesions, density, or lucency? How do the maxillary sinuses look? Is there a thickened lining or positive fluid level?

The multiplanar reconstruction (MPR) view, which has different names in different software, is the combination of the Axial, Coronal and Sagittal views. When the axes are properly aligned, this provides a quick assessment of overall symmetry and structure of the TMJ, cervical spine and all the sinuses (more than just the maxillary sinuses). Scrolling completely through each view is an efficient way to identify possible pathology and help prevent missed diagnoses.

After reviewing the image as a whole, dial in on the area of interest.

Preset note templates can help you hit all the common areas of the radiographic evaluation. Just make sure each area was evaluated. Consider it like a checklist. A preset note also can be damning if it is inaccurate. If you use presets, make sure they are accurate and updated for each patient.

Artificial intelligence is the future of radiographic evaluation. It may not ever be the definitive answer, but systems like Diagnocat AI will play a large role in diagnostic dentistry. They are impressive, powerful and simple. The algorithm is constantly learning and improving in its diagnosis. This can help avoid costly errors, potential litigation and hurting our patients' overall wellbeing. I am fascinated thinking about how far AI will advance our field.

Assumption and curiosity

Curiosity is easy to maintain when something is new or different. The more we see and learn, the easier it is to lose our curiosity. Be an artist, not an encyclopedia. It is more fun that way. I also believe it is better for us, our teams, and our patients. Convert assumptions into hypotheses. Assumptions are the death of learning. Hypotheses are only the beginning.

The evaluation begins with questions. It is populated through a system. And it culminates in a curiosity that is willing to learn new things. My patients teach me every day. And I want it to stay that way.

There are many other aspects of an evaluation worthy of their own systems. What questions do you ask every time? If your team did everything at your office except cut and sew, how would you teach them to approach these situations? Setting up consistent processes for your most common situations will improve efficiency and safety in your practice. Oral pathology, implants, third molars, exodontia, orthognathic, trauma, sedation and health history are examples of other such systems.

Pay attention to paradox in life and in surgery. It is an invitation into something truer than the obvious black and white. Setting up a system for evaluation threatens to lock us into our assumptions, but it also can open up the door to learning, allowing us the freedom to explore what we know and the vast universe of what we do not yet know.

Figure 3-36

POST-OPERATIVE PHONE CALL

I have an evaluation system in my practice for post-operative phone calls. I don't answer the phones at my office. Apart from after-hours calls that get forwarded to my cell, my team always evaluates patients when they call. The information they gather on these calls sets the stage for my evaluation. Out of necessity, I have established a set of questions my team asks every patient who calls with post-operative concerns. Sometimes, it may feel unnecessary to ask all the questions, but the routine of asking every question every time gives me confidence I will have the most critical information to determine what my patient needs. It makes everything safer.

Previous treatment and date: ______________________

____

Name of person and relationship who called: ________

____

Reason for calling: ______________________

____

Cell Phone #: ______________________

____

Pharmacy name: ______________________

____

Pharmacy phone number: ______________________

____

Comments: ______________________

____

____

____

____

____

Pain:

- How painful: (1-10) ______________________
- Where is the pain: ______________________
- Is it improving: ______________________
- Describe the pain: ______________________
- Pain medication: ______________________
- How much medication are you taking: ___________
- Is it managing the pain: ______________________

Swelling:

- Where: ______________________
- Is it improving: ______________________
- Is it spreading: ______________________
- Difficulty breathing: ______________________
- Difficulty swallowing: ______________________

Fever: ______________________

____

References

1. Gisondi M. Mise en Place, Teach the Sous Chef, Save the Patient [Internet]. ICE Blog. 2021 [cited 2023 Jan 11]. Available from: https://icenetblog.royalcollege.ca/2021/02/02/mise-en-place-teach-the-sous-chef-save-the-patient/
2. forceps | Etymology, origin and meaning of forceps by etymonline [Internet]. [cited 2023 Jan 1]. Available from: https://www.etymonline.com/word/forceps

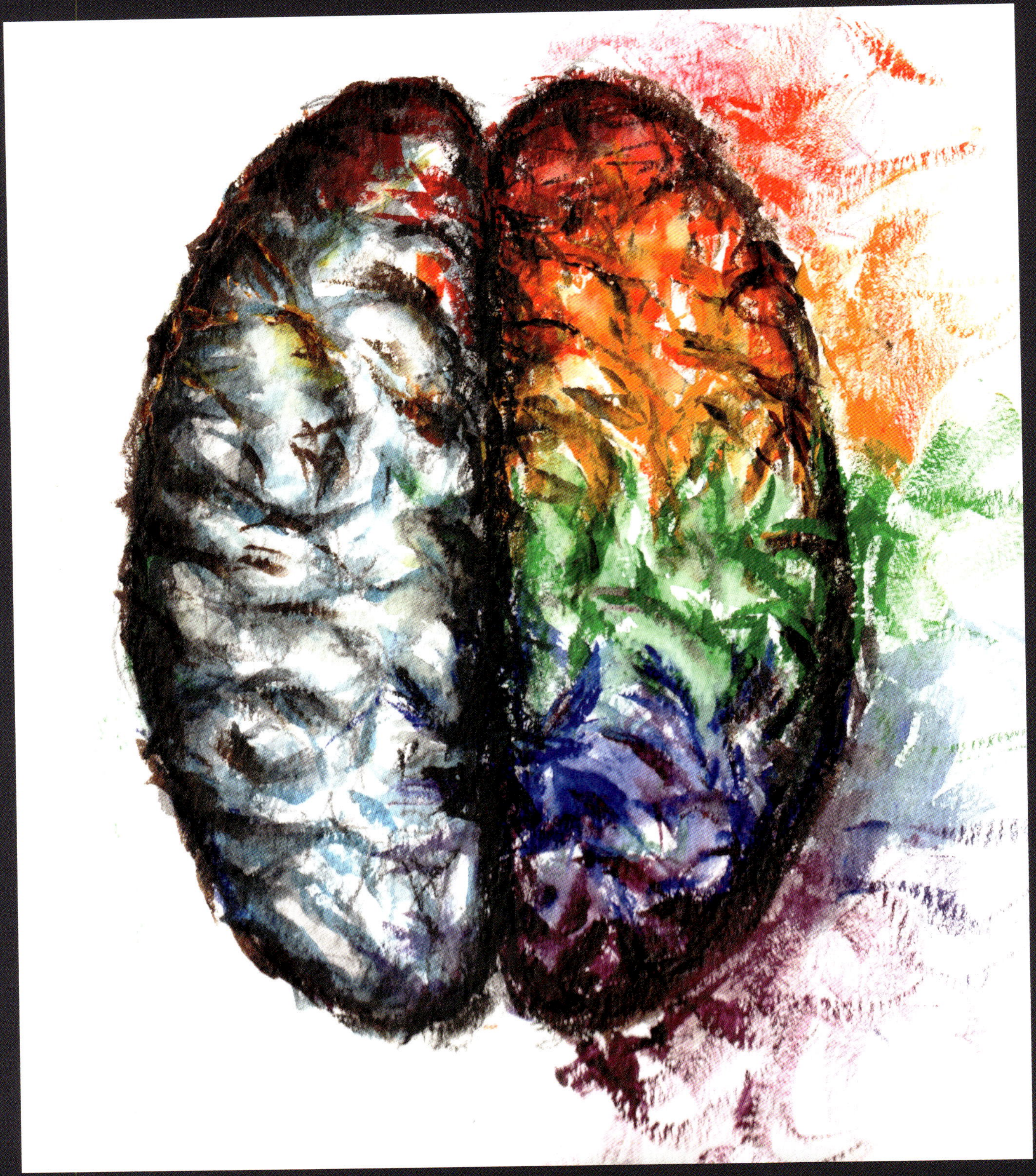

Living in Both Worlds. (Watercolor)
This book was born in the confluence of science and beauty. Logic and creativity don't compete; they complete the picture.

CHAPTER 4

THE ART OF EXODONTIA

The tooth you remove will cause no pain or swelling after the extraction. It will neither contribute to infection nor alveolar osteitis. It is the remaining hard and soft tissue that will bear witness to the extraction. They will tell the story. It is their mark that your patient will remember and retell. As Randy Travis sang, “It’s not what you take when you leave this world behind, it’s what you leave behind you when you’re gone.”

While the procedure is typically considered a tooth extraction, I would invite you to instead consider it as the development of an extraction site. If in your mind you are merely trying to get the tooth out, you can get in line with everyone else performing exodontia. Even a baseball bat can do that. If you want to master the art of exodontia, think about preparing the soft and hard tissue to heal well.

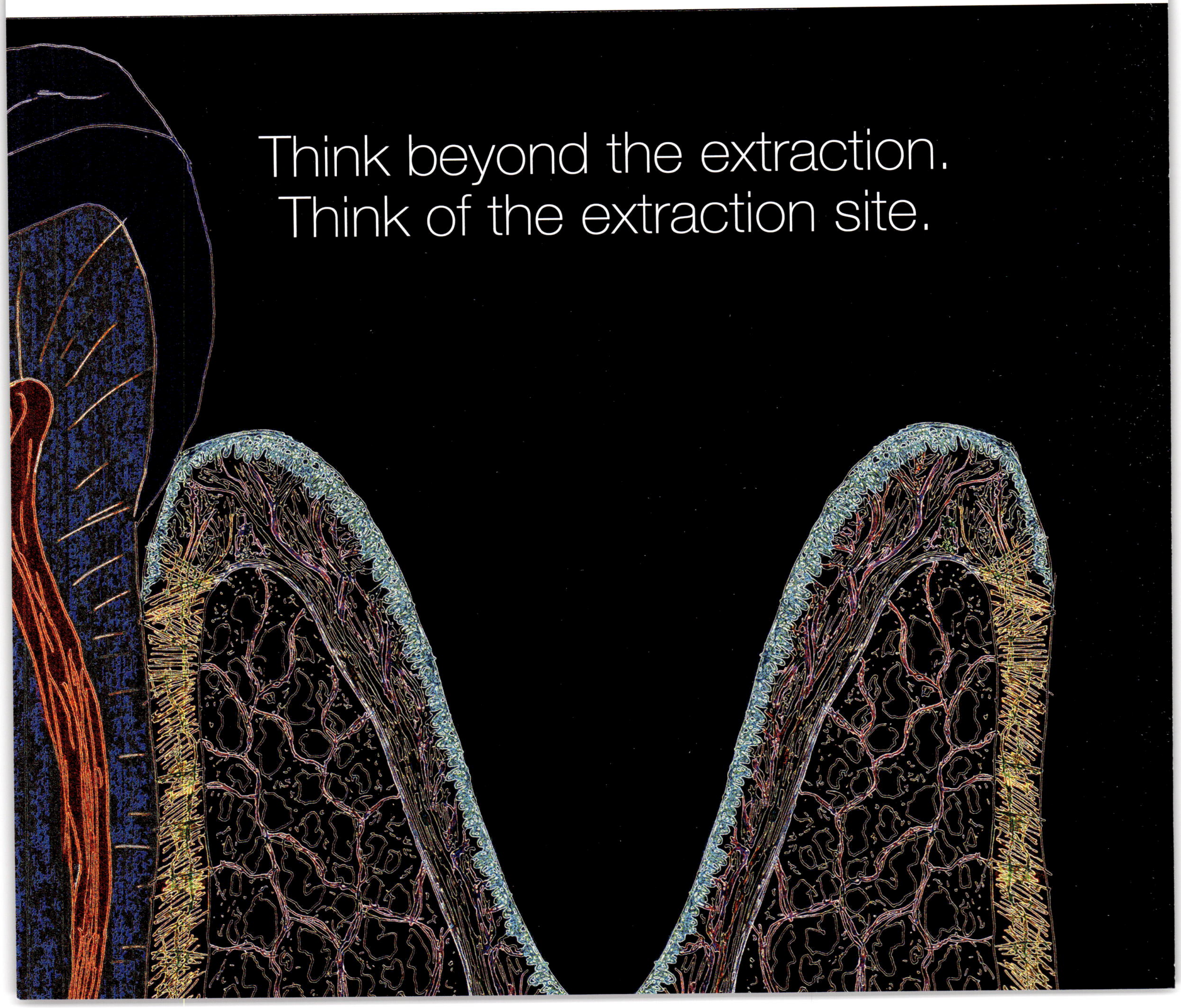

Natural Tooth Retention

What keeps teeth in place? The better we understand the mechanisms of retention, the better we can remove a tooth. Everything that makes a tooth harder to extract is actually good for the patient, unless, of course, you need to extract the tooth. Generally, teeth aren't supposed to come out. They are retained both mechanically and biomechanically. The bone surrounding the tooth mechanically holds it in place. It is a rigid structure tightly formed around the root. While the bone itself retains the tooth, it also serves as the foundation and framework for the biomechanical retention: the periodontal ligament. It is the periodontal ligament that provides the primary, dynamic and lifelong retention of a tooth. The bone and periodontal ligament are inextricably dependent on each other for retaining a tooth. Separating the principles of mechanical and biomechanical retention in your mind creates a systematic process for evaluating, envisioning and executing the extraction. Think about how the bone and periodontal ligament are working together before and during the extraction. Plan accordingly. And when a tooth is putting up a fight, evaluate them both independently. Think about how the bone is retaining the tooth and how the ligament is retaining it.

Mechanical retention: bone

The bone surrounding a tooth provides mechanical retention through the properties of matter and friction. This is how a dry skull retains teeth. As a property of matter, the tooth and bone cannot occupy the same space at the same time. The tighter the bone hugs the tooth, the more friction there is keeping the tooth in place. When the tooth is tightly embedded deep within dense bone, it will mechanically resist forces of exodontia with more rigor than if there is a wide socket in soft bone.

Friction between the bone and root structure also retains the tooth. This may be an oversimplification, but it is helpful for me to think about it this way during extraction. More root structure rubbing harder against the bone increases friction. Thus, root shape also influences retention. A root with any bit of curve will resist extraction more than a straight root. The tooth and bone cannot occupy the same space. For a curved root to traverse past the surrounding bone, it will either need to displace the bone, be sectioned into smaller pieces, or physically move around the corner.

This truly comes to life when removing a tooth with a big old curve on the root. It can be quite frustrating, especially when the radiograph doesn't accurately show the anatomy. It is much easier when you see the curvature beforehand and can tailor the surgery to accommodate for it. A luxator moves the tooth around the curved roots by using the adjacent tooth as a fulcrum. Rotating the instrument lifts the tooth out around the curvature.

Dilacerated roots were originally described as teeth with a severe bend in the root form due to trauma in the developmental stage of the tooth, leading to a sharp change in the developing root's angulation[1]. The term dilaceration, which means to tear up, is commonly used today to describe severely curved roots[2].

◂
Figure 4-1 This is how I envision a tooth (*blue*), periodontal ligament and crestal fibers (*gold*), alveolar bone, periosteum, sulcus, and gingival tissue (*aqua*). The inverted colors help me visualize the different structures. These are the main considerations in exodontia. They each play their own role. And the goal is to develop the extraction site (*right*).

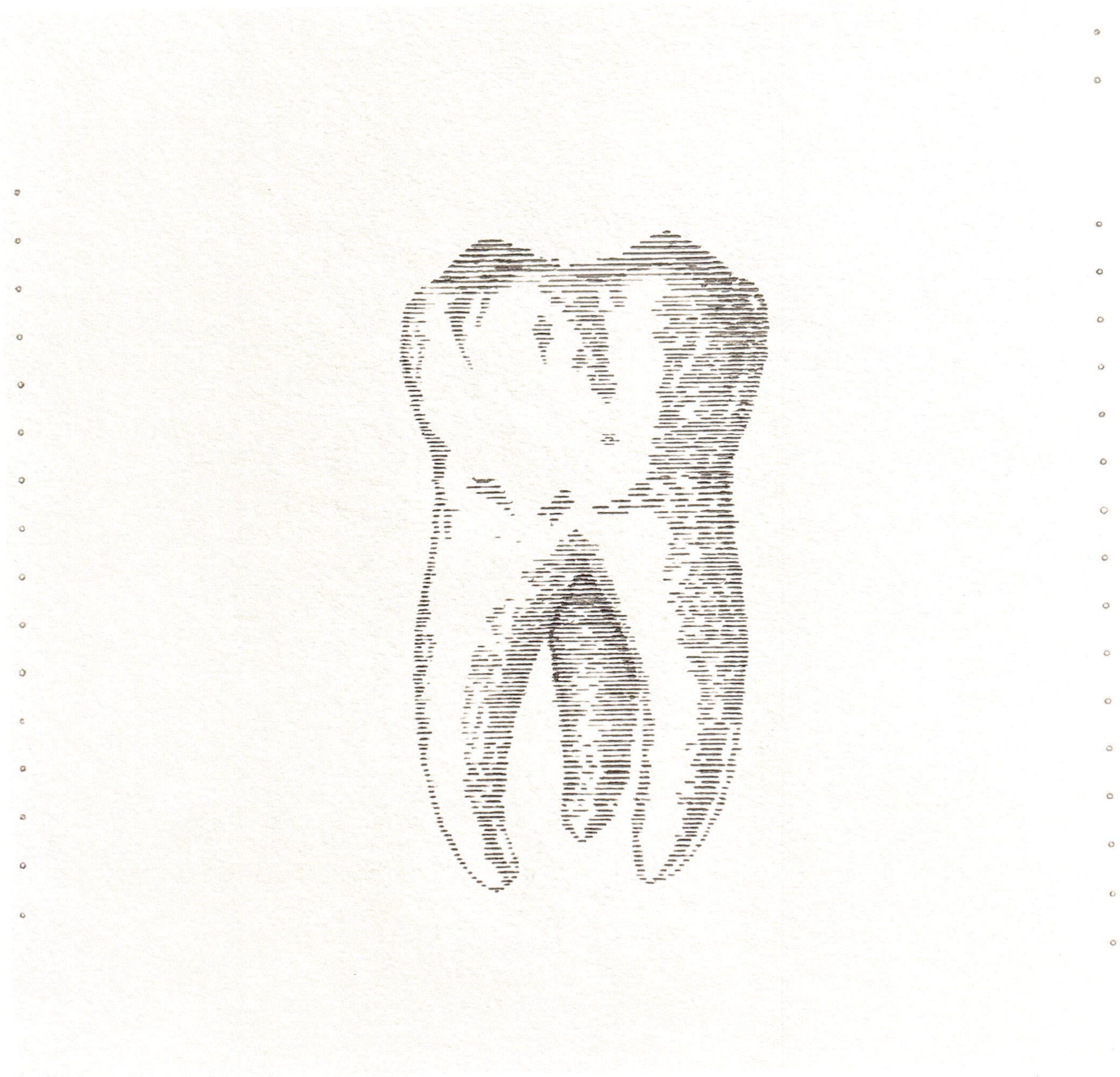

Figure 4-2 You can read a tooth line by line, but putting all the lines together brings the picture to life. It can be helpful to think about the individual components, but don't lose sight of the big picture. (Artwork inspired by Agnes Martin.)

Biomechanical retention: periodontal ligament (PDL)

This fascinating structure serves its whole career guiding the eruption of teeth, ensuring their maintenance and position during development and growth. It maintains tooth stability in a grueling environment subject to tremendous bacterial and mechanical burdens. And then, in its retirement, it ensures its legacy by contributing significantly to the extraction socket's healing. It is surely an unsung hero marked by a life of service. (I feel like we should give it a round of applause. Bravo, my little friend). If we could only be so inspired in our own lives.

It is helpful to understand some properties of the periodontal ligament when learning how to manage it. The periodontal ligament is a very specialized band of dense, flexible fibrous connective tissue inserting into the cementum of a tooth on one side and the surrounding alveolar bone on the other. It is composed mainly of type 1 collagen and water.

It is about 70% water. The water is thought to provide a significant amount of the absorptive properties that sustain the ligament during mastication. It holds the tooth in constant sprung suspension, always under tension. Sharpey's fibers of periodontal ligaments are the entheses, the end of the ligament that attaches to the cementum on one side and the lamina dura of the alveolar bone on the other. Its most basic responsibility is to retain teeth in the bone.

Sharpey's fibers are embedded in the bone and extend through the periosteum to join with the ligament. The ligament itself spans across the gap where it embeds into the surface of the cementum with another layer of Sharpey's fibers. To remove a tooth, this complex must be destroyed in at least one of these components.

Biology flashback: I am fascinated by how ribosomes in a cell can translate RNA into long peptide chains of amino acids. With the help of Vitamin C, these chains are modified to form a triple helical structure that is transported by the Golgi apparatus and secreted from the cell. Once outside the cell, a whole host of events transpire, organizing the collagen molecules into fibrils and ultimately into collagen fiber. About 90% of the collagen in our bodies is type 1 collagen. This is all constantly taking place microscopically in our cells. How amazing!

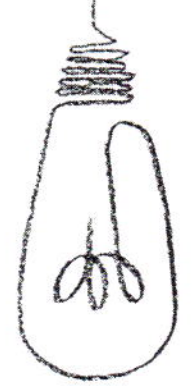

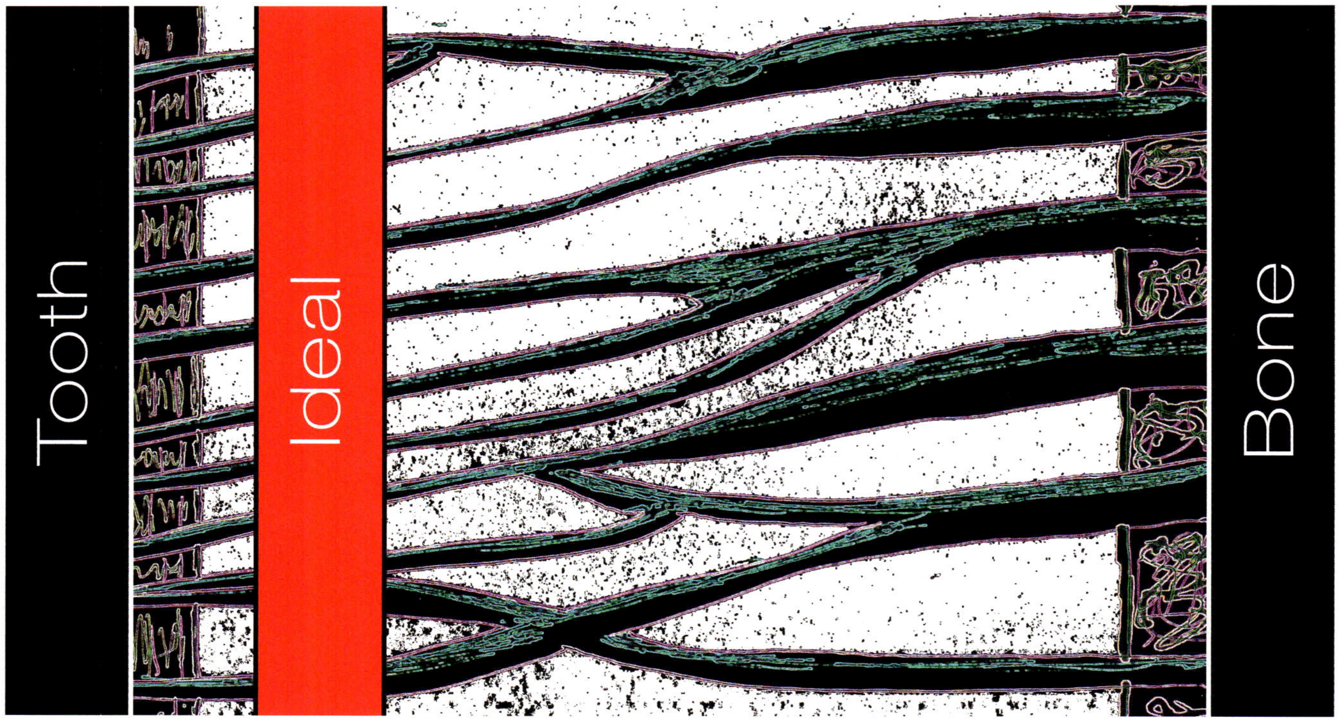

Figure 4-3 Sharpey's fibers insert into the cementum (*left*) and the alveolar bone (*right*) as they span the ligament space (*center*) to retain a tooth. Ideally, we would sever the Sharpey's fibers immediately adjacent to the tooth, preserving most of the ligament within the extraction site.

In an ideal, theoretical world, we would be able to sever the ligament precisely at the junction with the Sharpey's fibers on the cementum side of the ligament. This would preserve the majority of the ligament and all its regenerative assets within the healing socket. In contrast, the least favorable way to extract a tooth is removing the surrounding alveolar bone. This is much more destructive, and it sacrifices the benefits of the ligament in healing. In practice, we can try to preserve the ligament and bone during extraction by being aware of it and protecting it. This seems contradictory. We want to preserve the same structure we need to break? That's right. We want to keep as much of the ligament on the bone side of the equation after the extraction as possible. Extraction is a form of ligotomy: the cutting of a ligament.

Successful exodontia occurs when the mechanical and biomechanical retention of a tooth and its ligament is overcome. The art of exodontia is both theory and performance. Canvas and paint. And mastery of the art.

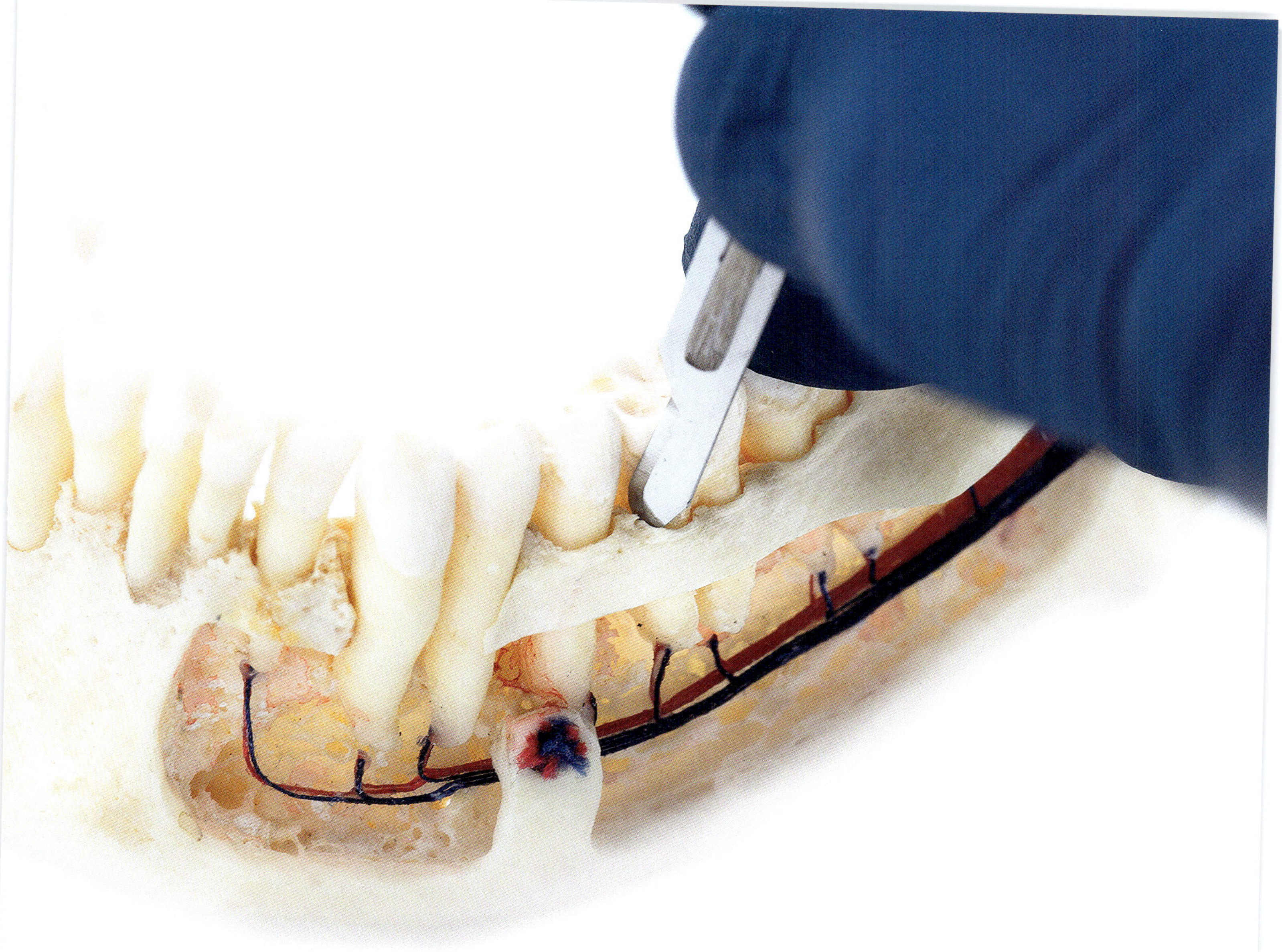

Figure 4-4 Extraction is a form of ligotomy, the cutting of the periodontal ligament. A scalpel can be the first instrument to cut the ligament.

Exodontia Evaluation

What you look for determines what you will see. Take the time to look before you cut. Keep the bone, periodontal ligament, tooth, and soft tissue in mind when evaluating a tooth for extraction.

Bone

Plain film radiographs can give you a general sense of the bone around a tooth. A periapical or panoramic image shows mesial and distal bone levels and general root contours. You can get a sense of the bone density, which can impact mechanical resistance during extraction. Pay attention to the curvature of the tooth roots as well. Envision the movement while looking at the image. Make the image come to life in your mind, almost like it is animated.

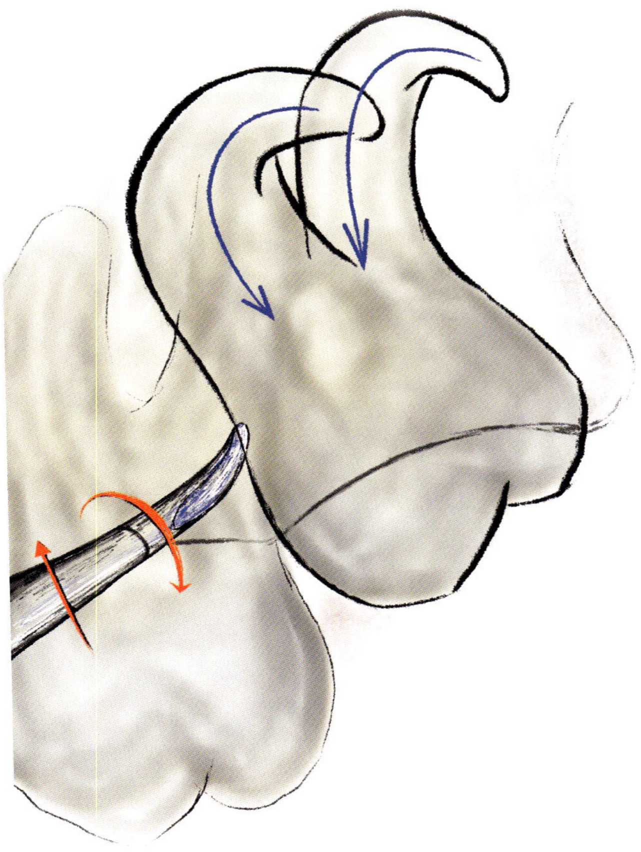

Figure 4-5 A luxator can elevate the tooth around the curvature of the roots. Rotating the instrument (*orange arrows*) lifts the tooth out around the curvature.

Three-dimensional imaging provides significantly more information. If you already have a CBCT image, take a moment to review it right before picking up an instrument. It is always better to learn about the challenges before surgery than during surgery. A CBCT's cross-sectional images may reveal where the bone is denser or less dense circumferentially.

Visualizing bone density can help you determine which direction to elevate. It can also provide insight on the best position for the elevator. If the bone appears quite dense, proceed with a higher level of caution during initial elevation. A decision to section the tooth or possibly remove bone early on may be rewarded if the dense surrounding bone is far more stubborn than the tooth. Understanding bone density may help optimize the progression through the surgical protocol from simple elevation to sectioning and bone removal.

Pay attention to the proximity of the adjacent teeth and structures to avoid harming them while drilling. For instance, there may be inadequate interproximal clearance for bone removal near the crest, but farther apically it may be safe. This is helpful to know prior to surgery and as a reference during surgery.

Expect increased bone density when you see exostoses, signs of parafunctional habits, or a thick ridge. These clinical clues may encourage earlier or more aggressive sectioning or bone removal.

During surgery, you can use a periodontal probe or scalpel for bone sounding. By advancing the instrument in the sulcus, you can attain a lot of information about where the bone may be thin or recessed. Capitalize on areas of thin bone to more easily elevate and deliver a tooth.

Periodontal ligament

Evaluating the ligament space radiographically is also beneficial. A well-defined, wide space may indicate an easier extraction as there is more space to luxate the tooth. It can be manipulated farther in each direction, stretching and rupturing the ligament more extensively. In contrast, a narrow or non-existent ligament space indicates very limited room for manipulation. The tooth has nowhere to go, so you can't stretch the ligament very much.

Sometimes, a radiograph shows a complete lack of periodontal ligament space. While not necessarily diagnostic for ankylosis, this certainly indicates a potentially more difficult extraction. In truly ankylotic teeth, there is no periodontal ligament, and the bone is fused directly to the cementum. In these cases, the bundle bone will come out with the tooth. Intentional bone removal can be performed to direct fracture patterns of the surrounding bone, improving the outcome of surgery and optimizing the healing site. A difficult extraction is not necessarily an ankylosed tooth. Truly ankylosed teeth are not nearly as common as a difficult extraction with a limited periodontal ligament. In my experience, it has been painfully obvious when the tooth was truly ankylosed, which has only happened a handful of times.

Wider periodontal ligament space = easier. Less likely to section or remove bone.
Narrow periodontal ligament space = harder. More likely to section or remove bone.
No periodontal ligament space = possible ankylosis. More likely to act like ankylosis with resulting fracture of surrounding bone.

Tooth

To extract a tooth, you need to be able to apply enough force on the tooth to disrupt the periodontal ligament. The tooth's overall condition directly impacts your ability to apply such forces. Clinical and radiographic tooth evaluations can help you visualize the extraction. How will the tooth respond to elevation? Where can I get a good purchase point? Will this elevate straight out, or do I need to bring the roots around a curve?

Radiographic evaluation of the crown's condition can help predict how the tooth will respond to extraction forces. Know the crown's condition and where to elevate. It is difficult and quite unproductive to elevate against soft, mushy caries. Pick a different spot. The image will often help identify the best place to elevate.

Understanding the curvature and overall anatomy of the roots can be advantageous in determining where and how to elevate. A lower molar with converging curved roots and dense bone is not likely to elevate out in one piece. It may be helpful to section it right away to preserve the bone and expedite extraction. An upper molar with divergent roots may also benefit from sectioning. This also can preserve the more fragile buccal plate. Extra roots can complicate the extraction or be retained unintentionally. Don't just assume the lower molar has two roots. Look for signs on the radiograph and then check the site upon extraction.

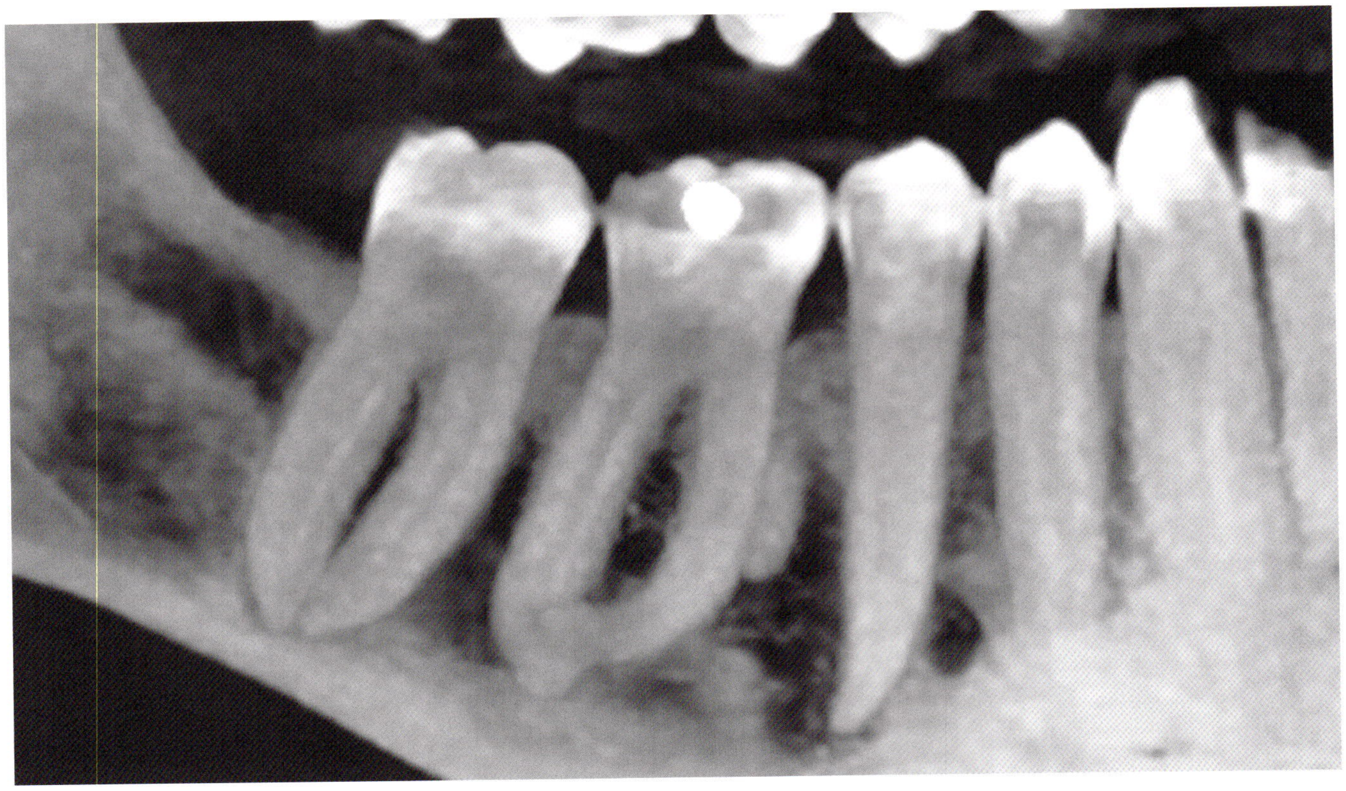

Figure 4-6 A lower first molar with long curved roots like this is not likely to elevate out in one piece. This could be sectioned to allow elevation around the curve of the roots. Also note retained primary tooth roots that are asymptomatic and unlikely to cause complications.

Endodontically treated teeth

Does gutta percha sometimes seem like it is made of kryptonite to you? It feels like all my best moves can be thwarted when that stuff is inside a tooth. The tooth fractures like a dry twig and there is no help from the periodontal ligament because it has turned into cement. Chemical irritation of the endodontic treatment protocol and limited blood supply change the properties of the tooth and ligament.

Blood supply is a collateral network of vessels feeding all the tissue in the body. This incredible design builds in redundancy to ensure perfusion in the event of injury. It also increases the ability to regulate end organ supply. Teeth and their surrounding structures have their own extensive vascular network supplying the tooth, periodontal ligament, alveolar bone, and surrounding soft tissue. Venous congestion within a tooth significantly increases the intrapulpal pressure causing necrosis of the delicate tissue. This venous congestion can occur when reactive cementum is laid down as a defense mechanism, reducing the outflow of blood. Iatrogenic or accidental trauma also can cause inflammation that increases internal pressure, leading to pulpal necrosis. No matter the cause, the necrotic pulp no longer performs its role in collateral circulation. This starves the cementum of nutrients, causing changes in its structure. It also limits blood supply to the periodontal ligament, which undergoes sclerotic changes. With these changes, an endodontic tooth no longer behaves like a vital tooth when it comes to exodontia.

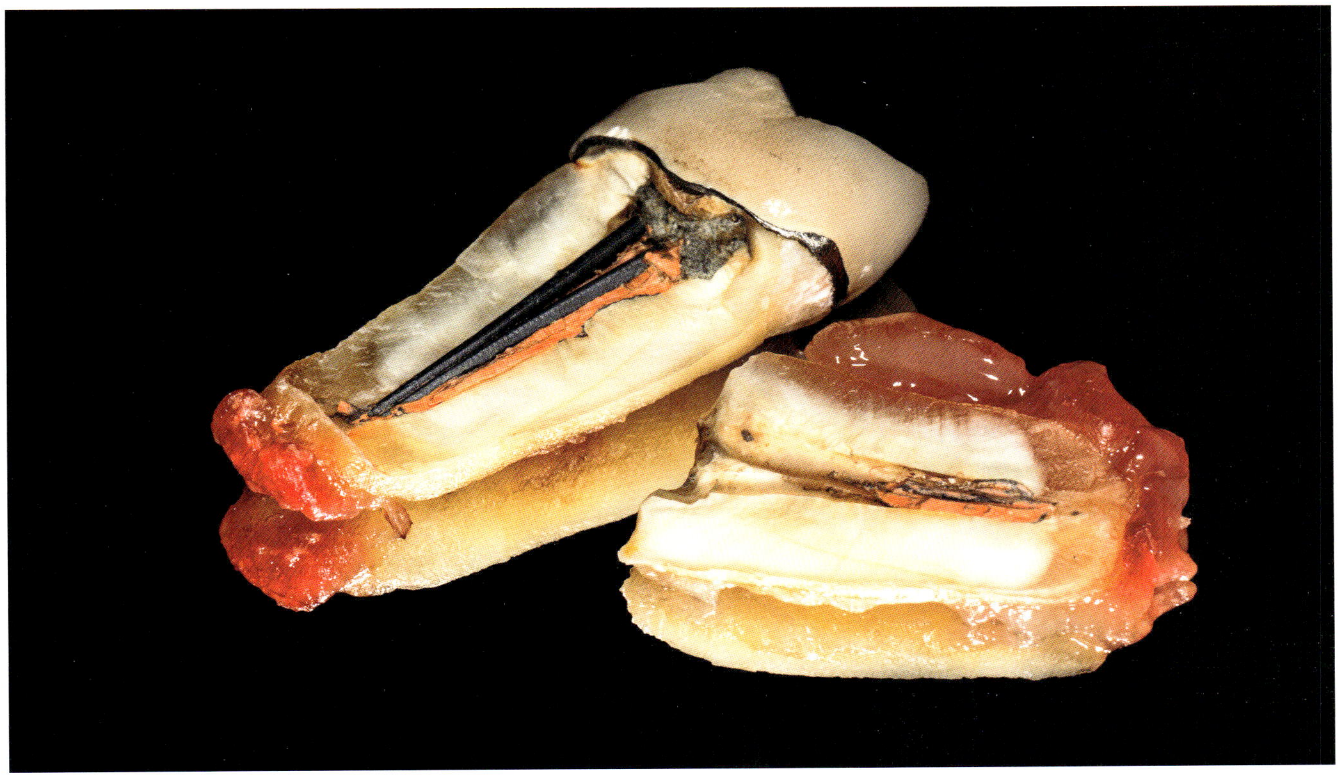

Figure 4-7 Fractured endodontically treated tooth. Notice the visible changes in the cementum and dentin. (Artwork inspired by Claes Oldenburg.)

We often like to think of problems according to their solutions. We separate endodontic problems from periodontal problems because they are treated differently and often by different people. But I am amazed at how interdependent everything is. In the same way that an endodontically treated tooth will have periodontal changes, it has been shown that chronic periodontitis has a profound impact on a vital tooth's cementum and pulpal tissue. It goes both ways[3].

Despite the challenges it brings, gutta percha has a hidden asset. It can serve as pale orange navigational beacons marking the root centers. This marker can guide the often-blind drilling deep within a tooth. When the tooth fractures repeatedly and requires the use of a surgical handpiece, look for the orange. This can be especially useful when sectioning a multi-rooted molar. Just keep the bur between the orange dots and you should end up with a reasonable split to elevate the roots independently.

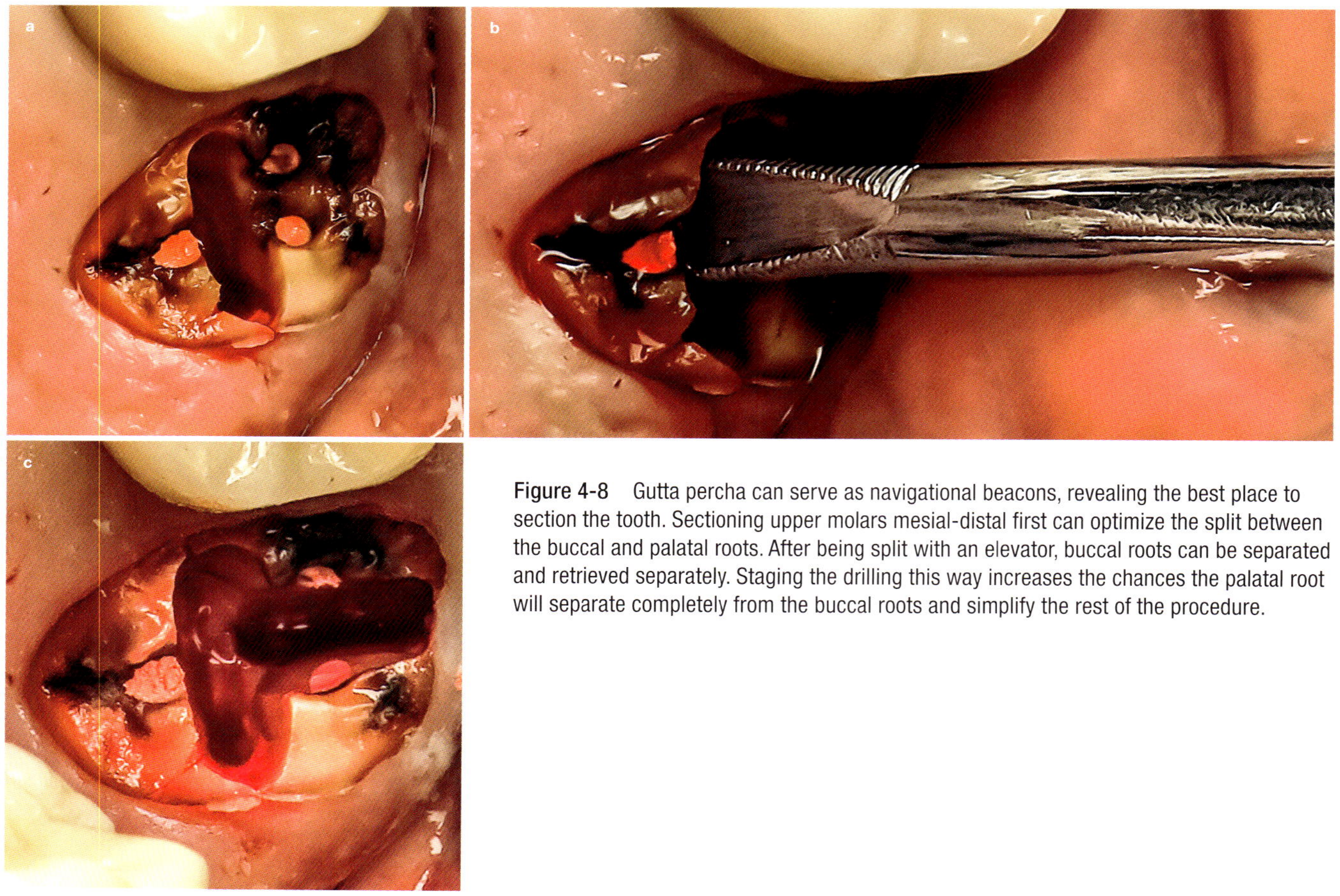

Figure 4-8 Gutta percha can serve as navigational beacons, revealing the best place to section the tooth. Sectioning upper molars mesial-distal first can optimize the split between the buccal and palatal roots. After being split with an elevator, buccal roots can be separated and retrieved separately. Staging the drilling this way increases the chances the palatal root will separate completely from the buccal roots and simplify the rest of the procedure.

Also consider the advantages of gutta percha with a single rooted tooth, such as an upper canine. It can be difficult to determine the long axis of the tooth, especially when the crown has fractured off. In such a case, it is comforting to see gutta percha. Follow the orange and you know you will be in the center of the root's long axis. Then you can swing the bur either to the mesial and distal or to the buccal and lingual to complete root sectioning—with a relatively high level of confidence your cuts will be effective.

Knowing the history of an endodontically treated tooth is also helpful. The longer a tooth has been endodontically treated, the more time it has had to undergo sclerotic changes. I move much more quickly to sectioning or bone removal when the endo treatment is years or decades old. I am also more aggressive with the drill. I favor removing more bone than tooth because I know the tooth structure is more brittle and the periodontal ligament is more sclerotic. This is in contrast to a vital tooth where I would favor removing more tooth structure and preserving bone structure.

Take your time. Endodontically treated teeth can be more stubborn, requiring increased patience balanced with deliberate and sometimes aggressive drilling. Visualization is key to pre-operative preparation. If you can visualize the upcoming challenges, you will be more successful.

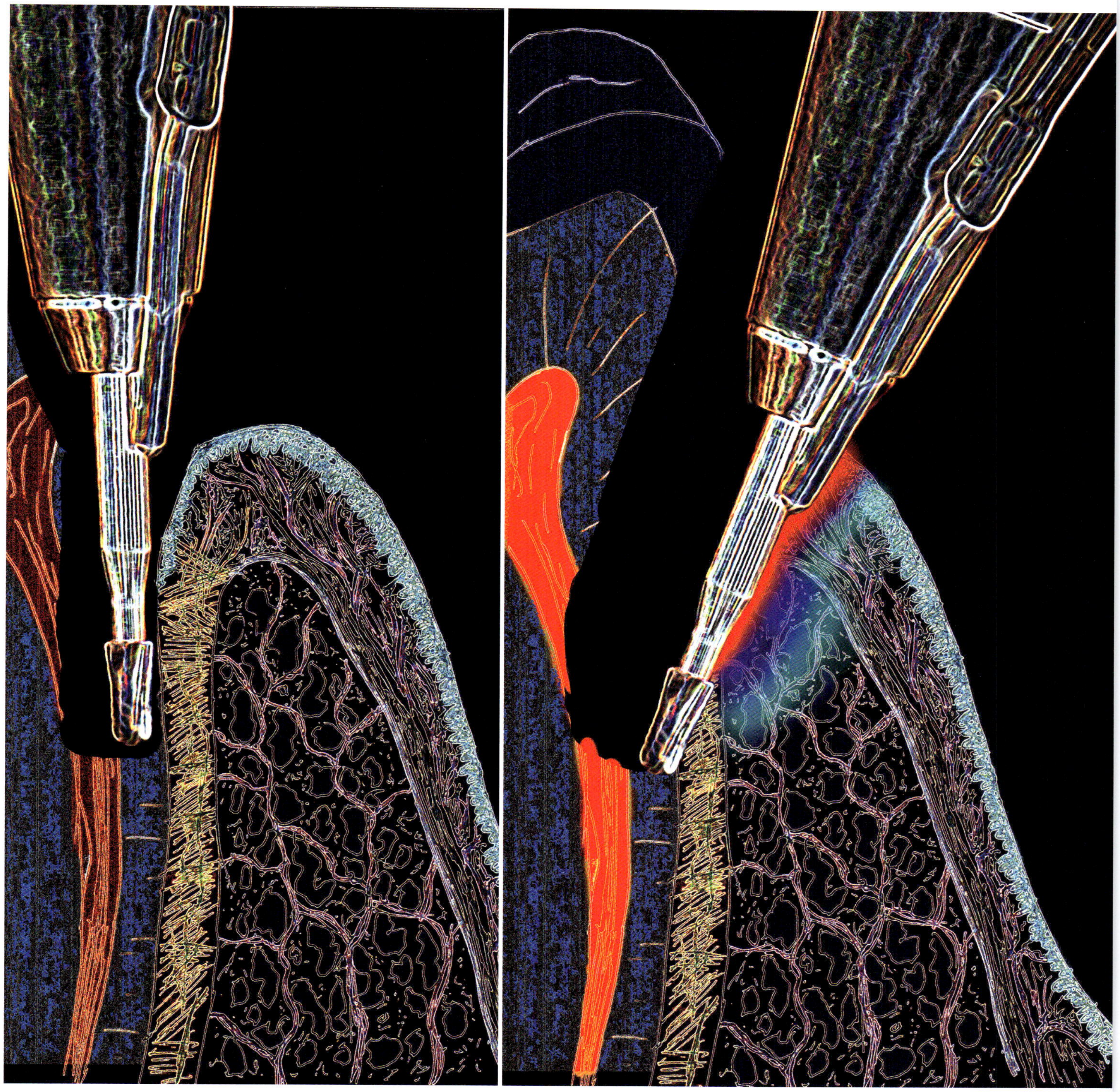

Figure 4-9 When a tooth needs to be sectioned, there is an advantage to preferentially drilling away tooth structure instead of removing the periodontal ligament and further injuring the surrounding bone (*right*). Endodontically treated teeth may benefit from more bone removal. Also note how this picture portrays the heat generated if the bur's shank is rubbing against the soft tissue and bone. Always make sure irrigation is adequately reaching the cutting edge and consider reflecting the tissue to improve visualization and irrigation.

People generally want to know things are going well. When procedures take longer than expected, patients worry that something must be going wrong. Pointing out the positive may be all they need.

You can say something like, *"Just want you to know things are going fine. You have nice, dense bone here, which means it should be more stable for the long term."* Patients appreciate any attempt at filling in the voids with positivity.

They might ask, *"Doc, does it look like an easy extraction? Will it take long?"*

Looking for reassurance and comfort, patients often ask the same thing we're asking the tooth: What's it going to take to get this tooth out? How long? What instruments will be needed? What techniques will work best? Will it come out whole or will it fracture? Will this put me behind schedule, or can I make up some time?

To our patients, it is a question of suffering. To us, it is a question of efficiency and productivity.

"I can only tell if it is an easy extraction after the tooth is out. It all depends on how the tooth cooperates." I often say this, hoping my candor will be endearing. We all have been surprised at least a time or two by how long it can take to remove a single stubborn tooth. There are ways to do it faster, but better sometimes takes just a bit more time.

Soft tissue

Before we get into extraction mechanics, we must first address the soft tissue. The tooth sulcus is where the tooth penetrates through the epithelium into the oral cavity. It is under constant attack by bacteria slimed with biofilm. With only 10 to 20 cell layers of epithelium separating the biofilm from the bloodstream, it is always a potential site of exposure to harmful bacteria. During an extraction, the risk of exposure becomes much higher. It must be handled with care.

Cleanly incise the sulcus. Circumferentially sever the tissue with a knife, Micro Buser or periotome type of instrument. This clean incision reduces collateral damage to the tissue and can help release the circumferential periodontal ligament attachment. Blunt tearing of this tissue results in increased exposure and inflammation. It also improves access for instrumentation with elevators and forceps. They can be positioned more favorably and with less trauma to the soft tissue.

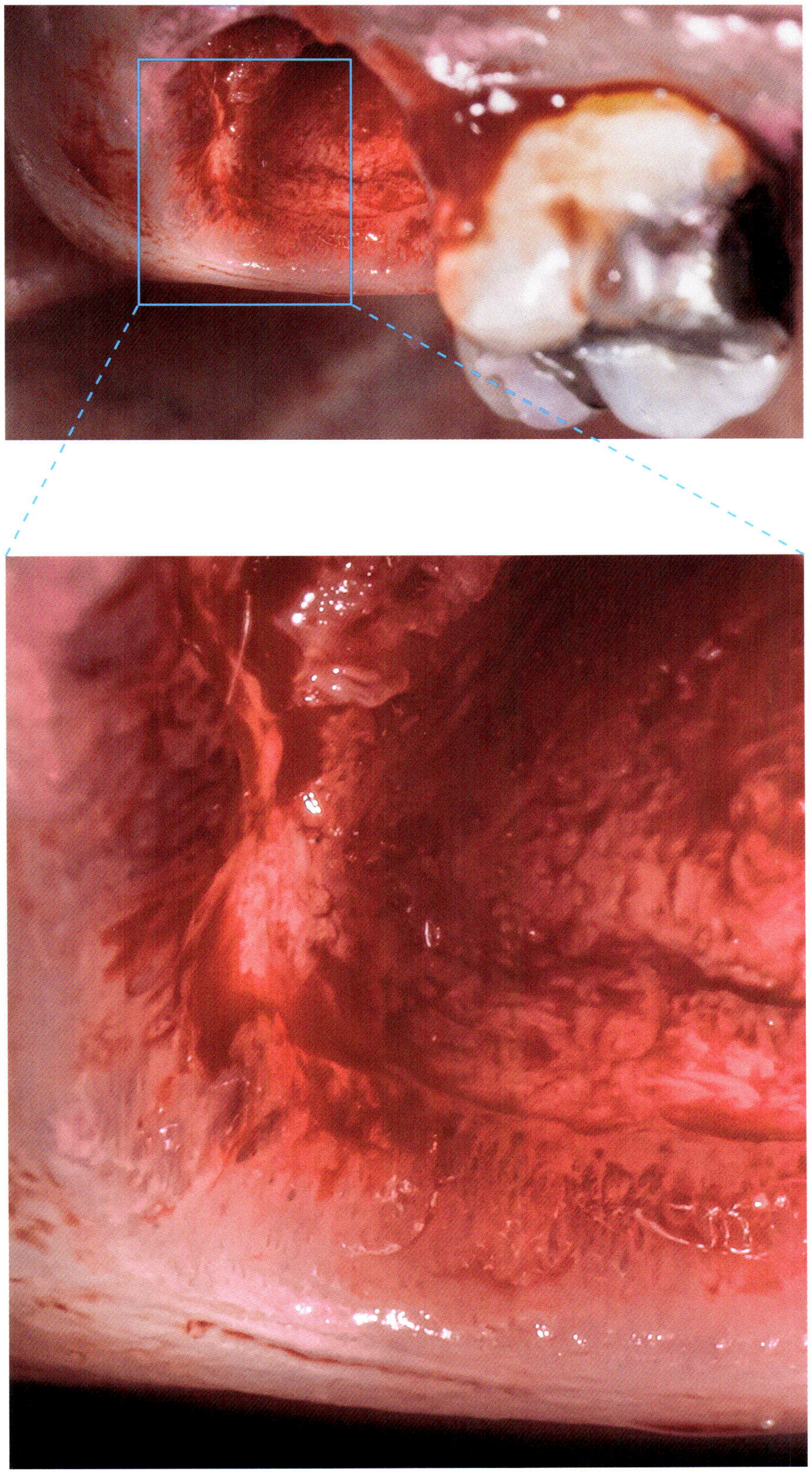

Figure 4-10 The tissue is very thin between the biofilm of the sulcus and the underlying bloodstream. This is exposed through extraction. Check out the periodontal ligament. Look for it when inspecting an extraction socket. It is fascinating to see and is a good reminder of the essence of healing.

Papilla

An elevator can crush, tear and make a mess of the papilla if it is not sharply incised with a blade and gently mobilized to make room for the instrument. Before you pick up an elevator, consider using a knife. This can protect the soft tissue from blunt trauma and improve visualization and access. While this is not always necessary, incised tissue heals better than crushed tissue. As I critically evaluate my own technique and procedures, I have found I don't always realize how much trauma I can cause the tissue when elevating.

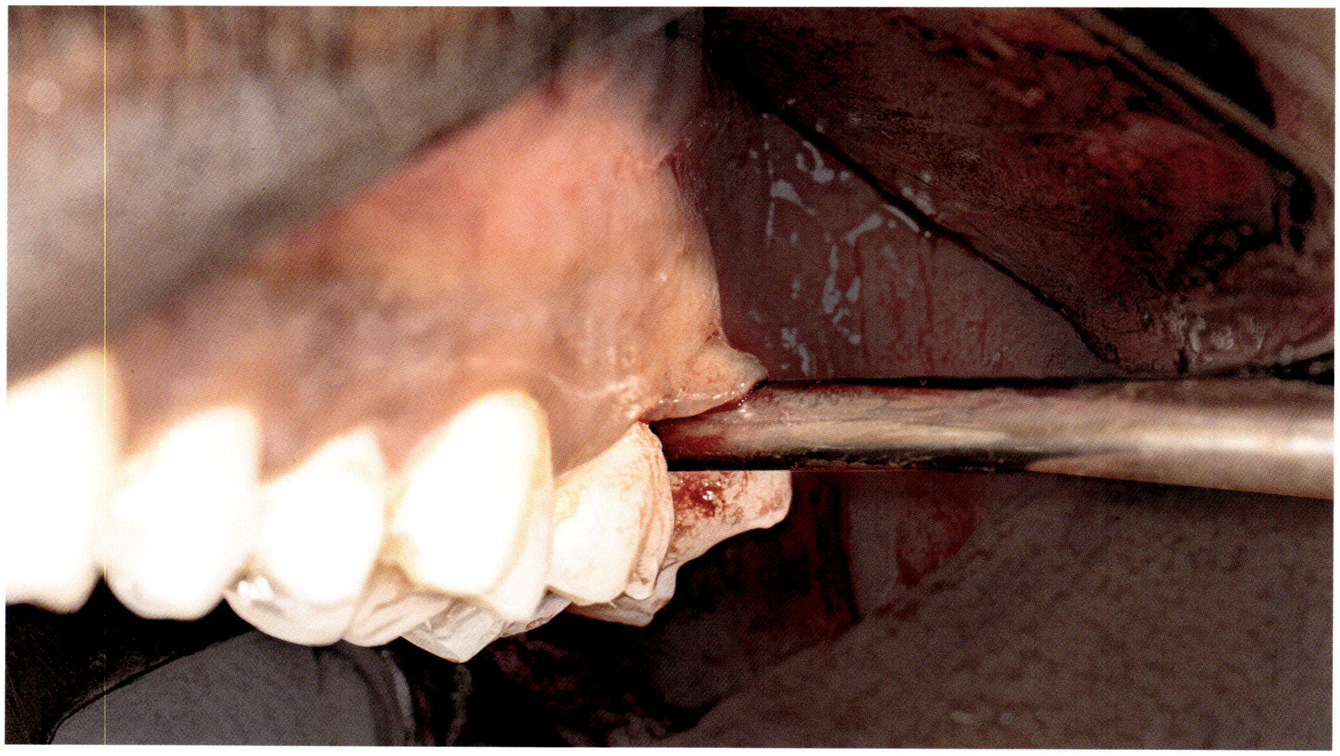

Figure 4-11 Incising and gently reflecting the papilla creates a safe space for instrumentation with elevators, like this small Bein luxator. This protects the papilla from blunt trauma, improving healing. The papilla still must be protected when elevating. It can be traumatized, even if it is reflected initially.

Flap design

At times, elevating a flap can make all the difference. It can protect the soft tissue and improve visualization and access when needed. The first thing I ask when struggling with an extraction is whether I have adequate access and visualization. Sometimes, I reflect a flap right away if I know it will be needed and helpful. It is important to become comfortable with a simple sulcular or envelope flap as well as performing vertical releases. The releasing incisions can really open up the access to the site.

Incisions should be made in good tissue, sloping away from the flap to protect the blood supply. When making a full thickness incision, envision cutting the bone with the blade. I often see the incision line in the surface of the bone after reflecting a flap.

Design the flap so you can see what you need to see. Think about the needs of the entire procedure. Then incise and reflect a flap that will help you do your best work and help the tissue do its best work during healing.

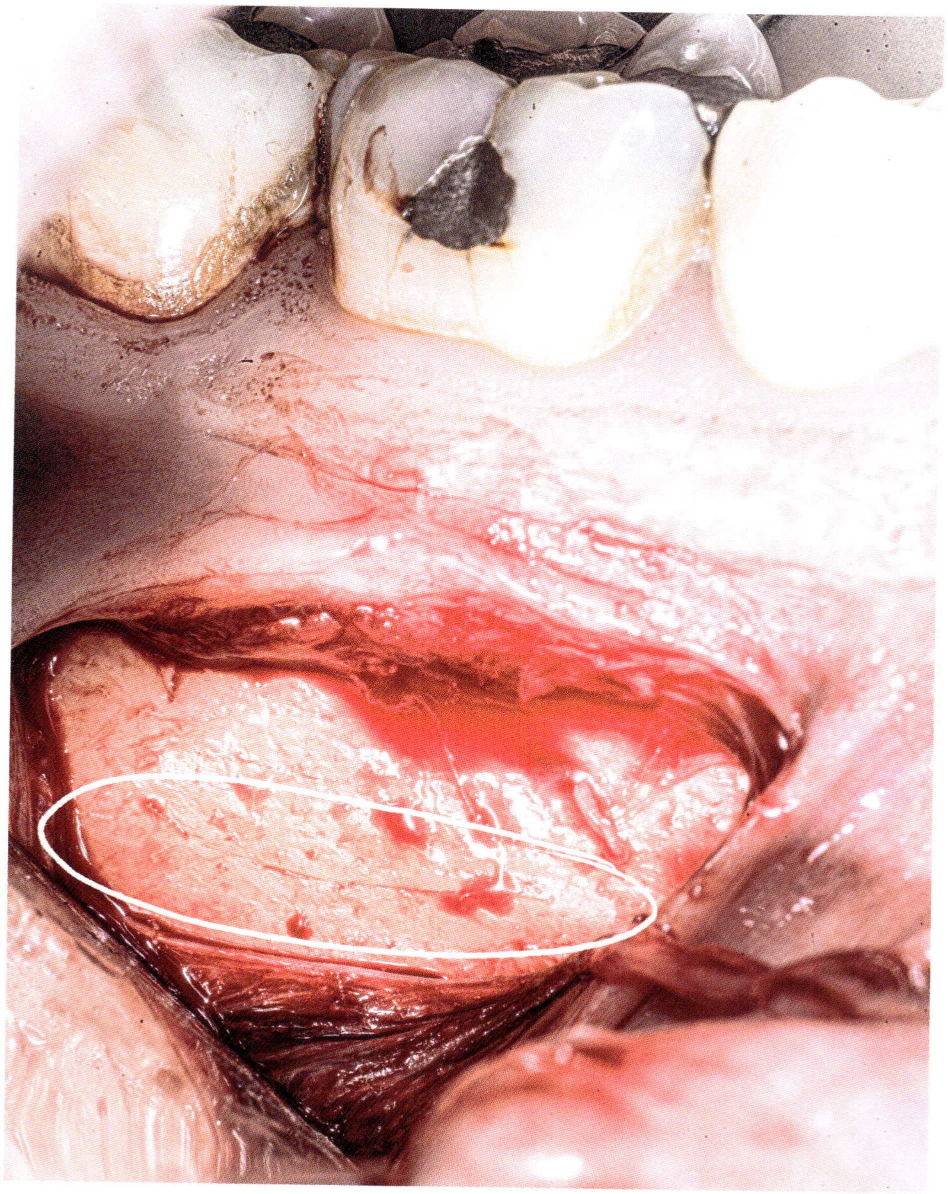

Figure 4-12 This flap was developed as access for an intraosseous biopsy. It shows the mark on the bone from the scalpel. Envision the blade cutting all the way to the surface of the bone to optimize the full thickness cut. This picture was taken after the flap was reflected. Note how the access can be developed above and below the initial incision. Also note how the periosteal access extends beyond the overlying mucosal access. Extending the periosteal incision after the initial dissection can significantly increase exposure without additional soft tissue trauma.

In trauma and orthognathic surgery, I always envision the site of the fracture or osteotomy and the hardware I plan to use before incising the skin or tissue. Dissecting through the layers one time is quicker and much better than fighting with inadequate access and having to extend the incision.

After making the incision, begin elevating the flap by turning the papilla out with a small tissue elevator. The papilla is denser and thicker, therefore it is often the easiest starting point. As the instrument passes along the incision, the flap is elevated. If it isn't reflecting easily, it may be helpful to cut it with the blade again. This helps avoid tearing the tissue. Always be kind to the tissue. Clean incisions and delicate tissue management are essential in the art of oral surgery.

Flaps often need to be sutured, typically with a single suture per papilla and at least one or two sutures at the release. Sometimes more are necessary. After sutures are placed, manipulate the tissue a bit and see how it moves. Make sure it will stay together after the patient leaves. Check your work. Now is your chance to make a difference by stabilizing the tissue well.

Vertical release tips:

- Avoid the esthetic zone. Place a distal release when possible.
- Avoid teeth with recession or thin facial bone. Avoid in thin biotype if possible.
- Extend the release beyond the mucogingival junction. This provides significantly more mobility and access.
- Reflect to the extent of the incision. Don't limit your access unnecessarily. Don't incise tissue if you won't reflect it.
- Two releases, both mesial and distal, can be made if greater access is needed or the flap needs to be mobilized and advanced.

Extraction

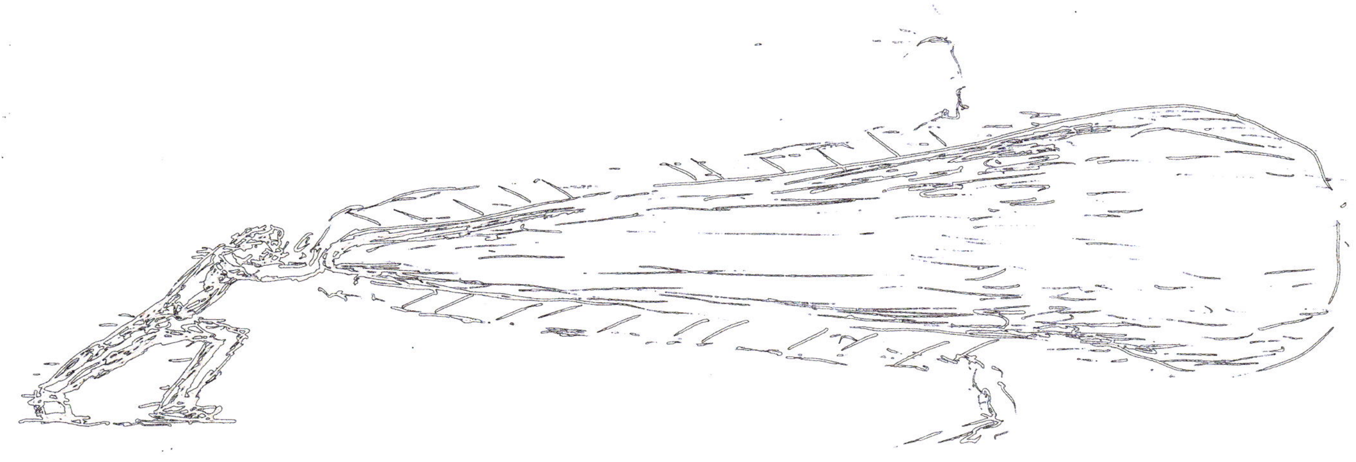

Figure 4-13 Sometimes you just need to figure out the best place to push. (Artwork inspired by Christopher Boffoli.)

Simple machines

Extraction instruments often have been described as simple machines: wedge, lever, and wheel and axle. (Contemporary Oral and Maxillofacial Surgery. Peterson et. al and other texts.) While these seem like clearly distinct principles and mechanics, I often find there isn't a distinct separation between them. They work well together and at the same time. There are many new variations and developments, but they generally all use the same principles.

Understanding these principles when visualizing the surgery helps direct the steps.

The purchase point itself seems to be a most critical piece in the puzzle. Either identifying or creating a safe purchase point maximizes success. The other mechanics all rely on this engagement of the tooth.

The purchase point

This is that immediate feature on a tooth that affords a desirable and intended force to be applied, most efficiently and effectively moving toward the desired end goal. More simply: The best spot to crank on the tooth. The engagement of an instrument on the tooth, or the friction point.

There may be many potential purchase points during an extraction. Pay attention to which one seems to be the best throughout the procedure. It changes. Identify the best purchase point by using an elevator (Micro Buser or small luxator) progressively in the most obvious, best positions first. If you get stuck with one purchase point, look for other potential options.

When you have no purchase point, consider establishing one or more with a handpiece in multiple different locations, such as mesiobuccal, distobuccal and mesiopalatal. Pick areas that are easy to see and that you can get an instrument into. This gives you multiple options to move between with different instruments, maximizing efficiency and minimizing the need to pick up the drill more. The more times you pick up the drill, the longer it takes.

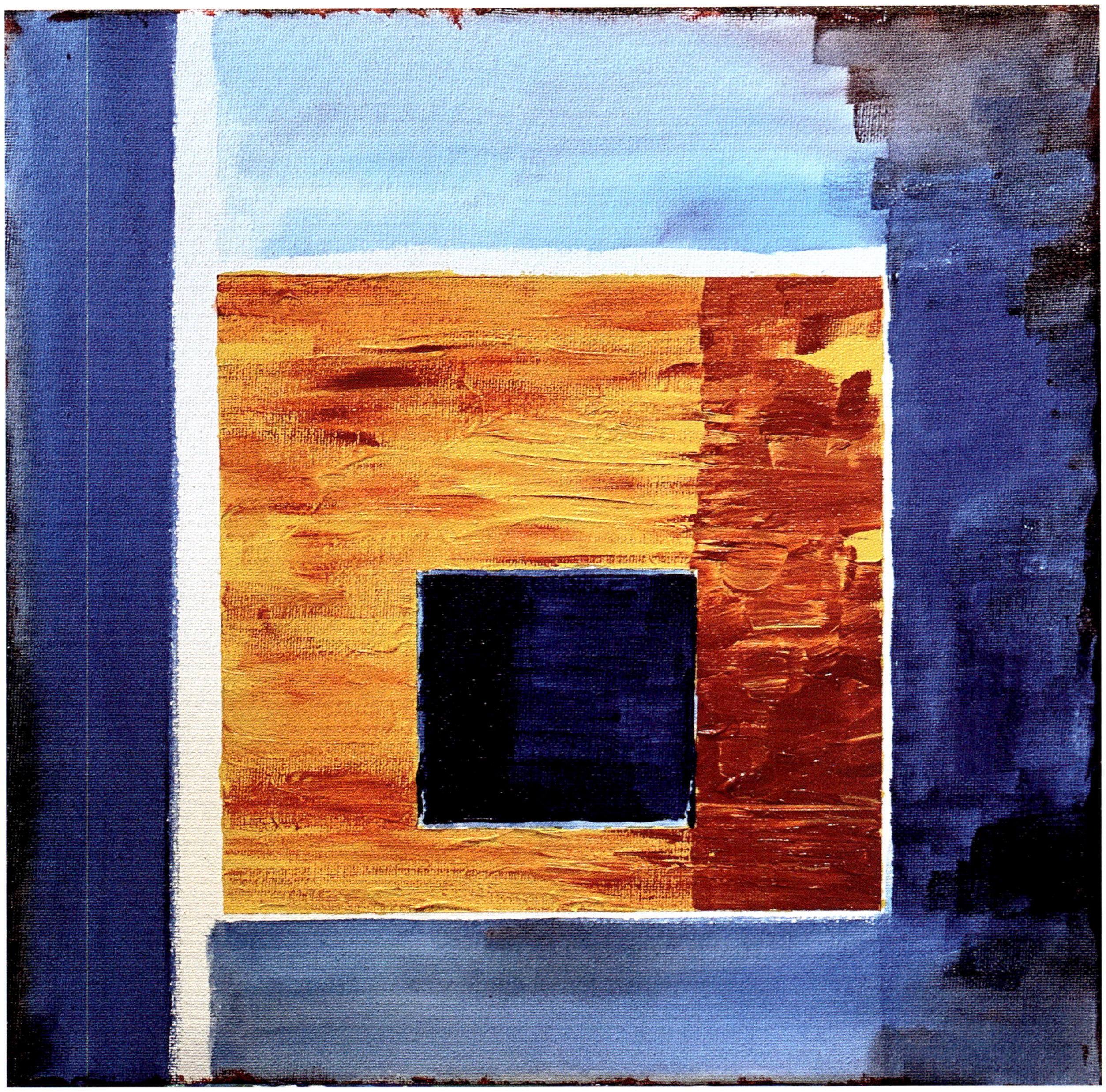

Figure 4-14 Work smarter, not harder. There is a fine line between faster and better. But they are not mutually exclusive. The line is more of a perimeter or a box containing varying shades and colors of faster and better. The art is in optimizing both within the box and then looking outside that box to continue to improve. Remember, there is always another box.

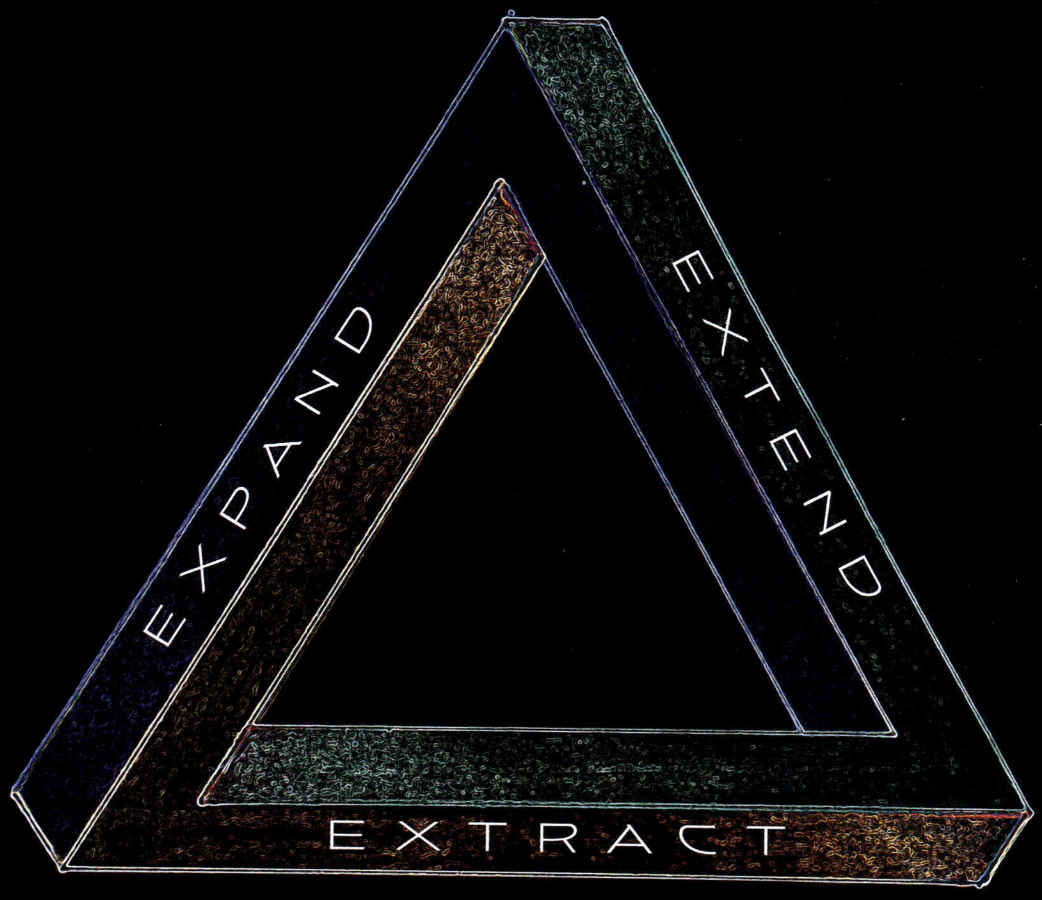

Figure 4-15 These all happen simultaneously. It is not a linear, stepwise process.

Extend. Expand. Extract.

Extend the ligament

The periodontal ligament is designed to sustain vertical and some horizontal forces during normal function. There is rarely any significant vertical force pulling on a tooth. Teeth are not naturally subjected to rotational forces either. That is why we use these types of forces to remove a tooth. The ligament is not designed to resist them nearly as well.

All forces applied to a tooth cause varying amounts of compression, tension and shear forces on the ligament. Increasing these forces ultimately ruptures the ligament. Work with the tooth. If it seems to be moving more in a mesial-distal direction, capitalize on that. I often find rotational forces to be my favorite. When I can achieve them, they seem to be kinder to the surrounding bone and more effective at straining more of the ligament at the same time. It feels more efficient and effective.

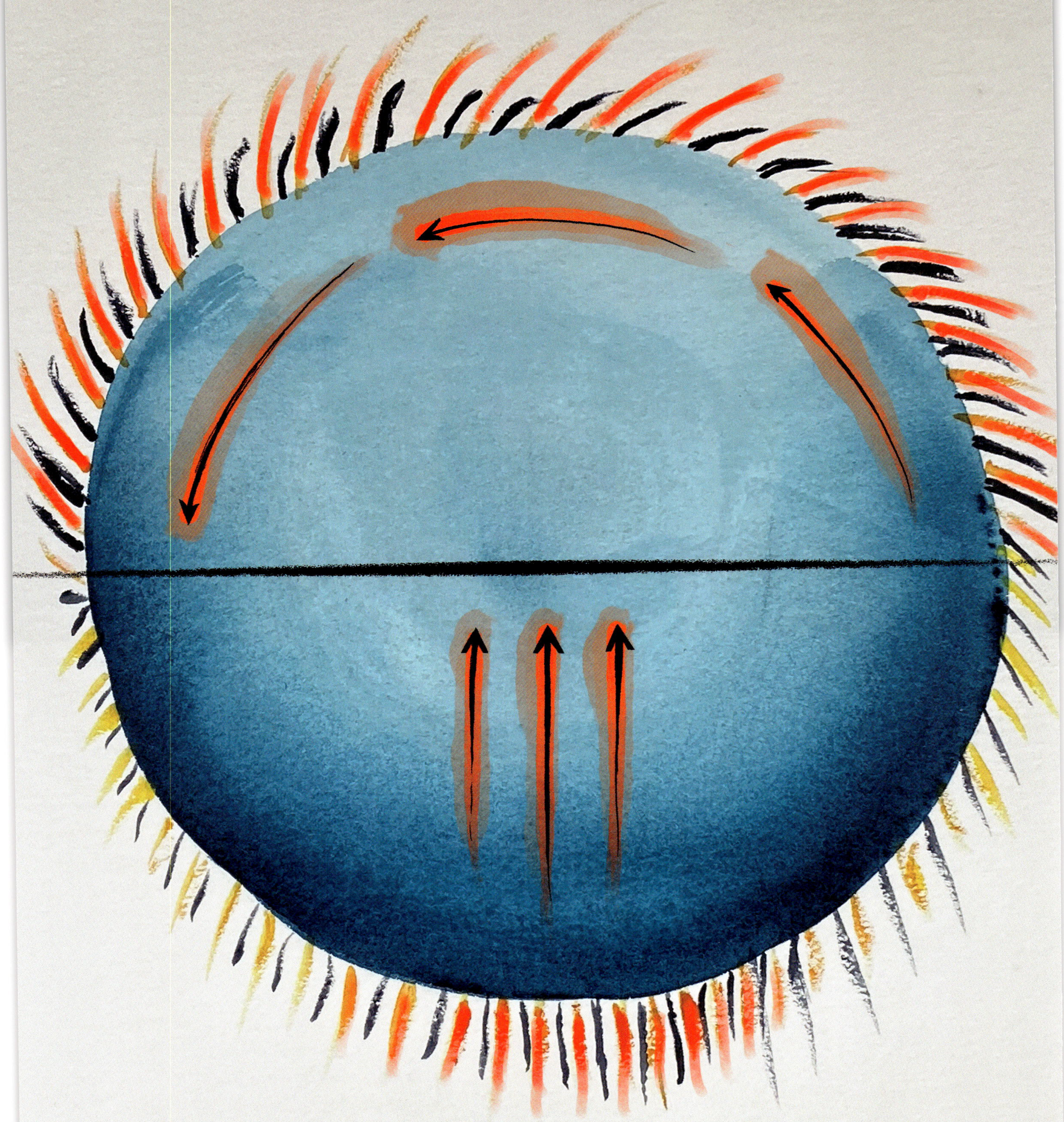

Figure 4-16 Straight lateral forces stretch some of the ligament (*bottom*). Rotational forces stretch the entirety of the ligament (*top*). The rotational forces are much more efficient at disrupting the ligament in an extraction.

The ultimate goal is to completely release the ligament. The crestal portion of the ligament can be partially severed with a sharp instrument prior to elevating on the tooth. Inserting a narrow blade, periotome, or small elevator circumferentially as deep as possible is a valuable step. This gains a lot of momentum in the extraction process.

The instrument is often inserted into the periodontal ligament space, actively incising portions of the ligament. It seems easiest to consider this in a two-dimensional model. In reality, it is a three-dimensional process with the vast majority of the forces being applied in tangential vectors, combining shearing, compressive and tensile forces.

Figure 4-17 Even with the cowhorn forceps, the motion is not purely buccal-lingual or pumping up and down. The figure eight motion is substantially more effective at disrupting the ligament, expanding the socket and extracting the tooth. I find this is true for almost every extraction.

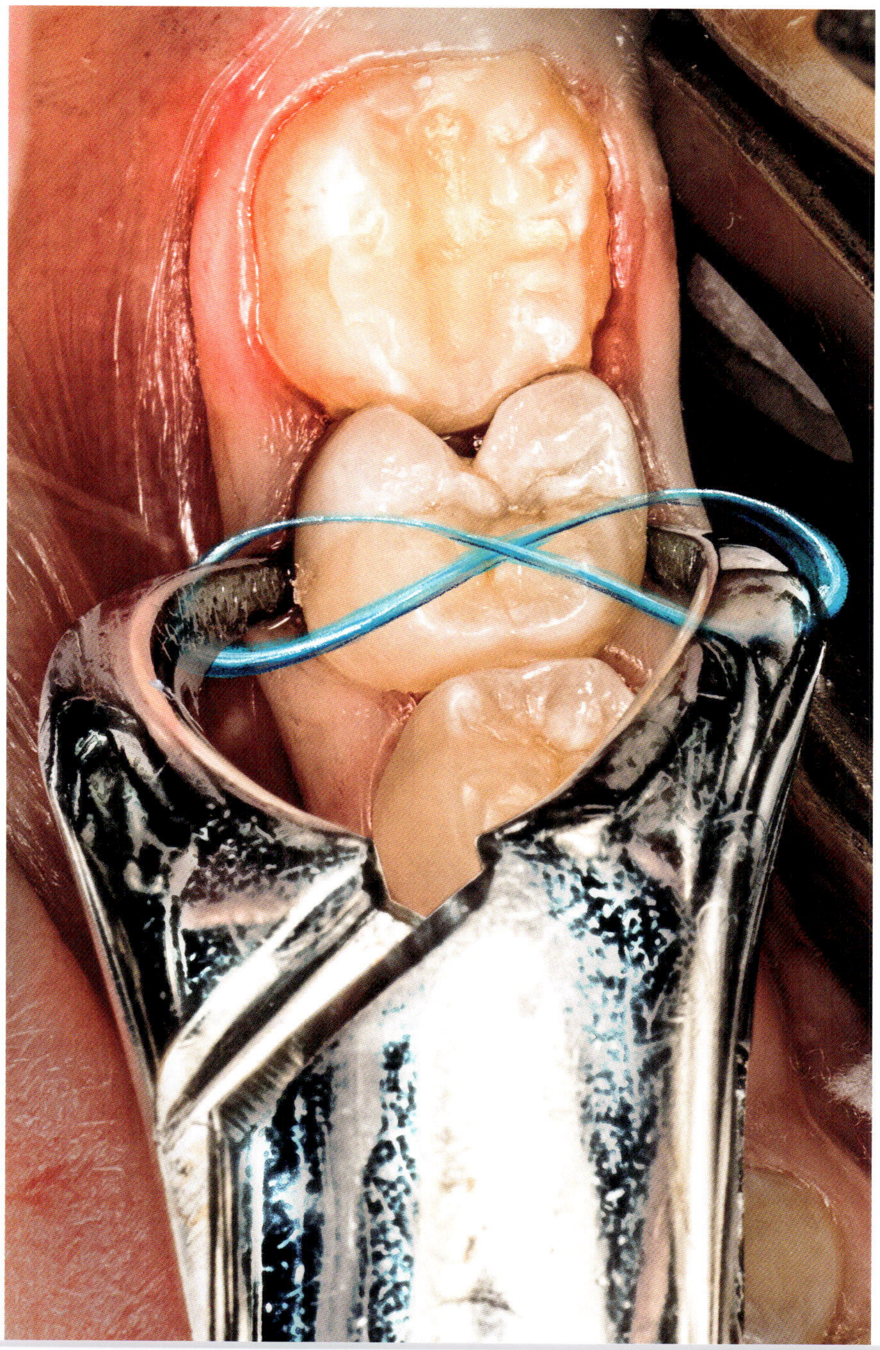

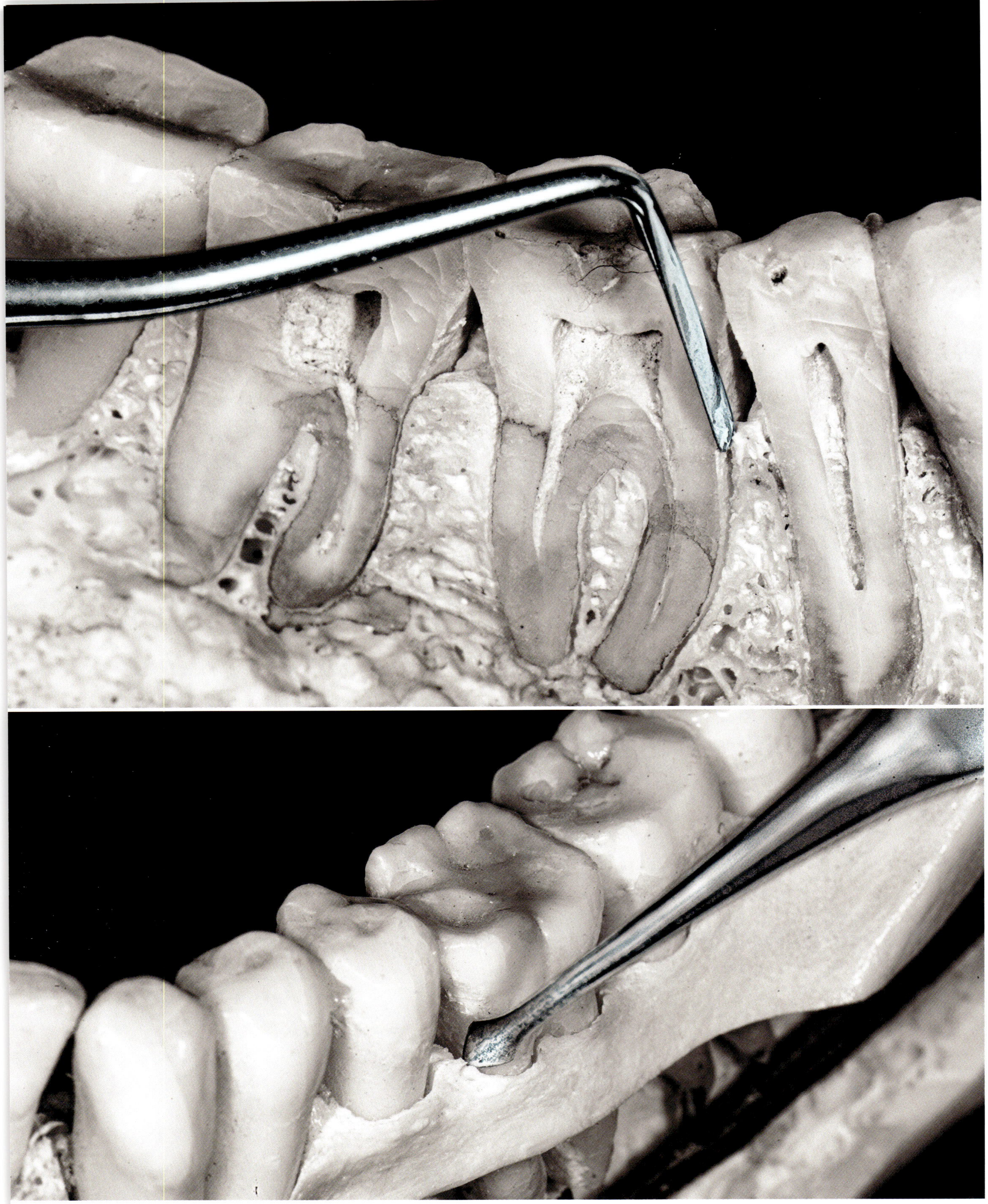

Figure 4-18 Periotome and Micro Buser can be used to extend and sever the periodontal ligament by advancing the tip of the instrument into the tight space between the tooth and bone.

Expand the socket

The socket itself naturally retains a tooth. Elevating a tooth causes microfractures of the surrounding bone as it presses outward. Progress is made as the socket is expanded with elevators or forceps. You can often feel the socket expanding, and you also can feel when it is not.

Extract the tooth

When all the retentive capacity is defeated, the tooth finally comes out. Sometimes this is achieved with an elevator popping the tooth out, but often forceps are needed. The forceps also expand the socket and extend the ligament.

Sectioning and Bone Removal

Before reaching for the handpiece, make sure you have a good sense of the tooth. Be patient. Give it some time. Explore ways to remove the tooth without cutting bone. If you have a reasonable purchase point or enough tooth structure to grasp with forceps, keep the pressure on for a while. It often just takes a few minutes. While this can feel like an eternity on a busy day, patience pays off.

Bone removal is a bit of a paradox. We want to save bone, but sometimes removing bone is the kindest way to remove the tooth and leave the site ready to heal. The wisdom is in being able to hold both as true, to find the balance between them in the moments of surgery. It is not either/or. It is both/and. Save bone and remove it.

When should you section a tooth or remove bone? When it will help achieve the best possible outcome for the patient. It should not be considered a last resort, only used when nothing else is working. The surgical handpiece is a wonderful instrument, useful in so many ways. It can create a better purchase point, create space to elevate, and separate divergent roots. It can preserve bone, protect adjacent anatomy, and expedite the procedure. But it must be respected as it can cause significant harm when used recklessly.

When sectioning a tooth or roots, it can be quite helpful to remove some bone to create space for the roots to elevate out. Sectioning and bone removal are often done simultaneously. There must be room for the instruments and remnants to move. Visualize the instruments you will use. Envision how and where you will use them. There must be enough space to insert the instruments, but not so much space that you compromise the leverage. If I am planning to use a spade next, I often remove minimal bone and make a narrow cut because the spade is quite narrow and pointed. If I plan to use a large luxator, on the other hand, I will remove more bone. You need adequate room to place the instrument tip deep enough and to activate and engage enough tooth structure to minimize fracturing the tooth and maximize the potential for the tooth to move. Knowing the relative size of the drill and instruments can help plan your cuts. It is helpful to know the length and width of the cutting flutes to avoid complications and effectively set up the site for the next instruments.

Consider cutting off the occlusal portion of the crown prior to sectioning a multirooted tooth. This creates space to luxate by cutting below the height of contour. It also improves visualization for root sectioning.

It's easier to remove a small fractured distal root than a mesial root. The distal root's view and angle are more favorable. Err on the side of sectioning more of the distal root in case a portion of it fractures unfavorably. You don't want to make it more difficult to remove the mesial root than it already is.

Troughing bone can be done more at the expense of the tooth than the expense of the bone. Kind of like a crown prep. Make sure you drill deep enough so you don't just fracture off more of the root structure. When drilling on tooth structure, remember your potential purchase points are being whittled away. Be aggressive enough to be efficient, but not so aggressive as to cause harm. Therein lies the balance. The finesse. The art of extraction.

Does crushed bone heal better than cut bone? It depends on the extent of the injury. The worse the injury, the worse the healing. When deciding whether to remove bone during an extraction, ask this question: *Will this heal better if I remove some bone or if I continue to elevate and expand the socket?* Sometimes getting some of the bone out of the way with a surgical handpiece creates a much better environment for healing than crushing the bone with an elevator

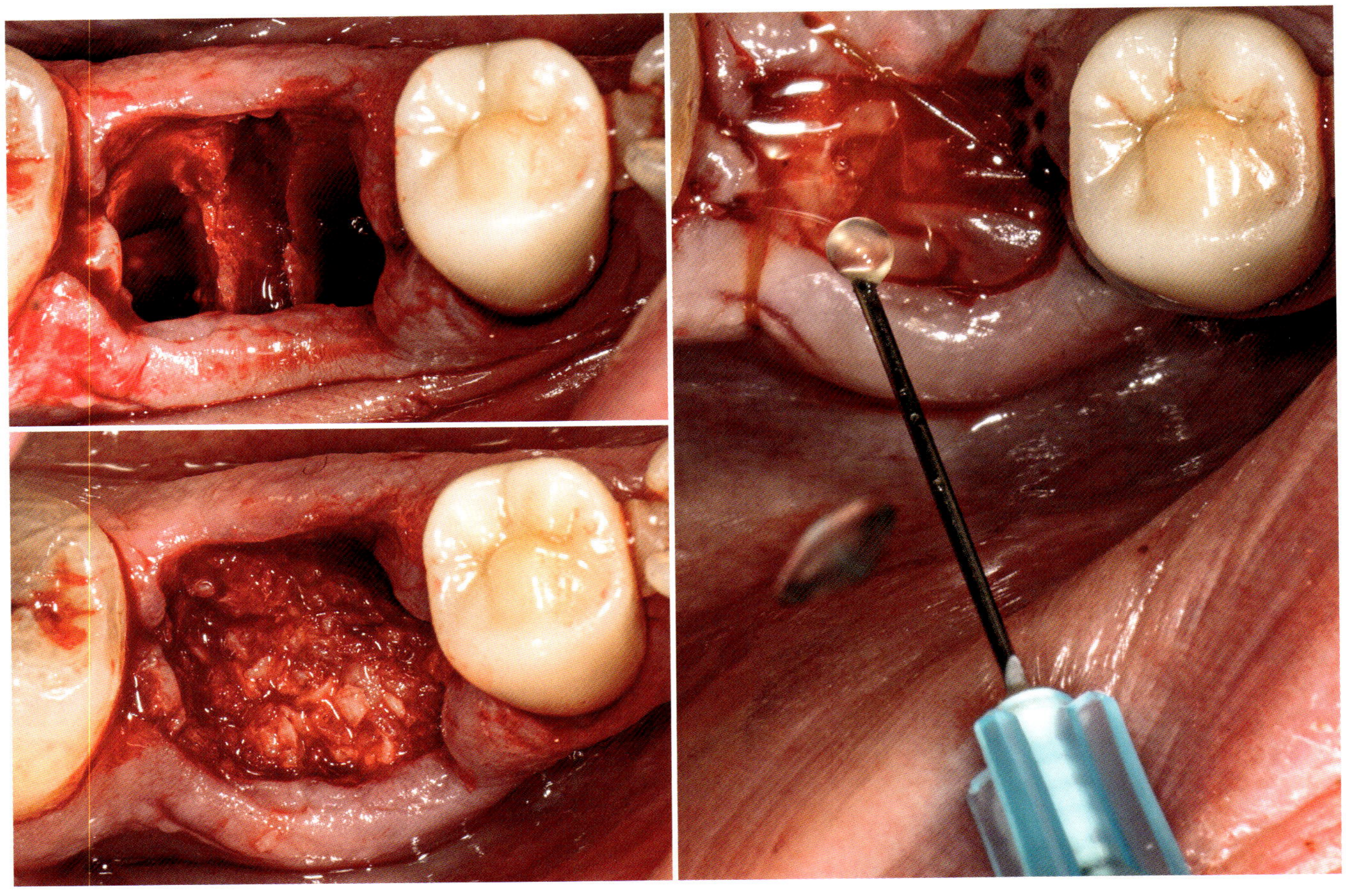

Figure 4-19 Sometimes drilling deeper can damage interradicular bone. In a case like this, the impact is likely nil. Ridge preservation was performed, covered with a PRF membrane, and retained with 4-0 chromic figure eight suture. The final step was to inject i-PRF within the graft site as well as apply it over the membrane (*right*). With good buccal and lingual bone, ridge preservation resulted in an excellent site for an implant after healing.

or fracturing the alveolus. Healing is dependent on the extent of the injury.

Elevators can disrupt a significant amount of bone. By design, their force is generated as a lever through a fulcrum. The fulcrum is either bone or an adjacent tooth. Removing some bone with a drill may ultimately cause less trauma to the bone.

It is important to protect the buccal plate of bone. But sometimes it is helpful to remove some bone on the mesiobuccal or distobuccal to create a purchase point. A small vertical buccal plate defect created with a well irrigated bur will heal better than a fractured buccal plate or troughing completely around a root. The osteoblasts from the adjacent bone can easily fill in a narrow gap. But if the entire plate is fractured, its blood supply and structural integrity are compromised, as is the healing potential. There is a lot more work to do in the proliferation and maturation phases of healing.

It can be frustrating to fracture off a crown, but sometimes it is helpful because it opens up the space to work. You have different angles to see what remains of the roots. There may be a different purchase point you can use to elevate the tooth that didn't exist before it fractured. Look for the opportunities to turn frustration into fascination.

Nuances of Exodontia

Extractions happen step by step. Sometimes the steps run together. Sometimes it feels more like a sidestep. And sometimes steps can be skipped. Here are some specific sidesteps to consider when removing teeth.

Retaining root fragments

Chasing a small fragment of a posterior maxillary root may sometimes displace it into the maxillary sinus—and that changes everything. If you cannot immediately retrieve the piece from the sinus, further dissection and exploration may be necessary. It is better to remove the tooth in its entirety than to retain a portion as a future liability—and better yet do it without the complication of a displaced root tip. There is no perfect formula for this. The tooth structure, size, condition and the patient's overall comorbidities and anatomy all play a part in the decision. Plan A is usually to remove the tooth entirely. In these situations, I need to convince myself it is better to retain the piece than to keep trying to remove it. Herein lies the art of oral surgery. It is an art form in and of itself.

Retaining a root fragment is an intraoperative decision (sometimes unknowingly) to retain a small portion of the root when it seems that further attempt to surgically remove the remaining piece will cause more harm than good. This is different in some ways from a coronectomy, which is a planned crown removal and retention of a portion of the root to decrease the chance of harming the inferior alveolar nerve. In comparison, the decision to retain a root tip is made when further surgical trauma will likely increase the risk of sinus perforation, damage to adjacent teeth, or damage to the inferior alveolar nerve.

Sometimes, there is no distinguishable periodontal ligament, making it impossible to detect where the tooth stops and the bone begins. It all looks the same. If the piece is less than 5 mm, it may be safer to retain it. A piece that small will likely become encased in vital bone with good blood supply and a low chance of infection[4].

When a root tip is knowingly retained, discuss it with the patient. Patients seem to be quite receptive and appreciative when they know why you decided to leave some of the tooth behind. Typically, a small piece less than three millimeters doesn't even need antibiotics.

As always, documentation is quite important. I usually document it something like this:

"A small portion of the palatal root fractured during elevation and was retained after an attempt to retrieve due to increased risk for sinus complications. Discussed with the patient and informed of potential complications. Patient indicated understanding. Questions were sought and answered."

Figure 4-20 This root tip fractured and came out with the mesial root after sectioning and splitting the tooth. If retained, a piece this size would have a high likelihood of revascularizing and healing without complications.

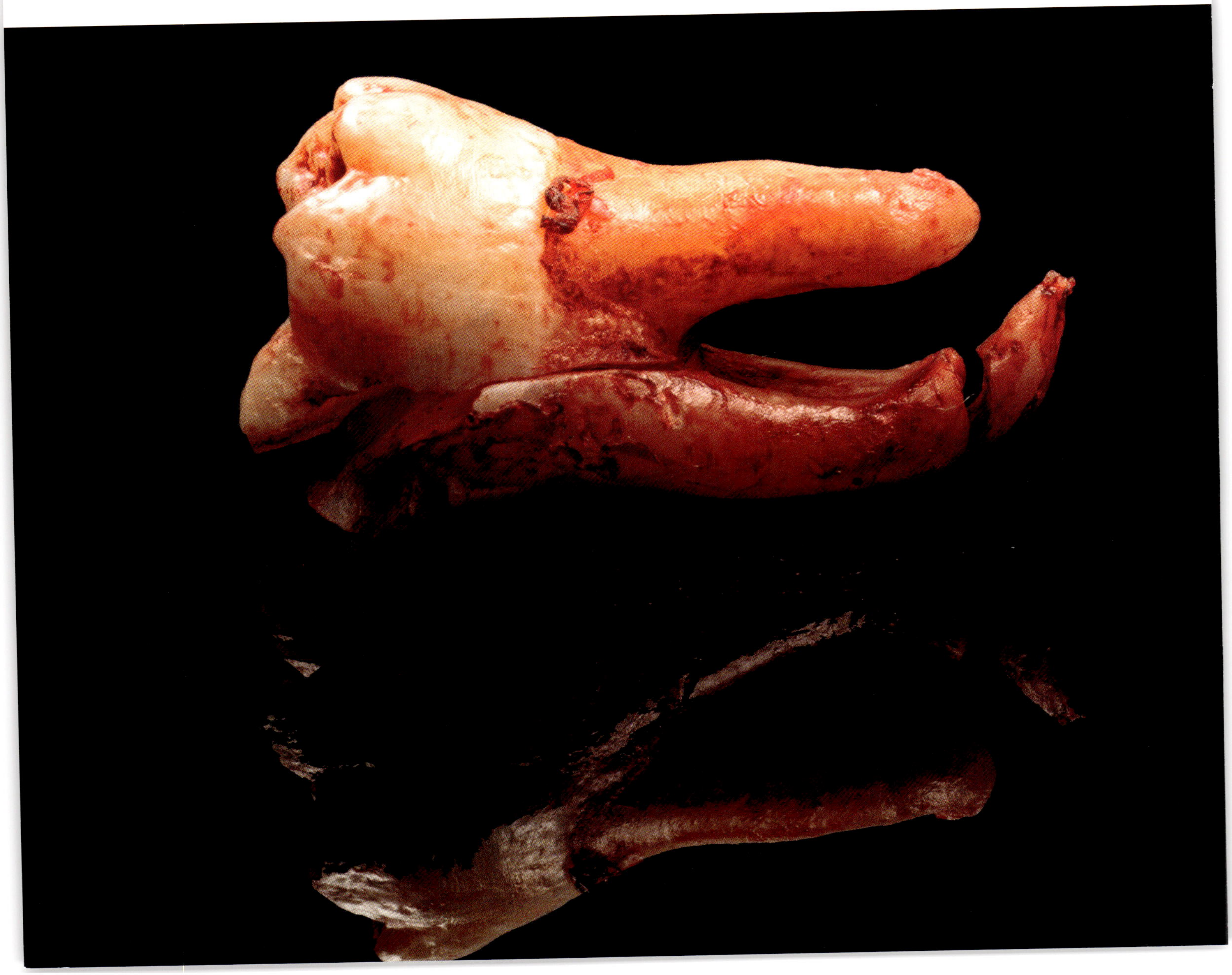

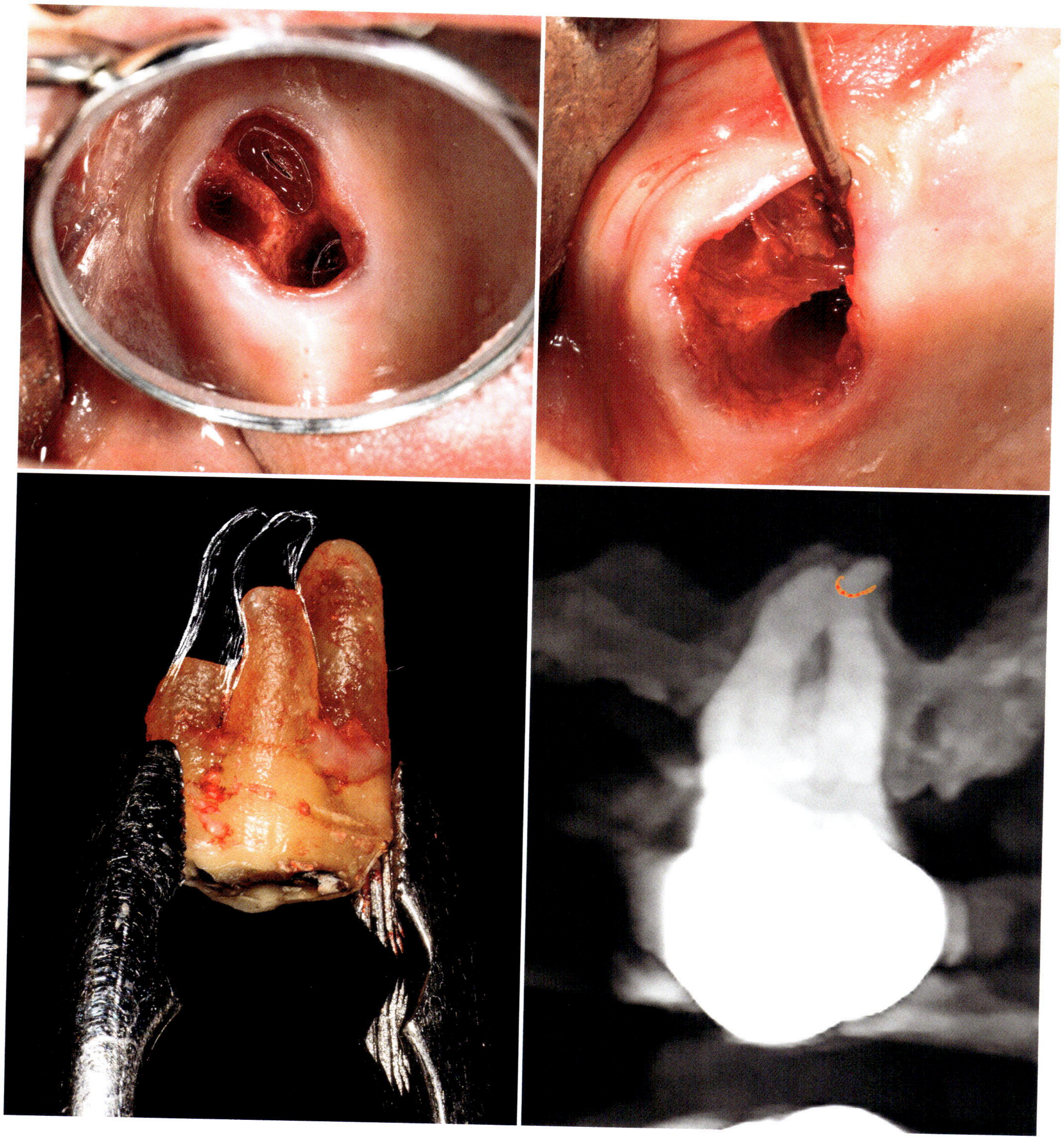

Figure 4-21 Two of the long, curved roots of this upper molar fractured. They were elevated out with a Micro Buser without sinus perforation. It is helpful to inspect the removed tooth as it can be difficult to see the retained roots in the socket (*upper left*). If the fractured tips were much smaller or I had trouble removing the roots, I would consider retaining a piece. But these pieces are too large in my opinion to retain without just cause. If it were small, like the tip outlined in the lower right picture, I would be a bit more likely to retain it if it didn't come out easily.

"I can speed up if you'd like." I sometimes say this jokingly when a patient seems to be getting impatient. I have not yet had a patient take me up on my offer. Afterall, impatience is just an argument with the reality that it takes time to do a job well.

Elevating against adjacent teeth

Adjacent teeth can be a great fulcrum for elevating. But they can also come with a significant cost. Collateral damage can occur in the form of inflammation in the adjacent tooth's periodontal ligament, dislodged crowns or fillings, or even fracture of a healthy tooth. The calculated risk of potential damage to adjacent teeth or structures is part of proper informed consent because it is a known risk, even in the most ardent and skillful hands. But a crown on an endodontically treated neighboring tooth would not be a good fulcrum for elevating between the teeth. Also watch out for Class V restorations as these have little retention and are prone to dislodging even with subtle crown flexion. The elevator doesn't even need to touch the restoration for it to pop off.

When the adjacent tooth is the fulcrum, be aware you are potentially compromising a good thing. But when another part of the tooth being extracted can be the fulcrum, it is like double dipping. This happens when a multirooted tooth is sectioned and you can elevate between the roots. Both the lever arm and the fulcrum need to be mobilized. They are both being elevated or luxated at some capacity. This is much safer than elevating against an adjacent tooth.

It can be helpful to drill away some bone between teeth when performing multiple adjacent extractions. This improves the elevator's fulcrum and purchase point. When bone reduction is planned, like for implant supported hybrid dentures, that bone may need to be removed anyway. You may be able to speed up your surgery with no significant consequences by drilling between the teeth before elevating.

Protecting soft tissue

It takes time to carefully manage soft tissue. Reflecting the papilla or a flap without tearing it may add considerable time to a procedure that was planned to take only a few minutes. But suturing a torn flap takes longer. An extra little bit of time and attention at the outset will ultimately save time and improve healing. Consistently putting in the time on the front end pays in predictability and patient satisfaction.

Elevators can become dangerous when they slip or if the tooth fractures. Sometimes they have a lot of force behind them. The grip and the stop can help minimize slippage. The gauze and the tongue retractor can protect the tissue in case of slippage. Gripping the elevator closer to the tip with an extended finger stop can catch the instrument if its footing breaks free. It will still move, but the finger can keep it from impaling the tongue or palate. A tongue retractor and pharyngeal curtain can protect the underlying tissue from accidental assault like a backstop.

Removing more bone

The periodontal ligament is responsible for retaining teeth in the alveolus. Therefore, obliterating the bone that anchors the ligament ensures swift delivery of the tooth. This can be accomplished by rotary or hand instrumentation. Drilling out all the bone around a root may make the extraction easier and quicker, but not likely better. Similarly, applying uncontrolled forces with an elevator or forceps can significantly compromise the alveolar bone's integrity, though it may hasten the procedure. It all must be balanced.

In my earliest extraction training in dental school, the advice handed down to me was to use forceps in a straight buccal-lingual motion only. The tooth would "roll over" the buccal bone and voila! It would come out. It doesn't so much "roll over" as steam-roll through the buccal plate with this technique. The buccal plate still may be attached to the periosteum and thus seem to be intact, but the strict buccal-lingual motion seems to have serious limitations. Consider adding a rotational component to the movement. A figure eight motion with the forceps works very well in my hands. It strains the ligament more without expanding the socket as much.

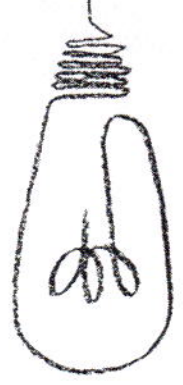

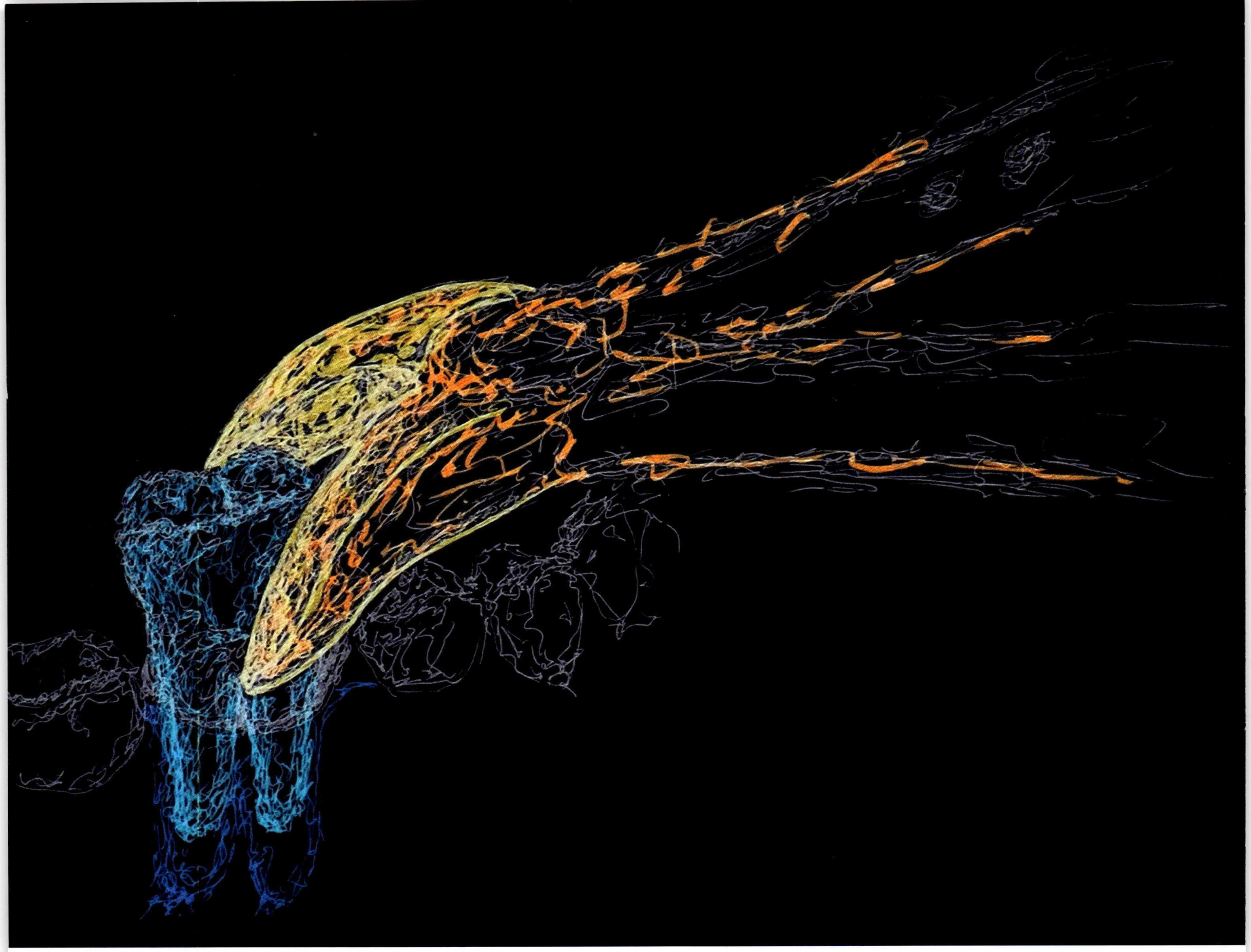

Figure 4-22

The cowhorn

Cowhorn forceps (#23 forceps) are a good example of an instrument that can make things faster but not always better. They can quickly deliver a lower molar by pumping them up and down while maintaining high compression in the furcation. The tooth often elevates vertically and comes right out. The furcation bone, however, may pay a hefty price for that quick and easy extraction. Worth it? Sometimes, maybe, but not always. In addition to potentially compromising the furcation bone, the horns also can fracture the tooth in a most unfavorable way: a clean, horizontal break just below a dense alveolar crest. Any chance of elevating the tooth for a simple extraction may be gone. However, with the crown out of the way, it may be easier to see where to section between the roots.

The horns are designed to function like a wedge and an inclined plane. As the converging beaks are forced together, they press along the cervical portion of the crown and into the furcation. As the tips move further into the furcation (seating), they amplify the force of the lever arms (handles) and drive the tooth outward. Sometimes, the tooth seems to just pump right out of the socket, much to the satisfaction of both the patient and the surgeon. When the bone and ligament are primed for the picking, the cowhorn forceps can quickly, effectively and easily remove a lower molar with minimal trauma.

The tooth and forceps provide helpful predictors that can easily go unnoticed if you aren't paying attention. Tactile feedback from the instrument tells the operator if the horns are seating into a furcation or deflecting interproximal. Are the horns seating deeper in the middle of the furcation, or slipping mesial or distal? If they deflect, they can harm adjacent teeth, easily dislodging neighboring restorations or teeth. If they don't seem to be seating deeper or the tooth is not moving at all, those pointy horns may just be squeezing the crown, ready to fracture it.

When the horns seat into the furcation, the classic "water pump" action can be used to extract the tooth. Pumping up and down on the handles of the forceps under compression can literally pump the

Figure 4-23 Pumping the forceps wedges the beaks into the furcation, forcing the tooth out of the socket.

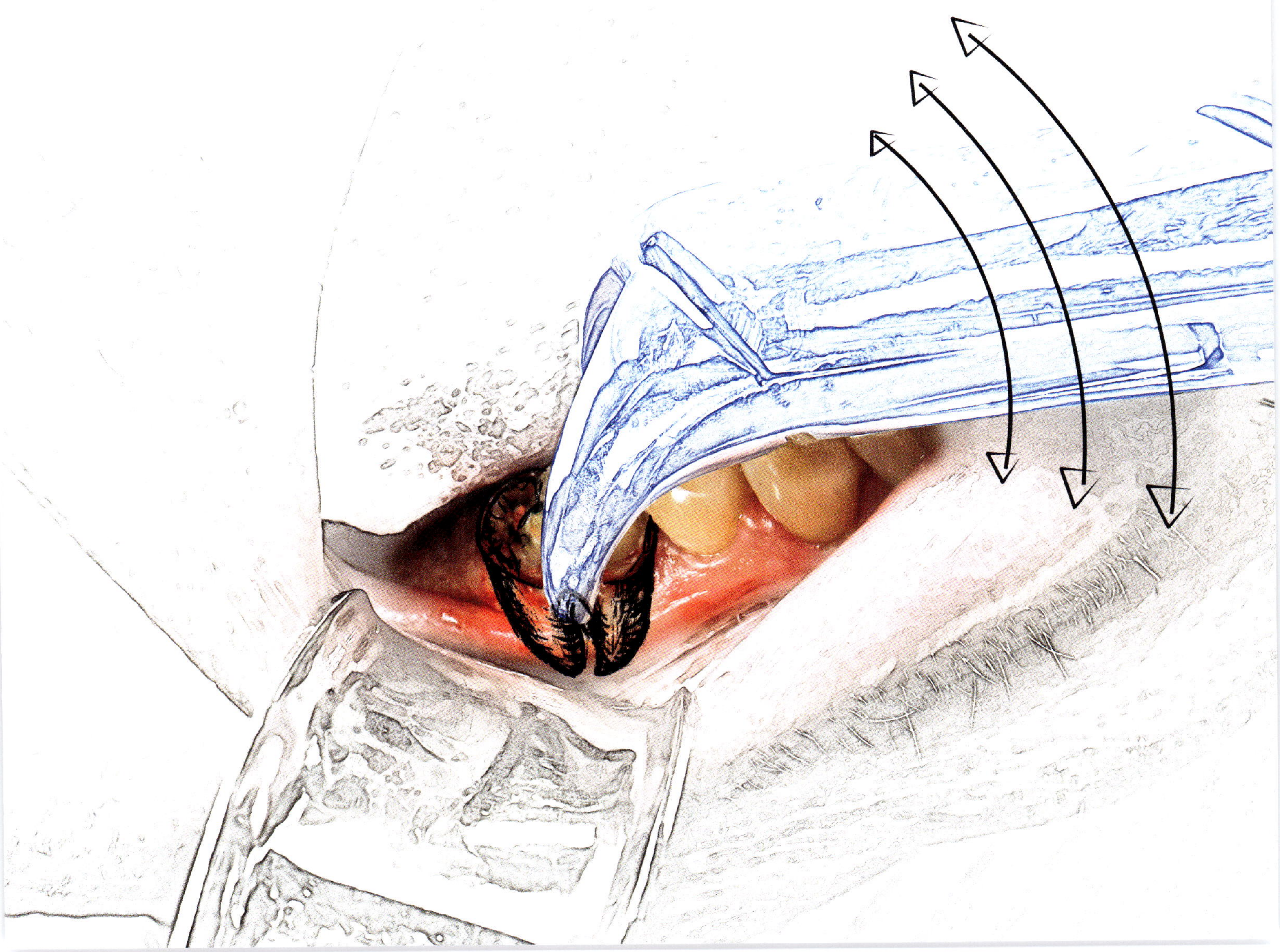

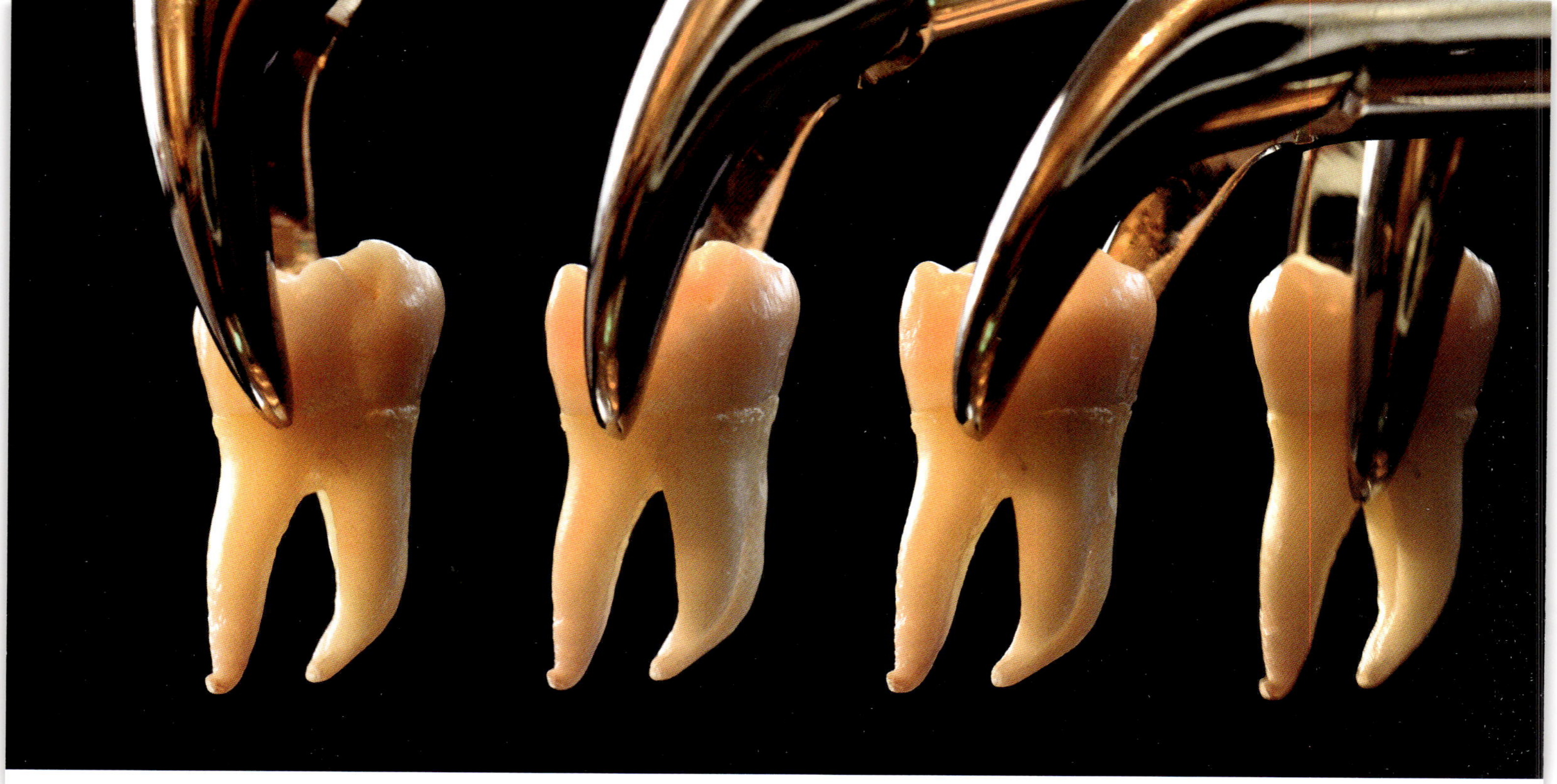

Figure 4-24 The pumping action seats the beaks into the furcation.

tooth right out of the socket. If this steady, firm action seats the forceps and the tooth still shows no signs of movement, that may indicate the tooth isn't interested in cooperating with this plan. How much force can be applied safely in this situation? Just a little less than it takes to snap off the crown. The beaks also can damage the bone in the furcation. This traumatized bone may heal poorly, with bone fragments working their way out over time. It also may be detrimental if an implant is planned in the site.

When the forceps seat and the tooth seems willing to cooperate, the simple vertical pumping can be transitioned into a circular or figure eight pattern. The ligament maintaining the tooth is circumferential and inherently functions to resist forces in all directions. Extraction forces need to overcome the retention forces in all dimensions. Pure buccal-lingual forces with this instrument leave a lot on the table in the negotiation with the tooth.

There is a distinct "unknown" in using these forceps. They have tremendous potential to simplify and expedite the extraction process. They have equally impressive capacity to complicate the extraction by fracturing the crown. I can only imagine how loud and startling this is for an anxious patient. It can be quite loud and piercing for the rest of us.

The patient's sympathetic nervous system, already on edge trying to protect its precious human, gets an enormous boost. Almost as if it screams, *"See, I was right! This isn't safe. I can't protect you if you keep sitting here with your mouth dangling wide open like this. GET OUT!"* it shouts as the epinephrine and norepinephrine are being dumped into the bloodstream. *"Those sound effects are pretty impressive and totally normal."* I often say, attempting to ease the blow to the autonomic nervous system.

When the crown fractures off with the cowhorn, the instrument falls on the wrong side of the balance sheet. A tooth that had a crown and multiple potential purchase points can get decapitated below the collar, leaving nothing but dense surrounding alveolar bone and a flat, subcrestal plane of cementum and dentin. Now there is little to get a hold of. A potential next step in this case would be to create a purchase point between the two roots by drilling through the furcation. A straight or angled elevator rotated in the newly formed slot will finish separating the roots and expand the socket if the bone isn't too dense. This will also strain the periodontal ligament and loosen the roots. Working back and forth between the mesial and distal roots with the elevator optimizes this purchase point. At times, this is adequate to mobilize both roots and deliver them individually. Other times, this only removes one of the roots or neither of the roots and further sectioning or bone removal is required.

Sometimes a root continues to fracture more and more. What seems like adequate bone removal and sectioning results yet again in a smaller stub of tooth clinging for dear life to the bone. This scenario may benefit from a circumferential trough. Consider cutting bone and periodontal ligament around the entire perimeter of the remaining tooth structure, or at least as much as is accessible with the handpiece. This requires adequate access and visualization. If you can't see where you are going, you don't know where you will end up. The often-faint line of the periodontal ligament may serve to guide the drill. Follow the line. This will remove some tooth structure and some bone. Consider using a small elevator or luxator. Clearly, the tooth wants to break as it has done multiple times already. If the tooth doesn't start moving with a little force, it is likely to break with more force. Use as much finesse as possible to work with the tooth. Losing more tooth structure now creates even more of a challenge.

When the tooth isn't cooperating, consider taking a little break and a periapical radiograph. This may shed light on a new angle or potential purchase point. Every once in a while, I find I am chasing bone, not root fragments. Sometimes, the tooth structure has been removed completely and what looks like tooth structure is the dense bone of the lamina dura.

The Socket

When the tooth is finally out, the work is not necessarily done. The socket and tissue should be inspected. Look and feel for residual fragments. Even if the tooth came out in one piece, it may be helpful to flush the site with sterile saline and get a small suction all the way to the socket's apex. Debris can be anywhere. Look for fragments of bone, pieces of soft tissue, or even calculus and fractured tooth segments. The debris may be loose within the socket, stuck to the socket walls or attached to the gingiva right around the site. Consistently removing this debris will reduce post-operative visits and improve patient outcomes. And it is quick to do. I have been surprised many times to find an accessory root or a fragment of cementum remaining after what I thought was a straightforward extraction.

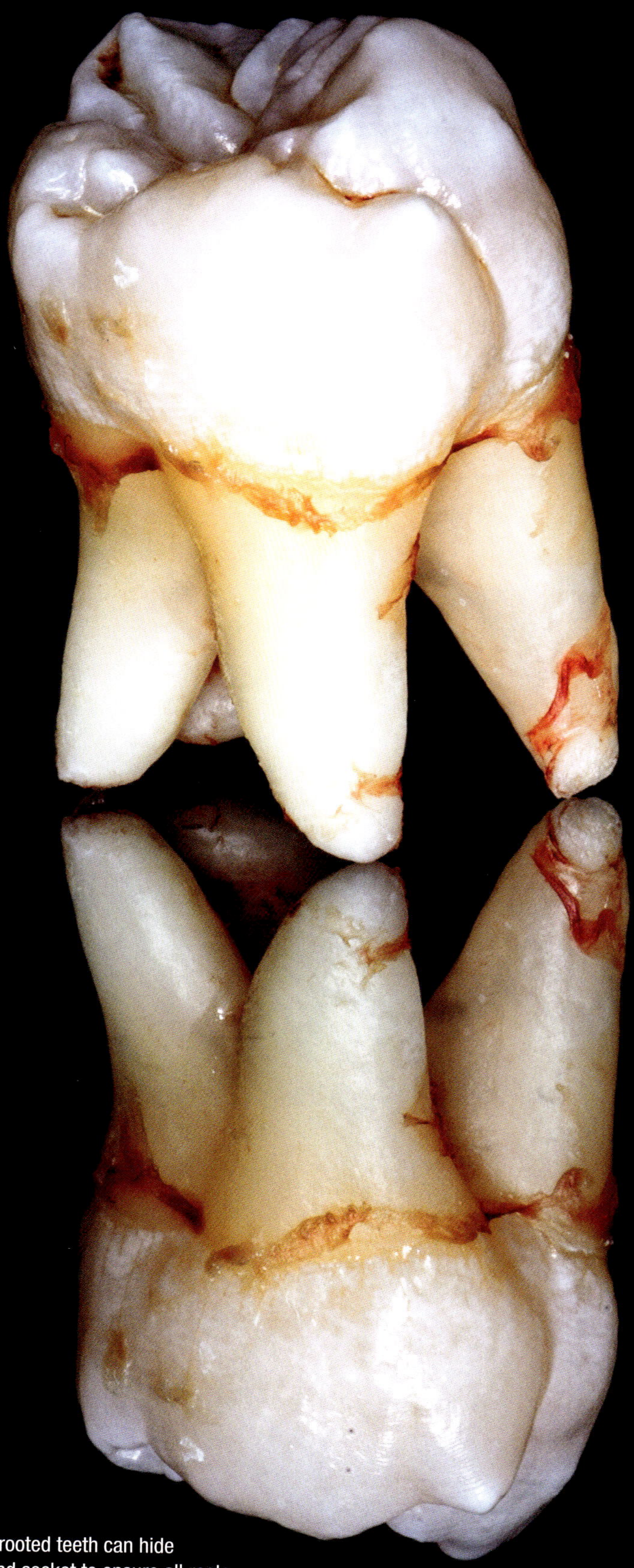

Figure 4-25 The socket of multi-rooted teeth can hide fractured roots. Inspect the tooth and socket to ensure all roots were entirely removed.

The inspection may also reveal bone fragments in the socket walls. Stable bone fragments provide a framework for osseous healing, whereas unstable fragments are a nidus for infection and complications. The line between them can be fuzzy.

It is obvious when a fragment is grossly mobile. It likes to flop around in the socket, chasing the suction. Those need to be removed. At times, the fragments are relatively stable. They could be moved with a curette, but they don't seem like they will freely move within the socket. Depending on the situation, these may be retained.

There are three questions that can guide whether to remove a bone fragment within an extraction site:

1. Will the stability promote bone formation? If not, the fragment becomes a foreign body, and the site will work to either expel the piece or take the time to break it down and resorb it. Neither of these is remotely as efficient nor easy as surgical removal. If the bone doesn't seem like it will move on its own, the healing process is likely to incorporate the bone and benefit from its presence.
2. Will the blood supply be adequate? When a fragment of bone is attached to periosteum, it has a much higher likelihood of healing well than when it is detached.
3. Will retaining the fragment improve the outcome? Consider if you need more bone in the site.

Apical pathology

The body tries to protect itself from the bacterial assault that ensues when a tooth becomes necrotic. An elaborate immune response fights the bacteria, and a defense system is set up to wall off or contain it. We have several names for this: apical pathology, periapical lesions, apical periodontitis, apical cysts, granulomas, or granulation tissue. Whatever we call it, we are taught to remove the apical pathology when removing the tooth. This seems logical. If it is pathologic, it should probably be removed.

I wonder if this axiom will change in the future. If the apical tissue is the host's own defense system, might there be some intrinsic healing potential we eliminate by removing it? Endodontic treatment is often quite successful without mechanically debriding this apical tissue. I don't want to undermine the importance and value of removing apical pathology. I don't like to leave pathology behind and routinely curette or debride this pathologic tissue in my own practice. I just hope to get you thinking outside the box.

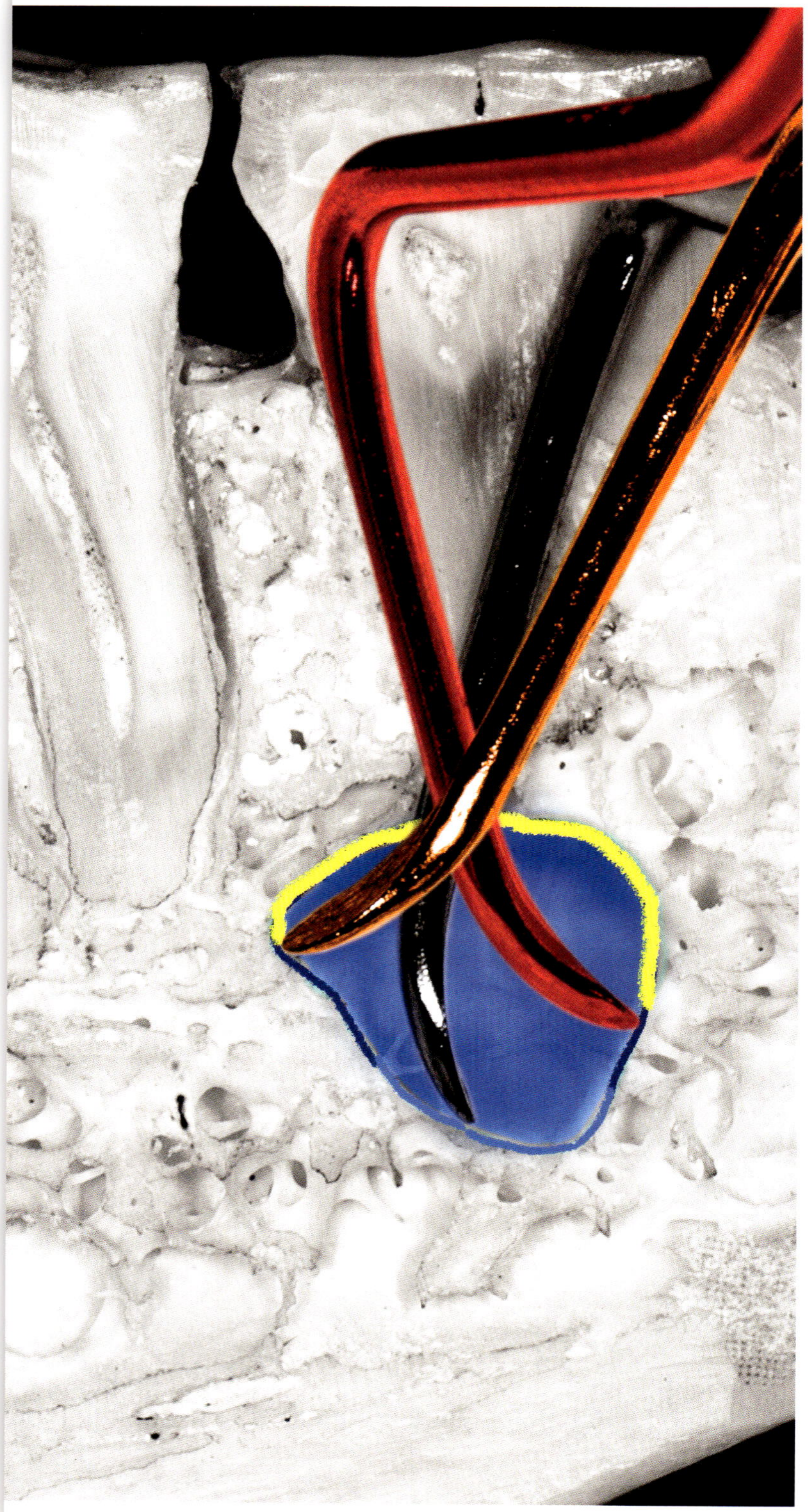

Figure 4-26 The undercuts can make it very tricky to completely remove the pathology (*yellow line*). (Artwork inspired by Andy Warhol.)

When performing ridge preservation, pay close attention to the apical tissue. If there is a cyst, this is the body's attempt to wall off and keep the bacterial invasion out. It must be completely removed for the body to best incorporate the graft material. When ridge preservation is not being performed, it may be counterproductive to thoroughly curette the apical socket. The cells in that area have been recruited to protect and heal the site from the infection. As long as the toxic debris is out, some remaining tissue may be beneficial.

Curetting pathology from the socket is more critical for ridge preservation or implant placement than for routine extraction. Epithelial remnants of a cyst can infiltrate the graft or implant surface where we need bone. Any remaining bacteria can contaminate the graft or implant surface. Depending on the anatomy, it can be quite tricky to completely remove an apical cyst or granuloma. They can be tenacious and difficult to access. But it is nonetheless important to try to completely remove the pathology to optimize success.

Removing apical pathology is a bit like peeling off a sticker. Sometimes it's quick, clean and easy; sometimes it's not. It may lift right off the bone and shell out, sometimes even remaining attached to the tooth. But sometimes it is like the sticker that rips and tears every time you get an edge lifted. It is like they applied the sticker with Gorilla Glue instead of Post-it Note adhesive. Generally speaking, the periradicular cyst will shell out more easily because it has an epithelial lining. The periradicular granuloma does not have the same peripheral barrier and it has a more infiltrative relationship with the surrounding bone. It is much more friable and tenacious. Either way, similar principles apply to removing an apical lesion as removing a sticker. Find

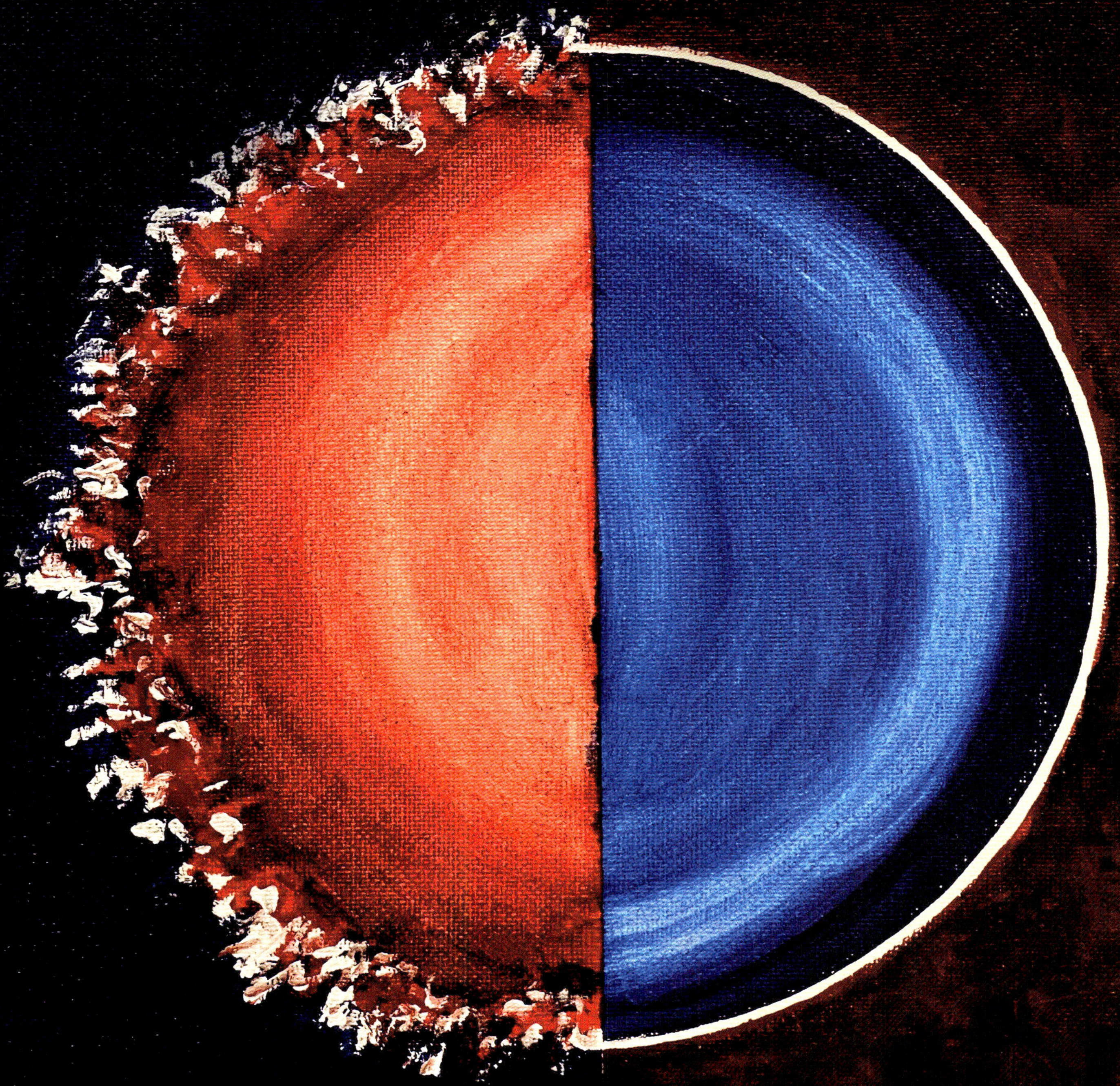

Figure 4-27 Apical pathology can have an irregular, infiltrative margin, like an apical granuloma (*left*), or a clean, cystic lining, like an apical cyst (*right*). The cyst tends to shell out easily while the granuloma can be more tenacious and difficult to completely remove. (Artwork inspired by Hilma af Klint.)

an edge or corner to start at. Peel it back slowly. If it begins to tear, try to get under that area to keep the tear from progressing or work around it from a different angle to get under it. It is easiest when it remains intact. Small remaining fragments can be difficult to remove.

When curetting apical pathology, look or feel for the free edge toward the coronal margin first. Find the easiest spot to access with the angled curette curving outward, toward the socket wall. Engage the wall and begin to peel the tissue off the bone. Work around the lesion, maintaining contact with the bone. If it is just tearing, consider starting in another spot. The curette works best with an acute angle on the bone, keeping the leading edge between the soft tissue and the bone. Similar to a sticker, it is easier to work with a broad edge. Go with the easiest spot. If the lesion doesn't shell out in a single piece, remove the loose portions to improve visualization.

Figure 4-28 Apical pathology sometimes comes out with the tooth. The site still needs to be examined and curetted. Note the area of disruption on the cyst's surface. This left some remnants in the site that needed to be removed.

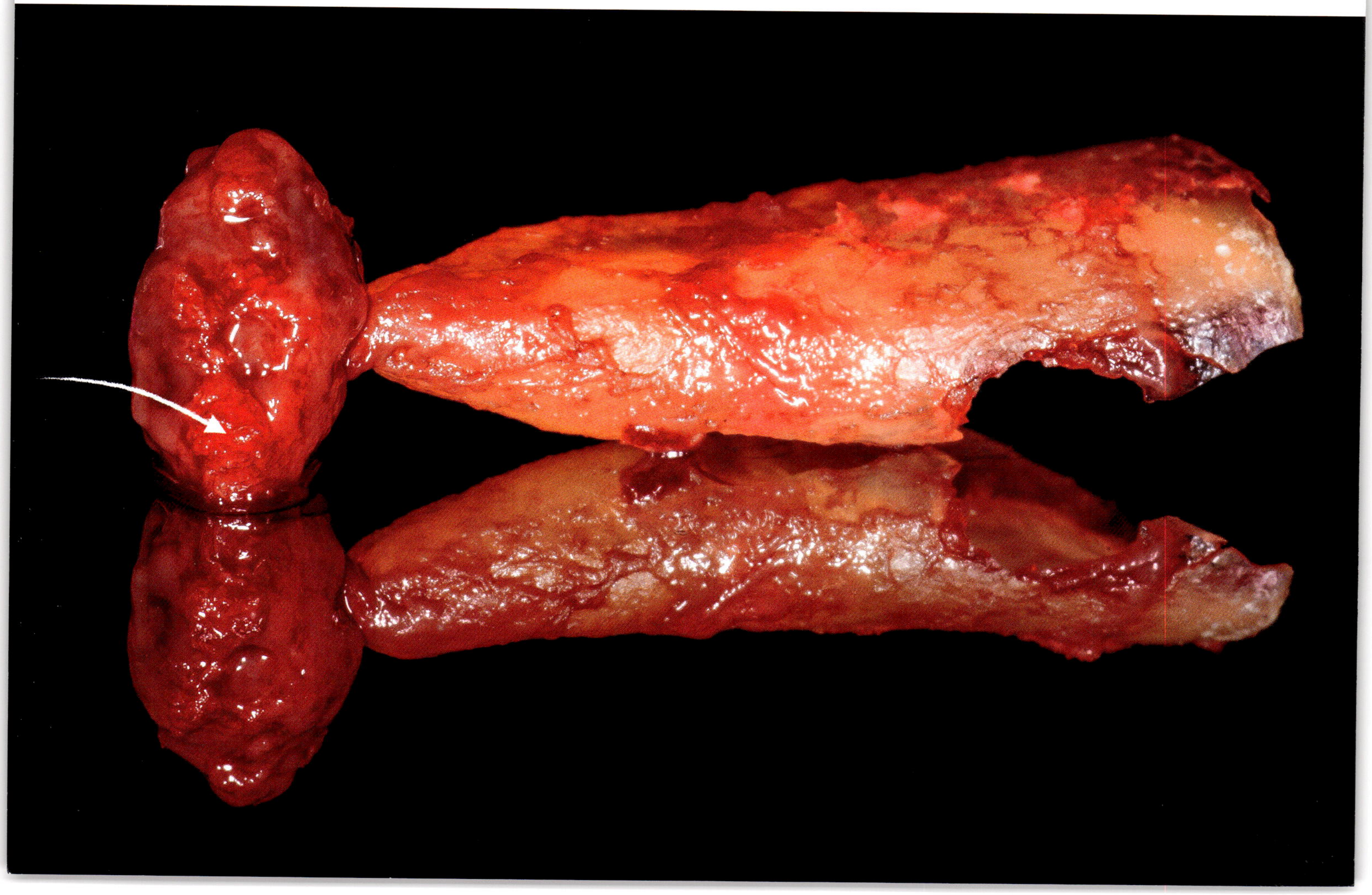

Depending on the orientation, a curette functions either like a scraper or a scooper. When angled away from the socket, it scrapes the walls. And when the tip points toward the socket, it is more like a scooper.

There is often radiographic evidence that gives clues about apical pathology. But it can be sneaky. It can easily go undetected or extend beyond the apparent radiographic margins in plain films. Pay closer attention when evaluating the socket if there isn't a CBCT available. Three-dimensional imaging helps to visualize the lesion and coordinate a game plan for success. Pay special attention to areas with difficult angles, like undercuts and lateral projections. Note the extent of the lesion and proximity to adjacent structures, such as the sinus, adjacent teeth, and the inferior alveolar nerve. Knowing the site improves the chances of successful curettage. If you don't know the lesion extends into an undercut, the site may look completely clean while harboring

Figure 4-29 The periodontal ligament is notable on this tooth's root. If the socket walls are curetted, the portion of the ligament that remains in the socket will be harmed unnecessarily.

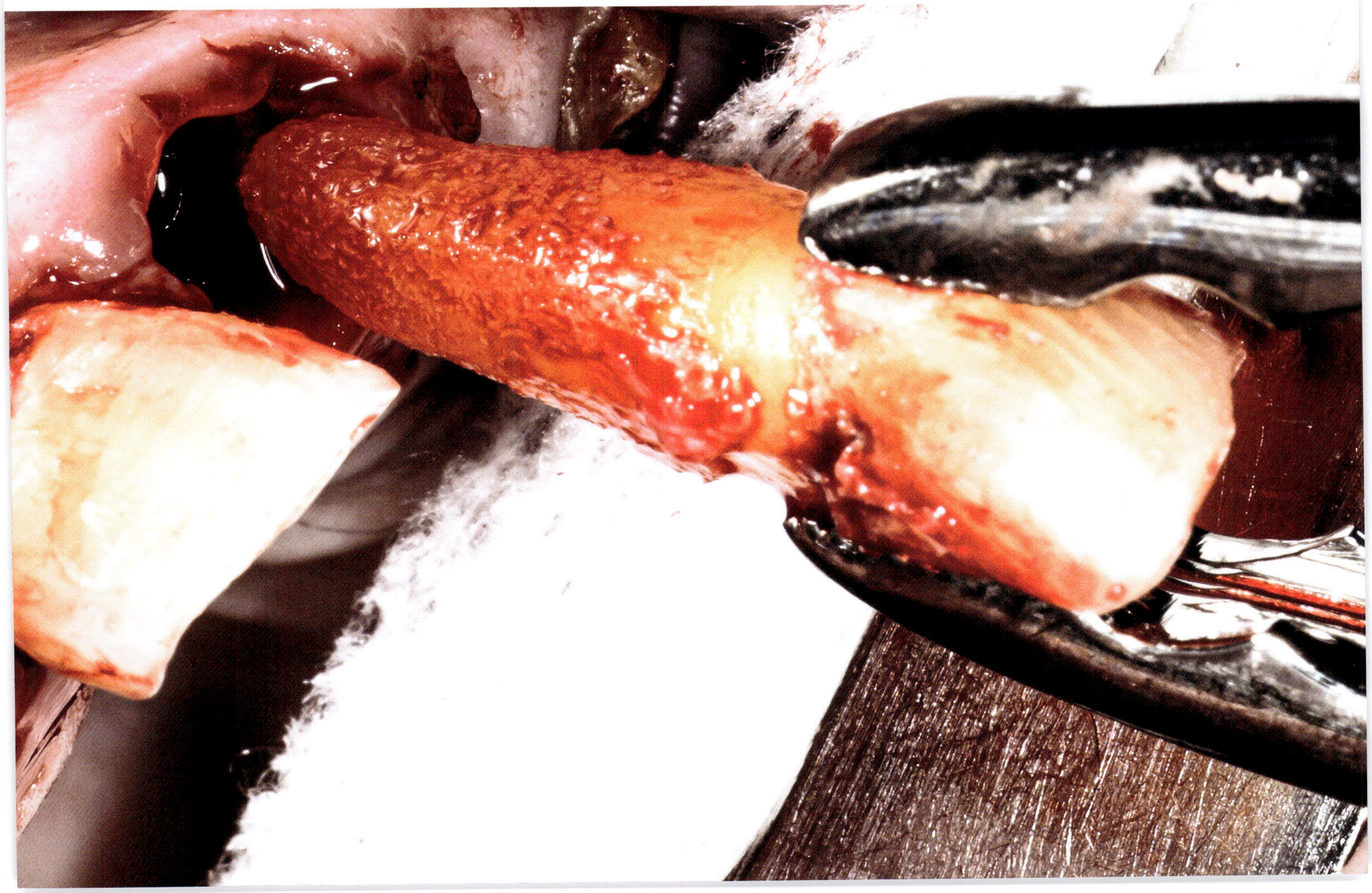

harmful bacteria and infiltrative soft tissue. It is also beneficial to know if there is a cortex of bone separating the abscess from the maxillary sinus. Even a thin cortex can be gently debrided. Without any cortex, it is very difficult to eradicate the pathology without compromising the sinus membrane. In a similar way, when the pathology approximates the inferior alveolar nerve without a cortical separation, there is significant risk of damaging the nerve during curettage, potentially causing temporary or permanent numbness. At times, the cyst extends around the apices of adjacent teeth. The acute angles and undulating anatomy can be difficult to access. Curettage is not likely to devitalize the tooth, but it is possible. It usually revascularizes, though it may test as non-vital for a while.

Do not curette healthy socket walls as this removes valuable periodontal ligament remnants and further traumatizes the bone. The remnants are tremendously valuable in healing, and they signal favorable cell differentiation. Removing periodontal ligament cells is harmful to healing.

A good saline flush of the socket will help you visualize and verify that the site is prepped to heal well. It also flushes out bacteria or debris that can inhibit healing. As they say, dilution is the solution to pollution.

When the tooth is out and the site prepared, healing begins. Our job as surgeons is to prepare the site as well as we can for healing. We are sculptors of the extraction site. We want to remove just enough and leave just enough.

Alveoloplasty

Healing is the goal of surgery. If the remaining alveolar ridge is punctuated by sharp shards of bone and littered with slivers and fragments, it will not heal as well. Alveoloplasty is a kind way to help the soft and hard tissue heal. What we can do in a matter of minutes with a rongeur and bone file can take many painful weeks and months for the patient's soft and hard tissue cells to accomplish.

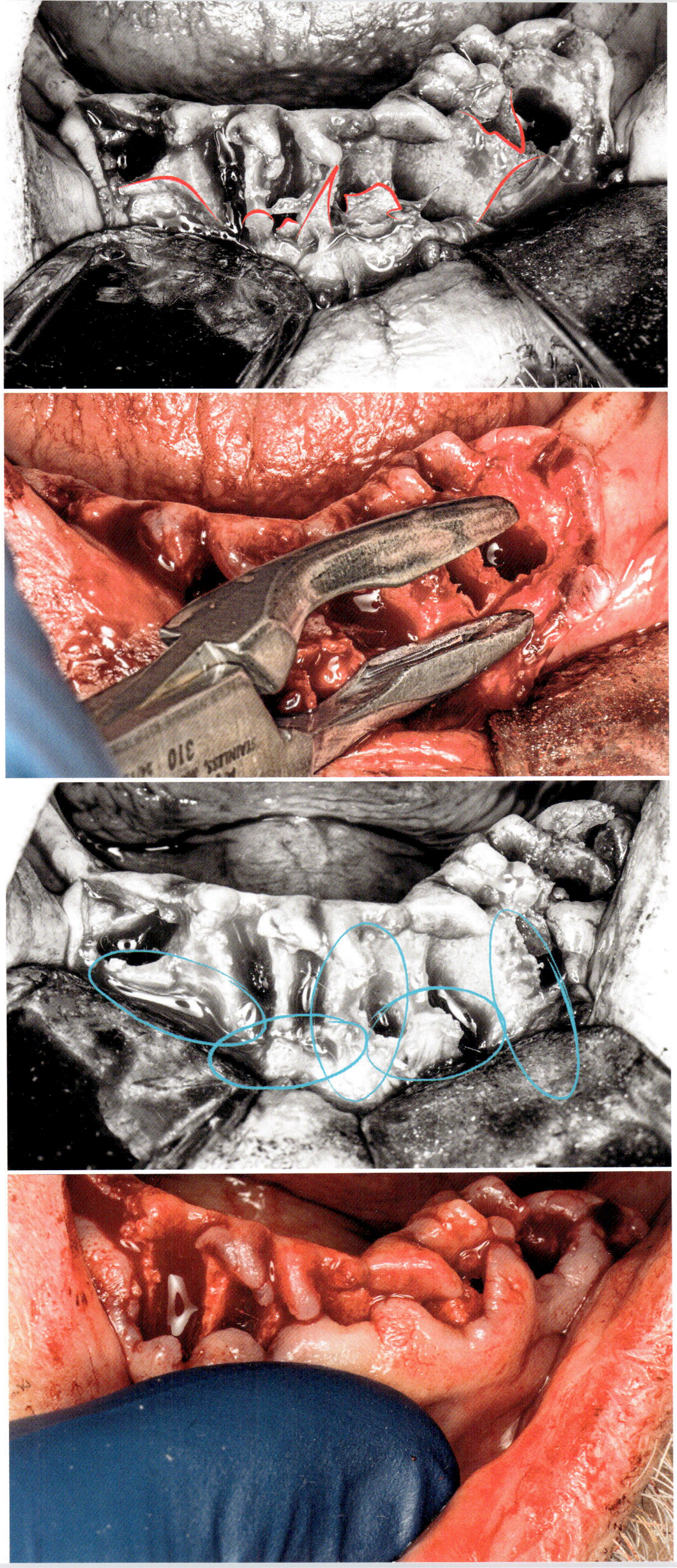

Figure 4-30 With the tissue adequately reflected, the sharp edges of bone can be trimmed with a rongeur, drill or bone file. The best way to evaluate progress is by palpating the ridge through the soft tissue. Pull the flap over the site and feel for sharp areas. Feeling with a finger over the tissue is the best way to evaluate progress. When it feels pretty smooth, inspect the area for loose fragments, flush the site to remove debris, and suture the tissue using caution to avoid excessive tension that can unduly harm the tissue.

Extraction Tips and Bailouts

Take a break. Have you ever struggled to get a jar open and then someone else helped and it popped right open? I think there is something to taking a short break. When an extraction doesn't seem to be progressing well, consider taking one. When you return with fresh eyes on the situation, you may be able to see beyond your previous limitations. There is also a theory that the periodontal ligament changes if you elevate and luxate for a bit and then let it marinate.

Reflect a good clean flap. If you can visualize the struggle, you can more likely overcome it. It is very difficult to defeat what you don't understand. It may take but a moment to reflect a flap, and it often pays dividends in being able to see your next move.

Get a different perspective. Sometimes there is a good purchase point or space in the periodontal ligament just around the corner and out of sight. Use a mirror, some irrigation and borrow the suction from your assistant for just a bit. This will often reveal a clue that helps facilitate the extraction, or at least helps you see what isn't working.

Change position. The instrument's angle is dependent on the position of the patient and provider. Changing the patient position and your position can open up new angles and new opportunities for success. Leverage and access can change by adjusting the chair a bit farther back or having patients tip their chin up a bit more. When working on lower extractions, sometimes sitting the patient up more is just what is needed.

Take an x-ray. A periapical radiograph is quick and simple, and it can provide tremendous insight into what remains and what is keeping you from success. Sometimes I discover what I was chasing wasn't a piece of root, but rather the surrounding bone.

Check the distal. It is easiest to elevate on the mesial of a tooth. Spend a bit of time with a periotome type of instrument separating the ligament on the distal. This can help create space for the root to be elevated from the mesial (which typically can deliver more force). As fragments of the tooth fracture, don't forget to recheck the distal. With each fractured piece, new real estate is potentially available.

Stay slow and steady. Hold a steady elevating force for 20 to 30 seconds. Even if you have been elevating or luxating a tooth without much movement, sometimes a bit of patience can disrupt the ligament more than a hasty elevation or repositioning the instrument after only 5 to10 seconds (which seems like a long time to some of us…)

Go big. A wide luxator can move the fulcrum farther away. This may open up other opportunities to use a purchase point that didn't otherwise have much value. It may also apply more force than a smaller elevator. Try using a bigger luxator.

Grab a curette. A small, curved curette can be a delightful tool at times when there is only a small portion of root remaining and the angles for the other straight instruments won't adequately engage the fragment. It is sometimes possible to slide the curette's leading edge into places other instruments simply cannot reach.

Add a dimple. Popping a small hole or dimple into the side of a root may allow for a better angle of engagement, facilitating a coronal vector of force. It often does not take much to get a purchase point.

Follow the canal. Tracking along the canal space with a bur provides a safe path for sectioning a tooth and protecting the surrounding bone. If you follow the canal, you will certainly be within the envelope of the root structure. This helps protect and preserve the precious surrounding periodontal ligament and bone. Sometimes the remaining root will even come out with the bur.

Check the perimeter. With a thin elevating instrument (like a periotome or Micro Buser), work your way around the tooth's perimeter, inserting the instrument tip into the PDL space. Search for another place to elevate and advance the instrument. Rotating or wiggling the instrument laterally can facilitate this advancement and further mobilize the root. If there is space, consider the advantage of using a small luxator or spade elevator in those places.

Check your work. Irrigating and examining the socket after extraction is a great habit. Fragments of a carious crown, retained granulation tissue, and extra root tips are much easier to address if you deal with them immediately. As I am sitting here writing this today, I had what looked like a routine impacted mandibular third molar that came out as planned. As I irrigated the socket, I noticed a small third root flared off to the buccal that I would have missed if I didn't look again.

References

1. A Course of Lectures on Dental Physiology and Surgery, Delivered at the Middlesex Hospital School of Medicine. Br Foreign Med Chir Rev. 1849 Jan;3(5):175-187.
2. Walia PS, Rohilla AK, Choudhary S, et al. Review of Dilaceration of Maxillary Central Incisor: A Mutidisciplinary Challenge. Int J Clin Pediatr Dent. 2016;9(1):90-98.
3. Li X, Hu L, Ma L, et al. Severe periodontitis may influence cementum and dental pulp through inflammation, oxidative stress, and apoptosis. J Periodontol. 2019 Nov;90(11):1297-1306.
4. Nayyar J, Clarke M, O'Sullivan M, et al. Fractured root tips during dental extractions and retained root fragments. A clinical dilemma? Br Dent J. 2015 Mar 13;218(5):285-290.

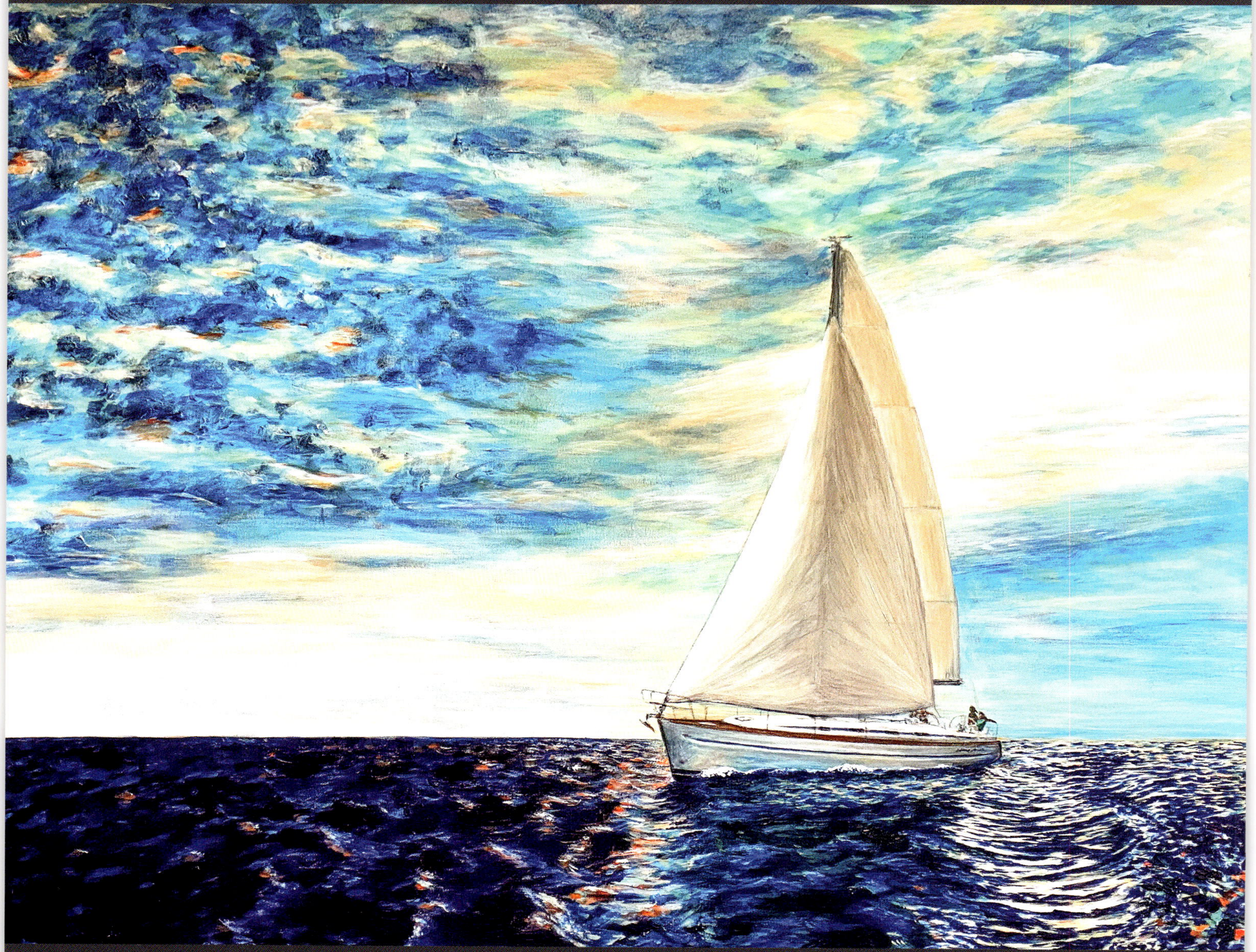

My Happy Place. On my boat (*A Frayed Knot*) on Lake Michigan with my family.
(40x60 inch acrylic on canvas)

CHAPTER 5

IMPACTED EXODONTIA

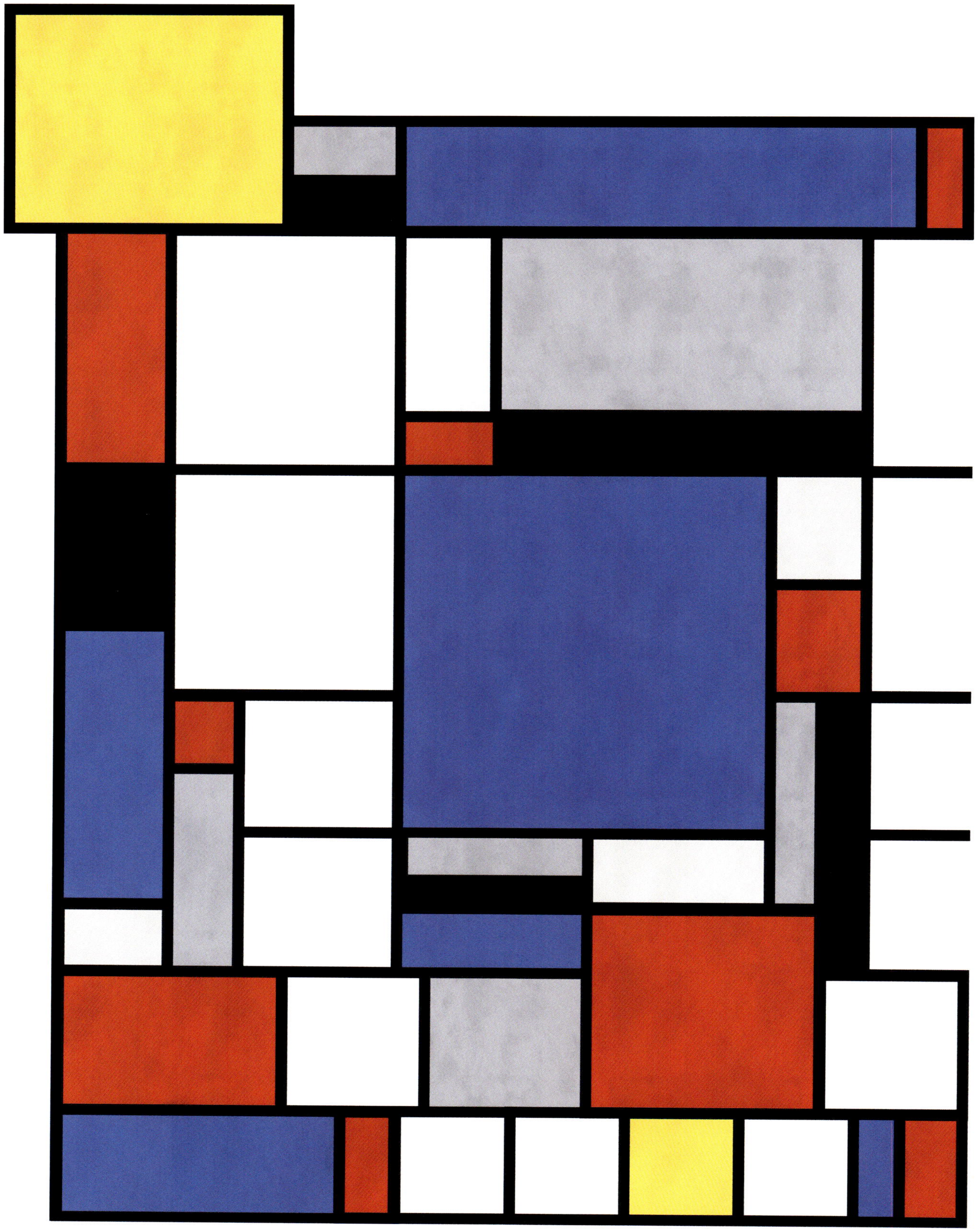

Figure 5-1 Sometimes, the art in our profession is very systematic and predictable. This piece portrays a dental arch in a Piet Mondrian style. Notice how the impacted third molar (upper left) may require you to think outside the box. The right side depicts the limited visualization common in extracting posterior teeth. (Artwork inspired by Piet Mondrian.)

Impacted teeth exhibit unique behavior. The general visualization, access and mobilization principles are the same for both impacted and erupted teeth, but each has nuances that, when understood, sometimes make removing impacted teeth easier than erupted teeth. That said, removing unerupted teeth is more challenging overall.

Unlike an erupted tooth, the periodontal ligament does very little to retain an impacted tooth. Rather, the mechanical retention from the contours of the overlying bone, the crown's snug fit and root architecture seem to be the retentive factors. The ability to accurately envision how the tooth and the bone will respond to drilling and elevating is critical to the procedure's success and how the patient heals. The general concept of visualizing the procedure is similar in any extraction.

Removing impacted teeth is a much more challenging artform. It requires significantly more finesse and technical skill. The risks are higher. The potential complications and morbidity are more severe. While it may not always be more time consuming, it is much less forgiving to technical errors or sloppy technique. Precisely and delicately handling the soft tissue while accessing and manipulating the hard tissue will significantly improve the patient's experience during recovery. Surgery sets the stage for healing. Keep the bone cool while you drill and be kind to it when you elevate. Protect the flap and the surrounding soft tissue.

Visualization

Visualization is critical to the outcome. Surgeons who can accurately visualize each step of an extraction in detail can control most of the extraction, even if they don't see the tooth until it is removed. In residency, one of my mentors said the first impacted third molar extraction you see is the first one you do. I find that a bit ironic because I still don't see most of the maxillary third molars I remove until they are out. Visualization can mean seeing it with your eyes or seeing it in your mind's eye.

Mental imagery is based on a combination of radiographic information and experience. Three-dimensional imaging can provide a clear picture of the tooth's position, adjacent teeth, surrounding bone and structures. With traditional two-dimensional imaging, there is certainly more information to fill in mentally. Upon reviewing the radiograph, experienced surgeons can already visualize the extraction subconsciously, knowing which instruments will most likely deliver the tooth with the least resistance. They no longer see Archer's or Pell and Gregory's classifications they learned in dental school. They just see the extraction and potential complications to avoid. These classifications provide a helpful framework to begin the visualization process. But visualization alone has never removed a tooth. Access and mobilization is where the rubber meets the road. This section primarily focuses on impacted third molars, but these principles can be applied to other impacted teeth as well.

Classification

Classifying the level of impaction from 1 to 4 (soft tissue, partial bone, full bone or complicated) primarily serves as a means of bookkeeping. We use codes D7220, D7230, D7240 and D7241 to determine reimbursement for our services. Indeed, this classification is important, but it does relatively little to classify a case's complexity or to describe the procedure. I don't usually think about the level of impaction until after surgery. I am focused on the actual work of removing the teeth, which doesn't necessarily coincide with this reimbursement classification system. In my current practice, my team provides patients with an estimate of their anticipated out-of-pocket expense prior to surgery. We try to be as accurate as possible with the estimate, erring on the high side. At the end of the procedure, they confirm treatment with me. This is the only time I really think about classifying the impaction level with dental codes.

There are a few main impaction classifications taught in dental school and residency, two of which are Pell and Gregory Classification, and Winter's Lines. While they provide a good starting point, both only capture one or two dimensions of the reality of the extraction. The two main factors in these systems are the depth of impaction and the tooth's angulation. These are very important. They provide the framework to build an understanding of the procedure. But they miss all other anatomical and patient-related factors that profoundly impact the procedure. Other main factors adding to the complexity include bone density, follicle size, root form, molar proximity, mandibular flare, patient age, and the work environment in the oral cavity. One of the biggest variables is patient cooperation. Whether sedated or awake, the patient's response to the procedure can add immense challenges.

My goal is not to introduce a new method for evaluating impacted extractions. Many useful ways have been described, each quite clever and helpful in developing an understanding of the challenges and complexities involved in removing impacted wisdom teeth. If you are interested, consider looking up Pederson's Difficulty Index[1] and the WHARFE Assessment[2,3].

The way I see it, the tooth's position sets a baseline for the extraction's complexity. It is the central framework. In my mind, all other factors are represented by the shades of black and white surrounding the central green, yellow and red matrix. These factors run the gamut and can make even a minimally impacted tooth quite complex. In practice, it seems impaction depth and angulation can be dealt with quite predictably. The techniques for each generally work well. Knowing how to access, where to drill, and how to elevate is discussed throughout this chapter. The true art is in putting all the factors together and setting the patient up for the healing that takes place after surgery.

Challenges increase as the impaction angulation deviates farther from normal. Vertical and mesioangular extractions have the simplest mechanics and trajectory. They are lined up the best for extraction. Horizontal and distoangular extractions are more complicated, requiring increased soft tissue exposure and drilling. Sometimes, distoangular impactions are the most difficult to remove. Buccolingual teeth can be awkward and challenging to remove because they are sideways to the extraction site. They can be particularly difficult to access when the apex is buccal and the crown is lingual or palatal. Inverted teeth are the farthest off course. They can be some of the most difficult to remove but are also not very common.

Extraction Complexity

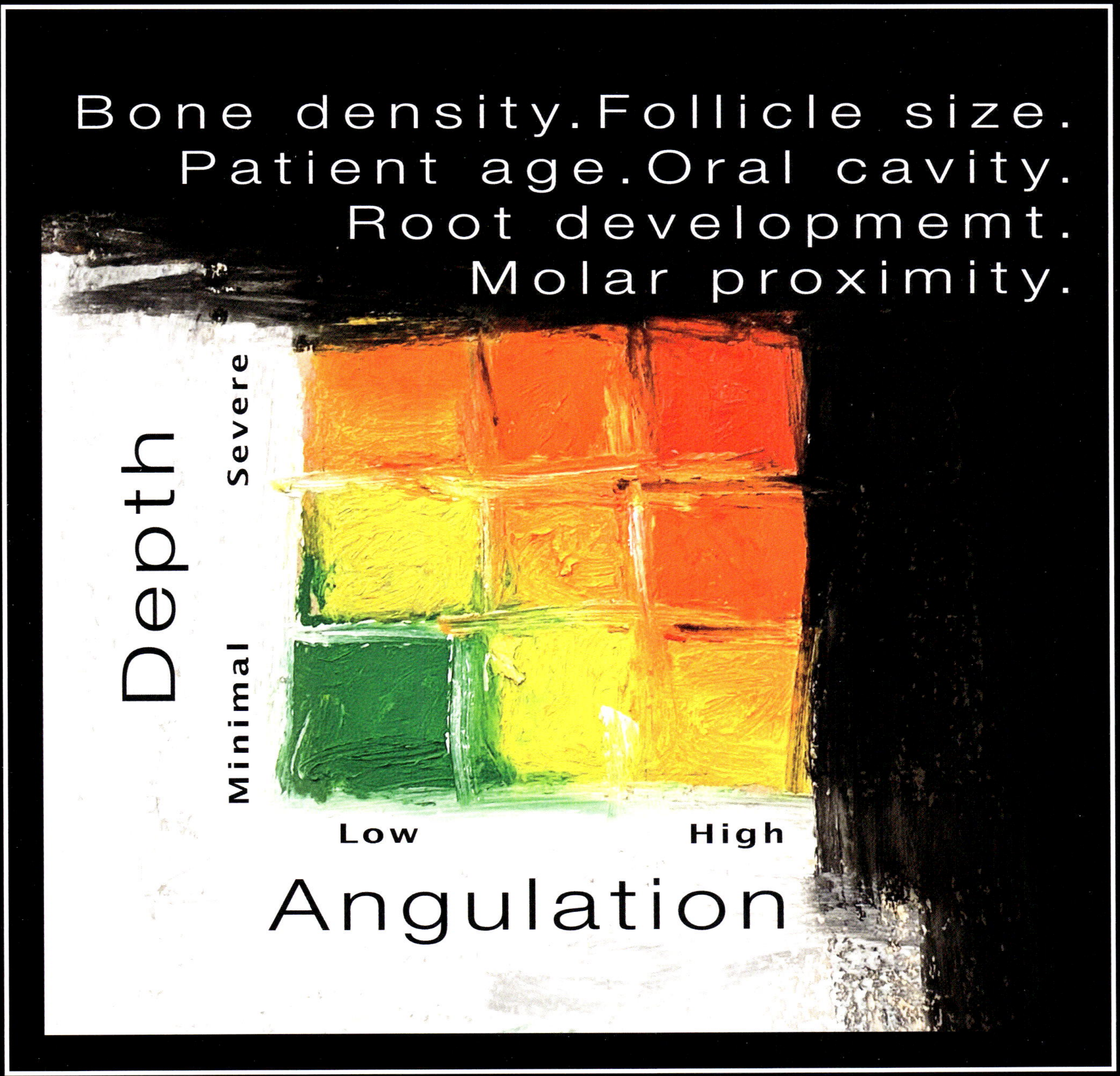

Figure 5-2 The complexity of extracting an impacted tooth is mainly based on impaction depth and angulation. All other factors play a part and can make a simple extraction much more difficult. These factors include bone density, follicle size, root development, molar proximity, patient age and the conditions of the oral cavity.

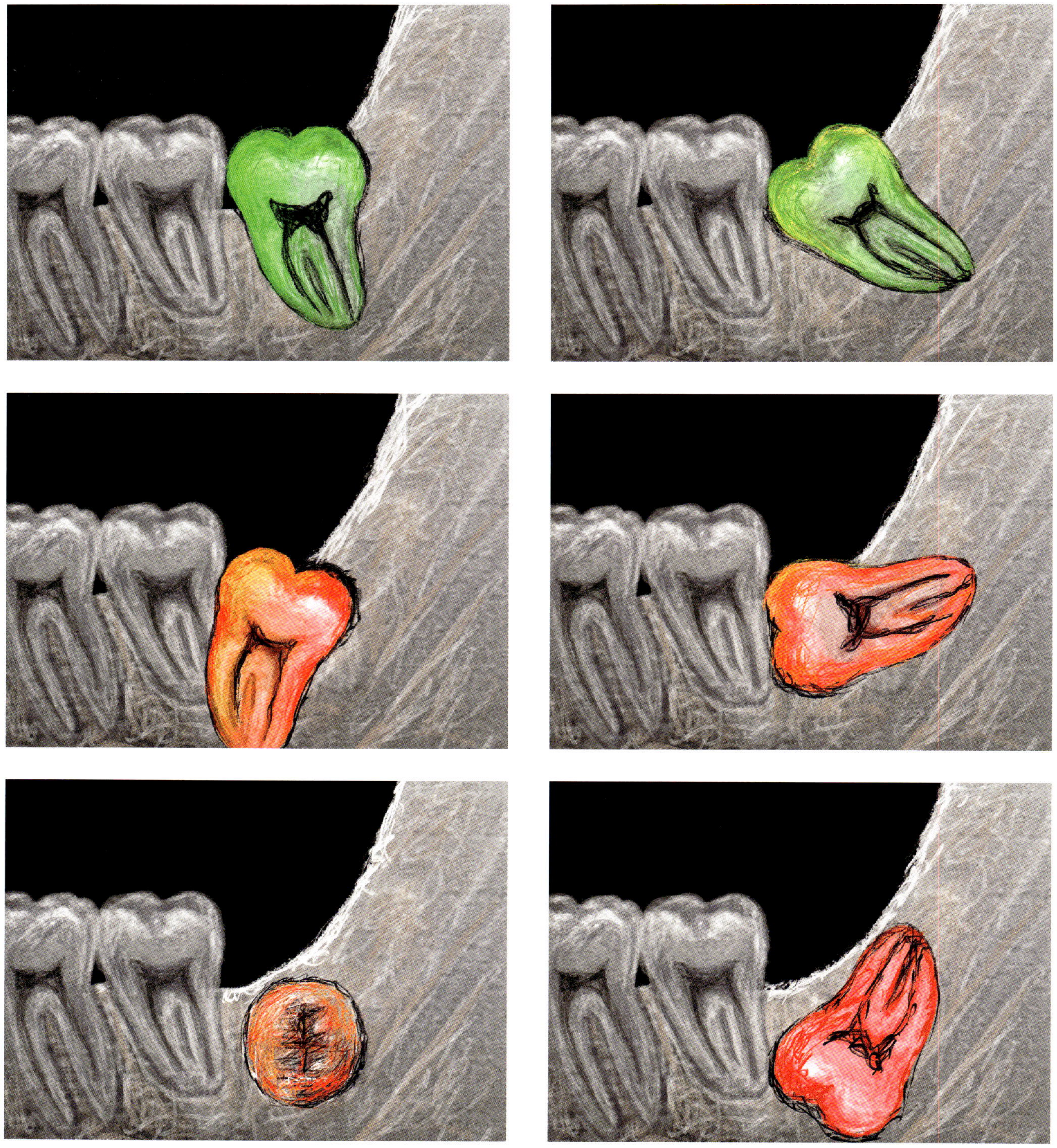

Figure 5-3 Angulation of impaction: vertical, mesioangular, distoangular, horizontal, buccolingual, vertical.

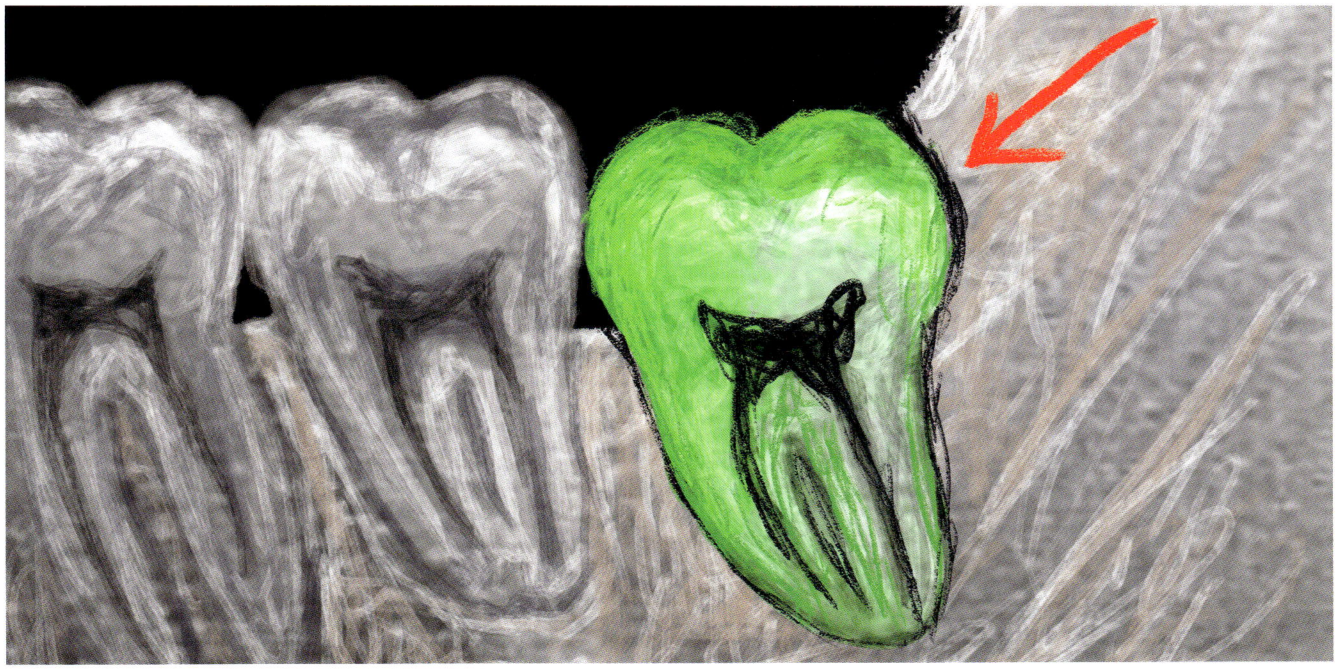

Figure 5-4 Vertical impaction. Pay attention to the distal bone. The ascending ramus can trap the tooth. It may need to be sectioned to remove the distal portion. Removing the crown's distal portion is often adequate to deliver the remainder of the tooth.

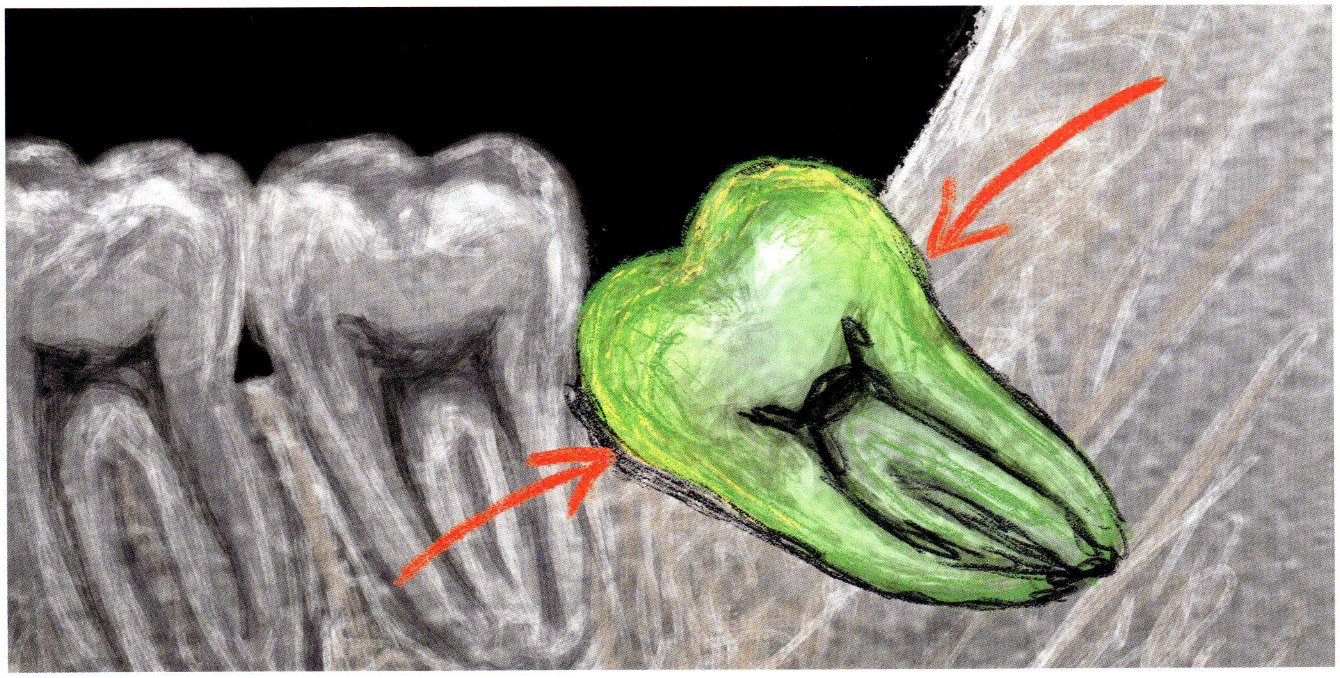

Figure 5-5 Mesioangular impaction. Pay attention to the mesial bone. There must be adequate access to place the elevator. Bone removal may be needed in this area. Also be aware of the distal bone. Like vertical impaction, there may be limited space for the elevation, especially if it is tucked under the ascending ramus.

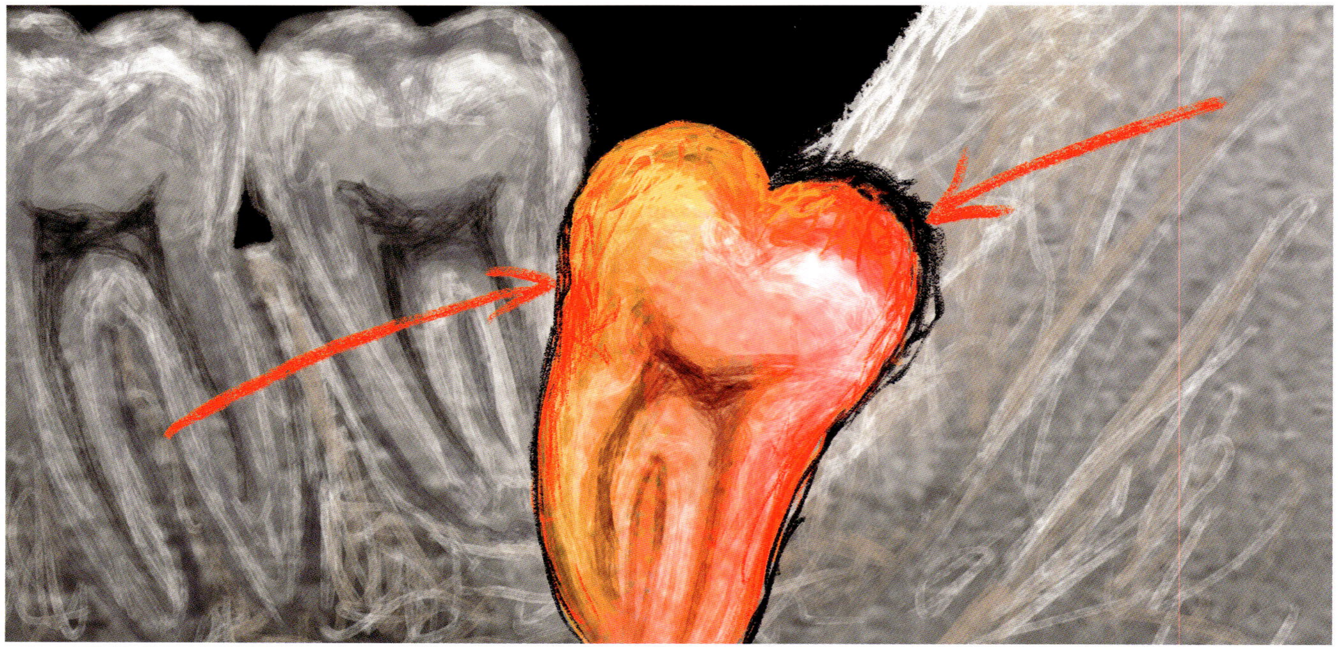

Figure 5-6 Distoangular impaction. Take note of the proximity to the second molar. These teeth are often very close to each other, making it difficult to position an elevator. The ascending ramus can make it impossible to mobilize the tooth without first removing the distal half or at least a portion of the distal crown. Removing the crown's distal portion is often adequate to deliver the remainder of the tooth.

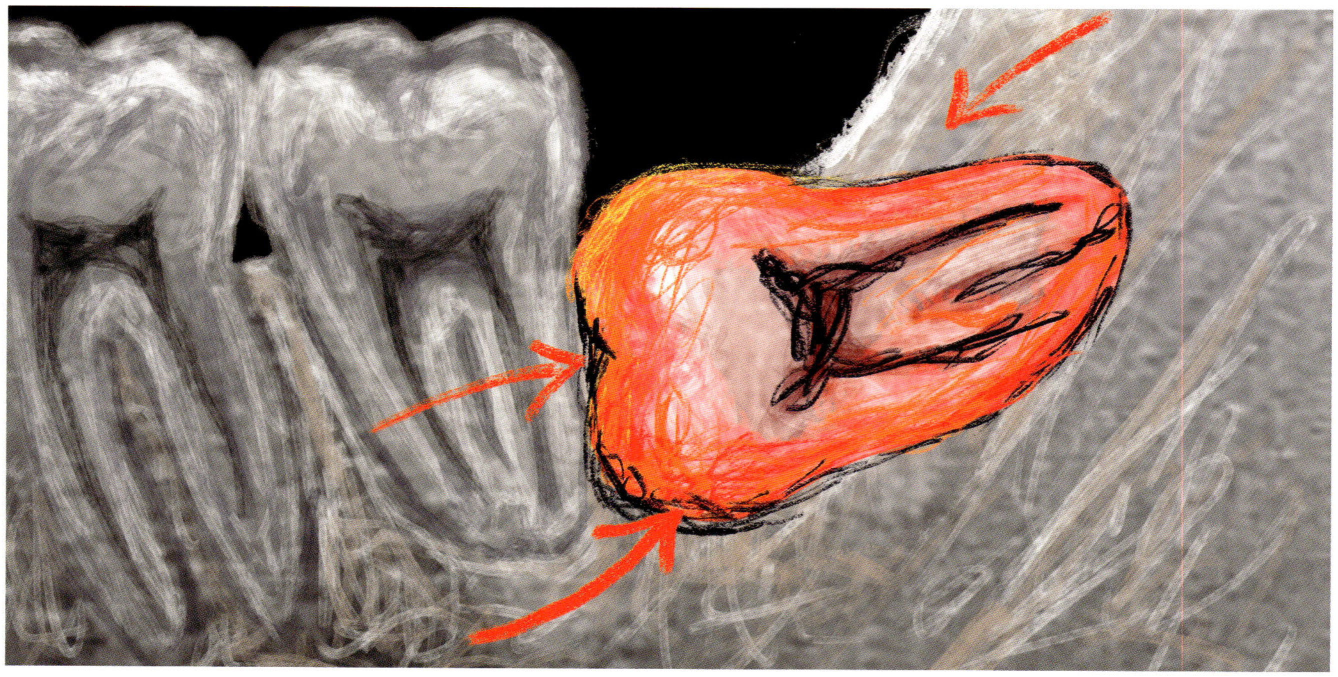

Figure 5-7 Horizontal impaction. Like the others, there is often limited space between the roots of the second molar. Elevating on the mesial can be a challenge due to the depth of the crown's mesial aspect. A generous buccal trough may be helpful if you cannot remove the coronal aspect first. The ascending ramus also can retain the roots and may require bone removal. Be aware of the angles of elevation on the tooth. The ascending ramus won't budge if you are elevating the tooth against it.

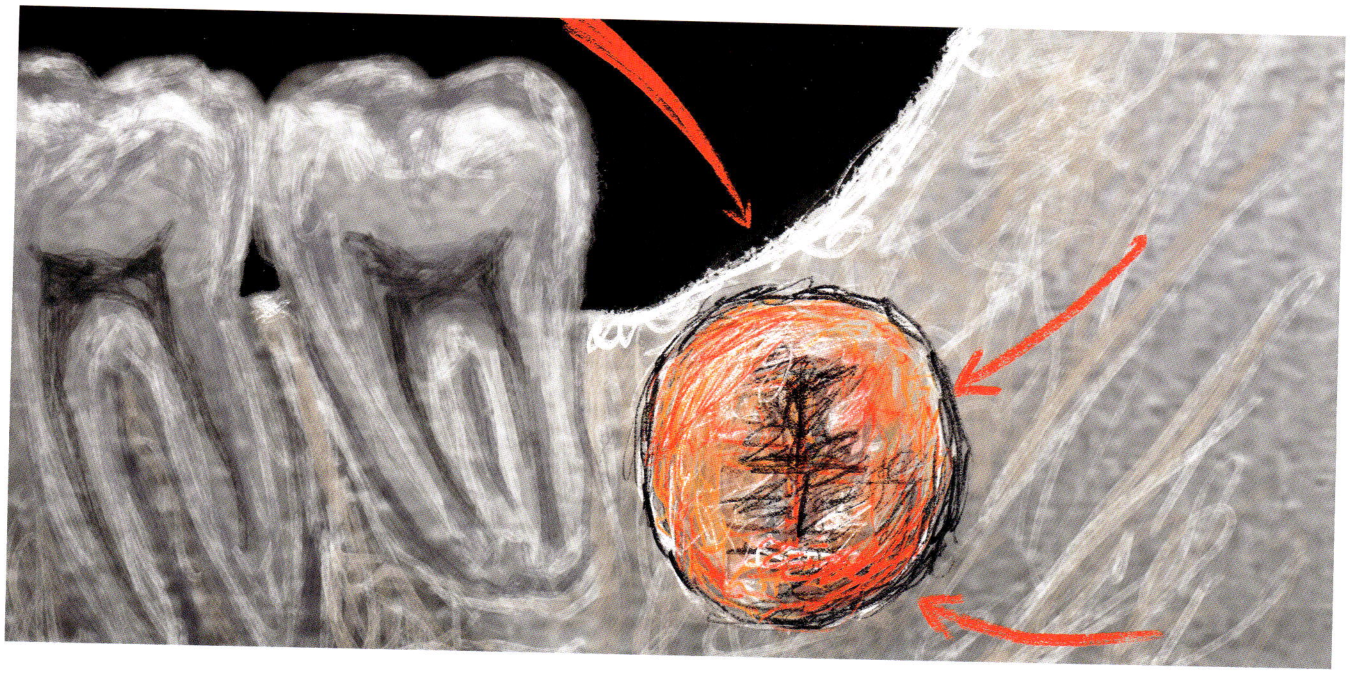

Figure 5-8 Buccolingual impaction. Three-dimensional imaging helps determine the orientation of these teeth. Be especially mindful of the lingual aspect. It may be protruding out the cortex of the mandible. It is helpful to know the anatomy. The most inferior portion of the crown can be difficult to deliver as it is often tucked in tightly within the dense cortical bone. The distal also can be challenging as it may be under the ascending ramus.

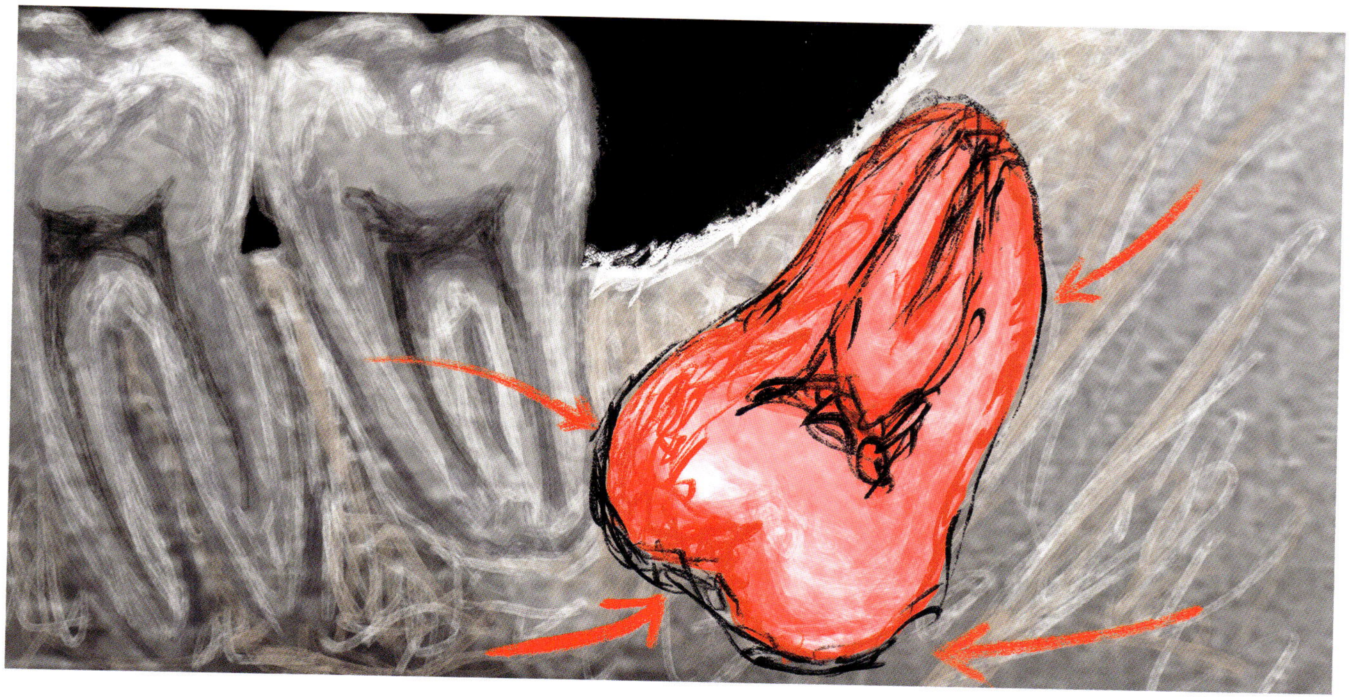

Figure 5-9 Inverted impaction. Everything about these can be a challenge. They don't know which direction is north. They often need to be harvested piece by piece. Particular attention should be given to the most inferior and posterior portions. It is easy to unintentionally retain portions when they come out in so many pieces and are tucked in so deep. Get plenty of access and expose the site well.

Impaction Depth

The depth of impaction amplifies or intensifies the nuances of the angulation. When a tooth is deeper, it requires more bone removal and sectioning. This is in part because of the amount of bone physically retaining the tooth. That is obvious. But a more subtle impact of the depth is on the point of elevation, the location where the elevating forces must be applied in order to deliver the tooth. The deeper this point, the more difficult the extraction. It requires more bone removal and likely more sectioning of the tooth. And it will take more for the patient's bone to heal.

Figure 5-10 Envision the point where the elevator would be to extract a tooth. It is under the mesial height of contour of the crown. Knowing the depth of this point of application will help you understand how difficult the extraction is. The deeper this point is, the more difficult the extraction. (Artwork inspired by Leonardo da Vinci.)

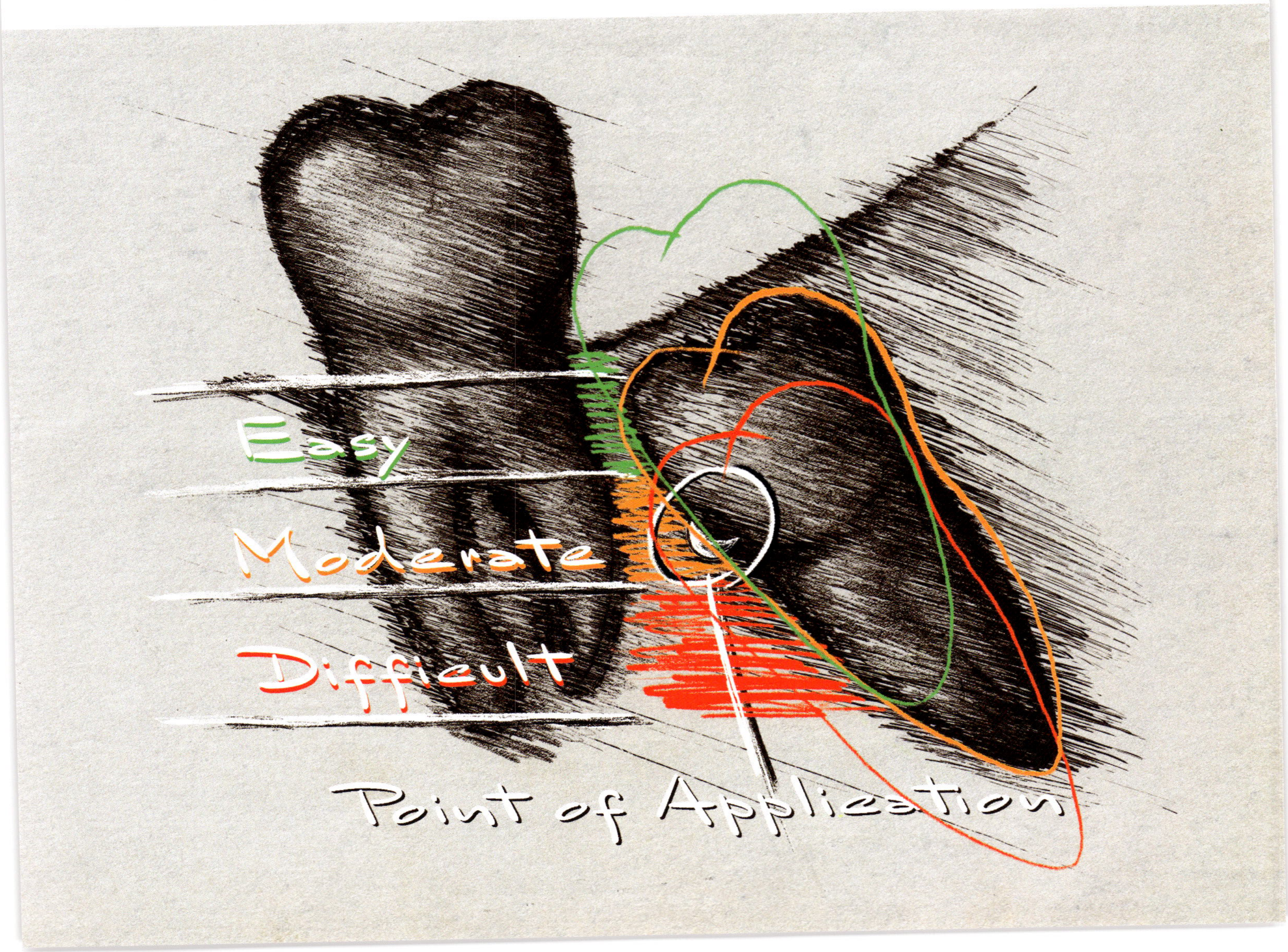

Table 5-1 Practical implications of impaction depth

Depth of impaction	Shallow	Moderate	Deep
Bone removal	Less, possibly hand instruments	Some, likely drill for access	Significant removal required to access and create space for extraction
Sectioning	Less likely	More likely	Necessary and likely into multiple pieces
Soft tissue access	Small incision, may not need to elevate full flap	Full thickness flap	Full thickness flap with significant exposure, possible vertical releases
Tooth or fragment displacement risk	Lower	Moderate	Higher
Overall healing	Easier recovery	Moderate	Potential longer and more arduous recovery

Follicle Size

A generous follicle is a wonderful thing. It provides more space for elevation and less mechanical retention of the tooth. Conversely, when there is limited or no apparent follicle, all the space for elevation must be created either by removing bone or tooth structure.

When the follicle is large, it may be possible to insert a small luxator between the mesial of the crown and the bone, even when there is some bone overlying. After reflecting the soft tissue flap, place the Micro Buser where you plan to place the luxator. You may find there is space for the luxator, and you may be able to proceed with elevation and delivery of the tooth. If the follicle space is limited or the overlying bone too dense, a buccal trough can be developed.

Bone Density

When the overlying bone is thin or less dense, there's a better chance you can remove or manipulate the tooth with hand instruments. You may see hints of this on the radiograph, but you won't really know until you engage the bone with an instrument.

It is sometimes possible to reflect the overlying bone with a tissue elevator, creating access to deliver the tooth. Other times, the small luxator or elevator can sneak between the mesial of the crown and the bone, elevating the tooth. This may displace the bone enough while simultaneously elevating the tooth out. In these cases, particular attention must be paid to manage the thin bone fragments displaced by the extraction. If they are retained with adequate blood supply and stability, they may heal fine. But, if there is inadequate stability or they have been stripped of the periosteal blood supply, they are likely to at least bother the patient if not cause a sterile subperiosteal abscess or an infection.

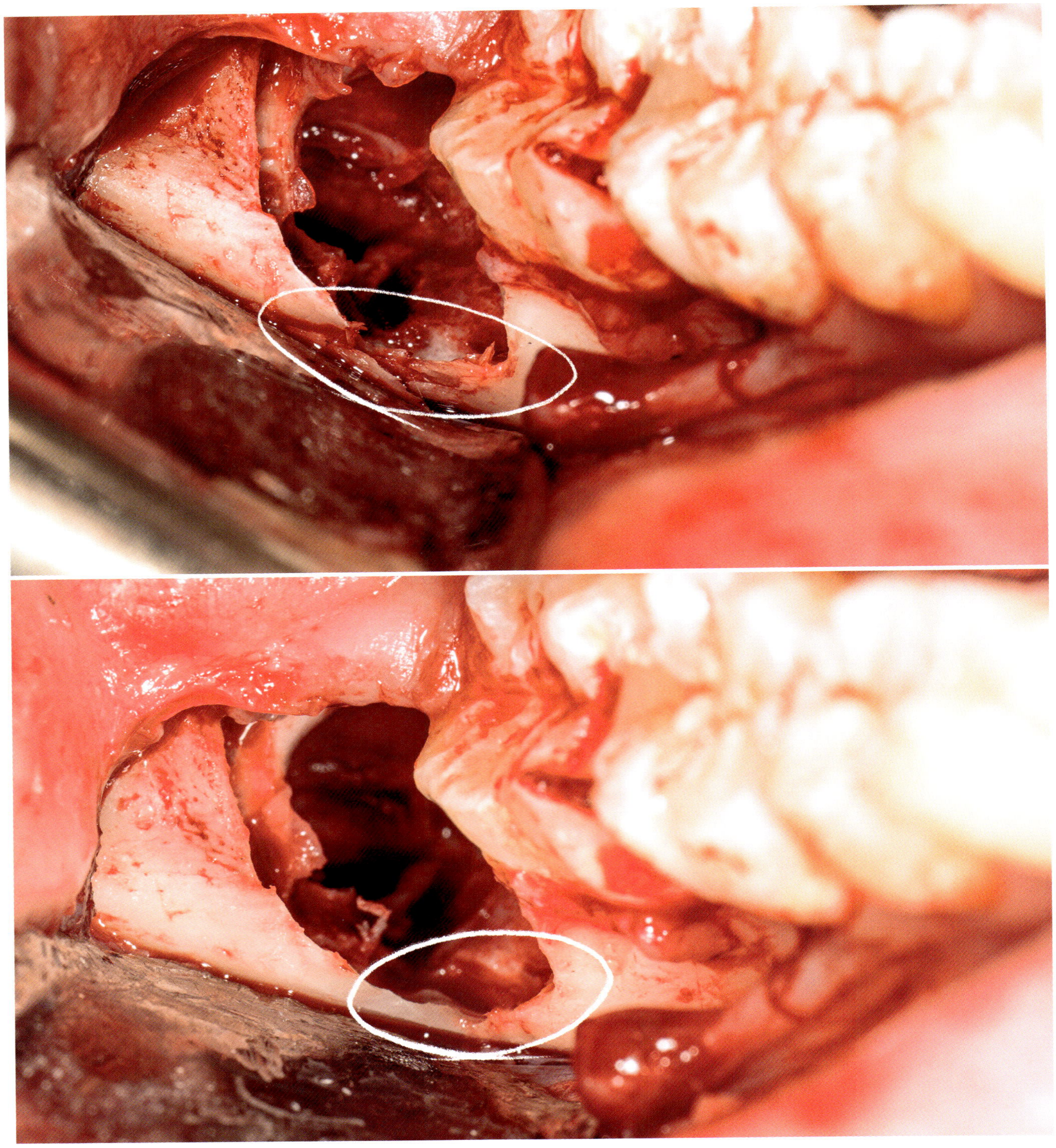

Figure 5-11 Fragments like these will likely cause problems. It is possible they will heal fine, but the body will likely either resorb them or get rid of them. Think about the size of these pieces compared to a macrophage. These pieces are between 1 to 4 millimeters. Macrophages are about 20 micrometers, which is 200 times smaller. It is much easier for a surgeon to remove these pieces than a macrophage. Set the site up for healing.

The art of oral surgery is in the practice of "just enough." Removing just enough bone to get the tooth out. Reflecting just enough tissue to access the site. Sectioning the tooth just enough to split it without perforating the lingual cortex.

Dense or thick bone can be very frustrating if it is not tended to adequately. It doesn't flex or displace with hand instrumentation. It requires proper attention with an appropriate bur and copious irrigation. Because the bone doesn't flex, the hole must be large enough for the tooth or tooth fragments to pass. The smaller the pieces, the smaller the hole. On paper, it might seem kind to the tissue to section the tooth into smaller fragments to avoid extensive bone removal, but smaller pieces can be much more difficult to manage. This can lead to extended surgical time and further trauma to the surrounding tissue.

In residency, I was encouraged to only pick up the handpiece once during the procedure. The process went like this: Remove adequate buccal bone, section the tooth so it splits right through the furcation, elevate the distal and then mesial segments. Presto. It looked so easy when my instructors did it. The challenge seemed to be making an adequate buccal trough, visualizing the ideal position and angulation for the bur, and going deep enough into the tooth to split it with the elevator (but not so deep that the lingual cortex was compromised). This is ideal, and it feels good when it all goes as planned. Over time, I have learned picking up the handpiece a second or third time is much better than trying to force pieces out through inadequate access. When the bone is dense, as it often is in the posterior mandible, the hole size must be adequate for both the pieces and the instrument delivering them.

The blood supply of bone is usually inversely proportionate to its density. Dense bone has less blood supply. It not only heats up quickly when drilling, but it also responds poorly to that heat during recovery. Keep it cool, especially in dense bone.

Saline is cheap. Use plenty of it when drilling, especially in the posterior mandible. Pay close attention to exactly where the irrigation is going. It is possible for the irrigation to be diverted from the cutting edge of the drill by the adjacent soft tissue, bone, or even the suction. If the soft tissue flap is not properly reflected and retracted, the irrigation may deflect off the tissue and never reach the bur. When drilling a deep trough or sectioning deep into the bone or the tooth, the irrigation also may be inadvertently deflected. The saline stream also can be diverted directly into the suction if not positioned well. While it is important to adequately evacuate the irrigation for visualization and to prevent aspiration, make sure it accomplishes its purpose before being evacuated.

Irrigation works best when it directly flushes the cutting edge of the bur. Depending on the system, the tip may be adjusted. When a shorter or longer bur is used, it may be worth adjusting the nozzle tip. When there is inadequate irrigation, the increased friction will generate more heat, the bur's flutes will jam up with bone, and you can plan on a more grueling recovery.

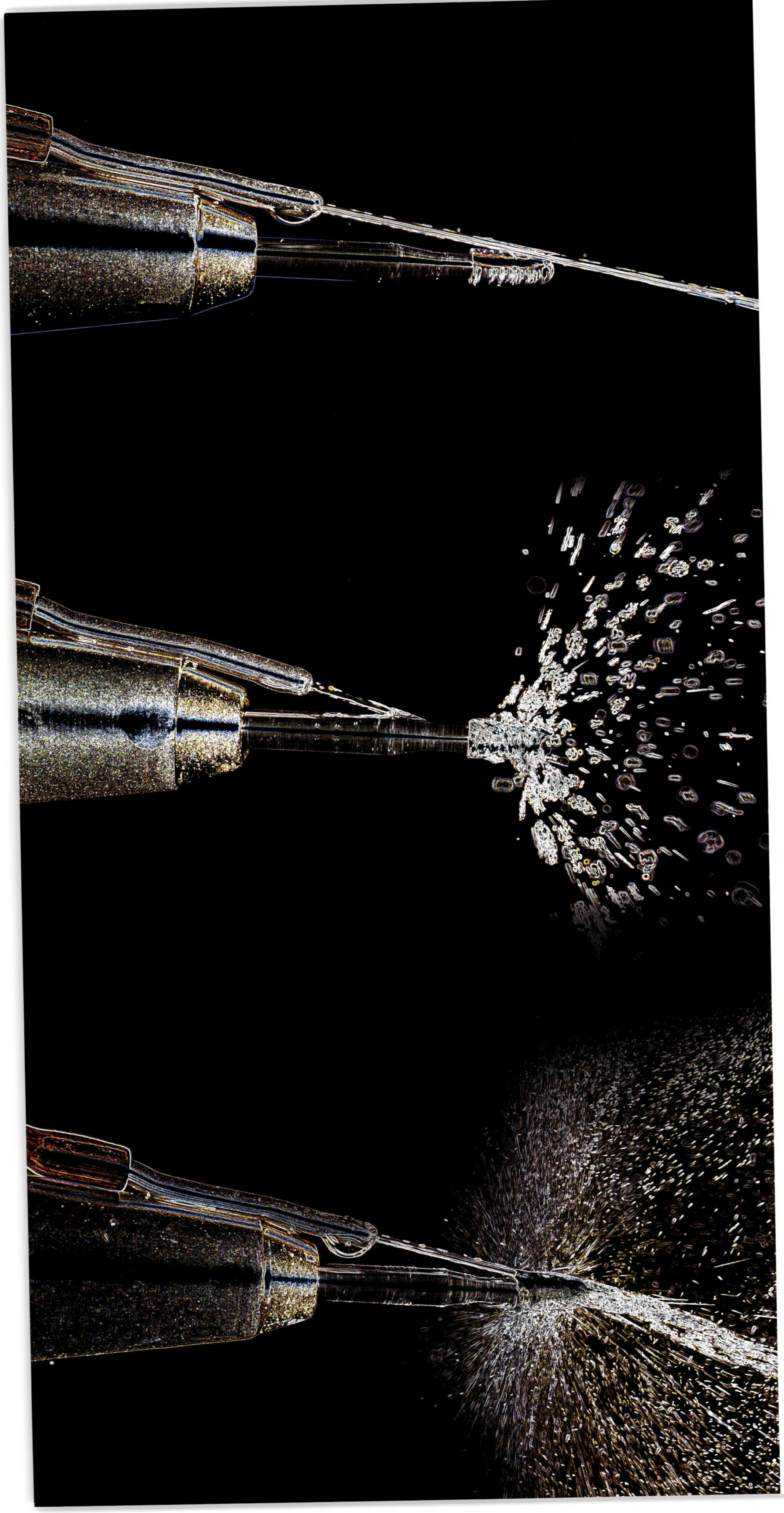

Drilling principles

- Reflect a good flap and retract it well.
- Orient the irrigation tip so it will direct the irrigation into the trough.
- Move slow enough to efficiently cut bone without generating significant heat.
- Position the suction to efficiently evacuate the irrigation after it has reached the bur.

These principles apply whenever using a drill, but they are increasingly important in the dense, vulnerable bone of the posterior mandible.

Figure 5-12 If the irrigation stream is too high (*top*) or too low (*middle*), the drill flutes will not clear as well. But when it hits the flutes just right (*bottom*), heat dissipates, and the sharp cutting edges remain exposed and effective. Don't assume the irrigation is effective just because it is flowing. Pay attention to how well the bur is cleared.

Root Form

There is a sweet spot in tooth development that is optimal for the harvest. This is usually between ⅓ and ⅔ root development. Premature removal increases the difficulty because there is more bone to remove, and the tooth is more difficult to manage within the follicle space. Late removal adds to the challenge because there is more root in the bone, complicating the elevation and increasing the chances of nerve or sinus issues. A tooth with a fully developed, dilacerated root also can be a challenge.

Fully developed roots

The challenges that come with removing a tooth with fully developed roots are quite the opposite of undeveloped roots. The same basic principles of visualization and access apply. Instead of chasing these around, it may be a struggle to get any mobility.

Visualization begins with a good radiograph. Knowing the general anatomy of the roots is critical. If they are bulky and bulbous, they may be less likely to fracture when elevating. But if they are slender and curved, precise elevation with ideal vectors of force will optimize success. Even then, though, there is a higher chance of fracturing off a small portion of the root tip if it is thin.

An ice cream cone shaped lower third molar is a treat. With converged roots, almost any force will be eruptive. Not so with the candy cane shaped roots. The moment you start to elevate, they break right in the middle of the hook. It is like that thin plastic wrapper is the only thing holding them together. Preemptive bone removal in key locations can improve efficiency and decrease surgical trauma by creating space for the roots to move. Retrieving a small, thin piece of root that is tucked around a tight, dark corner, surrounded in dense bone, with a nerve lurking somewhere just beneath the surface is more of a trick than a treat.

Root curvature

Whether impacted or erupted, the same principles apply regarding root curvature. Check out the beginning of Chapter 4: The Art of Exodontia for a discussion on how root curvature impacts extraction.

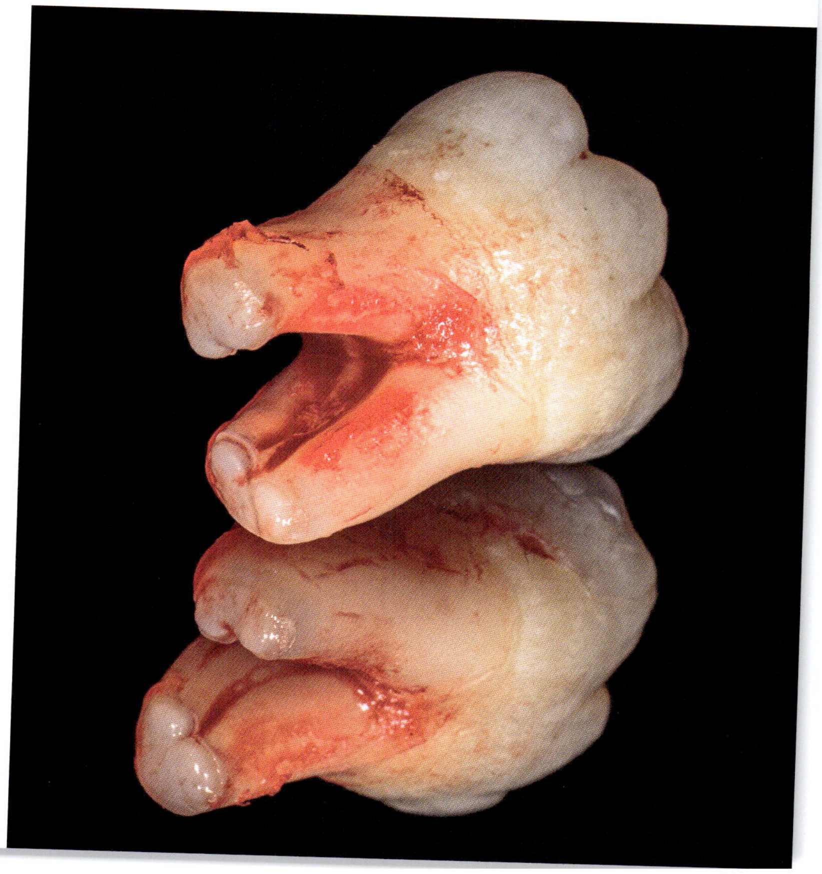

Figure 5-13 Incomplete development of the root apex makes for an easier extraction and lower potential risk of nerve injury. Note the developing apical tissue that acts like a bumper potentially protecting a nearby nerve.

Undeveloped roots

When removing a tooth with little or no root development, your access needs to be a little more generous. Create a proportionately larger osseous window, uncovering most of the crown. It may be possible to remove the entire tooth intact if the window is adequate, but remember the round shape of the tooth behaves much like a slippery marble. Therefore, sectioning it into at least a mesial and distal half is good. Sometimes it is beneficial to also section it into buccal and lingual segments before splitting or elevating it.

Try to make all anticipated cuts before splitting or elevating as the tooth is the most stable in the socket before fracturing and elevating. Even when the window appears adequate and the tooth has been sectioned, it still can be difficult to retrieve these small pieces. An elevator or luxator may do the trick. Angled curettes and curved hemostats also may come in handy when fishing out the pieces.

Sometimes, it can feel like you are chasing the pieces around the little socket with the drill or elevator. The instruments seem to repel the tooth as though they have the same magnetic polarity. With sufficient finesse and patience, the pieces will come out. If the tooth pieces are too large to retrieve through the access, first consider sectioning the tooth into smaller pieces. The tooth must be pinned into a stable position to section it, otherwise it will just bobble around the bur. Using the bur, try to pin the piece back in its original position. This is often the most stable spot. Then, gently release the pressure on the bur to allow it to start spinning before cutting into the tooth. If the piece jumps around, you may be able to pin it in a different location. It also may be beneficial to enlarge the access, but this does sacrifice more bone and increase surgical injury. Remember, there needs to be a large enough access for both the instrument and the pieces. These can be tricky little buggers, but with a well thought out and executed technique (and a bit of experience), they become quite predictable.

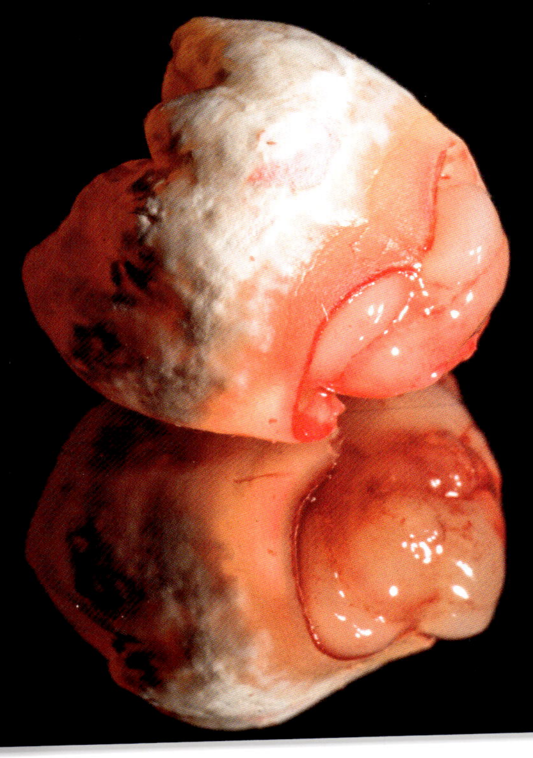

Figure 5-14 The matrix of the root structure is being laid down by the dental papilla and Hertwig's root sheath. Envisioning crown and root structure development informs the plan for removal. Although we don't routinely remove teeth at this early stage, factors such as unerupting second molars may be reason to do so.

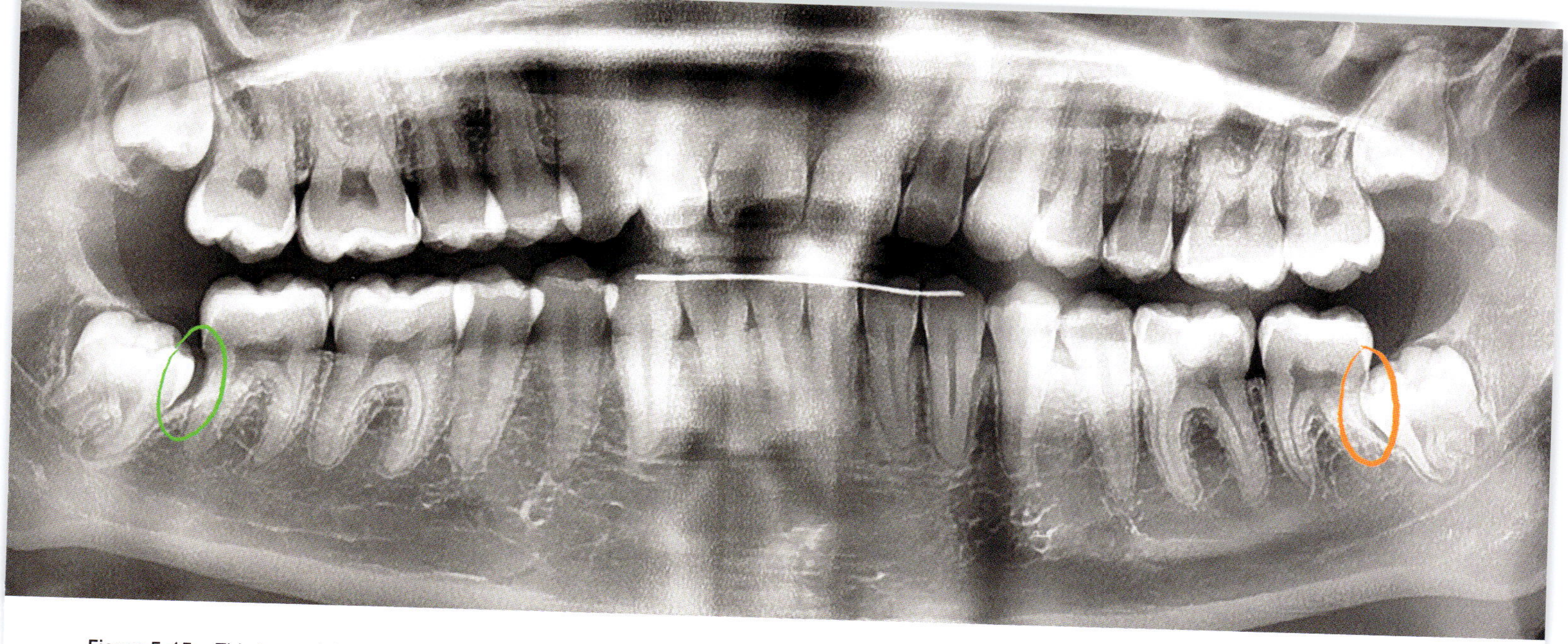

Figure 5-15 This lower right third molar (*green*) will likely be easier to remove than the lower left (*orange*) because of the space between it and the second molar. The right looks separated, and the left looks like it is overlapping. (Some of this perspective may be due to the angle of the panoramic radiograph, but I often find it predictive.)

Molar Proximity

Real estate is a main factor in removing lower third molars. When there is less room between the second molar and the ascending ramus, it is more difficult to develop the site and successfully remove the tooth. When the tooth is tucked in tight to the adjacent second molar, there is little to no space for an elevator or even a luxator to fit. Sometimes, you can sneak the fine tip of the Micro Buser or a slender luxator into this tight space to elevate the tooth. Be careful though. This is when instruments can break. There is nowhere for the crown of the tooth to move. The bone is very dense. The instrument is slender. A little too much force will break the tip, making the job significantly more challenging.

Picture the third molar's crown. Where does the tooth need to move? Up and back. So, there must be room for the elevator to fit below the height of contour on the crown's mesial. Clues on the radiograph can help plan for success. Look at the relationship between the two structures and picture where you will place the instrument and where the tooth needs to move.

Separated

There may naturally be adequate space for the elevator when the teeth are separated. As long as there is room for the tooth to move, bone removal and sectioning may not be necessary. This could be a pretty simple extraction with an elevator or luxator.

Nested

When the third molar crown is tucked under the height of contour of the second molar, bone must be removed more inferiorly and anteriorly to allow the elevator to be positioned under the height of contour of the tooth. This is relatively easy as the angulation of a surgical drill is in line with this area.

Intimate

If the teeth are in direct contact interproximally, great care must be taken to develop the access to protect the second molar. Consider creating a slightly more lateral path for extraction by sectioning the mesiolingual portion or removing the crown. This allows buccal positioning of the elevator as there is no space on the mesial. Cutting a buccal trough develops a lateral purchase point and space for the instrument.

Overlapped

If they are overlapped, the lower third molar is likely buccal to the second molar. Upper third molars may be buccal or palatal. The buccal trough can be extended around to the mesial of the tooth, avoiding the roots of the second molar. This usually becomes evident when developing the trough.

When the third molar appears overlapped radiographically, the mandible often flares significantly behind the second molar. This flared anatomy can occur without radiographic overlapping as well. Palpating the lingual aspect of the mandible in this area provides insight into the anatomy.

Patient Age

It is well documented that younger patients recover much better after impacted third molar removal[4,5]. Our inherent healing capacity dwindles as we age. Meanwhile, our alveolar bone becomes denser, more brittle and less vascular. Extraction techniques must be tailored accordingly.

Young bone is more pliable and forgiving. The socket expands easier and it can sustain significantly greater force before fracturing. A luxator may be able to do the work in a 15-year-old that would require a drill in a 40-year-old. In general, if a patient is older than 25, consider sectioning the tooth and removing a little more surrounding bone earlier in the process. I have a lower threshold for drilling in older patients. But older bone also tends to generate and retain more heat. Take it slow and keep it cool. It is worth the extra effort.

Oral Cavity

My grandpa taught me to set up my work environment for success. When I spent time with him as a young boy in his woodshop, we would turn on the bright lights, get all the materials for the bird house ready, and bring the step stool up to the workbench before any of the good stuff happened. We worked in his garage, not a mouth. In oral surgery, we are tasked with far greater environmental challenges than a well-organized woodshop. (I can only imagine how funny it would look trying to build a birdhouse if we had a big tongue and floppy cheeks with stringy saliva all over the place, working under the workbench with no space or light.)

Sometimes, a procedure that should be so simple is terribly frustrating and takes way longer just because of the work environment in the oral cavity. If we could do our work on a bench top, like in the prosthodontic lab in dental school, everything would be easier and much more predictable. The fact is, we can't remove the tongue, cheeks or the patient's gag reflex before removing the tooth.

We can be intentional about ensuring we have optimized the lighting, tongue and cheek retraction, and other patient factors throughout the procedure. For instance, if the throat pack becomes saturated or is obstructing the view, replace it. Placing an isolation device, like a throat pack or pharyngeal curtain, is non-negotiable. It is a standard of care. At any time, the tooth could fracture or a segment could launch into the abyss behind the tongue. Protecting the airway must always be top priority. If the gauze is soggy and crowding the drill, replace it with a fresh piece. The pharyngeal curtain and tongue retractor also help protect the patient from inadvertent injury if an elevator or drill should slip.

Bottom line, sometimes the oral cavity can make a simple case very challenging. Use a well-positioned tongue retractor over the pharyngeal curtain, a Minnesota cheek retractor (not a dental mirror) and a good surgical light. (Sometimes it feels like a bull ride, like you are just trying to make it all 8 seconds.)

Table 5-2 Factors making extraction easier and harder

	Easier	Harder
Angulation	Vertical or mesioangular	Distoangular, buccolingual or inverted
Impaction depth	Shallow	Deep
Bone density	Soft and malleable	Dense and unforgiving
Follicle size	Large	Non-existent
Root formation	1/3-2/3	Closed apex
Root shape	Conical	Severely curved
Molar proximity	Spacious	Tight
Patient age	15-25 years	Older than 25 years
Oral cavity	Generous and accessible	Overcrowded and active

Soft Tissue Management

Managing the soft tissue is the first act of surgery. There must be an adequate passageway developed to access and deliver the tooth. Soft tissue can stretch some, but bear in mind there is a limit to how much the tissue will give before being harmed. A torn flap is messy and painful, but it happens at times. When a tooth is partially erupted, it can be tempting to begin elevating before adequately addressing the soft tissue. It can look like it will pop out. An incision may not be necessary, but should always be considered. This happens more often in the maxilla than the mandible. **Attend to each step, though at times, each step needn't be taken**.

It seems to me the periosteum in the maxilla is more forgiving than in the mandible. For that matter, the maxilla overall is generally more forgiving than the mandible when it comes to extractions. Periosteum is tough and relatively immobile. It must be definitively incised or reflected for safe and effective manipulation. The overlying connective tissue and mucosa is much more flexible than the periosteum. The dense periosteum is the limiting factor in flap mobilization. If a full thickness incision is made perpendicular to the bone, the connective tissue and epithelium can be mobilized much more than the periosteum. When passing the blade through the superficial tissue, extend it a bit to make the periosteal incision slightly longer. This provides improved access and decreases complications and post-operative pain.

Flaps provide the access for surgery. They are a means to an end. They are part of the surgery, but they are not the purpose of the surgery. Not all flaps are equal. Some need to completely expose the surgical site, allowing access and visualization for bone removal and sectioning. And sometimes they simply need to provide a passage for a tooth to be delivered, like a trap door.

The incision sets the stage for the flap. To be effective, it must be well designed and completely through the periosteum along the entire incision. It can be helpful to think about cutting all the way to the bone when you're making an incision. This will help ensure a full thickness cut. In areas where the periosteum was not adequately incised, either the surrounding tissue will tear, or the dissection plane will become supraperiosteal or partial thickness. In either case, the flap is more difficult to manage and tissue trauma is increased. The incision should be performed with a decisive and steady hand. Picture the blade passing completely through all layers of the soft tissue including the dense tissue of the periosteum all the way to the surface of the underlying bone. Full thickness.

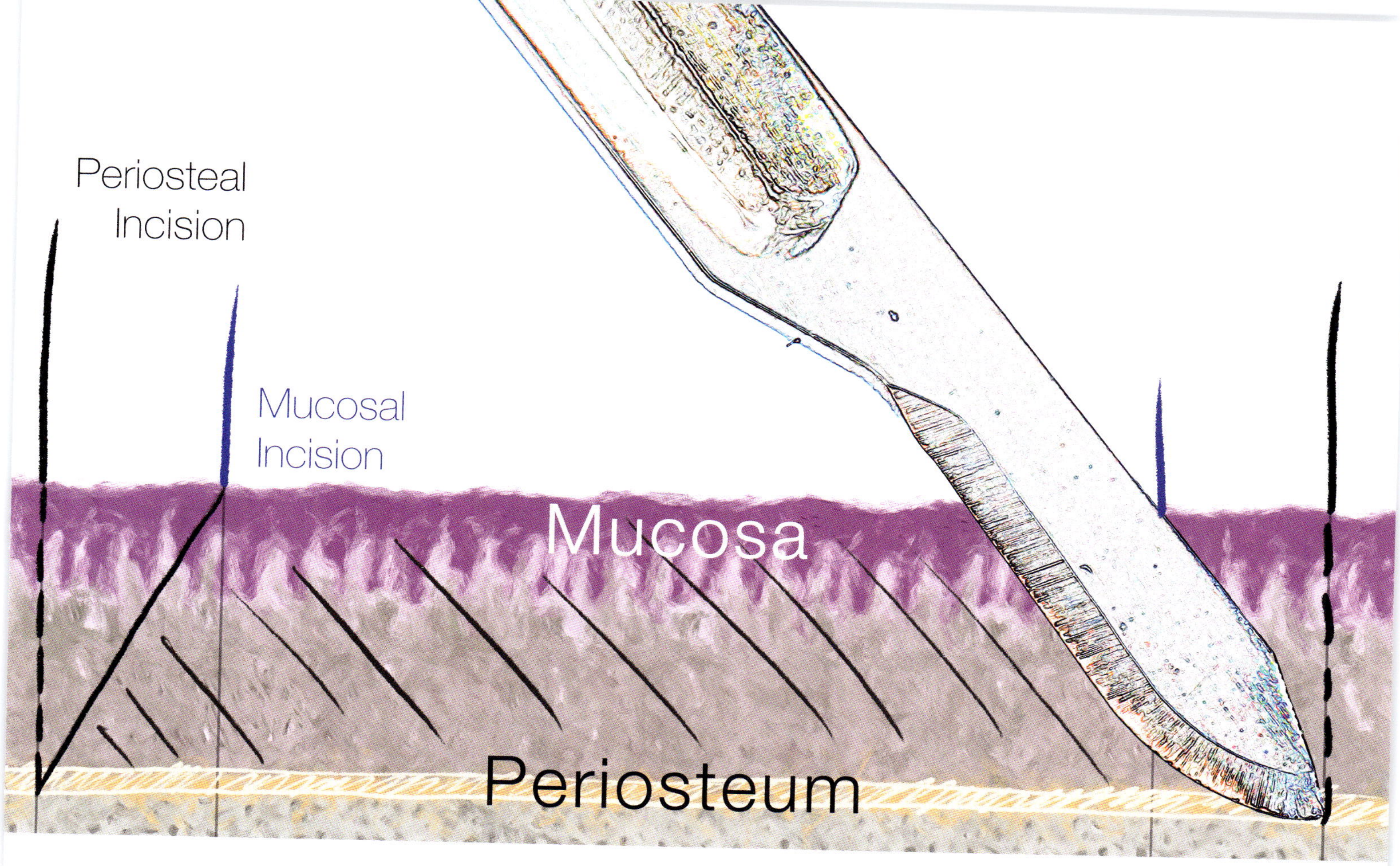

Figure 5-16 Extending the periosteal incision farther than the mucosal incision increases the access of a flap. The periosteum is much less flexible than the mucosa, so the periosteal incision must be longer to achieve the same exposure.

Flap design

When something has been extensively researched and published, it is usually very important and/or controversial. Surgical flap design is one such thing[6,7]. The flap directly impacts access to the site and tissue manipulation. It also directly impacts the recovery process. There are countless variations of intricate flaps that have been described for different surgical procedures: full thickness, split thickness, rotational, tunneling. Flap design can get quite creative. For removing impacted teeth, the flap is relatively simple, and is always full thickness. With one general incision line, the envelope flap is the simplest. It is a workhorse in oral surgery. When more exposure is needed, a releasing incision can be added on one or both ends of the flap, greatly increasing exposure. Flap design will depend primarily on the position of the impacted tooth. If a tooth appears to be a more challenging extraction, consider a more generous flap vertically as well as possibly extending it one or two teeth mesial to the extraction site. Fighting for exposure can turn an operative challenge into a miserable battle.

A mathematical argument for a shorter incision could be made. Fewer traumatized cells = less recovery. On my general surgery rotation during residency, I was taught long incisions heal as fast as short incisions. This principle is taught because a shorter incision can result in increased tissue trauma from retracting more forcefully while fighting for access instead of just starting with a longer incision. But an incision that is longer than necessary will hurt more and increase inflammation. In the mandible, for example, extending the incision distally results

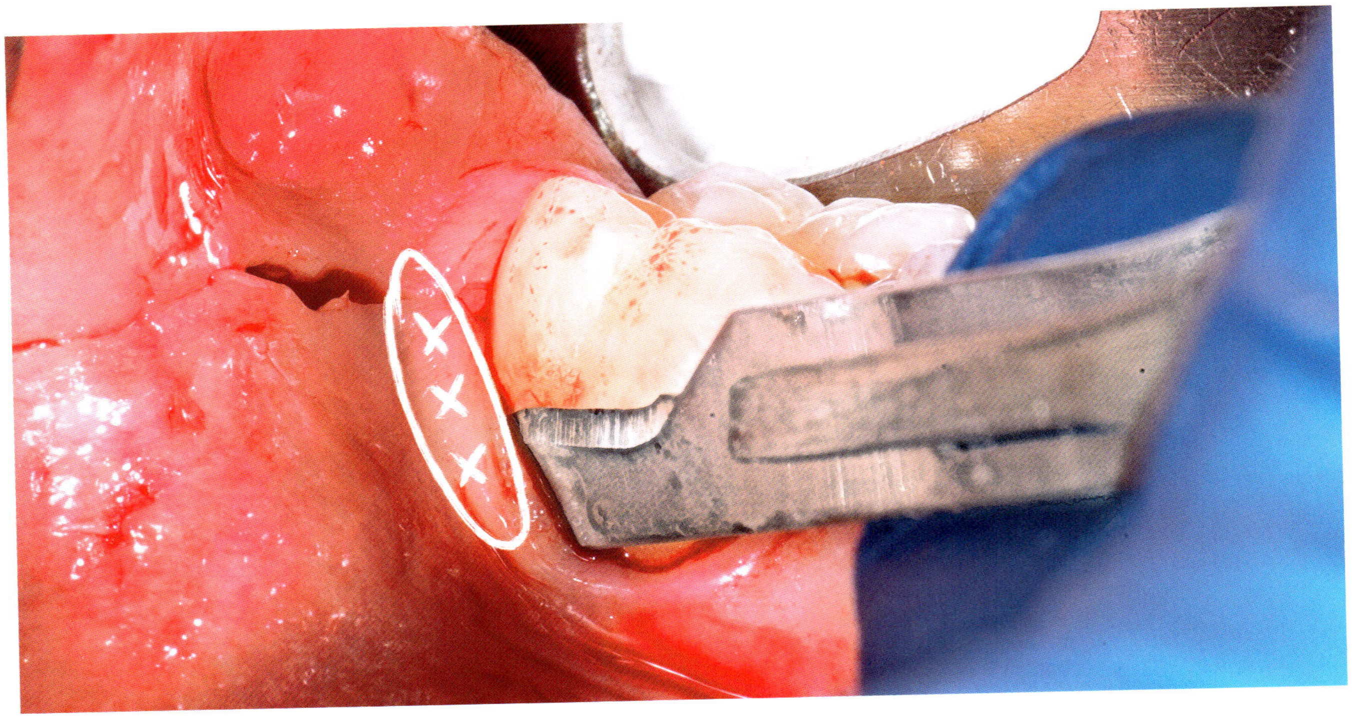

Figure 5-17 The point where the follicle of the impacted tooth meets the periosteum is the most tenacious tissue. This needs to be sharply dissected to protect the less durable overlying mucosa from tearing when reflecting the flap.

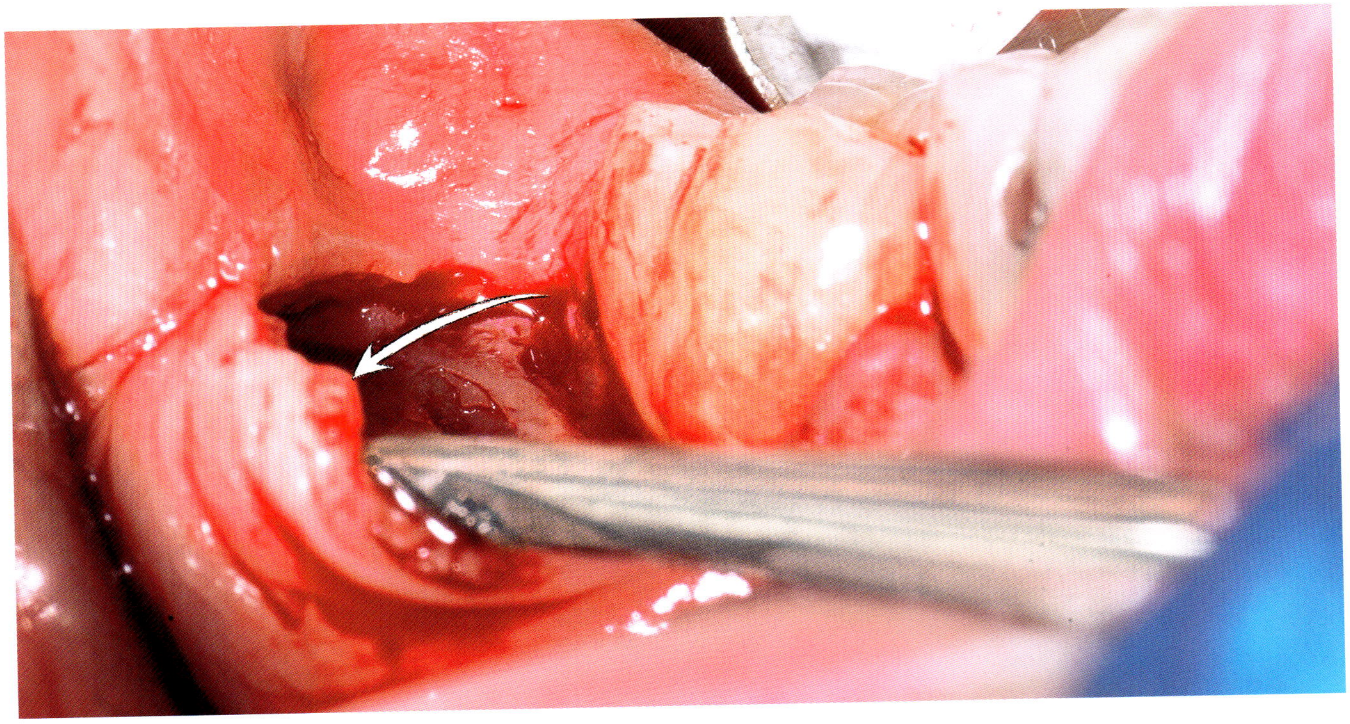

Figure 5-18 Make sure to get under the periosteum right at the corner. When this is reflected, the rest of the flap usually reflects easily.

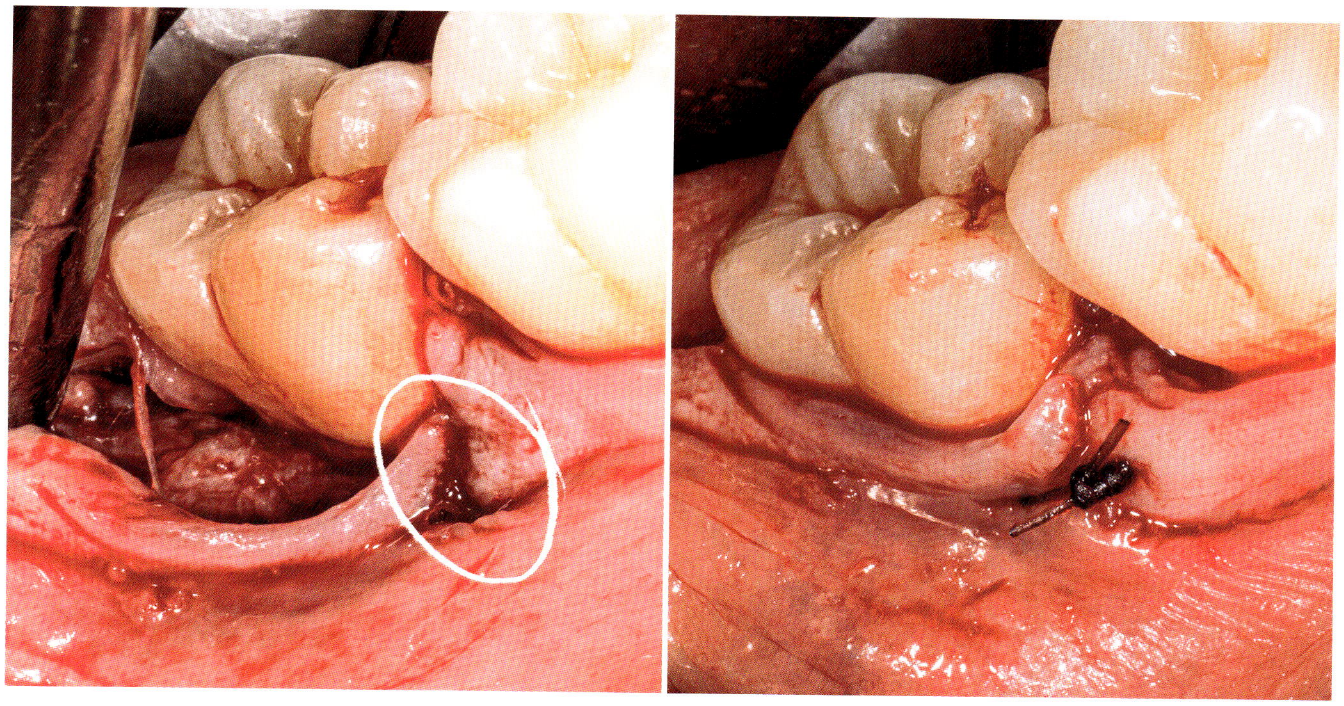

Figure 5-19 Gingiva doesn't stretch. A small tear in the buccal tissue usually can be avoided by developing an adequate flap. It still may tear from retraction during the extraction. This can be easily repaired with a single resorbable suture.

in greater trauma to the muscles of mastication. This leads to increased pain and trismus. Longer incisions also may require more sutures, adding to surgical time. Make sure the incision is long enough to safely access the site, but be prudent, knowing you might be causing further harm if it gets too long.

Periosteum

In my mind, the periosteum is the MVP in third molar healing. It has an incredible combination of blood supply, innervation and regenerative potential. Its blood supply nourishes the area. The osteogenic cells stimulate and directly act to heal. And the innervation directly influences post-operative pain. But it will turn against you if it's not treated with proper respect and care. The blood supply, surrounded by dense tissue, can become compromised and run dry if damaged. The innervation will revolt if macerated, and the cells responsible for stimulating new bone formation may be so tattered they recruit fibrous tissue instead.

Periosteum is composed of three main layers. The outer fibrous layer is mainly collagen fibrils. Most cells and osteogenic potential are located within the inner layer, which directly lines the bone. And the middle portion houses most of the vasculature. In total, it is less than 100 microns thick. But this thin tissue holds the keys to the kingdom of impacted exodontia. Through it, we access the underlying teeth and bone. Without its allegiance, the potential for healing is dismal[8,9].

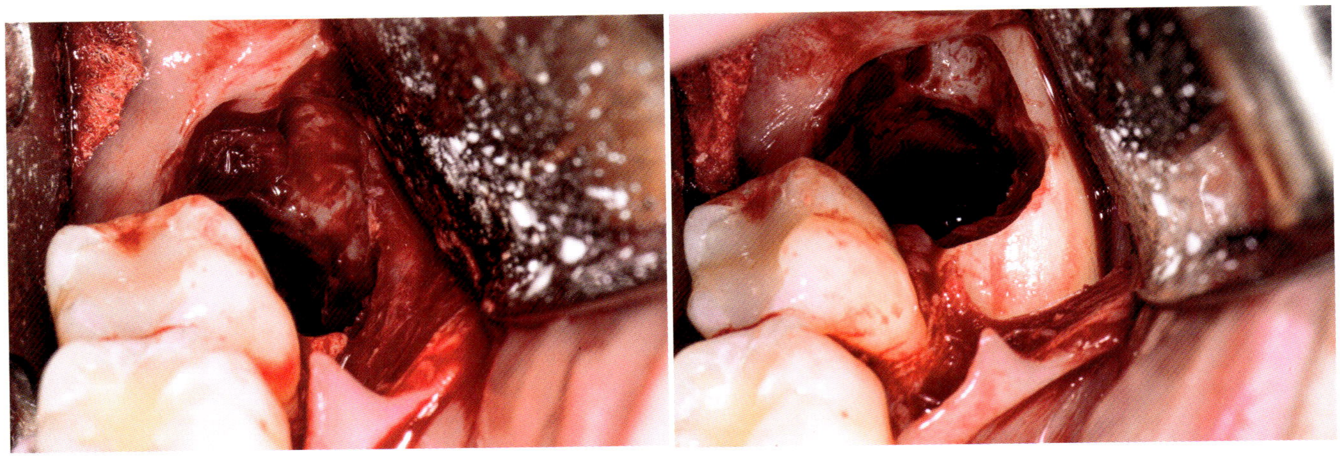

Figure 5-20 Protect the periosteum. It is easy for the tissue to slip under the retractor and get pinched between the bone (*left*). The tip of the retractor should be maintained on bone throughout the procedure to keep the tissue retracted and protected (*right*).

Maxillary third molars

Impacted upper third molars have a remarkable tendency to travel posterior and superior when elevating. It is almost like they are inherently attracted to the infratemporal fossa, which is a dangerous place for a tooth to go. This risk can be mitigated through incision design, retractor position and elevating forces.

When the tooth is elevated, the periosteum can capture it if the incision isn't long enough or if the incision isn't completely through the periosteum. The tooth will move out of the bone but stay under the periosteum and slide right up into the infratemporal fossa. Make sure the incision is full-thickness and that it extends far enough up the tuberosity. When a tooth is palatally inclined, the incision may swing more palatal, but the best access is routinely going to be from the distobuccal. When the impacted tooth is high, it also may be necessary to reflect the papilla between the first and second molar, or even place a vertical release at the distobuccal line angle of the first. The vertical release should be made mesial to the papilla, including the papilla in the flap. This improves flap mobility during surgery and makes suturing easier. A single stitch in the papilla may be enough. If the vertical incision is still gaping open, suturing the papilla first lines the tissue and helps stabilize it while suturing the vertical incision.

The Minnesota cheek retractor can help divert the tooth away from the infratemporal fossa and out into the mouth. Firmly position it in the vestibule between the extraction site and the fossa. Don't push too hard. The tip of the retractor can damage the tissue. While retracting, elevate the tooth down and out. If it feels like the tooth is moving up, change the elevator angle or the rotation. As the tooth moves, watch the tissue. If it is moving a lot but you can't see it, it may be moving toward the infratemporal fossa. If the soft tissue on the lateral aspect begins to bulge outward, you run the risk of tearing the flap. While it is often impossible to see the tooth until it is out, pay attention and look for clues on how and where it is moving. Sometimes, the flap needs to be extended or developed more. Other times, some bone removal is needed to get a purchase point or to guide the tooth into the mouth.

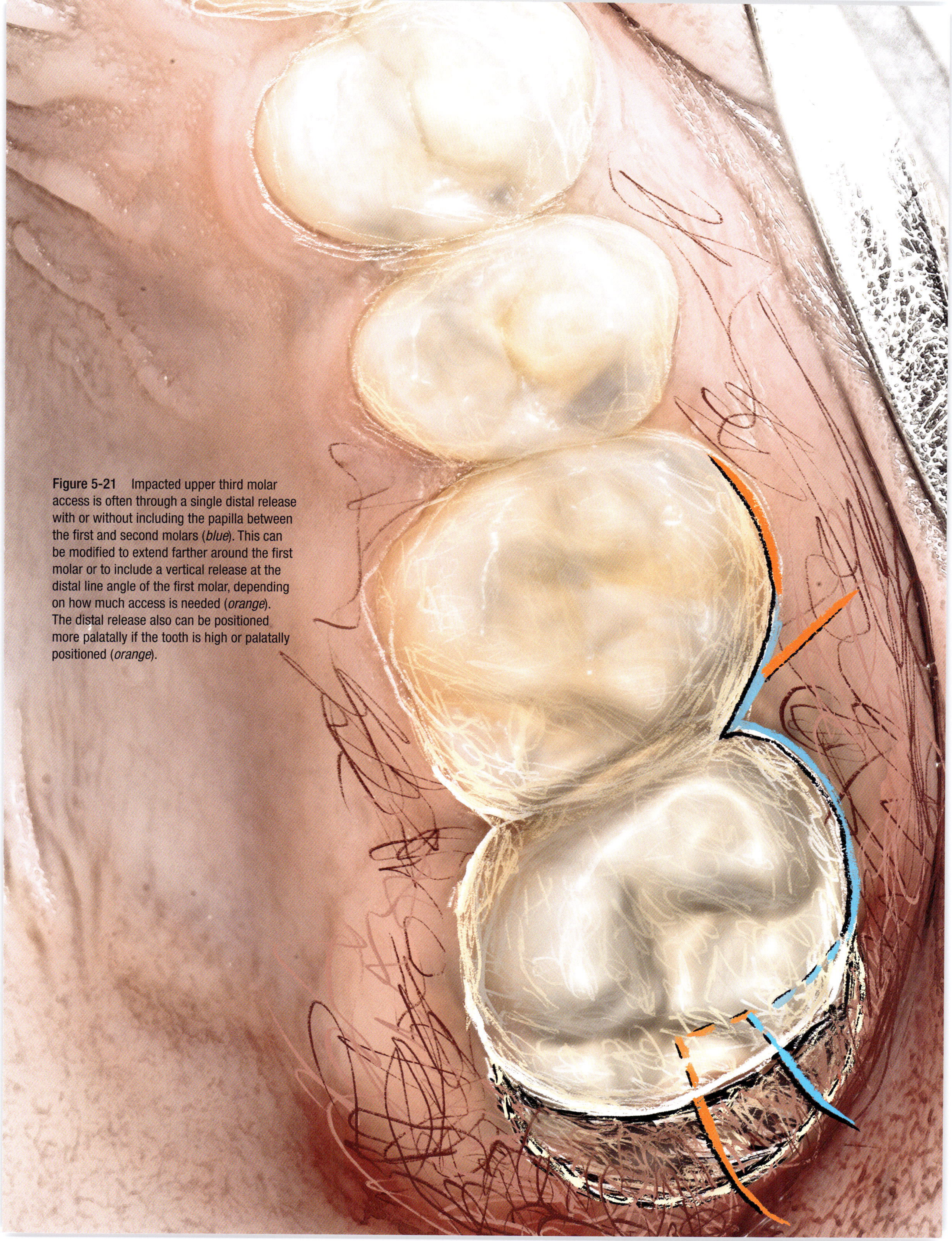

Figure 5-21 Impacted upper third molar access is often through a single distal release with or without including the papilla between the first and second molars (*blue*). This can be modified to extend farther around the first molar or to include a vertical release at the distal line angle of the first molar, depending on how much access is needed (*orange*). The distal release also can be positioned more palatally if the tooth is high or palatally positioned (*orange*).

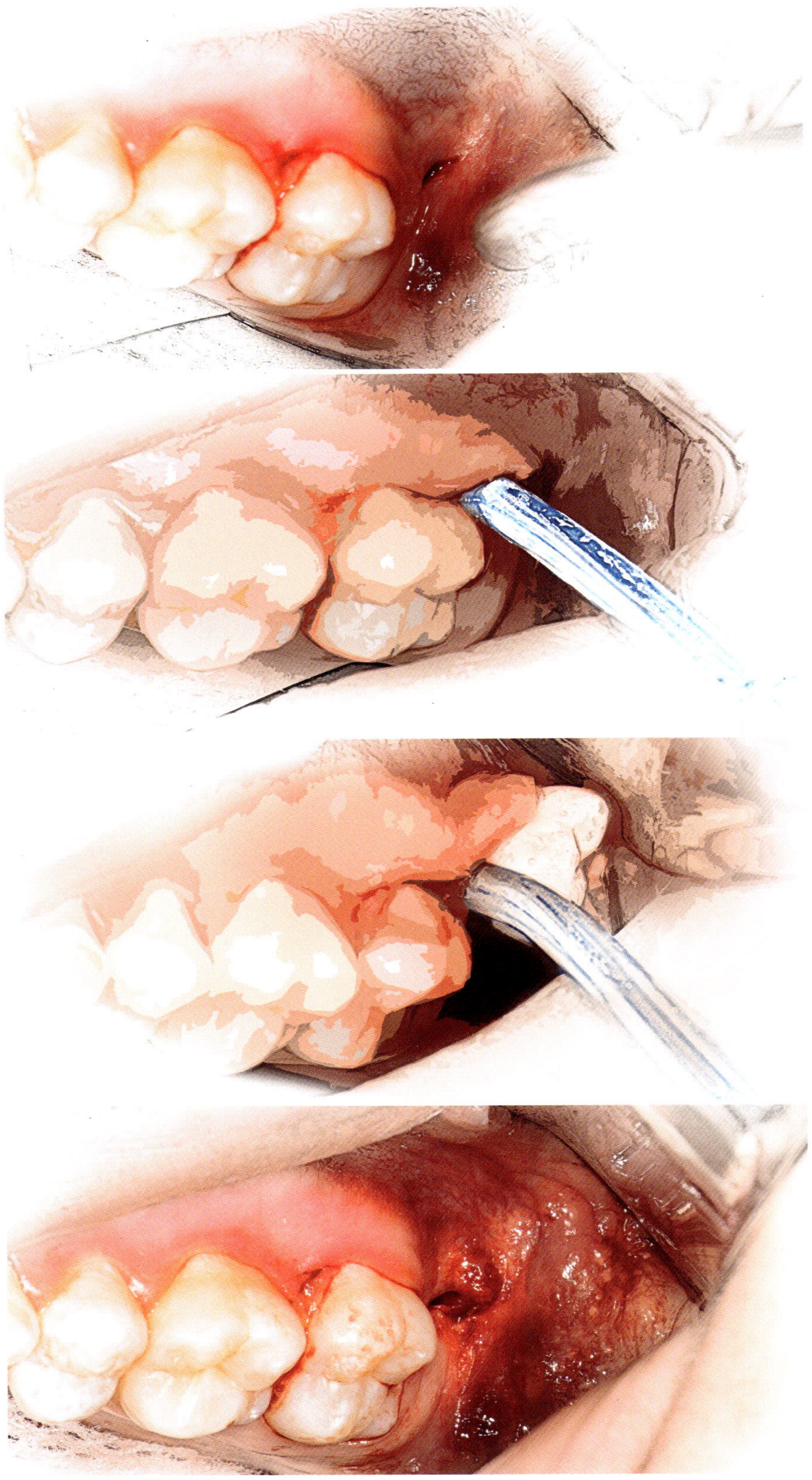

Figure 5-22 Distal incision provides access to an impacted upper third molar. A small elevator was used to mobilize the tooth and deliver it through the incision with minimal soft tissue elevation. The tissue stretches some but sustains limited trauma.

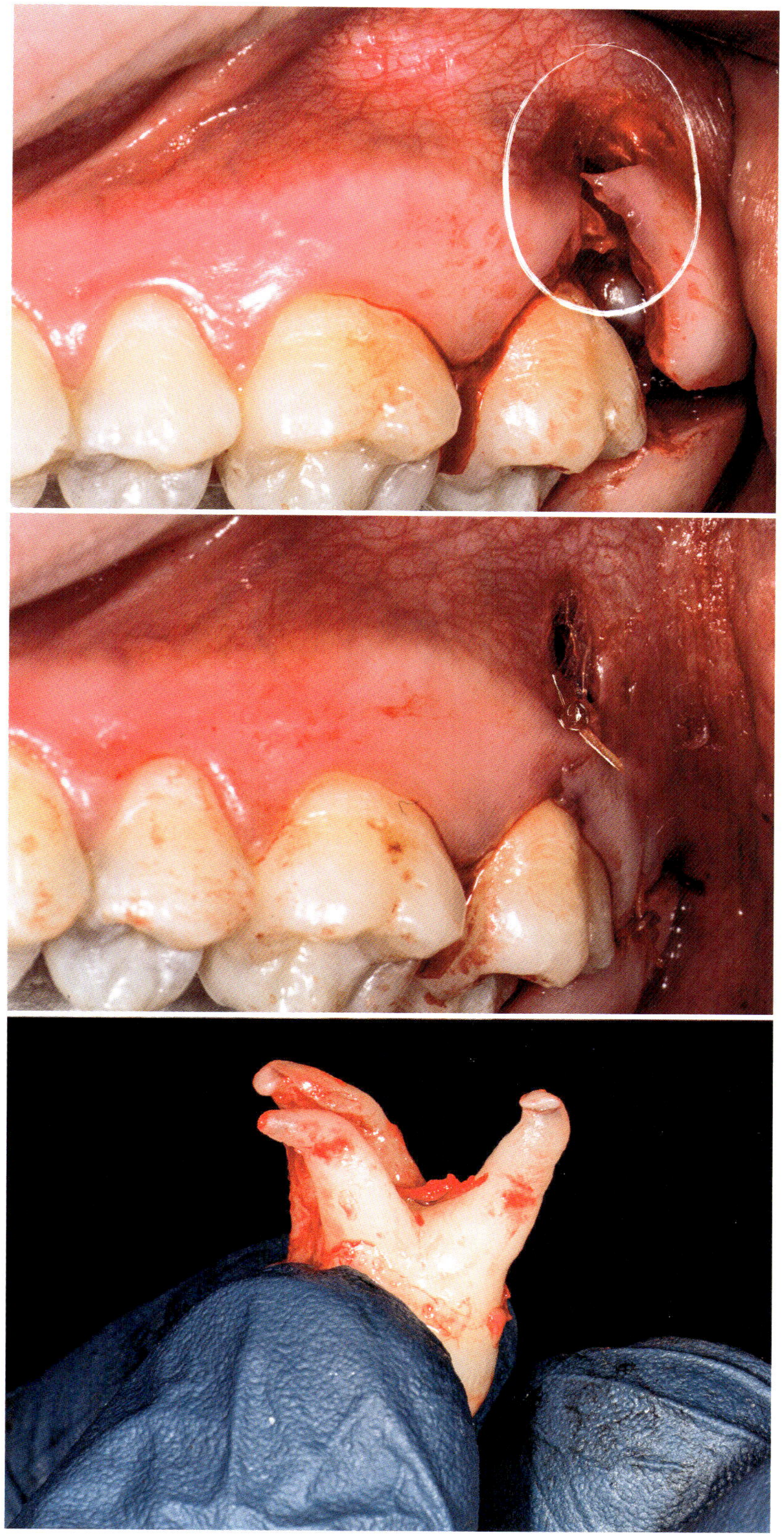

Figure 5-23 The tissue can tear if it is not adequately released or reflected before removing the tooth. The crown can get caught under the periosteum and unintentionally tear the buccal tissue. This takes extra time in surgery to suture and prolongs recovery. Note the torn tissue appears friable and may not need to be reapproximated completely. When the retraction is released, this tissue will fall into place nicely (*middle*). This tooth had flared roots, which contributed to the risk of tearing the tissue (*lower*).

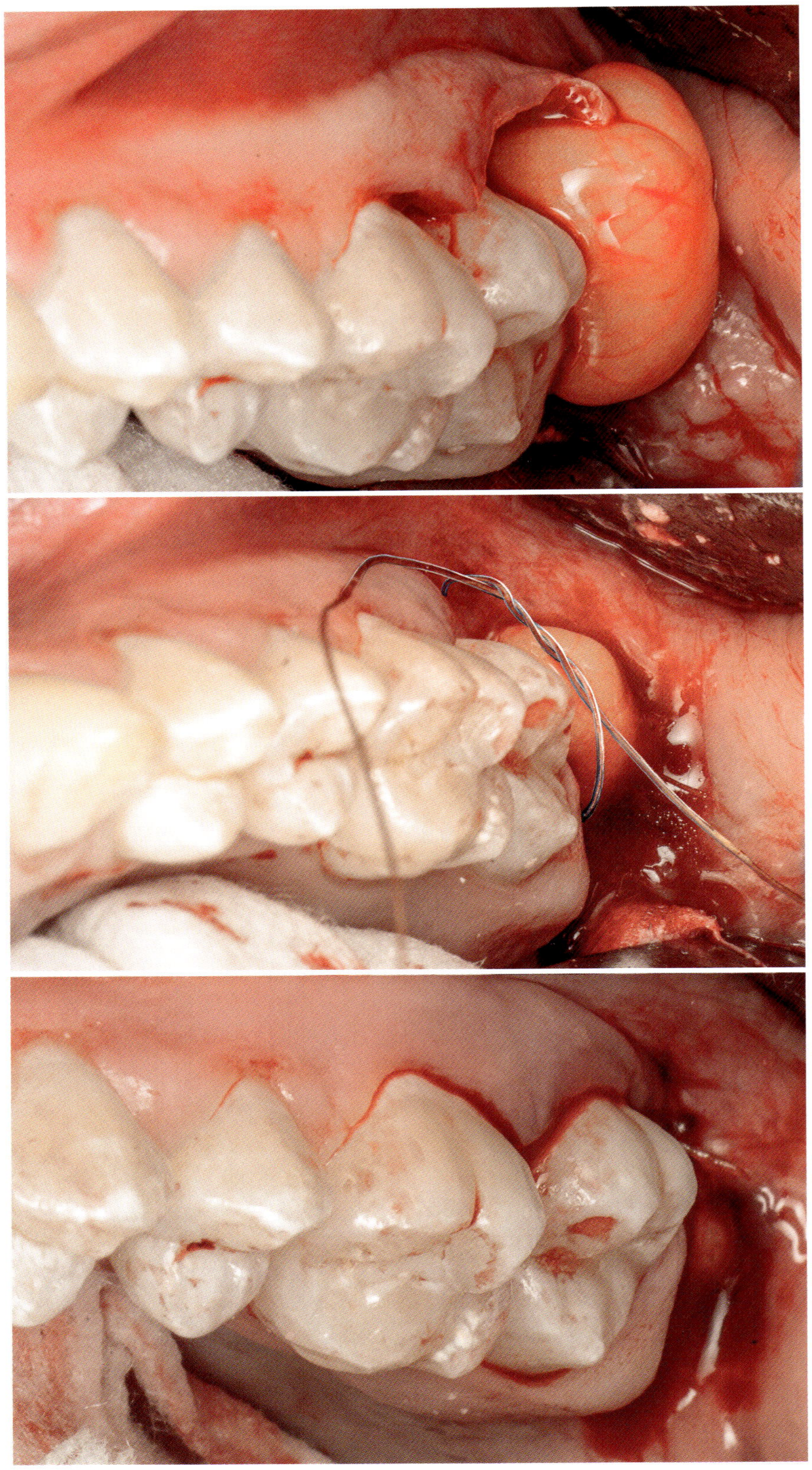

Figure 5-24 The fat pad sometimes pops out right away before you even elevate the tissue. In this case, the retractor restrained the fat pad until the extraction was complete. It was then secured with a single resorbable stitch.

Buccal fat pad

The buccal fat pad is an unwelcome visitor that comes unannounced and crowds the space. It is just beyond the periosteum, toward the superior and lateral aspect of the maxillary tuberosity. It is almost like it is under pressure, being held captive by the periosteum. Sometimes it tries to escape with the smallest access. It must be managed immediately. If not, it will continue to push out more and more.

Buccal fat pad management:
1. Minimize exposure.
2. Reduce the tissue.
3. Retain the tissue.

Minimize exposure

The buccal fat pad is directly in line with the typical upper third molar incision. The higher and deeper the incision, the more likely it is to be involved. But remember, the risk of displacing the tooth into the infratemporal fossa increases with a smaller incision. It is a balance. Part of the artistry.

Avoid liposuction. Fatty tissue seems to have a terribly high attraction to a suction cannula. A small amount of exposed fat can turn into a huge blob in an instant if it connects with the suction tip. The assistant will not be able to see this transpire until it is too late and the fat is herniating into the site. Let your assistant know you see the fat popping to avoid further exposure.

Reduce the tissue

Tuck it in. The fat pad can be tucked back in with a periosteal elevator, hemostat, or any other instrument able to push it back into where it came from. This can be very tricky when a large portion of the fat is herniated.

The fat pad can be so boisterous at times that it can't easily be put back into place and a portion of it may need to be removed. When this is the case, carefully stabilize the fat with tissue forceps or a hemostat, but avoid pulling on it. Tugging on the fat pad will entice more to herniate. The goal is to remove enough so the rest can be tucked back in. A portion can then be excised with scissors, scalpel or laser.

Restrain the tissue

When the fat is tucked back in, it may be temporarily restrained with a retractor or more permanently with a suture. Simply retracting the fat pad may be sufficient if the surgery is almost done and if the fat seems to be cooperating. Otherwise, a resorbable suture at the site of exposure may be well worth the effort. Struggling with a herniated buccal fat pad can be exacerbating and time consuming.

Mandibular third molars

Incision

One of the main concerns unique to mandibular third molar incision design is the lingual nerve. It is generally lingual to the mandible in this area. But it is above the bone sometimes. The design of a distobuccal releasing incision allows adequate access to the surgical site while respecting the danger zone distal and lingual to the second molar. It has been described as a hockey stick incision because of the shape.

The best place to make the distobuccal incision is an area between the insertion of the temporalis and buccinator. This helps reduce the pain and bleeding from cutting muscle. To identify the site, place some tension on the tissue with the Minnesota retractor. The whitish area is your guide to where the incision goes.

Reflecting the tissue can be quite challenging if it has not been sufficiently incised, especially at the junction of the periosteum and the follicle of an impacted tooth. If the flap is not elevating easily, it

Figure 5-25 Applying tension with the Minnesota retractor can help identify the best place for the incision.

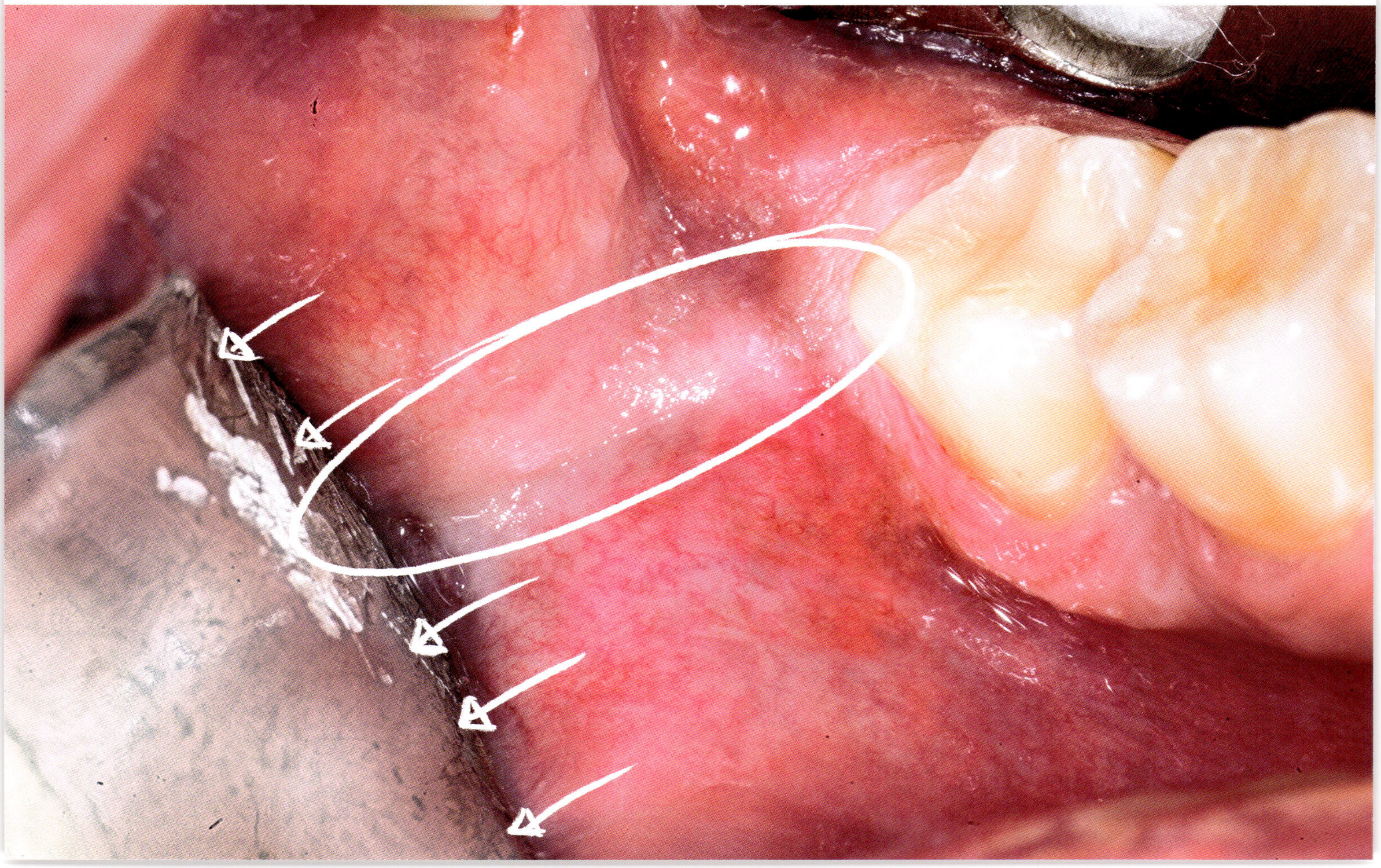

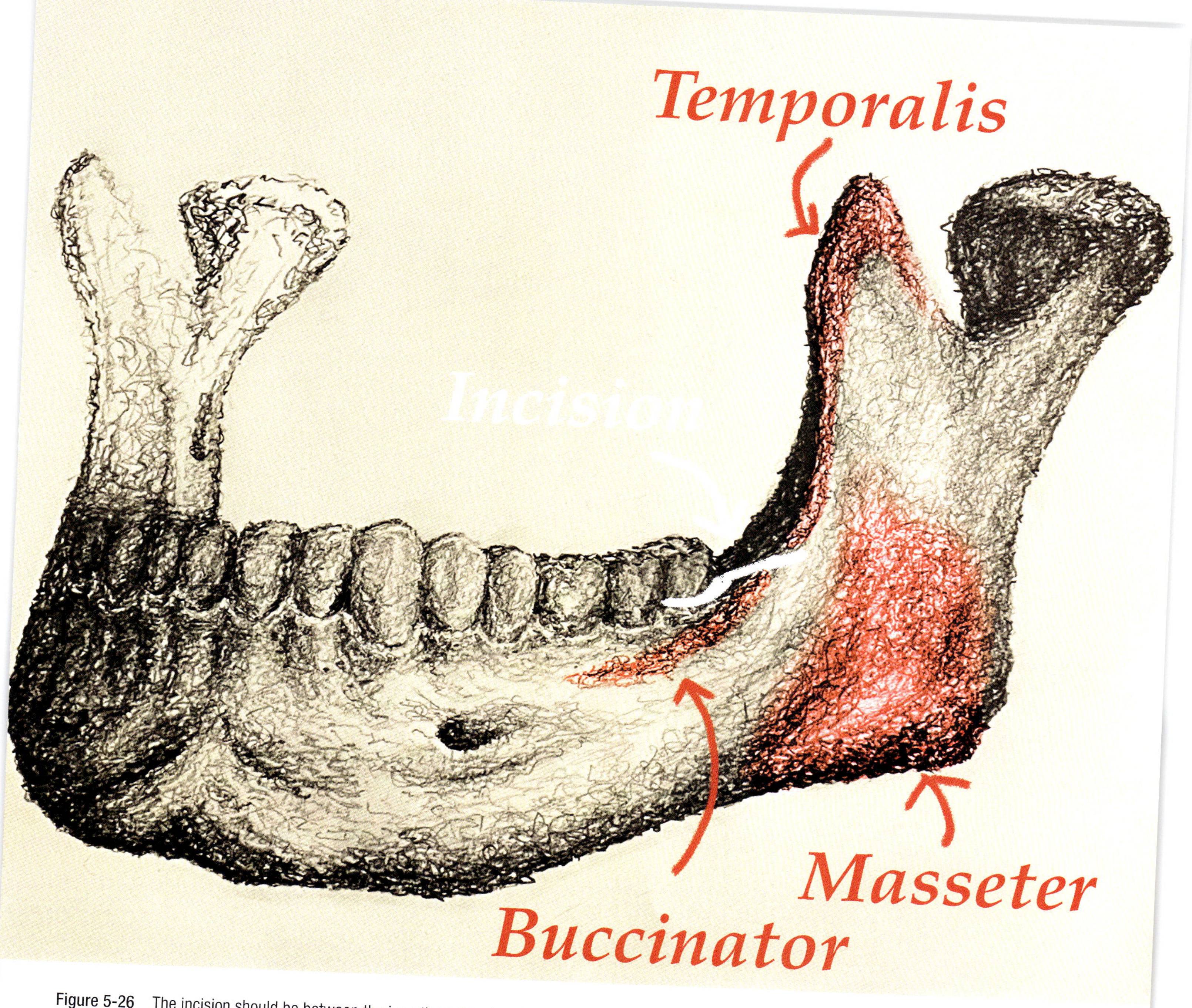

Figure 5-26 The incision should be between the insertion of the buccinator and temporalis to reduce pain, inflammation, bleeding and trismus. (Artwork inspired by Leonardo da Vinci.)

is often because of intact periosteum. Try retracting the tissue with the tip of the Minnesota retractor to identify the tissue that is holding on. While under tension, use the scalpel to release the tissue that is holding on. This seems to be especially helpful at the follicle-bone interface. A little work with a blade can go a long way toward making your job easier.

Be on the lookout for a small perforating vessel when elevating the flap. You may be able to work around it. Or you may choose to cauterize it, put a stitch in the soft tissue, or crush the bone around it to improve hemostasis. These small vessels can slow surgery down and cause issues post-operatively.

Mandible shape

Mandible shape varies significantly around third molars. It can generally be described as V or U shaped when looking in the axial plane. The amount of flare behind the second molars can be quite impressive. This can impact the potential lingual nerve position, lingual plate thickness and lateral positioning of the impacted tooth.

Lingual nerve location → **Incise buccally, elevate cautiously, drill skillfully**.

The lingual nerve has been shown to be in contact with the lingual plate of the mandible in 25% to 62% of patients studied and above the alveolar crest in 10% to 17%. It was all the way up in the retromolar region 0.15%[10–12]. Most of the studies reference the position of the nerve in relation to the mandible. When the mandible curves out sharply, the lingual nerve could be even more lateral relative to the second molar. Thus, the incision must be more buccal to avoid the nerve. With a less-flared mandible, the incision may more safely favor the distal of the second molar, improving access to the tooth. Caution is key.

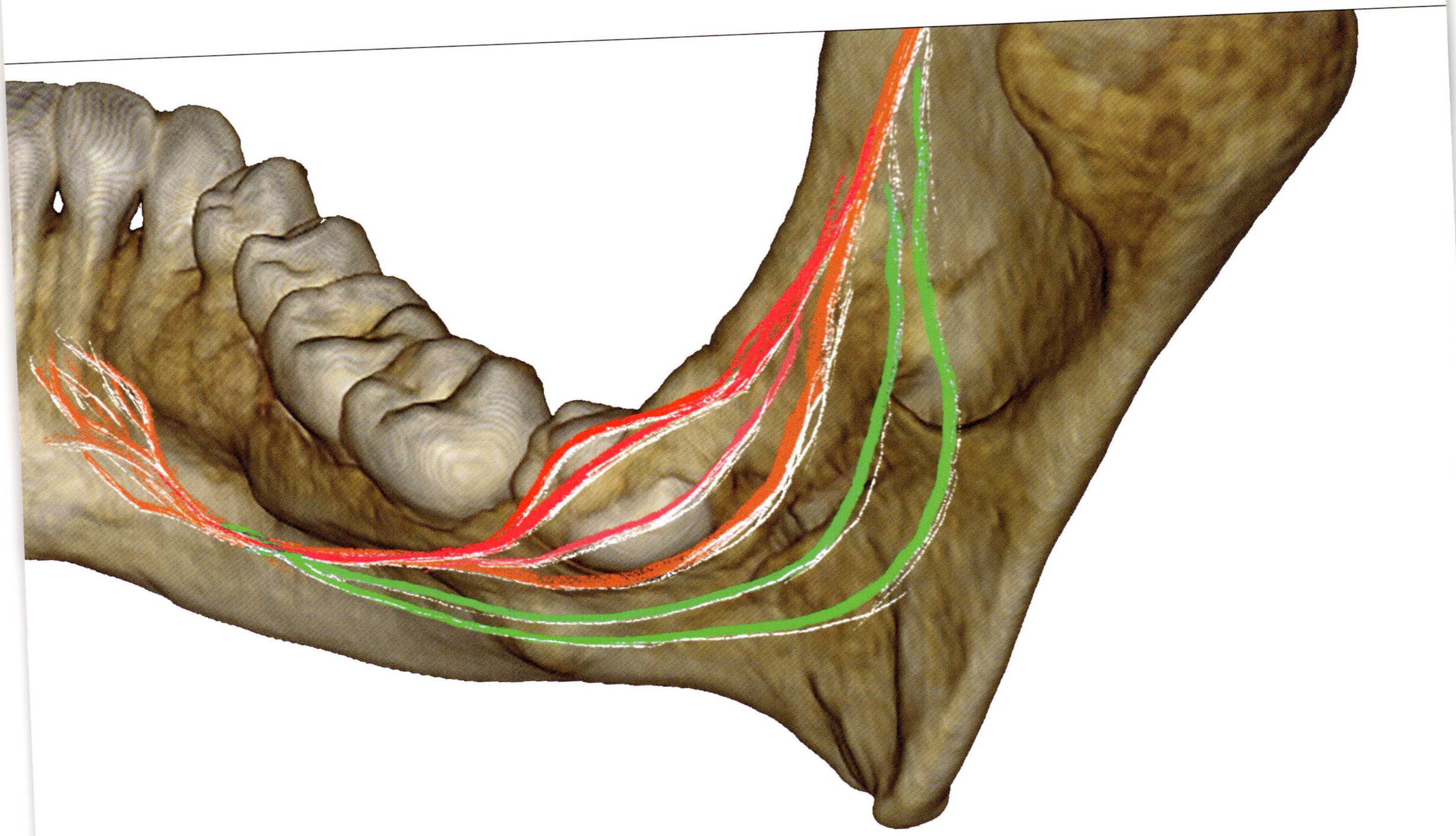

Figure 5-27 The lingual nerve can travel above the alveolar crest, directly over an impacted lower third molar. Great caution should be exercised to avoid damaging the nerve when incising, reflecting, drilling and elevating.

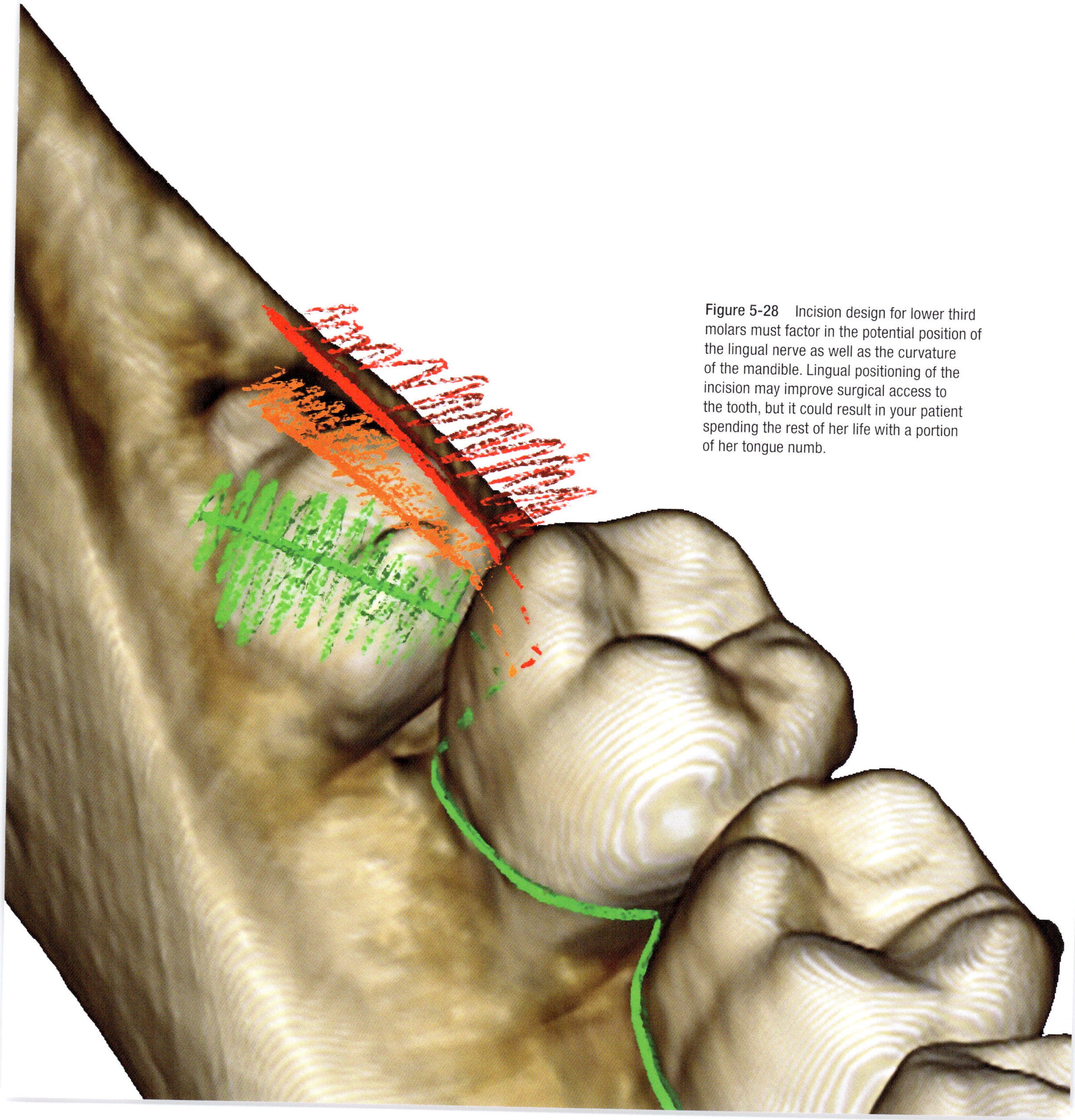

Figure 5-28 Incision design for lower third molars must factor in the potential position of the lingual nerve as well as the curvature of the mandible. Lingual positioning of the incision may improve surgical access to the tooth, but it could result in your patient spending the rest of her life with a portion of her tongue numb.

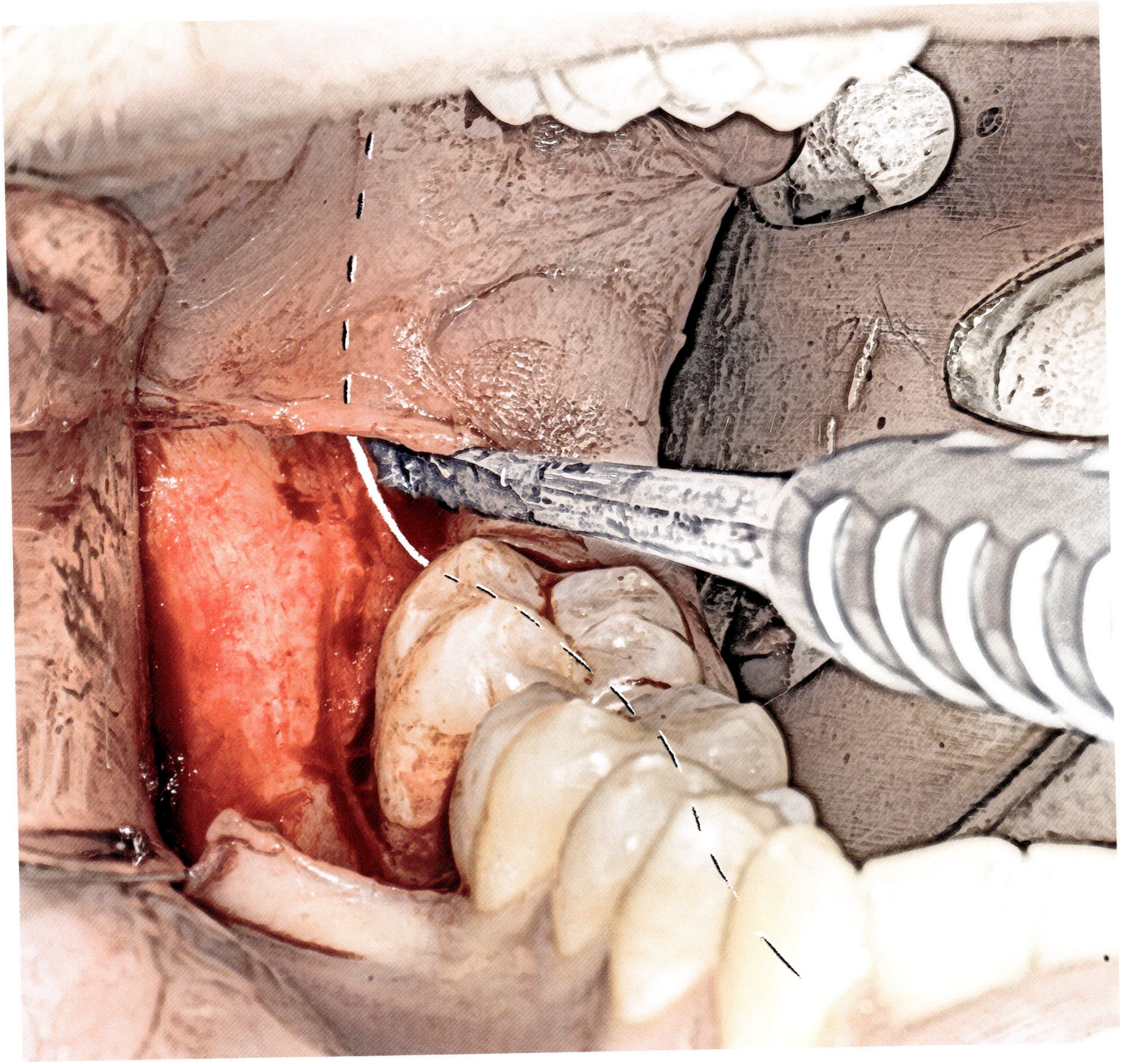

Figure 5-29 With the lingual tissue retracted, you can see how flared the mandible is here. It is almost in line with the buccal aspect of the second molar.

Lateral position of the tooth → **retract adequately**. The impacted third molar may have a more lateral position when the mandible is flared. In this case, access is optimized when the soft tissue flap is reflected, exposing the external oblique ridge and slightly down the lateral aspect of the mandible. This protects the soft tissue as the drill is more likely to pass outside the protection of the bone when developing the distal portion of the trough.

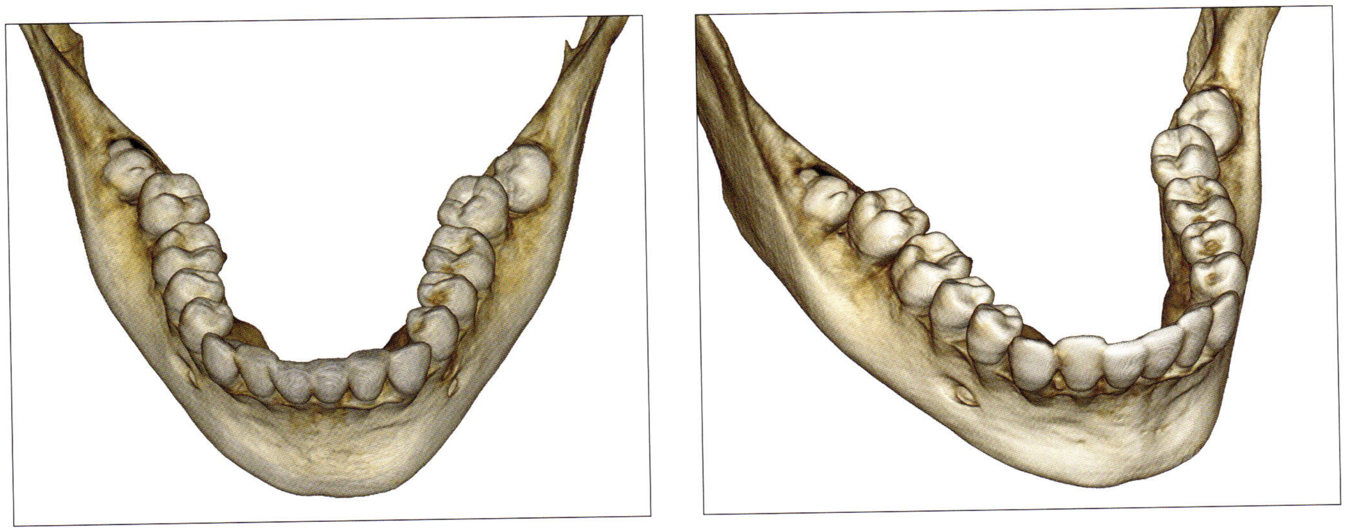

Figure 5-30 Lower third molars are often more lateral than the adjacent second molars. This is amplified when there is a flared mandible. The purpose of the incision and flap development is to access the underlying tooth. When the tooth is more lateral, the incision also should be more lateral and the flap may extend more toward the buccal.

Lower third molar tips:

- Incise buccally.
- Elevate cautiously.
- Drill discerningly.
- Retract adequately.

Tissue closure

The oral cavity is a unique surgical ecosystem. Open wounds are left to heal by secondary intention whenever teeth exfoliate or are removed. This contradicts the general surgical principle of passive primary closure, which is often unnecessary and may even be detrimental in the oral cavity. There are times, such as in some grafting procedures, sinus closures, or orthognathic surgery, when passive watertight closure is critical. But for routine extractions, even impacted extractions, it may cause more harm than good.

The way I see it, the tissue must be stable enough to heal but loose enough to negotiate the wet and dirty environment. It must be reapproximated well enough to know how to heal. It cannot be left blowing in the breeze. (It is similar to raising children. They need enough guidance to know how to succeed, but not so much that they can't.) I think primary closure can sometimes entrap what the body needs to get out. This can be food debris or even debris from the healing tissue.

When suturing a flap for third molars, I want to guide the tissue to heal. This may involve suturing a papilla when it is reflected. When a typical distobuccal incision is made for lower third molars, the most important thing is to restore underlying muscle fibers. This is often at the middle or toward the end of the release. Muscles complain when they are injured. A single suture approximating the muscular component of the distobuccal incision will often satisfy the blurry balance between tissue approximation and the ability to adapt during healing.

Eye opener. I recently read a study that compared suturing third molar sites with excising a wedge of tissue and leaving it open. The short-term results favored the tissue excision while the long-term results were inconclusive[13]. This isn't to say you should bail on suturing and leave it all to heal however it may. But it should make us stop and think about why we do what we do and how we can improve upon it. This sometimes takes the shape of new and more elaborate techniques and sometimes it means pursuing greater simplicity.

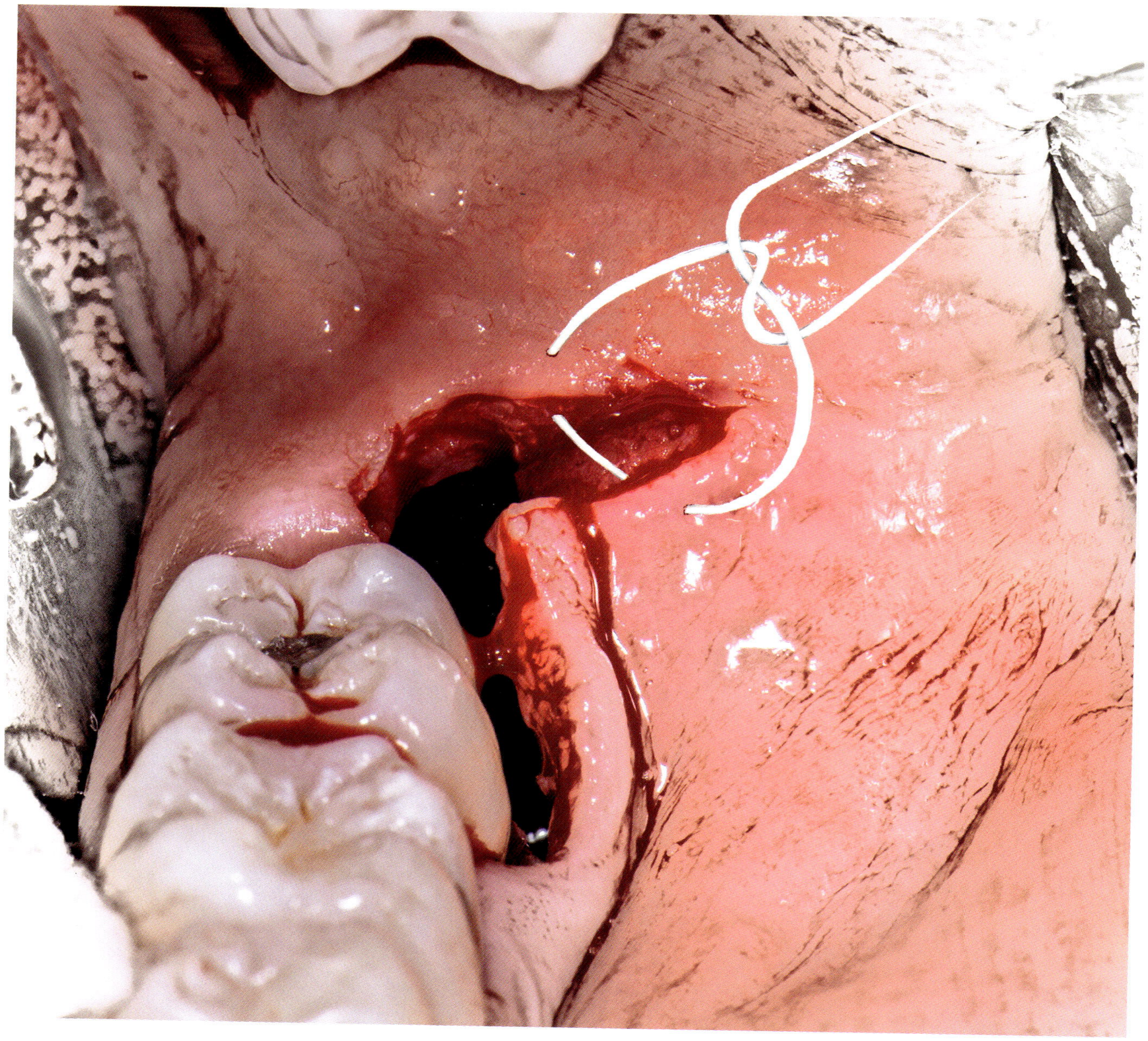

Figure 5-31 Reapproximating the muscle of the distal release is important for healing. This area can cause significant discomfort post-operatively if left open. A single suture in this area is often sufficient for the entire flap, depending on how much was exposed.

Hard Tissue Management

Lower third molar hard tissue

The lower third molar extraction site is ready and waiting for you to make a mistake. And it will hold it against you. Finesse and balance are the keys to success. Let's look at the process of removing a lower third molar. Each juncture is a decision, each intervention has a shape, and the whole thing is a balancing act designed to move and change. There is no perfect way through. See figures 5-36 and 5-66 for visual representations of the steps on the following pages. Surgery consists of a series of choices. It is dimensional. It is fluid. We can make it so complex, yet it is so very simple. Look for the simple.

Hand instruments

Elevate mesial

When there is an adequate purchase point and enough room to elevate, it may be possible to remove an impacted lower third molar with hand instruments alone. If a slender luxator can fit in the mesial below the height of contour of the crown, try to rotate the instrument with a lifting motion on the tooth. See how the tooth responds. If it is not moving, don't push it too hard. You can damage the bone with the elevator, increasing the chances of a subperiosteal abscess or delayed healing. After the tooth is out, it is wise to inspect the bone at the site of elevation for fragments or crushed pieces that need to be removed.

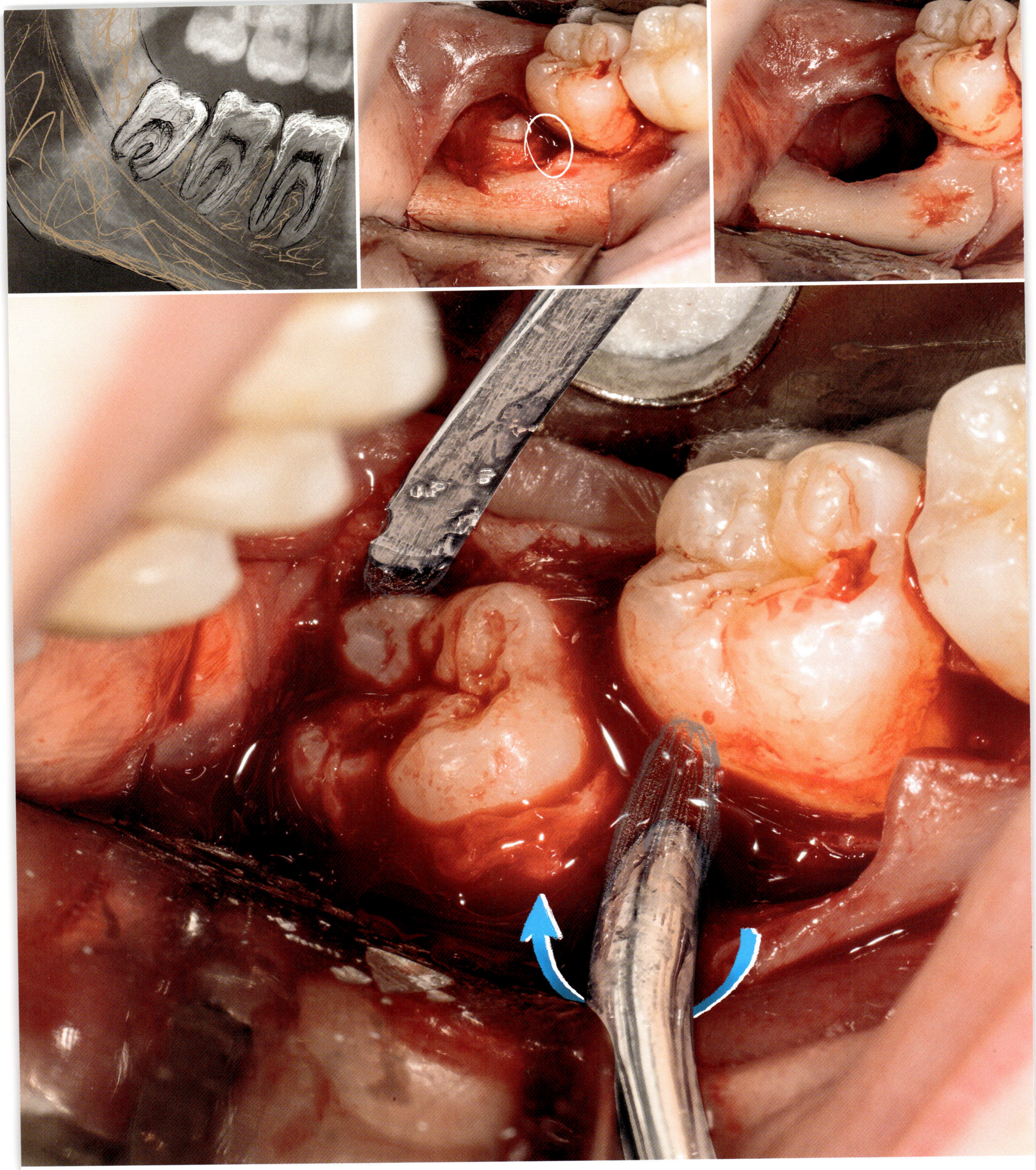

Figure 5-32 Impacted lower third molar. Exposure of the site reveals space for a small elevator. Retracting the lingual tissue and elevating the tooth allows atraumatic delivery. This socket is ready to start healing. The bone at the mesial where the elevator was placed does not appear damaged.

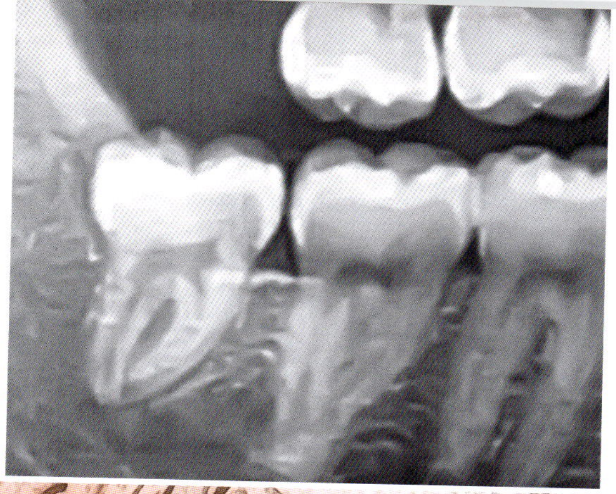

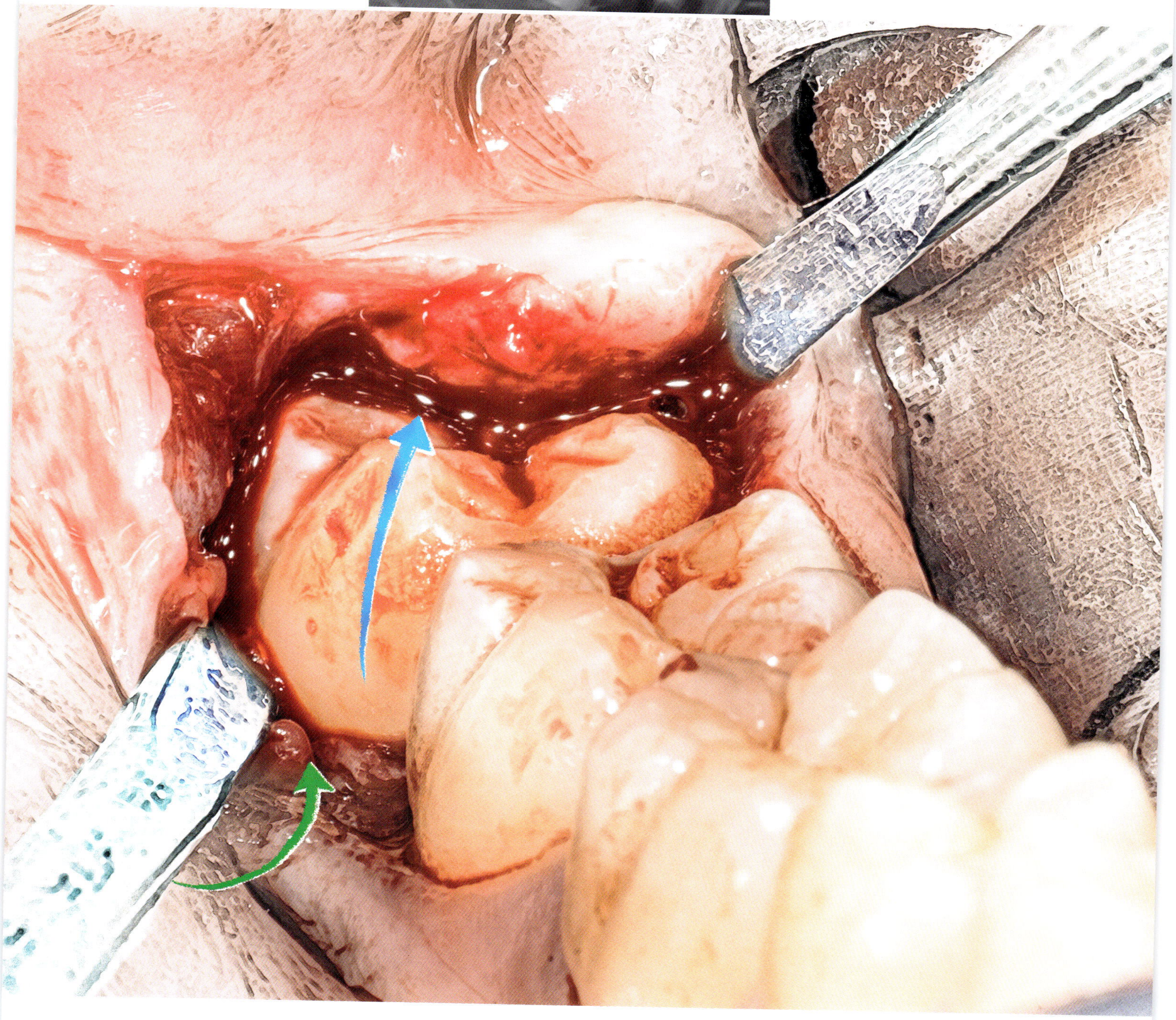

Figure 5-33 Reflecting the lingual tissue allows this third molar to be elevated out with a small Bein luxator. The instrument is wedged below the height of contour on the buccal aspect using the buccal bone as the fulcrum. Be careful of the lingual tissue. Elevating this way can stretch and tear it easily. Retracting it can protect it, but it can also risk damaging the lingual nerve.

Bone removal

When there is a thin layer of bone over the mesial and buccal, a small sharp hand instrument may be able to peel that bone away. Wedge the blunt end of the Micro Buser under the thin bone at the mesial aspect to test it. It may give and flake the overlying bone off, exposing the tooth and speeding up the extraction. If not, a drill may be necessary to access the tooth. This can create an access point for the elevator to be placed below the height of contour either on the mesial or buccal. Sometimes it is that simple. Other times it is not so simple and drilling is needed.

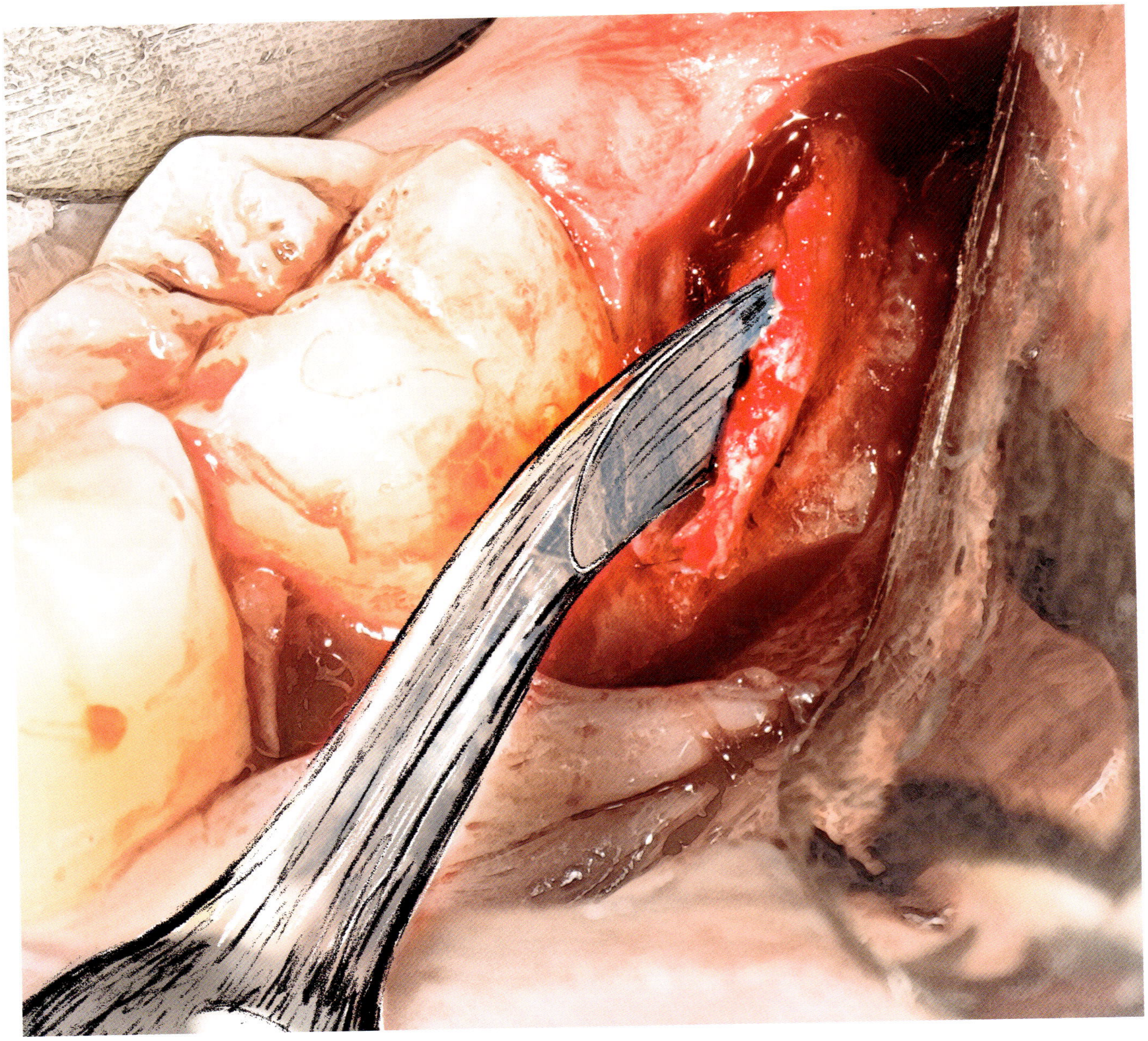

Figure 5-34 Thin buccal bone can be peeled off with the round end of the Micro Buser. This may allow adequate access for an elevator without drilling bone away. Bone removal is not always performed with a drill.

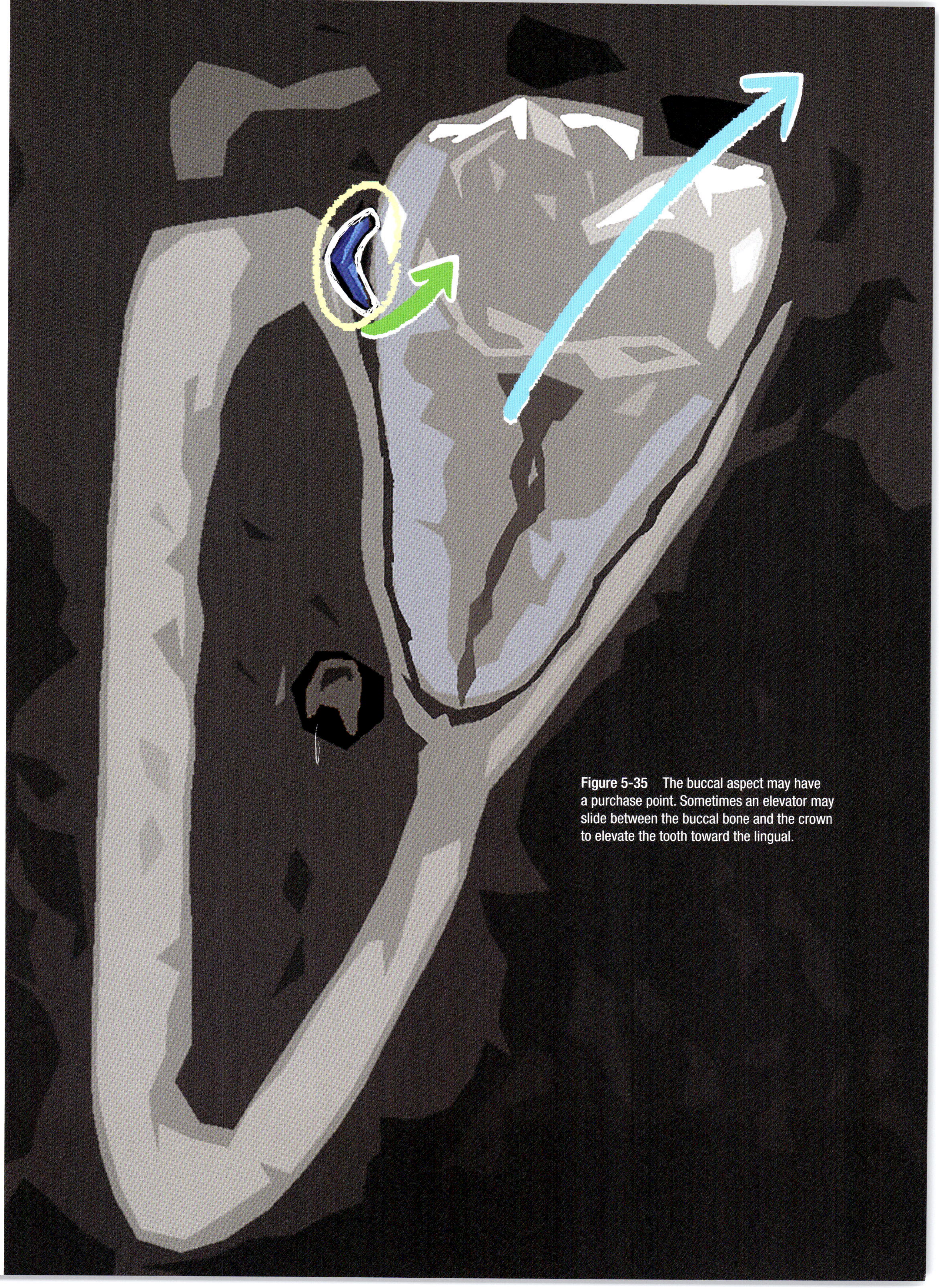

Figure 5-35 The buccal aspect may have a purchase point. Sometimes an elevator may slide between the buccal bone and the crown to elevate the tooth toward the lingual.

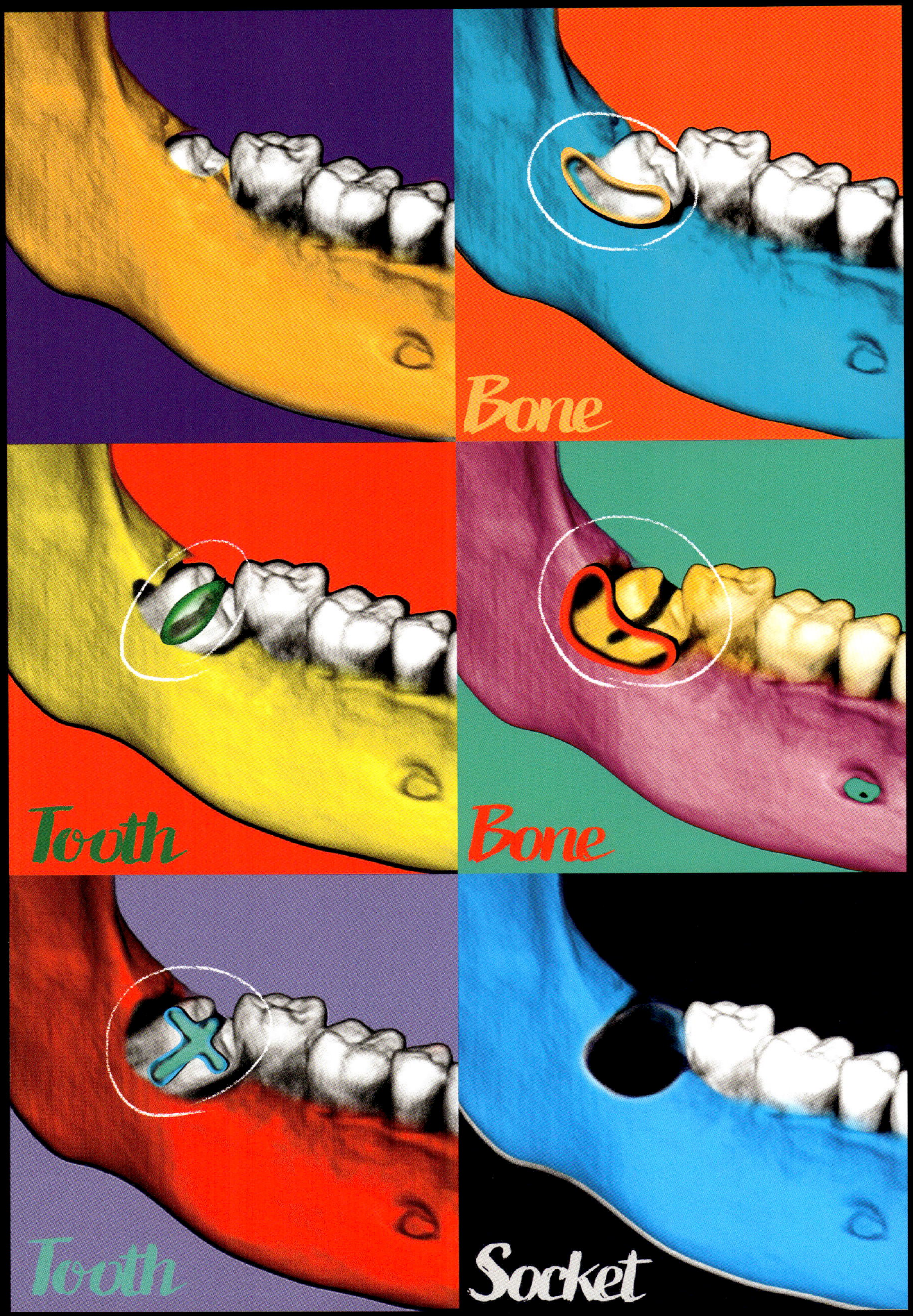

Figure 5-36 Basic drilling steps. Drill bone first. Then tooth structure. If needed, drill more bone and section more of the tooth. After the tooth is out, check the socket to make sure it has clean edges. (Artwork inspired by Andy Warhol.)

Drilling

Power tools make things easier. A drill removes bone and sections teeth much better than the old mallet and chisel. The purpose of the drill is to create access and establish a purchase point by removing bone and sectioning the tooth.

Bone removal

In preparation for drilling, ensure the soft tissue flap provides adequate access to the entire area needing bone removal. Blindly drilling beneath the distal flap increases the risk of damaging the lingual nerve as it travels in the adjacent soft tissue. Remember, the mandible often flares out behind impacted third molars. Drilling without adequate visualization may result in perforating the thin lingual bone and transecting the lingual nerve. In addition, drilling under the flap also increases thermal bone injury. Irrigation cannot sufficiently cool the bur or clear the flutes if it is not reaching the bur. Mobilize the flap to make it easier on you and the tissue. Begin with the end in mind.

With adequate access and visualization established, begin removing bone on the buccal ridge to locate and uncover the tooth. Let the drill's tactile feedback guide you. Bone cuts easier than enamel. While drilling, if you hug the crown with the bur you can get a pretty good idea of the location of the tooth. The distal extent of the trough may extend slightly past the line angle toward the distal to create space to deliver the tooth. But be extremely cautious to avoid drilling through the lingual cortex.

The mesial extent of the trough must allow adequate access to place a luxator or elevator. If it is not extended far enough, it can be quite a fight to mobilize the portions of the tooth. It may be possible to elevate the tooth after removing bone. But most of the time I section the tooth as well before elevating.

Sectioning the tooth

Make sure you can see enough of the tooth and the anatomy to orient your cut. Even after doing thousands of these, I sometimes find the angles disorienting. It is easy to get overly confident and stray off course in the depths of a lower third molar site. Clear away enough buccal bone so you can get perspective on the crown anatomy. Buccal bone is a cheap price to pay to be able to cleanly section and elevate a lower third molar, but it isn't free. A quick glance at the radiograph improves predictability. With the anatomy visualized, plan the cut to separate the tooth through the furcation. Splitting it through the furcation makes removing the roots much easier. You don't need to drill through the entire crown. Just enough to split the tooth through the furcation.

Common purchase points to look for or to make: mesial (mesiobuccal), interradicular (after sectioning), buccal (with or without trough).

Figure 5-37 Drilling a slot part way through the middle of the crown creates space to fracture the tooth with an elevator. Ideally, this fracture goes through the middle of the furcation, splitting the tooth mesial-distally. Splitting the tooth right down the middle is best. The arrow is pointing to the space created on the mesial to later insert the elevator.

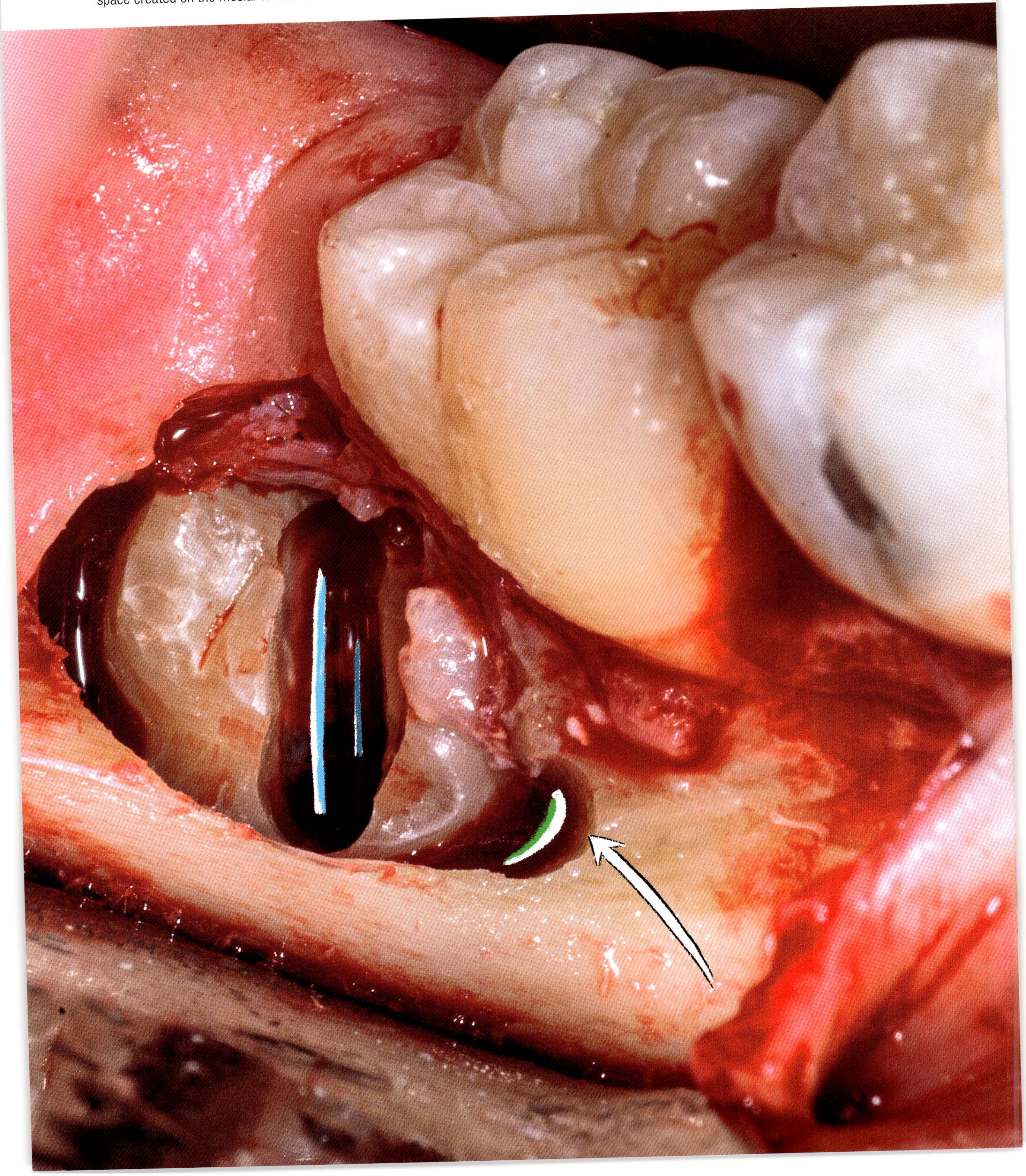

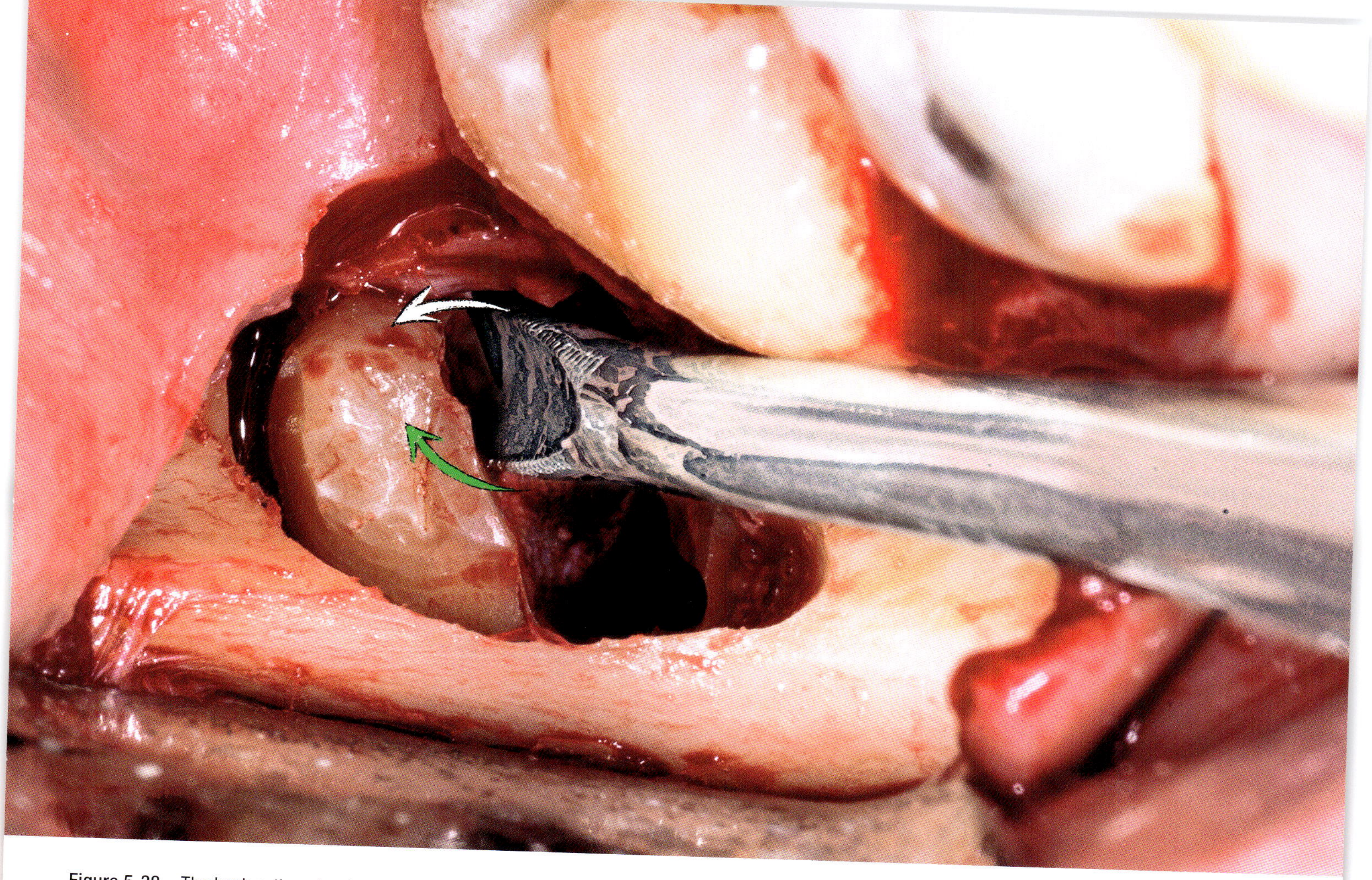

Figure 5-38 The back action elevator is inserted and torqued to complete the fracture (*white arrow*). Then it is rotated opposite to deliver the distal portion. The tip of the elevator can often engage the pulp chamber to provide lift out of the site (*green arrow*).

Rotating a back action elevator at the depth of the cut finishes sectioning the tooth and the distal portion is elevated out. Sometimes, the elevator can be repositioned to engage the pulp chamber as a purchase point. This improves the lift and helps protect the lingual and distal soft tissue. Pay close attention to where the tooth fractured and how much of it came out. This helps guide the next steps.

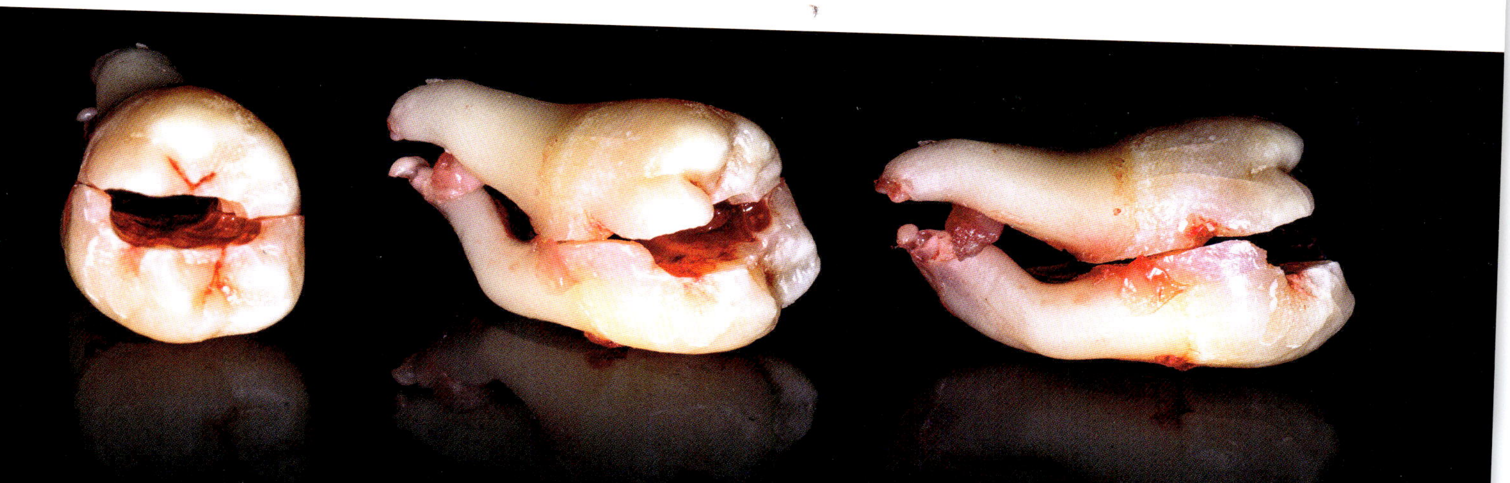

Figure 5-39 A well oriented cut splits it through the furcation. You don't need to drill completely through the crown.

Removing the distal portion of the tooth creates space to elevate the remaining mesial portion. Either the back action elevator or slender luxator can be placed beneath the height of contour at the mesial aspect to elevate the remaining mesial piece out.

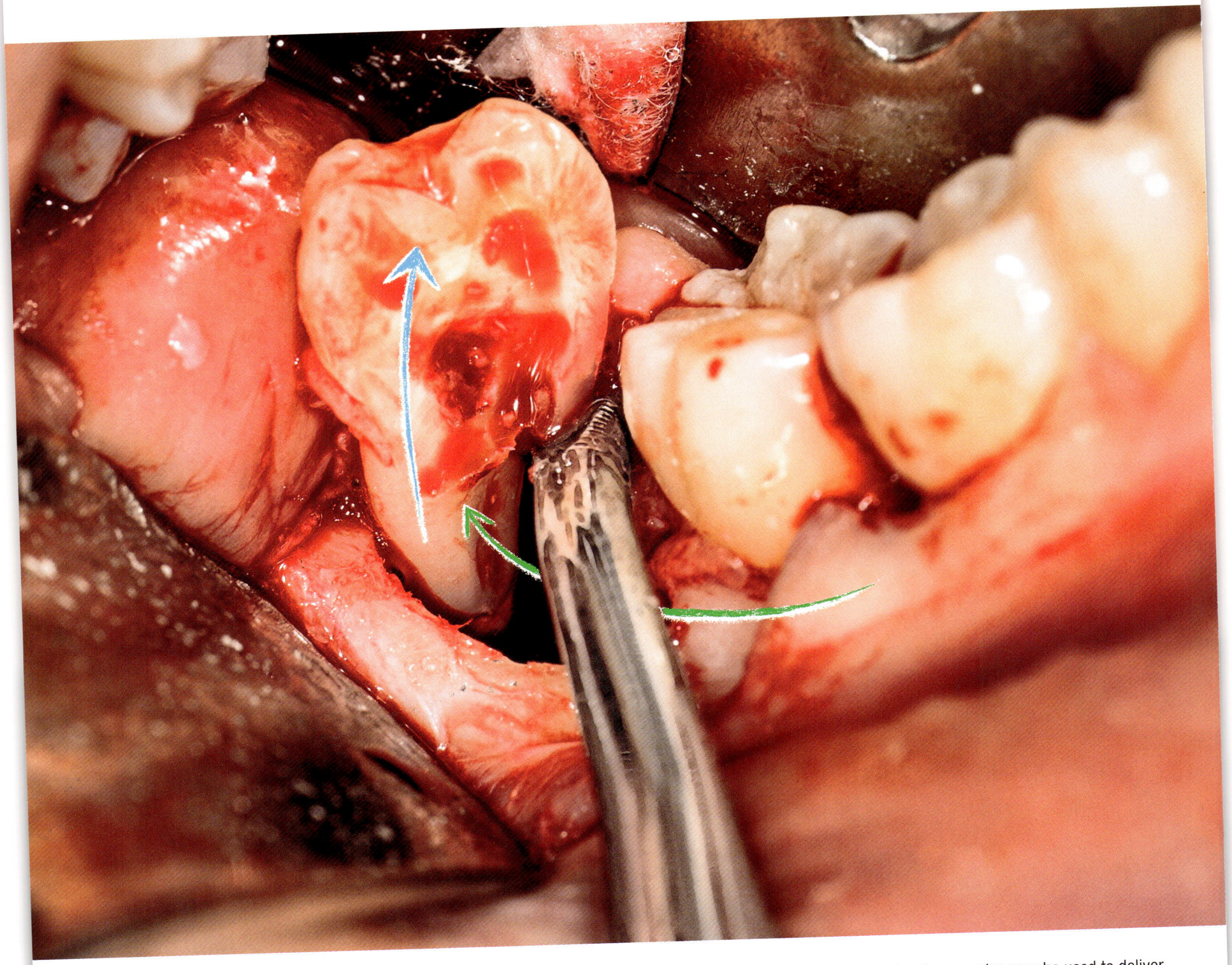

Figure 5-40 The back action elevator can sometimes complete the removal of the distal portion. A hemostat or forceps also may be used to deliver it from the socket.

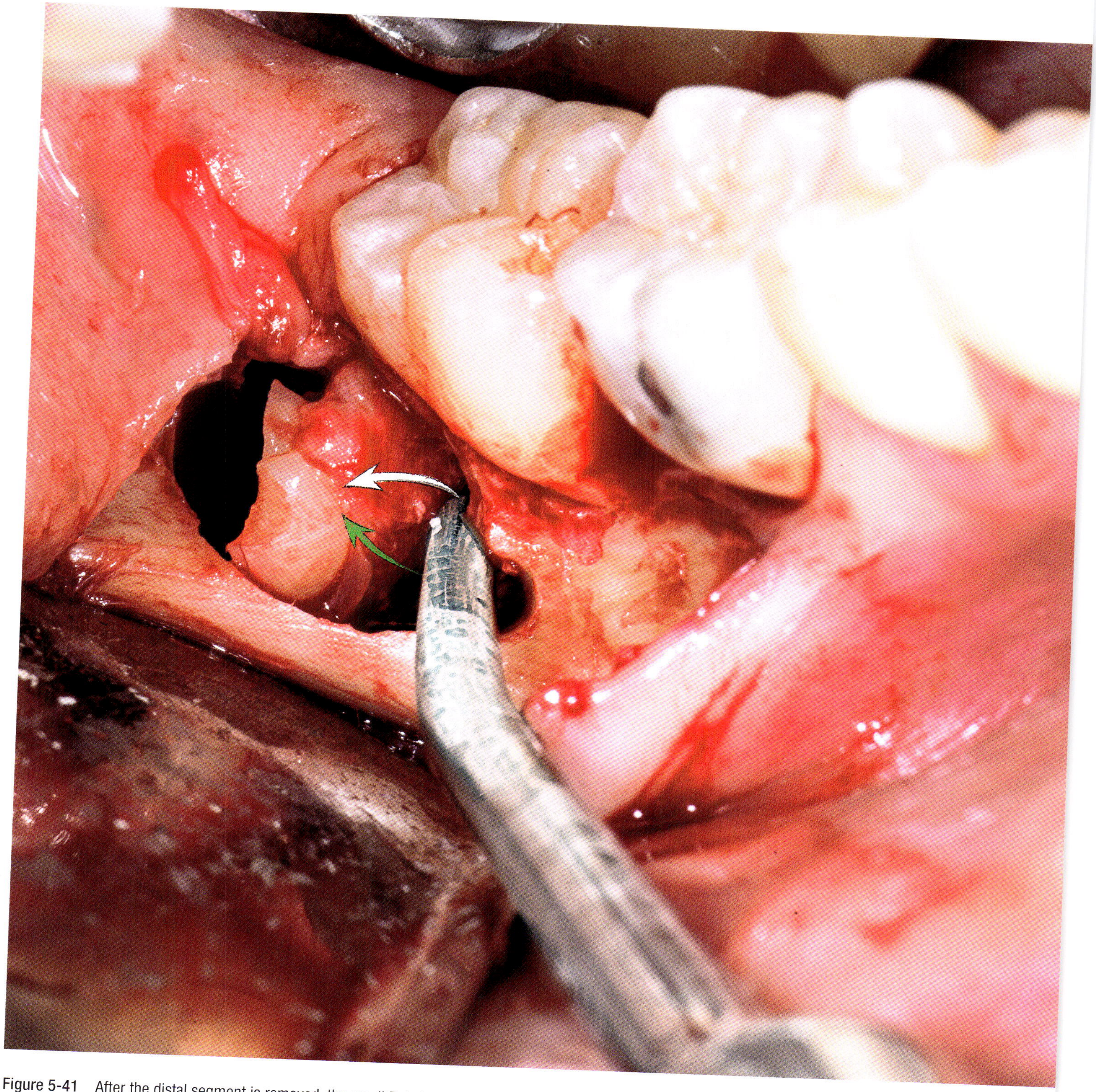

Figure 5-41 After the distal segment is removed, the small Bein luxator is inserted into the space created on the mesial. It is rotated first to displace the tooth distally (*white arrow*). It is then rotated opposite to deliver the segment (*green arrow*).

More drilling

When the tooth doesn't cooperate after the initial bone removal and sectioning, think again about improving access and establishing a purchase point. This can be done by either removing more bone or further sectioning the tooth.

Bone removal

Removing more bone can open up space either for the tooth to elevate out or to access a different purchase point. Be intentional with the drilling. Think about exactly what you are trying to accomplish with each move, visualizing the next steps. Removing more bone toward the buccal and around the distal can create space for the tooth to move. A shell of bone over the distolingual can sometimes prevent delivering the tooth. But be very careful drilling back there. It is a dangerous place to drill blindly. The lingual nerve is very close. Make sure you can either see the bone you are removing, or you know the three-dimensional anatomy from a CBCT before drilling there.

Sectioning the tooth again

When a portion of the crown comes out, examine it closely to better understand what is left. It is easy to assume the distal half of the crown is out when it may only be the distobuccal aspect. The remaining distolingual aspect of the crown may be lodged under the ascending ramus. When this is the case, typical elevating forces are in vain because you are pushing against the stout ascending ramus. In contrast, when the entire distal portion is out, there is space to elevate the tooth successfully. Pay attention to the pieces when they come out. They are guideposts for the next steps of the journey.

What remains determines how and where to further section the tooth. If the split didn't go through the furcation, drill deeper and at a steeper angle to separate the roots. If the distolingual portion of the crown remains, try to get around the corner to separate that piece. If the tooth splits through the furcation but the distal segment is stuck, consider splitting that distal segment into smaller pieces. And if the distal is out and it seems like the mesial is trapped under a lingual roof of bone, try sectioning that mesial segment diagonally into pieces. The options of where to drill make the shape of a plus sign. Keep it simple. Look at the remaining pieces and figure out which of these seems like the best place to drill.

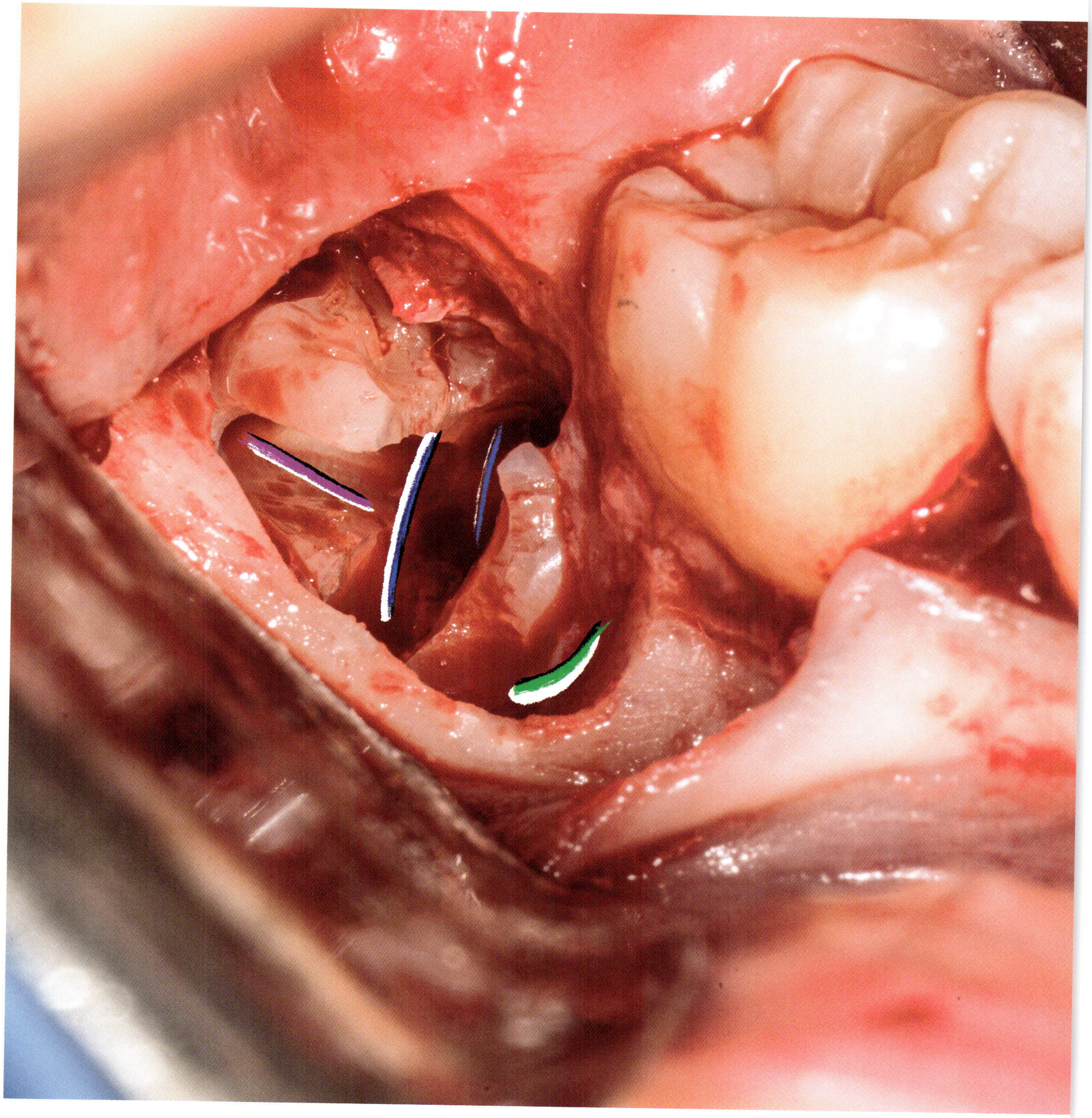

Figure 5-42 After the initial vertical cut, a second horizontal cut may be necessary to segment the distal portion of the crown to safely remove the distal half of the tooth. Note the trough extends to the mesial to elevate the mesial portion.

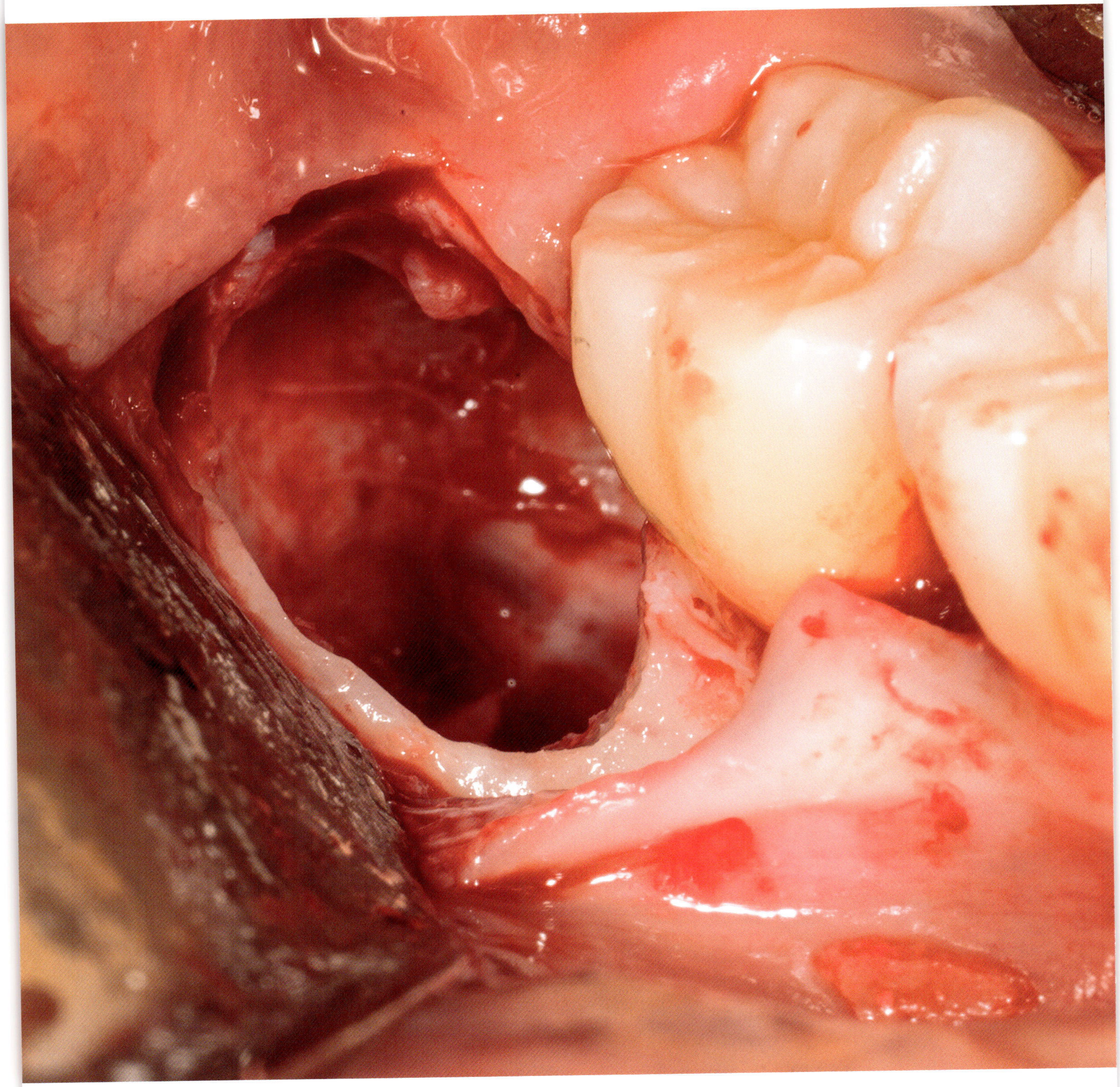

Figure 5-43 After the tooth is removed, the site is curetted to remove the follicle, thoroughly irrigated, and inspected for retained debris before suturing.

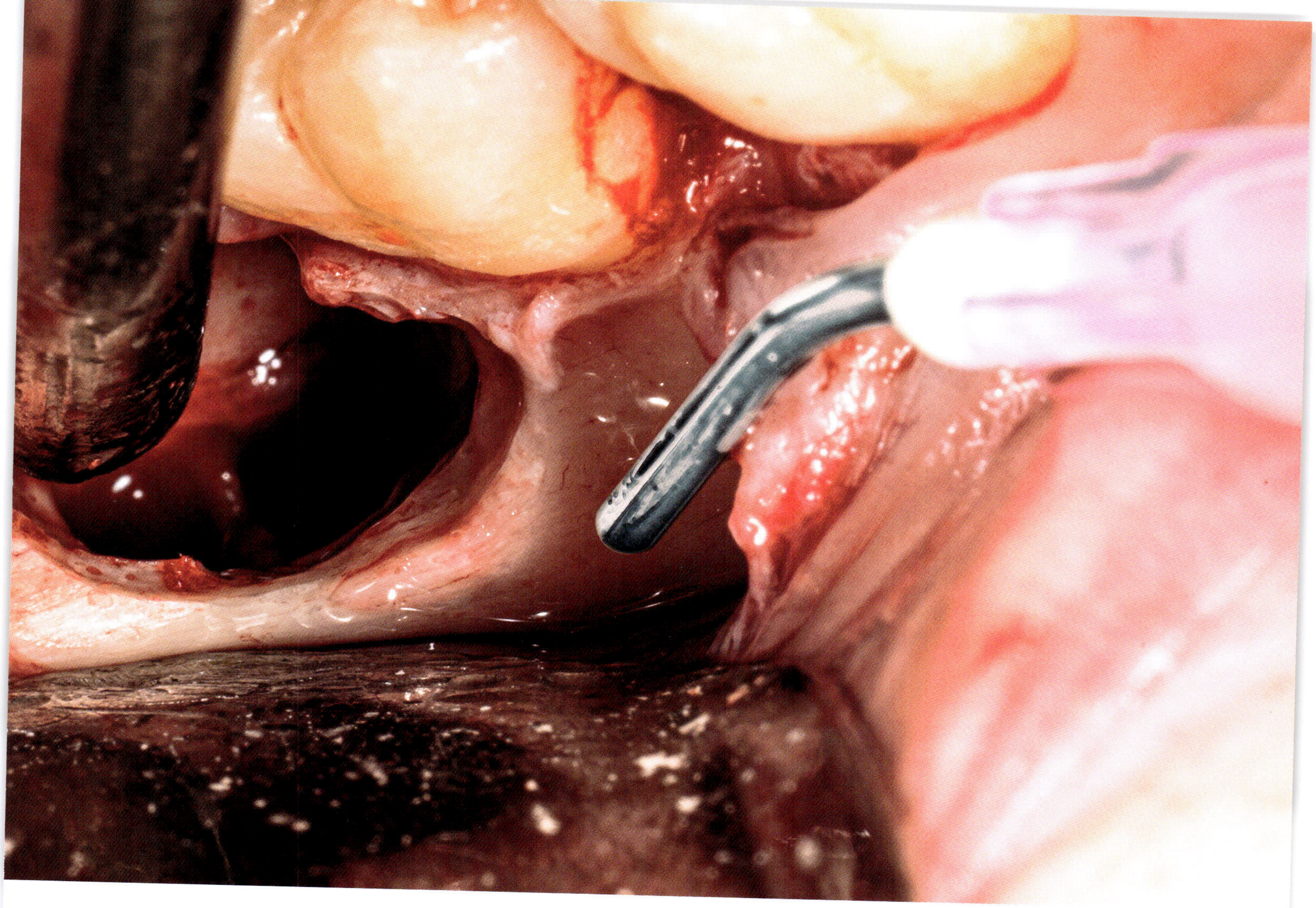

Figure 5-44 Direct the irrigation under the flap. This is the most common area to collect and retain debris that will later cause a subperiosteal abscess. Thoroughly flush between the periosteum and the bone.

Soft tissue

The soft tissue can get in the way of the extraction. A well-designed flap should maximize access, minimize risk and optimize healing. Sometimes this results in tissue holding the crown in over the lingual. Elevating and retracting this tissue will protect it from tearing and help guide the tooth out. After positioning a periosteal elevator, your assistant can hold it while you elevate. But be careful to watch the lingual tissue while it is being elevated. Even when it is retracted, a tear is possible. This maneuver of retracting the lingual tissue is a source of debate in the literature. My perspective is the lingual nerve is safest being retracted to avoid permanent injury.

The lingual cortex is a thin curtain of bone deserving respect. The space on the other side of the bone may seem like an abyss if a root tip gets displaced beyond its protection. And when the bone remains intact, the lingual nerve is completely safe from the drill. Ideally, nothing should penetrate the lingual cortex. Unfortunately, sometimes the anatomy is such that there is little to no lingual cortical bone present. This seems to occur most often when the mandible flares out behind the second molars. In these cases, it is much easier to accidentally displace a root (or even the whole tooth) into the floor of the mouth with an elevator or inadvertently drill beyond the tooth endangering the lingual nerve. Palpating the lingual tissue can reveal the shape of the mandible in the lower third molar areas.

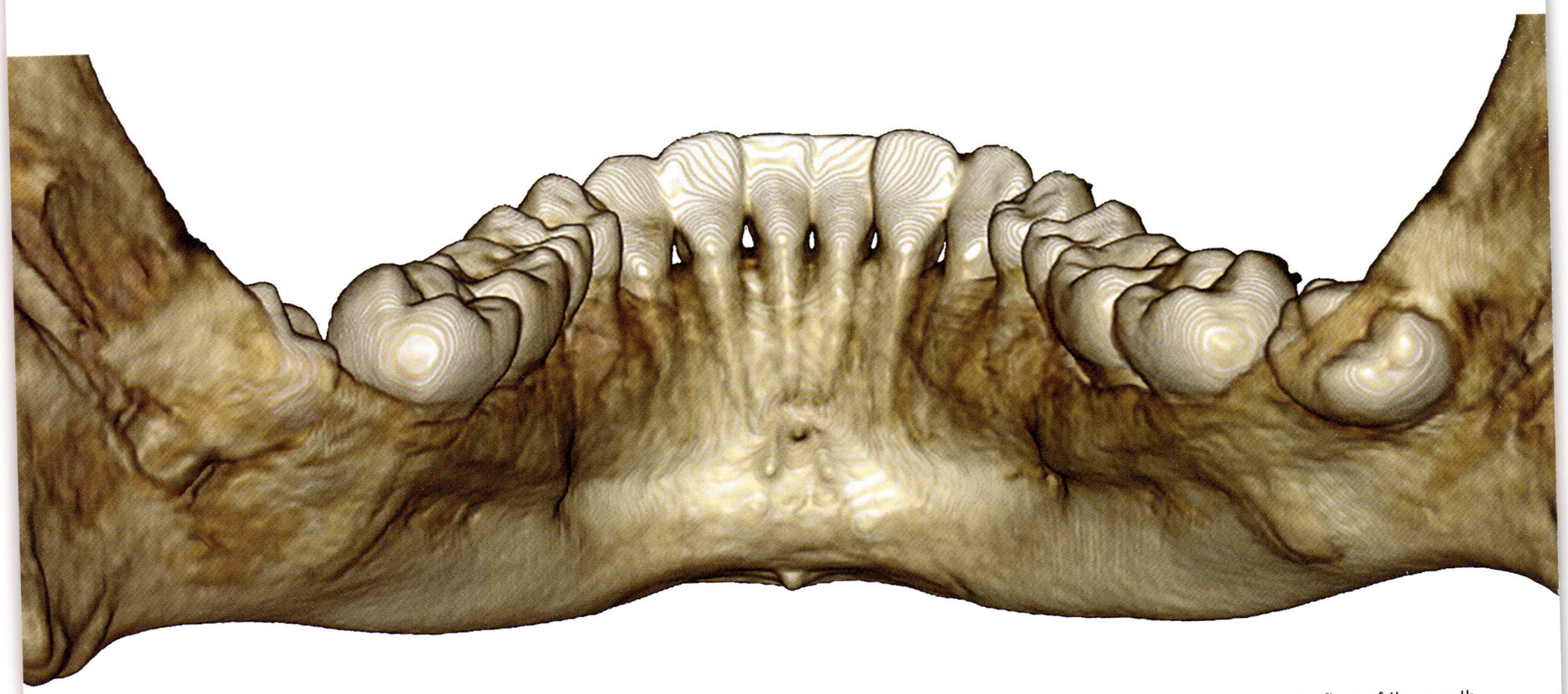

Figure 5-45 Look at how thin the lingual bone is over these third molars. There is a very thin curtain of bone between them and the floor of the mouth.

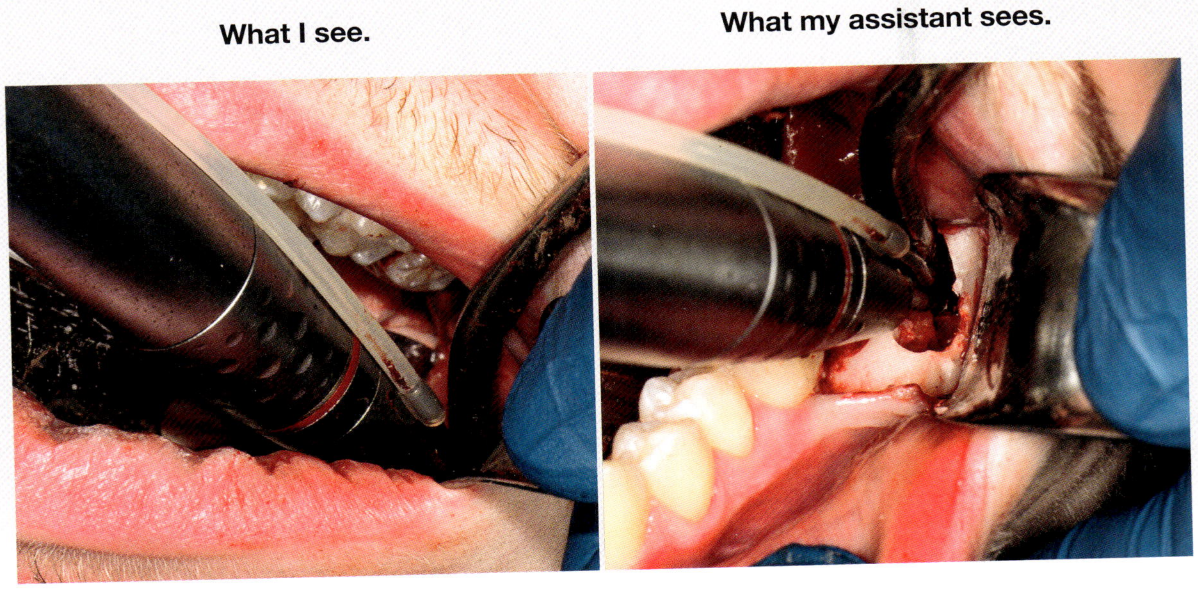

Figure 5-46 Sectioning a lower third molar can be difficult to see (*left*) especially when the irrigation pools. The assistant has an even harder time seeing (*right*). Our assistants have an incredible ability to know and do things without direct visualization.

When it comes to techniques for removing third molars, there are so many variables within my own practice and amongst surgeons around the world. I encourage you to find your own balance. Identify your own decision points. Pay attention to the details we have discussed. It will help you get better at what you do and also can help your team better understand your process.

Complicated impaction patterns

There are a few specific types of impactions that have variations in drilling protocol.

Horizontal impaction

There are clear steps to sectioning a horizontally impacted lower third molar. Bone removal is typically required. The steps can be completed in different orders, but they always include sectioning the roots, removing the crown and then delivering the roots. I find it easiest to section the tooth through the furcation when the tooth is intact. This way, I can orient myself better. After cutting through the crown toward the furcation, finish the split with an elevator. Then cut the distal aspect of the crown and deliver it. When sectioning the tooth, plan to leave enough structure to get a good purchase point. If you section too much of the coronal segment off, there may be no purchase point remaining. Then you are committing to more bone removal and a more complicated extraction. With the distal aspect of the crown out, the distal root can be elevated and removed. Sometimes the mesial root can come out with the crown intact. Other times, the crown and root must be separated. As always when drilling, make sure you know the anatomy of this specific case. Protect the nerve, adjacent teeth and lingual tissue.

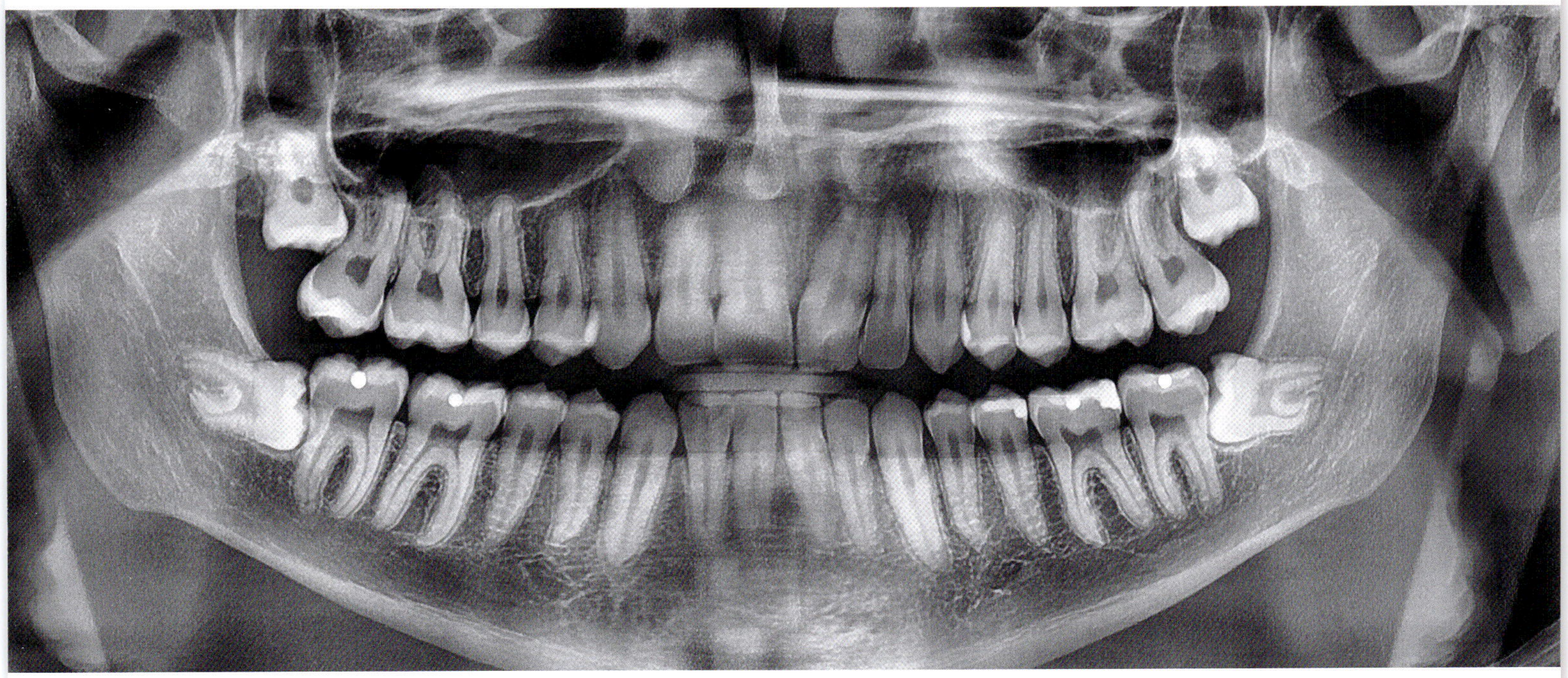

Figure 5-47 Horizontally imacted lower third molars.

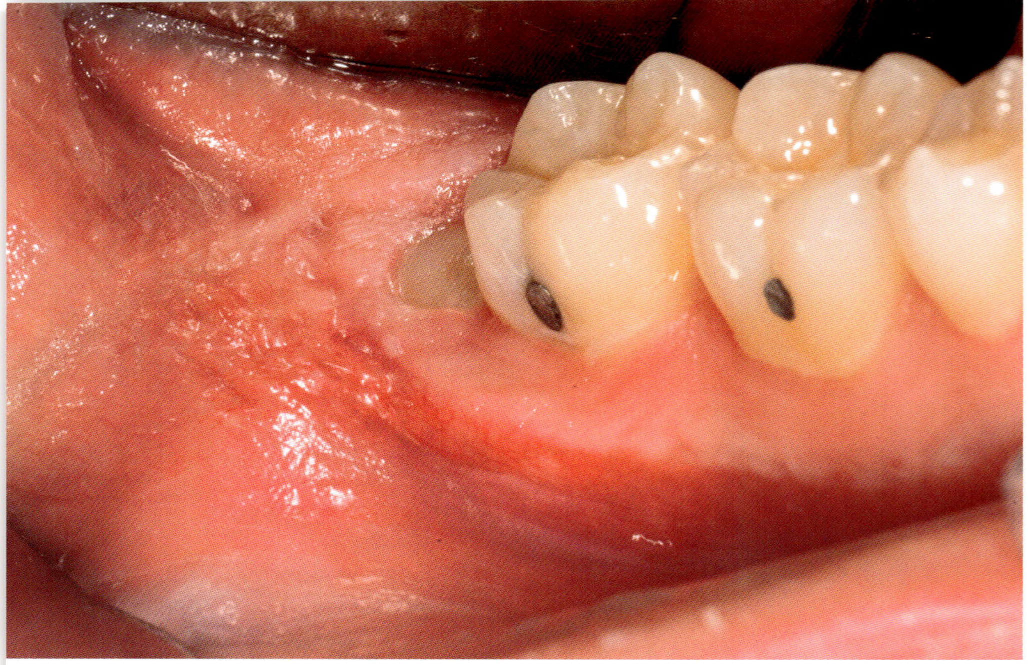

Figure 5-48 The third molar crown is peeking out. Hygiene is impossible to maintain around a tooth like this, compromising both the second and third molars.

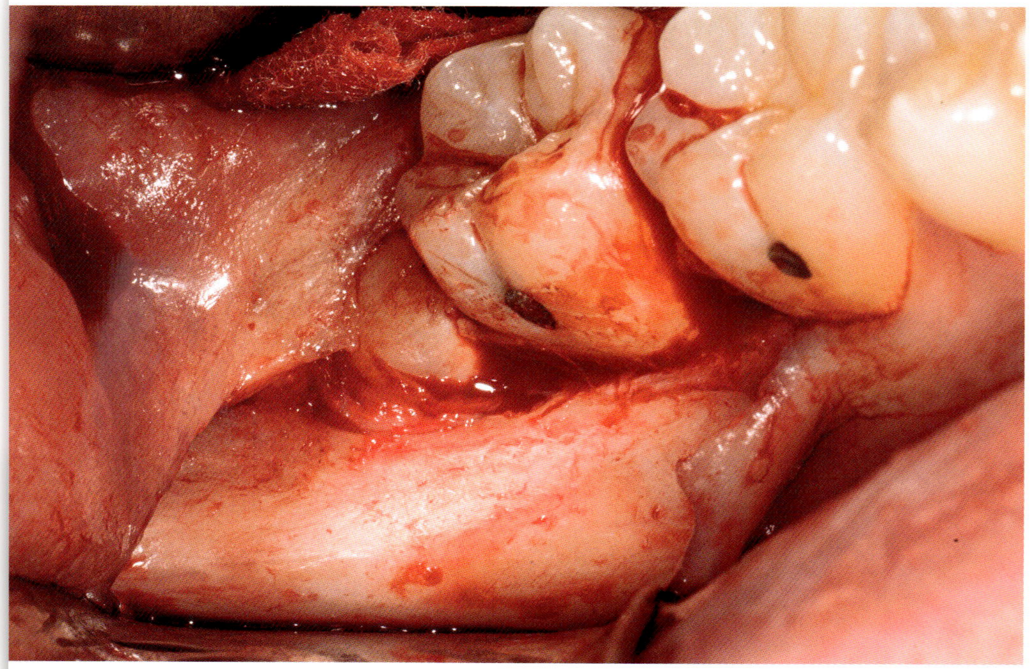

Figure 5-49 Generous exposure is needed to ensure the tissue is protected and the access is optimal.

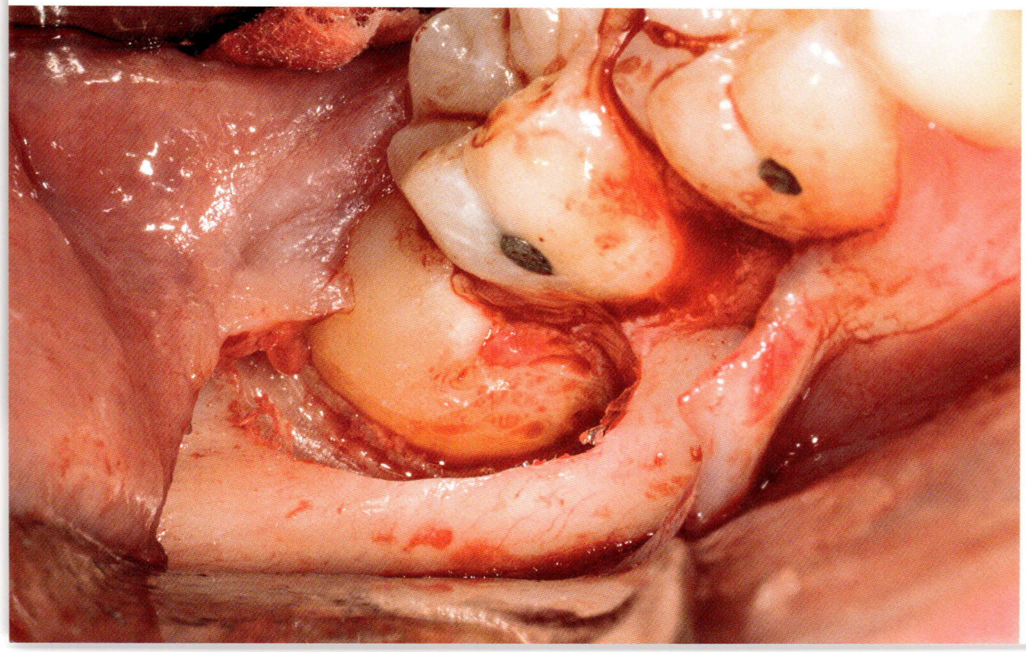

Figure 5-50 Bone removal should extend around the mesial line angle of the tooth to make space for the elevator. It should also expose enough of the crown to identify the position of the furcation.

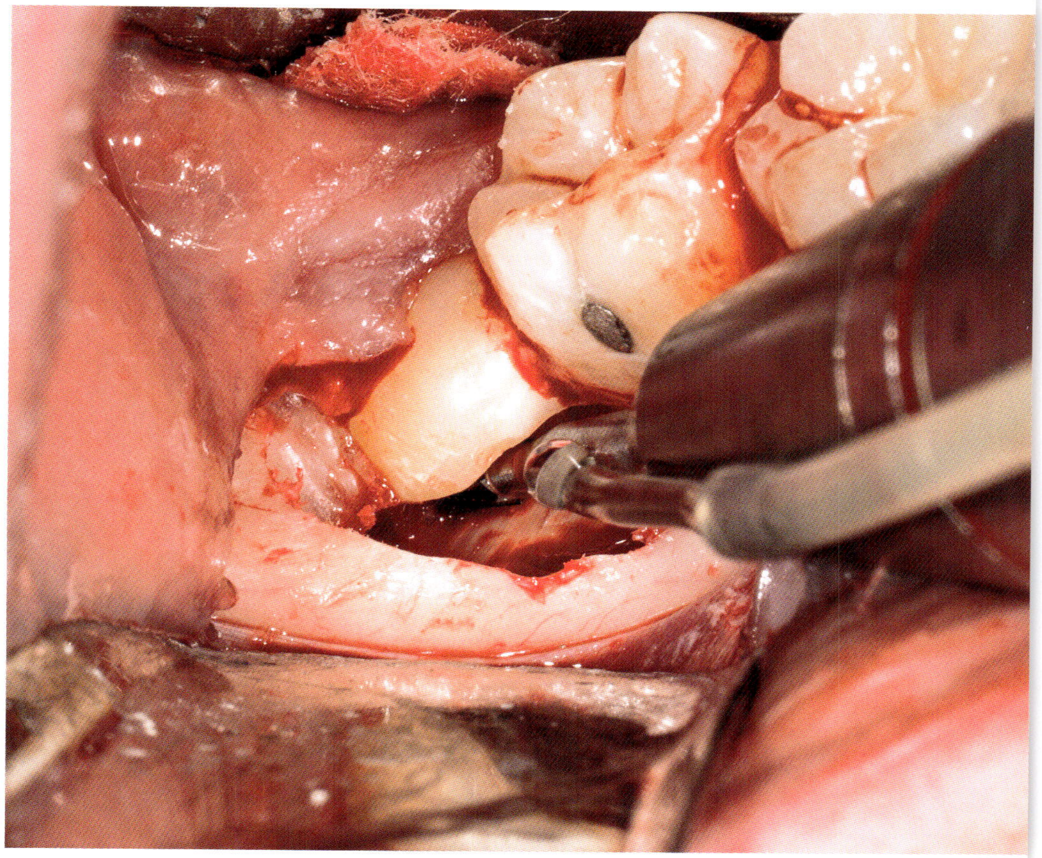

Figure 5-51 The goal of the initial drilling aims at splitting the tooth through the furcation. Estimating this angle is aided by looking at the panoramic radiograph and positioning the drill according to the occlusal plane. Completing the split with an elevator at this point maximizes the chances of splitting the tooth through the furcation.

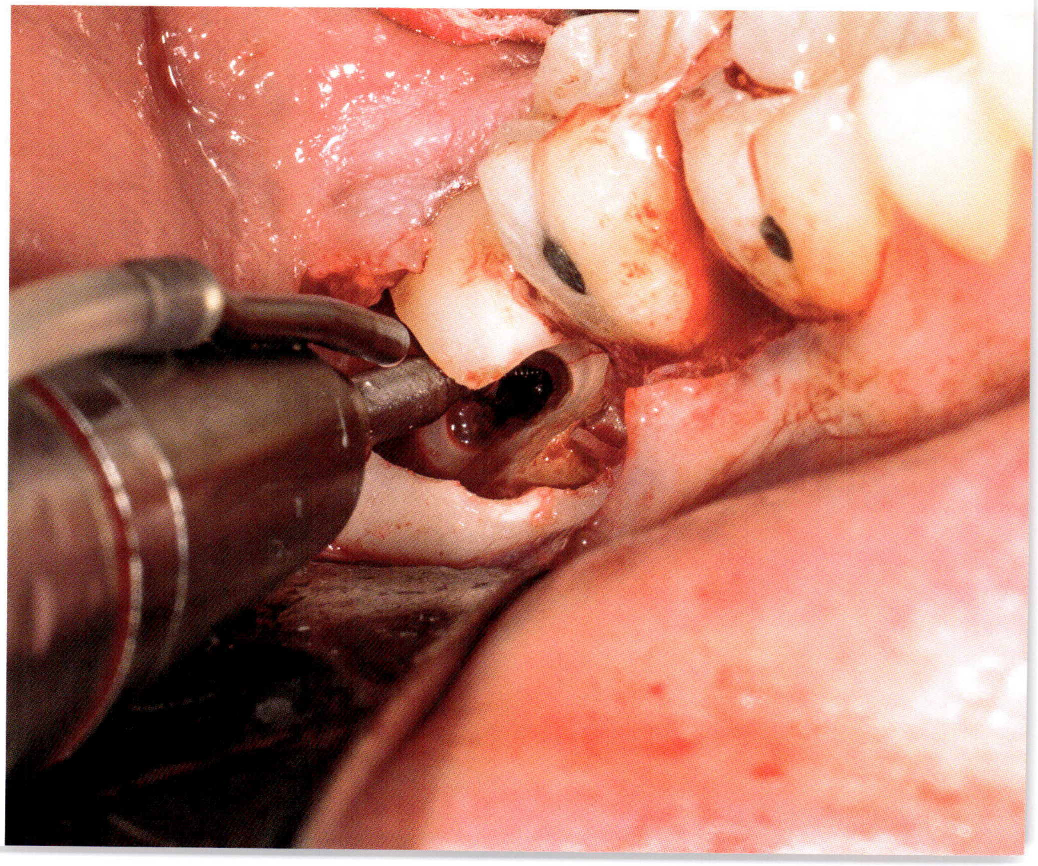

Figure 5-52 After the initial split, the distal portion of the crown is sectioned to be removed. This cut can extend through the mesial portion of the crown as well, depending on the angulation of the tooth. If it looks like the mesial half can elevate around the corner of the second molar, this cut may not need to extend through the mesial root. Note the hairline fracture in the occlusal of the tooth. This can help determine the path of the split.

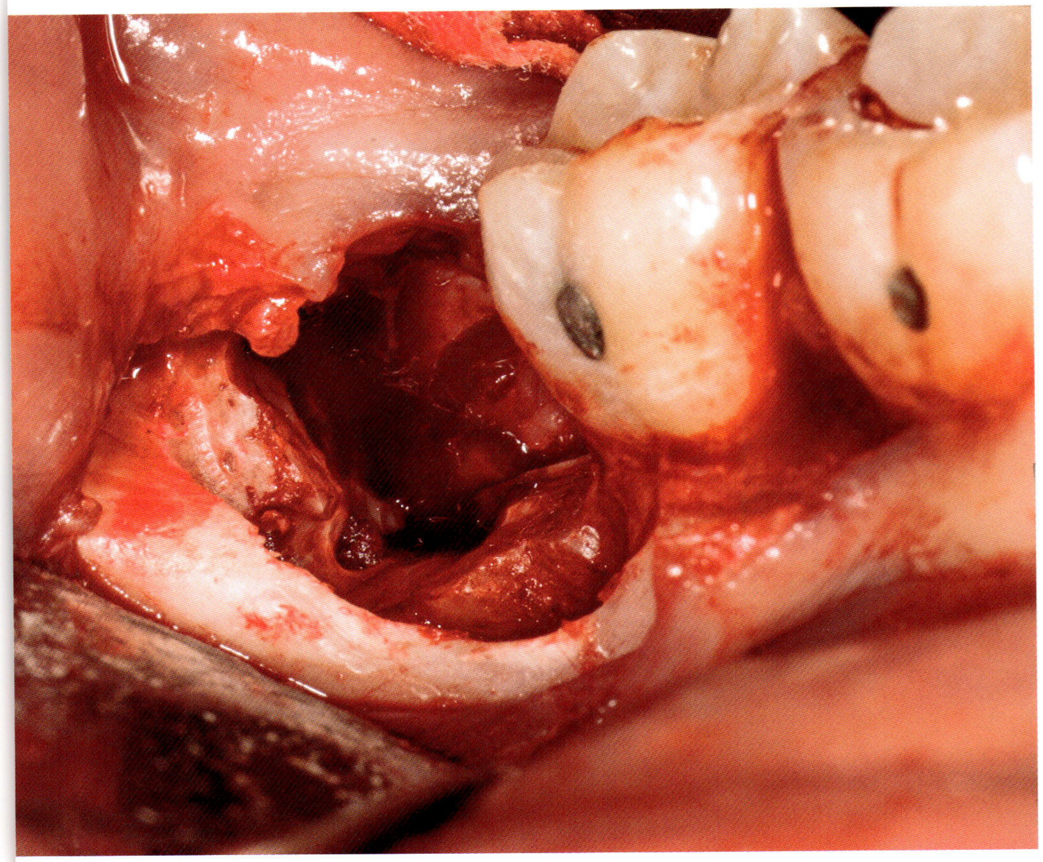

Figure 5-53 After the distal portion of the crown is delivered, either the distal root or mesial half of the tooth can be removed. Further bone removal or sectioning may be necessary. When the buccal trough is designed well, there is space for the elevator to engage the mesial portion of the crown.

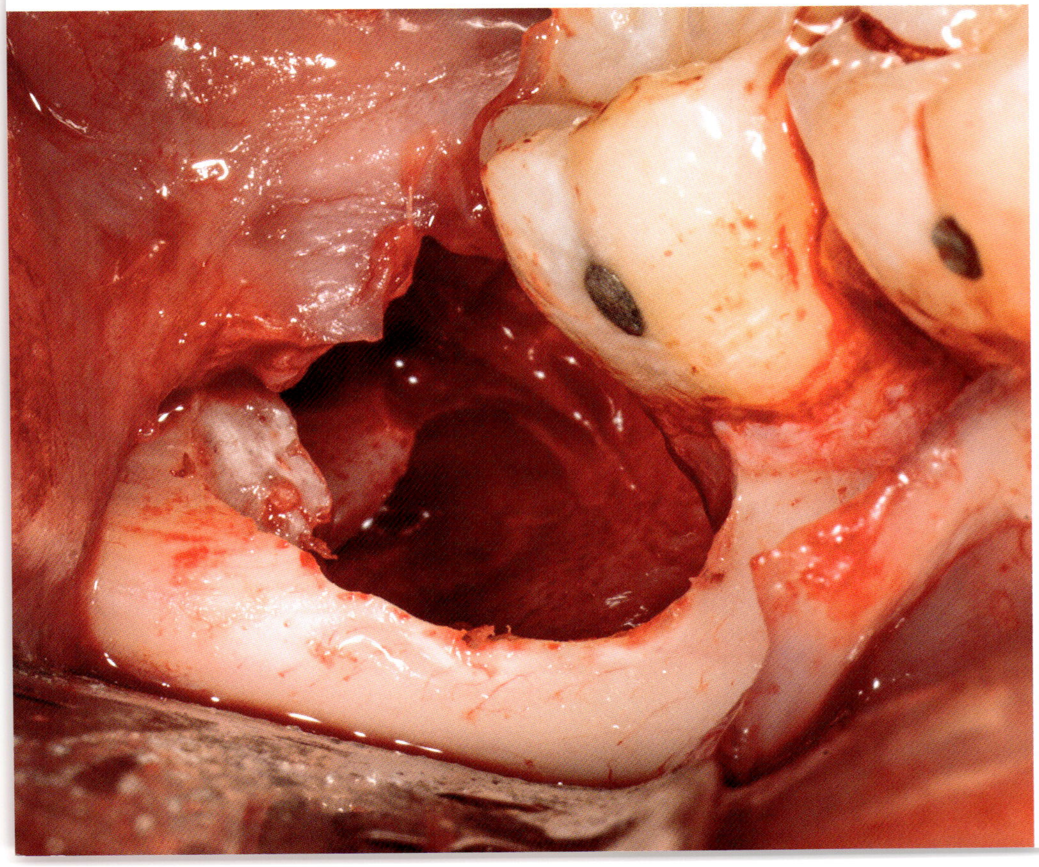

Figure 5-54 Upon successful removal of the tooth, the distal of the second molar should be examined. There is often follicle tissue or periodontally involved inflammatory tissue that should be curetted or scaled.

Distoangular impaction

Distoangular impacted lower third molars are lodged in tightly below the ascending ramus. And they are usually snug up against the second molar. This can make them quite stubborn to remove. Instead of trying to section these between the roots at the furcation, consider first removing enough of the distal aspect of the crown to mobilize the roots. Once they are mobilized, it is much easier to piece them out and remove the segments. The challenge is in removing enough of the distal of the crown (including the lingual aspect) to enable movement to either deliver the roots or section them further to deliver all the pieces more easily and less traumatically. In addition, it can be quite difficult to find a purchase point to elevate as these teeth are usually really close to the second molars.

At some point, if the struggle continues, you may need to remove more bone to make things easier for yourself and the patient. You have to find the balance, but you also need to get the job done. Sometimes, you just need a good, sharp, high-speed bur with copious irrigation to clear the path and remove the tooth. The beauty and art is in the balance.

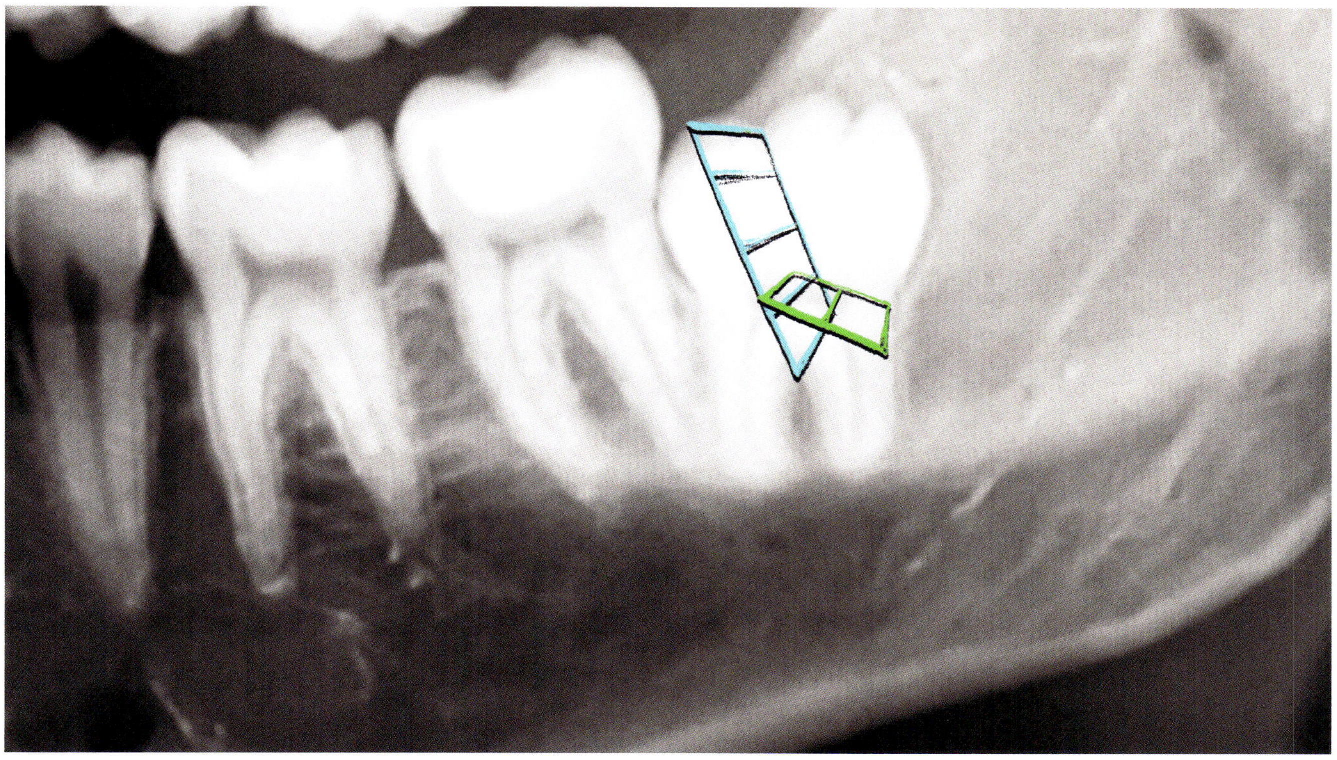

Figure 5-55 This is a representation of how the actual cuts and splits went in this case. Blue represents the first cut and split. Green represents the second cut to remove the distal portion of the crown before delivering the remaining distal and mesial portions.

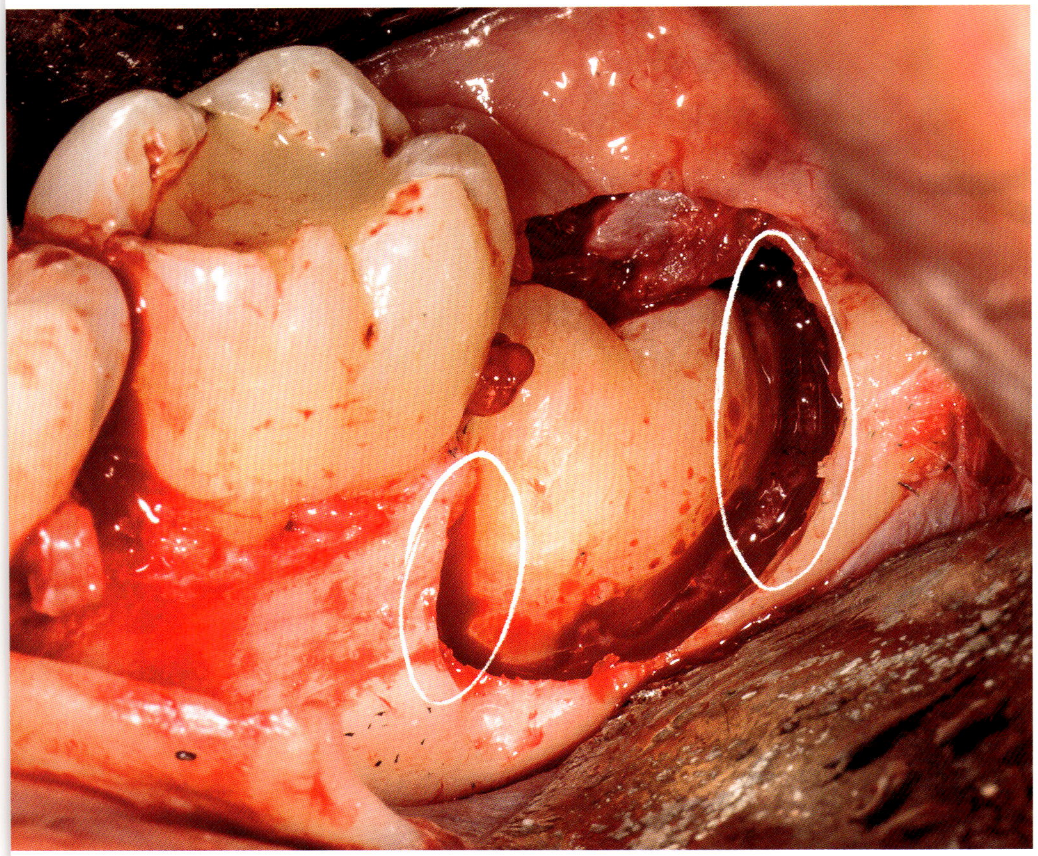

Figure 5-56 Bone removal provides access along the buccal, extending to the mesial and distal.

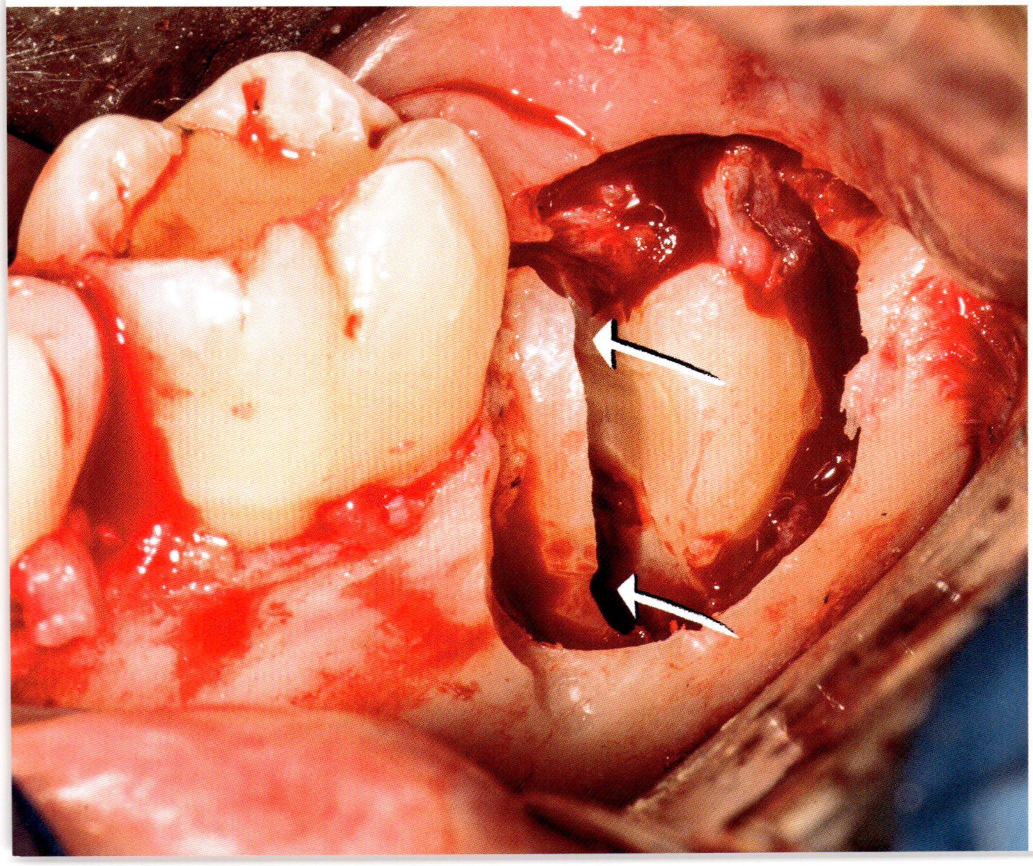

Figure 5-57 Sectioning the tooth initially into mesial and distal portions.

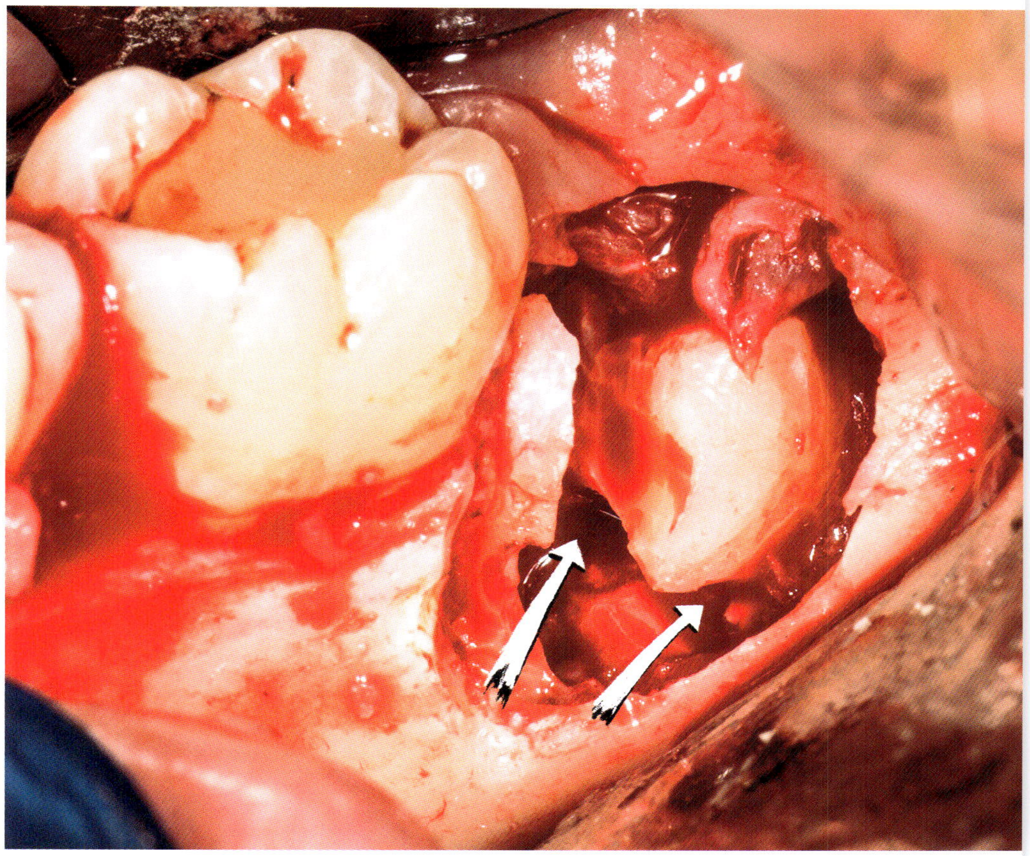

Figure 5-58 If the tooth cannot be delivered, the second cut is to remove the distal portion of the crown to create space to remove the distal and mesial roots.

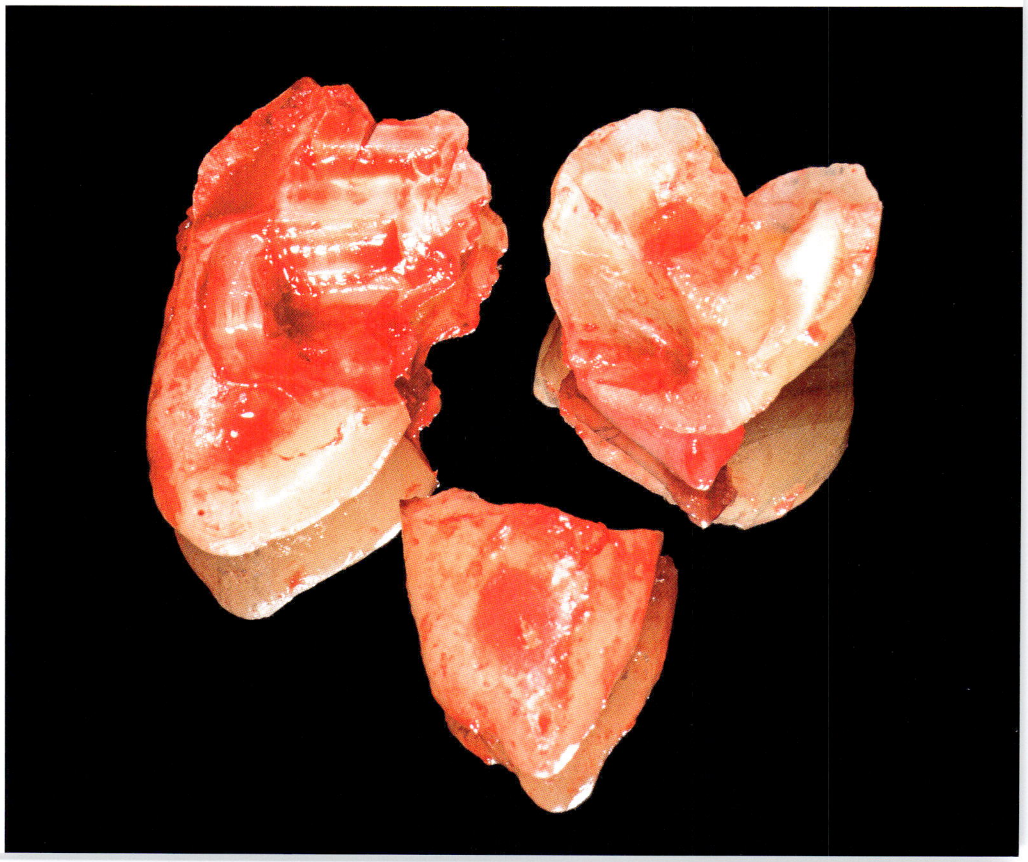

Figure 5-59 This shows the mesial portion and the two distal portions of this tooth.

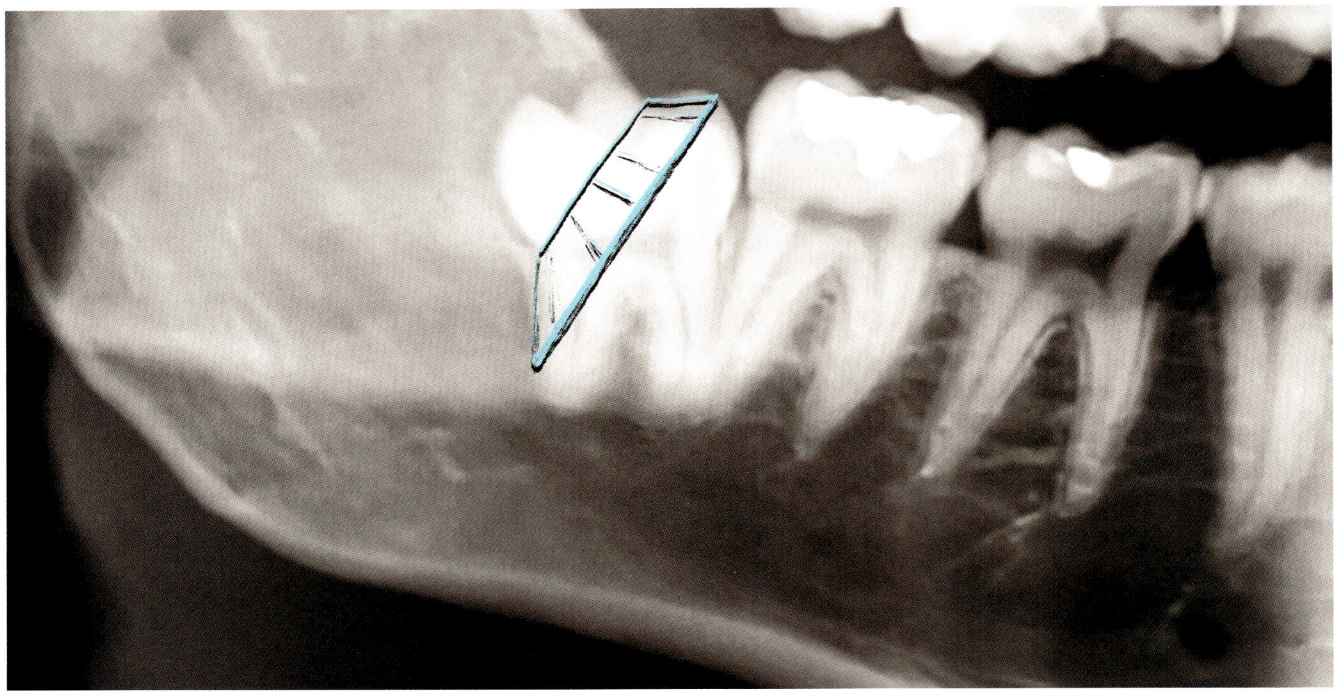

Figure 5-60 This is the approximate plane of where I sectioned the tooth.

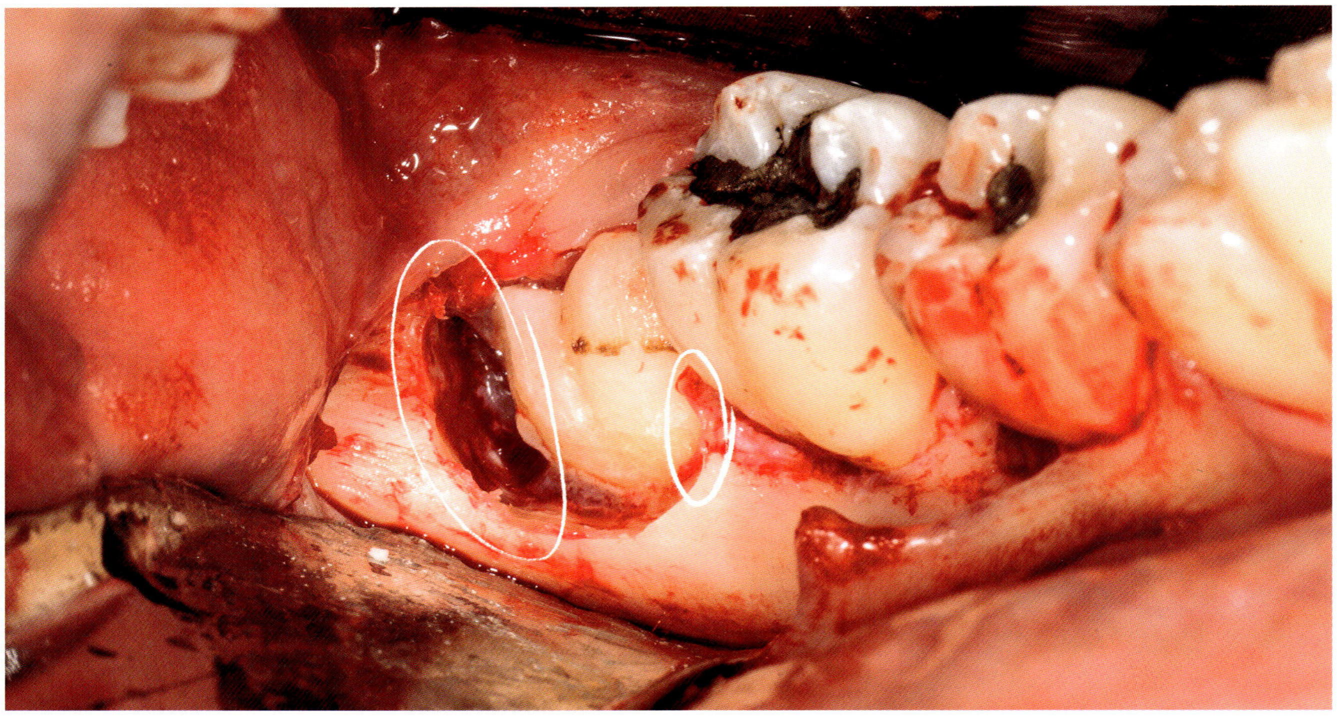

Figure 5-61 Bone was removed at the distal and mesial to create adequate space to elevate.

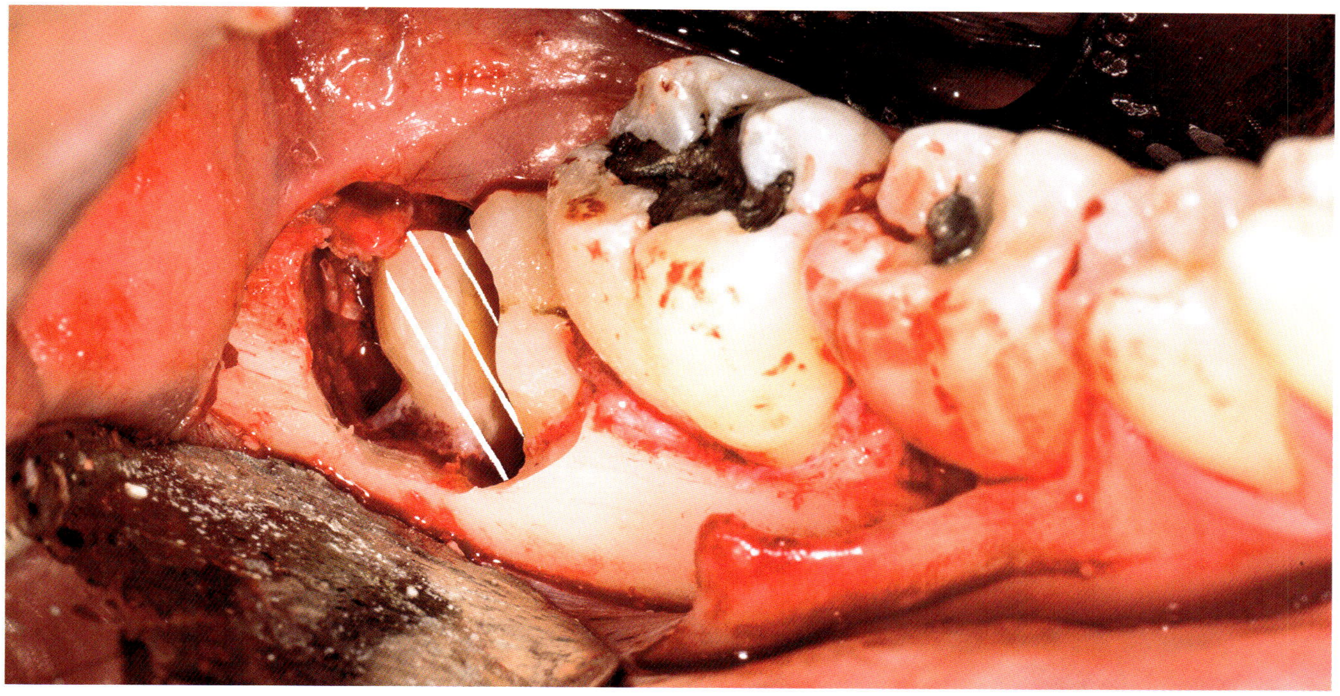

Figure 5-62 After the tooth is sectioned, the distal portion of the crown is mobilized and removed.

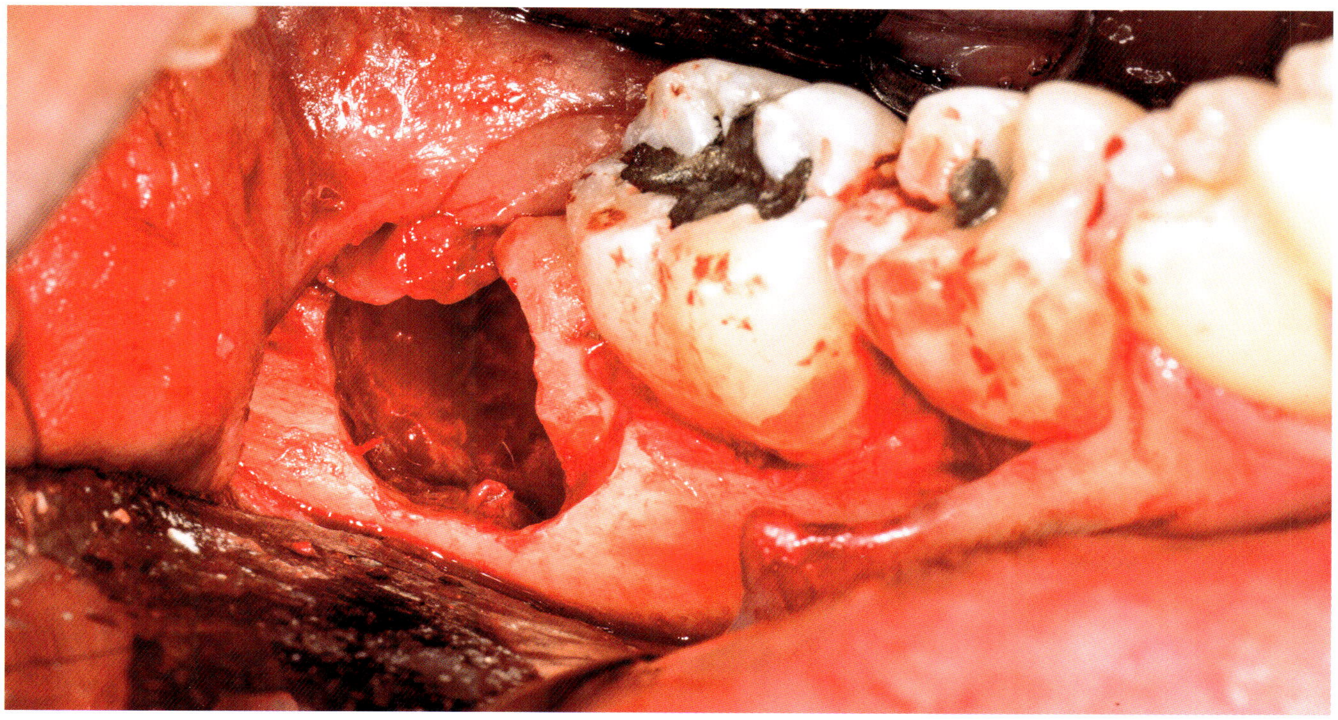

Figure 5-63 The mesial portion of the crown remains intact with both roots retained. A Bein luxator was used to elevate out the remaining crown with the roots intact.

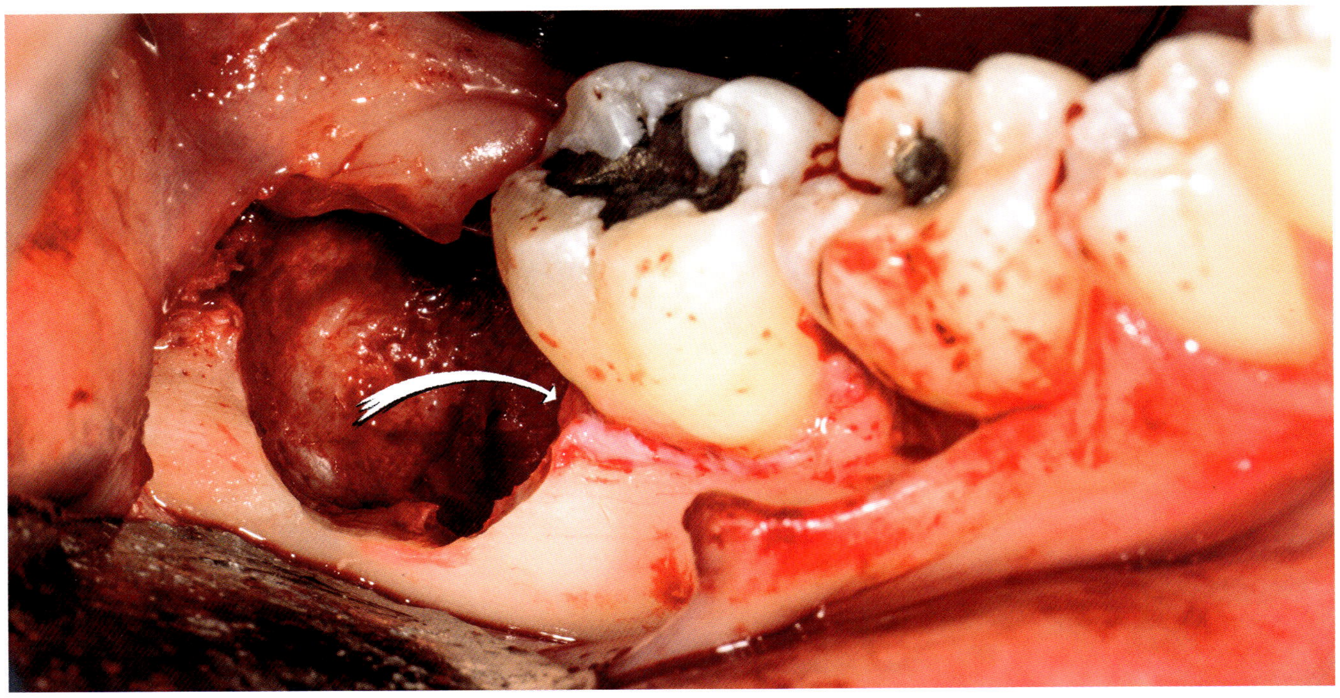

Figure 5-64 Check the distal portion of the second molar. It may need curettage prior to closure. There is often a periodontal defect to debride.

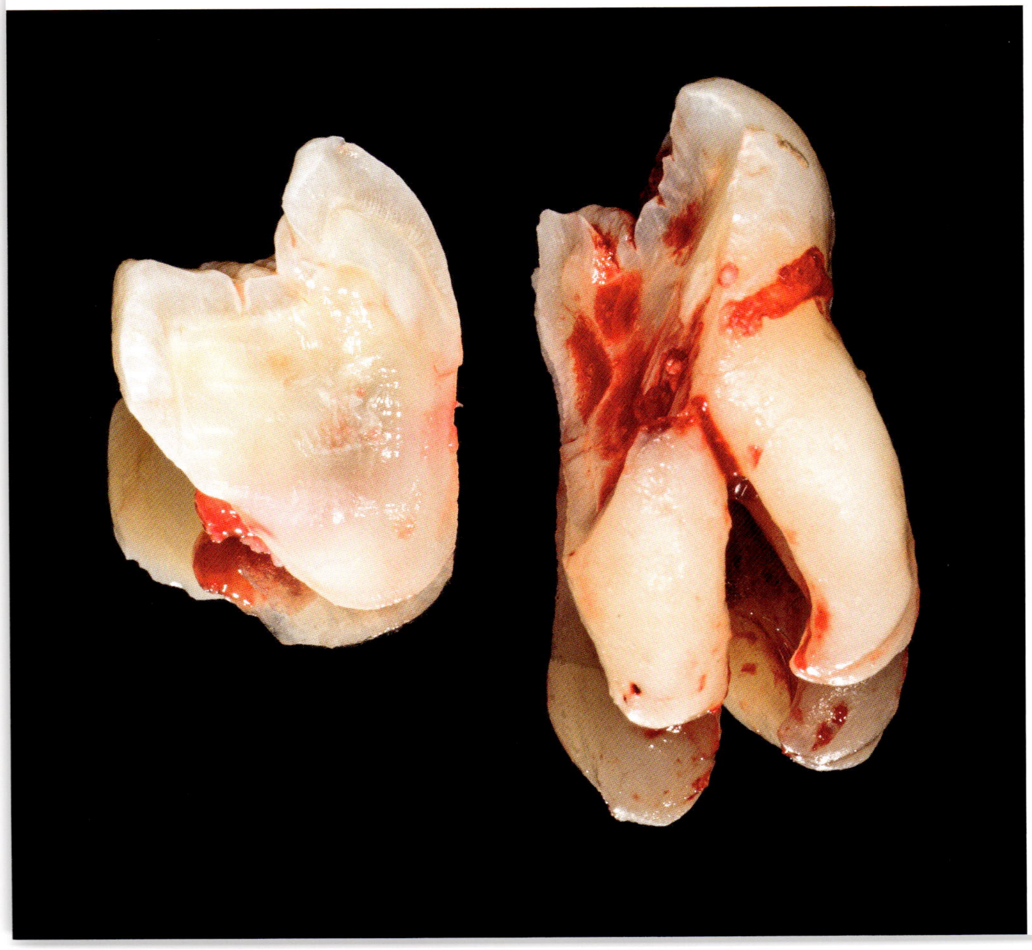

Figure 5-65 Inspecting the pieces as they are removed helps identify what portion of the tooth remains as well as confirms complete removal. You can see the distal portion of this tooth was removed and the mesial portion came out with the distal root.

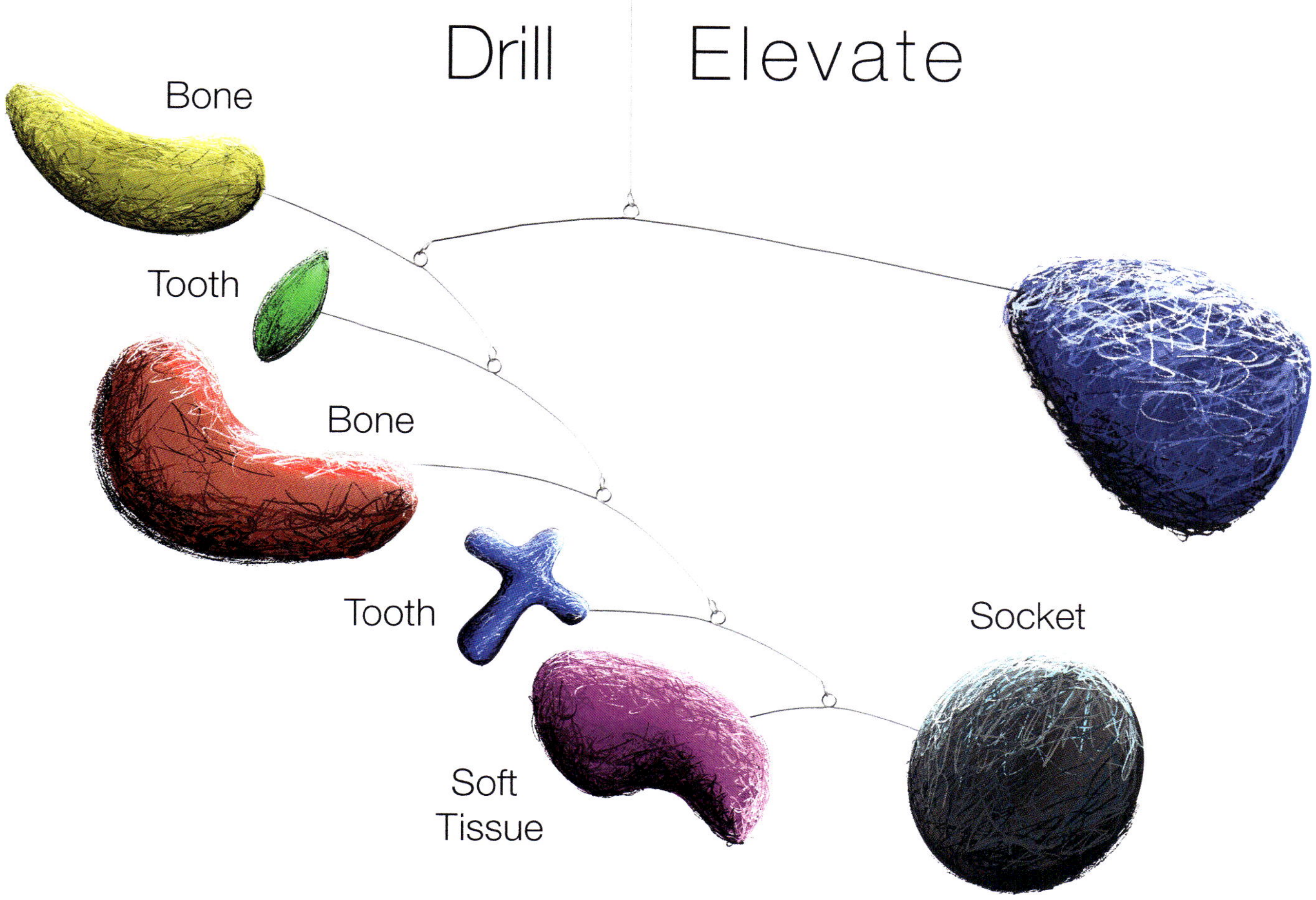

Figure 5-66 This picture sums up the steps for extracting a lower third molar. Sometimes, the tooth can be elevated out without drilling. When a drill is needed, start with bone removal (*yellow*). Then section the tooth (*green*). More bone removal may be necessary (*red*). Consider sectioning more vertically or adding a horizontal cut (*blue*). Make sure the soft tissue is adequately retracted (*purple*). And then evaluate the socket (*gray*). In my mind, it is like a mobile. (Artwork inspired by Alexander Calder.)

ART BREATHES LIFE INTO THE MUNDANE

It was mesmerizing. I was caught almost in a trance as I pondered the enormous mobile hanging from the ceiling in the Alexander Calder exhibit at the Museum of Modern Art in New York City. It is dimensional. It is kinetic. It is fluid. It is so complex yet so very simple. The balance. The flow. The shapes. *"This is surgery,"* I thought. Each fulcrum is a decision point. After the options are all weighed, another step is taken on this journey. Alexander Calder's mobile captures the essence of *The Art of Oral Surgery*. It is life breathed into the classic decision tree model. I now see Calder's work when I remove lower third molars.

Upper Third Molar

In removing upper third molars, there's a fine line between having control of the position of the tooth and losing control. It can feel good to push the envelope when things remain in control. But it's an altogether different experience when you lose control and don't know how to regain it. I'd like to share some tools and tips I've learned along the way on how to maintain control as well as how to regain control when things get tricky with upper third molars.

Principles of access are quite similar with hard and soft tissue. You need enough access and room to deliver a tooth and any fragments successfully. In the maxilla, hard tissue access can usually be created with hand instruments, but a drill can be necessary at times. The softer bone overlying a fully or partially impacted upper third molar of a teenager may often be reflected with a hand instrument. At times, the tooth itself displaces the bone during luxation and elevation. The movement of the tooth can expand the bone and create the access. The trick here is to make sure the elevator is inserted above the height of contour of the crown so you maintain positive control of the movement of the tooth in a favorable direction.

A slender luxator or back action elevator works well for upper third molars. The Minnesota cheek retractor should be positioned firmly on the superior and lateral/posterior aspect of the site. This helps prevent the tooth from being displaced superiorly into the infratemporal fossa. Impacted upper third molars are adept at sneaking around the corner in the subperiosteal plane as discussed previously in the soft tissue management section.

Sometimes, the overlying bone, minimal follicle space, or close approximation to the adjacent second molar prevents placement of a luxator. In these situations, when you can't blindly elevate the molar safely, soft tissue access must be increased before addressing the bone. First, consider making a distobuccal incision, elevating a simple envelope flap. Retract the buccal soft tissue to evaluate the overlying bone. If the tooth is high or the overlying bone is dense, the incision can be further extended to include the papilla between the first and second molars. Reflecting this flap will provide increased access to both identify what is impeding progress as well as safely deliver the tooth. We want to provide an easy path to bring the tooth toward the oral cavity instead of displacing it up into the no-man's-land of the infratemporal fossa.

It is sometimes possible to outfracture the overlying buccal bone without sacrificing it. Similar to the lower third molars, the blunt beavertail end of the Micro Buser can peel off thin overlying bone. If the follicle is near the crest or the bone is soft enough, gentle lateral pressure of this bone may displace it enough to create space for the luxator, and the extraction process can proceed. The lateral pressure can be controlled by fulcruming the instrument on the bone or sometimes cautiously engaging the adjacent tooth. This maneuver may completely fracture off the overlying bone to provide access to the underlying tooth. Care should be taken with this maneuver as it is easy to unintentionally fracture a large segment of the alveolar bone around the second molar. If the mobilized bone seems stable enough and with adequate blood supply, it may be preserved and pushed back into place manually after the tooth is out.

If the bone is too thick or too dense to remove with a hand instrument, use a drill to develop the access. The flap of soft tissue must be protected as usual. It can be tricky to manage the irrigation in this position. Try using a very low speed drill without irrigation just to get access through the cortical bone. The bone in the posterior maxilla doesn't heat up nearly as quickly as dense mandibular bone. When performed cautiously, this can be kind to the bone and allow you to develop ideal access to elevate the tooth successfully without drowning your patient.

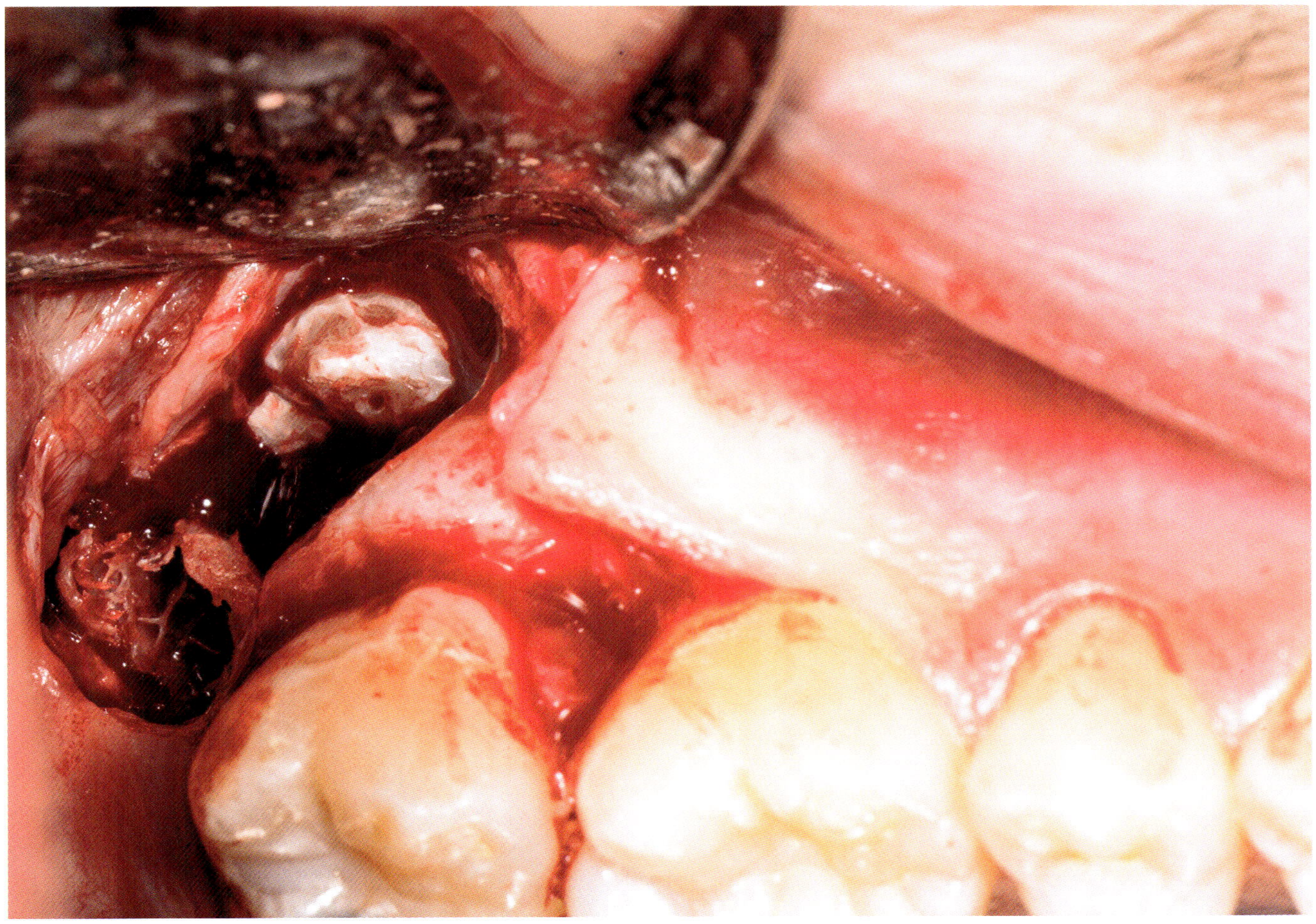

Figure 5-67 Accessing this impacted upper third molar required drilling to remove bone.

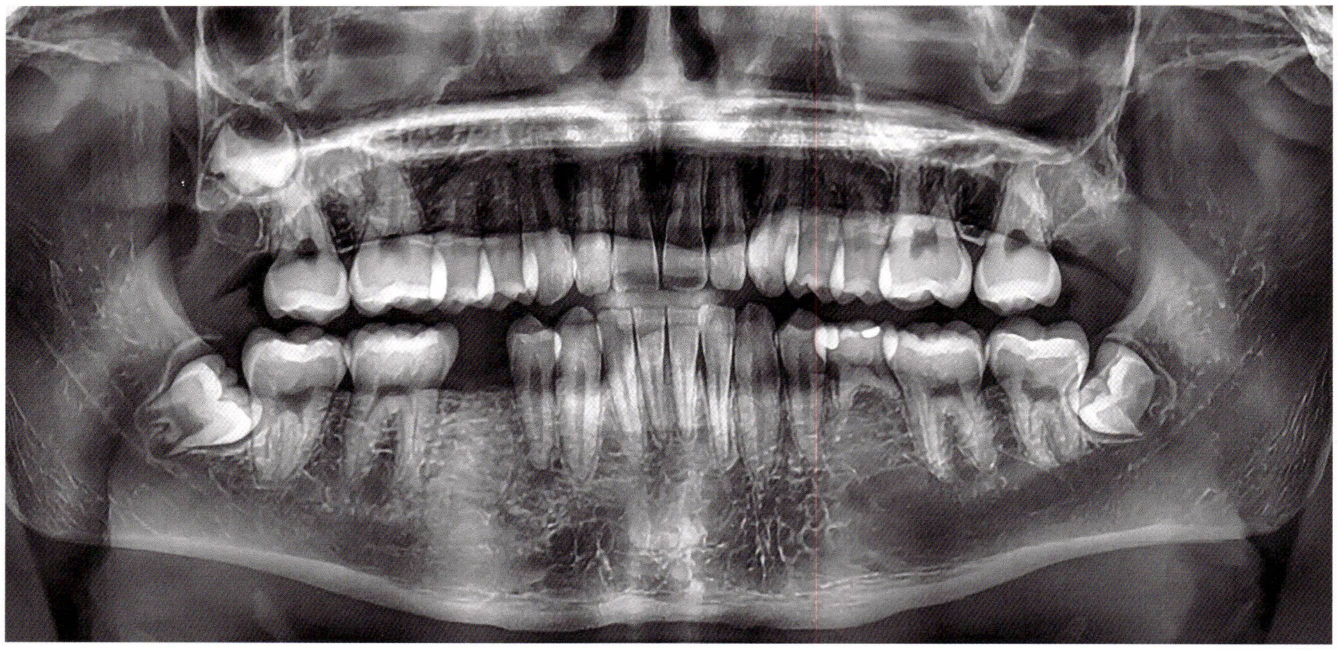

Figure 5-68 Bone removal with a handpiece may be necessary to access an impacted upper third molar such as this. Adequate flap reflection is important. When you remove bone to access the tooth, remember to remove bone in the path of delivery of the tooth as well.

After establishing a stable purchase point, if the tooth doesn't cooperate with elevation, it is often the distal or palatal aspect of the tuberosity overlying the tooth that is preventing the extraction. This bone is tucked out of sight beneath the soft tissue flap. One way of evaluating and addressing this is to slide a spade elevator or the blunt end of the Micro Buser toward the distal aspect over the occlusal of the tooth. Either of these instruments may be effective at both identifying and repositioning the overlying bone. The bone doesn't necessarily need to be removed. It may just need to be outfractured in order to create space to deliver the tooth. If you don't reduce that displaced boney roof, it can be terribly irritating to the palatal tissue during the recovery. Make it a practice to palpate the buccal and palatal aspect of any extraction site. During the surgery, any protruding fragments of bone can easily be reduced, optimizing the healing.

Impacted maxillary third molars can be complicated by dense bone or severely dilacerated roots. In these situations, generous access is critical, and the tooth may need to be sectioned. If I have been struggling for a while with an upper third molar and find five or six roots splayed out in all directions, I feel a sense of validation. These can be tough and require patience and close attention to detail.

Impacted upper third molars can be exceedingly difficult to section successfully. The angle and position of the tooth makes it difficult to fracture through the furcation. More frequently it results in sectioning off portions of the distal crown. Sometimes it results in fracturing the entire crown off. This can leave you with a tangled mess of roots hiding out of sight around the corner, very difficult to access with any instruments. And these roots seem to have a particularly high affinity for the maxillary sinus. Retrieving these fractured roots must be approached with great caution and an even broader access. Use a mirror, suction, small instruments, and as much time as you need. Impatience can cost a lot in these situations.

In general, the instrumentation to remove impacted upper third molars is the same as any other extraction. One additional instrument that seems to have a unique set of strengths here is the Potts elevator. The near 90° angle and curved tip can be leveraged with the T handle to elevate a high impacted upper third molar from the palate out toward the buccal. It also can be directed in the follicle space over the occlusal onto the palatal to leverage it laterally. At times, it can reach around the mesial-superior aspect delivering a tooth inferiorly and laterally. These are helpful tools, but they also have great potential to cause problems. They can apply significant force with the T handle and may easily, and unintentionally, displace the tooth superiorly or damage adjacent soft or hard tissue. They are usually used with more complicated high impactions. All the more reason to proceed with caution. Upper third molars can be a delight to extract, but they also can be very challenging.

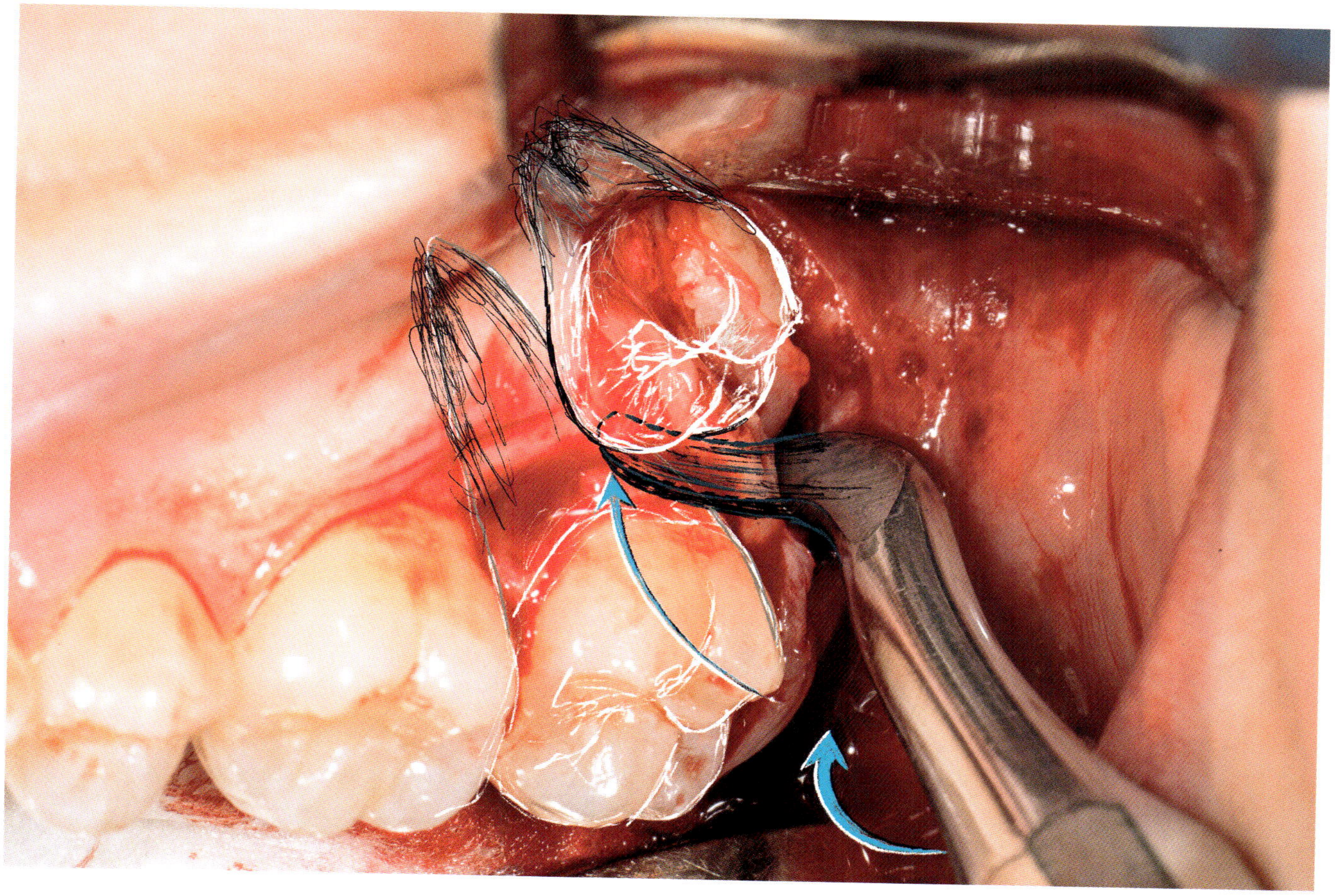

Figure 5-69 The Potts elevator provides a unique angle of elevation on upper impacted molars. Think about using this with a high impaction or if the force needs to be more buccal or palatal. The angle of the tip can hook around the crown to purchase points other instruments can't reach.

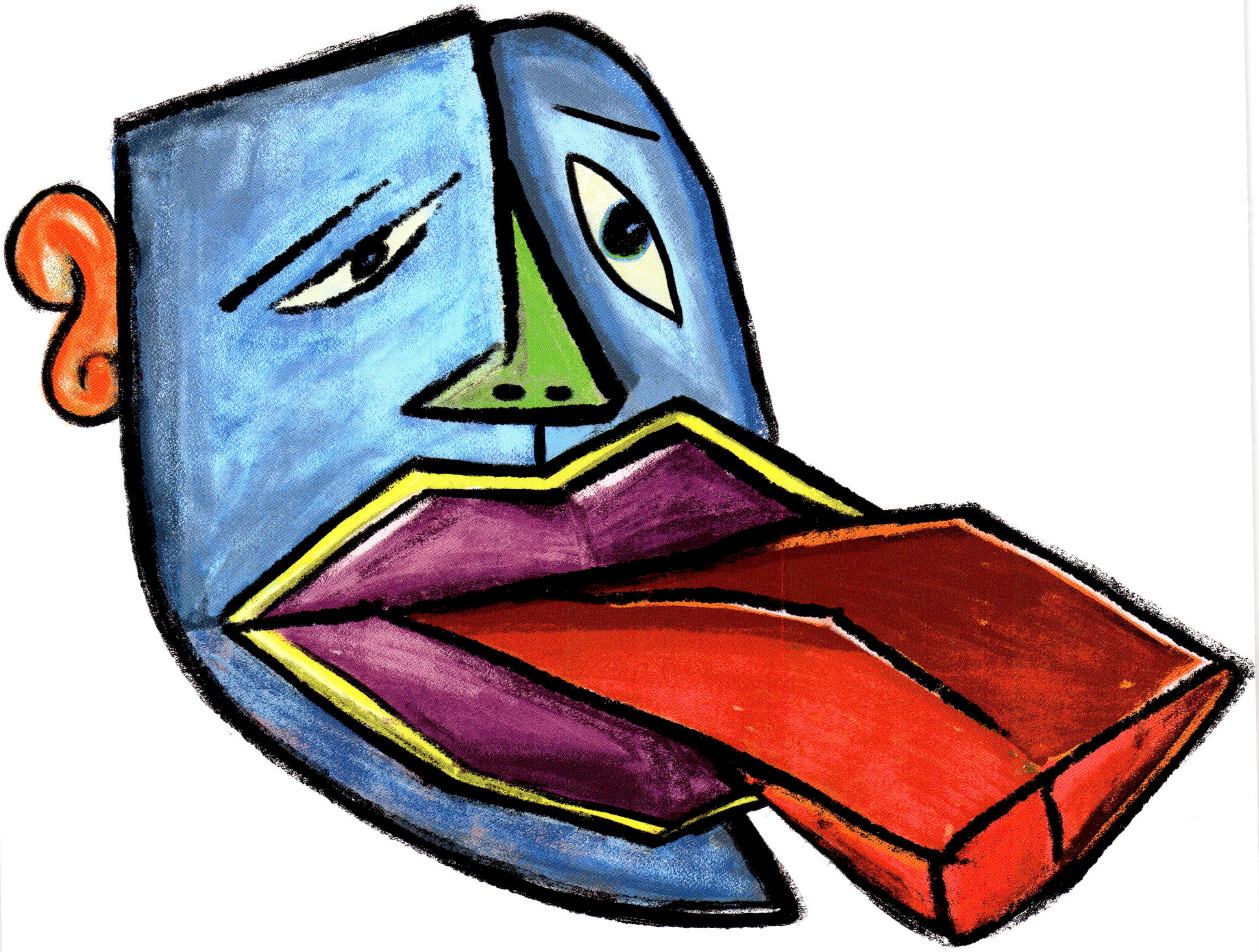

Figure 5-70 The lips and tongue have some of the highest somatosensory input with more area devoted to them in the neocortex than almost anywhere else. Their sensation is amplified, as is their silence in the case of nerve trauma.
(Artwork inspired by Pablo Picasso.)

Coronectomy

We seldom appreciate what we have until it's gone.

No one likes to be numb. It doesn't feel good. Each sensory nerve has its own, individual place in the brain, which somehow keeps track of about 250,000 afferent sensory nerve fibers. When a group of them goes silent, the brain tries all sorts of tricks to make sense of it because the brain doesn't like the silence. We don't do well with it. As we age, we slowly lose about 5% to 8% of our sensory innervation per decade. And we don't even like it at that pace.

Primum non nocere. First, do no harm. This core principle in medical ethics, commonly called non-maleficence, implores us as surgeons to work to reduce the incidence of surgical nerve injury as low as possible. We certainly want it below the reported 1.3% to 5.3% risk for removing lower third molars[14]. To do this, we must identify high risk patients and work to develop tools and techniques to mitigate the risk.

The mental nerve. Yeah, it's important.

Functional: Every word we speak and meal we eat is impacted by the sensation of our lips.
Our speech relies on the sensory input of our lips to enunciate words. Every bite of food or drink of liquid passes through our lips.

Pleasurable: The wonderful experience of eating can be hijacked by a numb lip. The intimacy and connection of a kiss is transmitted through the sensation of the lips. Think about the incredible action of the dopamine and oxytocin released with a kiss. That innervation is great!

Protective: If you can't feel it, you can't keep it safe. Innervation is a primary defense mechanism for the body. It is one of the initial alarms that something is not right.

Vanity: People think about their faces. They want to feel good about themselves. A numb lip can cause psychological and emotional stress. That precious little nerve even helps protect us from the embarrassment of having food on our face.

Evaluation

The anatomical relationship between the nerve and the root determines the risk for nerve injury with lower third molar extractions. The potential for recovery is impacted by the level of damage and the patient's age. The combination of these two factors, along with the technical execution of the procedure, determines the likelihood of temporary or permanent deficit. How can we reduce the risk? We cannot change the patient's age or anatomy. But we can always work to improve our technique and skill.

Anatomy

How close? And how involved?

The closer the nerve and root live, and the more intimately involved they are, the higher the risk of injury. A two-dimensional image is a useful screening tool to identify higher risk cases. But it is impossible to really understand the three-dimensional relationship with a two-dimensional image. When a panoramic or periapical radiograph shows deviation of the canal, darkening of the roots over the canal, or if the apex of the root extends beyond the canal, a cone beam CT scan should be considered. In my mind, if it looks like the nerve could be harmed during the removal of the tooth, the patient deserves a more thorough evaluation with a CBCT.

A cone beam CT image should be high quality. But even with an excellent image it can be difficult to identify the path of the nerve through the medullary bone. I find it extremely valuable to be able to see multiple angles simultaneously on the same screen. This helps my brain build the mental imagery needed to evaluate the risk of the procedure. There is obviously a higher risk when the image shows the roots invade and restrict the mandibular canal space.

While reviewing multiple angles on a CBCT, ask yourself how the nerve would get injured if the tooth were surgically removed. How close are they? Are the roots curved around or beyond the nerve? What would or could happen to that nerve? Would it suffer a compression injury? Tension? Tearing? Laceration? Could a sharp piece of bone get displaced into the canal space?

Some of the industry's "top of the line" CBCT machines produce far superior images than others. When purchasing a unit, do your own due diligence. Check out some real images of real patients from various machines. The differences may be subtle, but they can make all the difference. Compare the definition of the canal and the periodontal ligament space. I have found these two structures are good indicators of image quality.

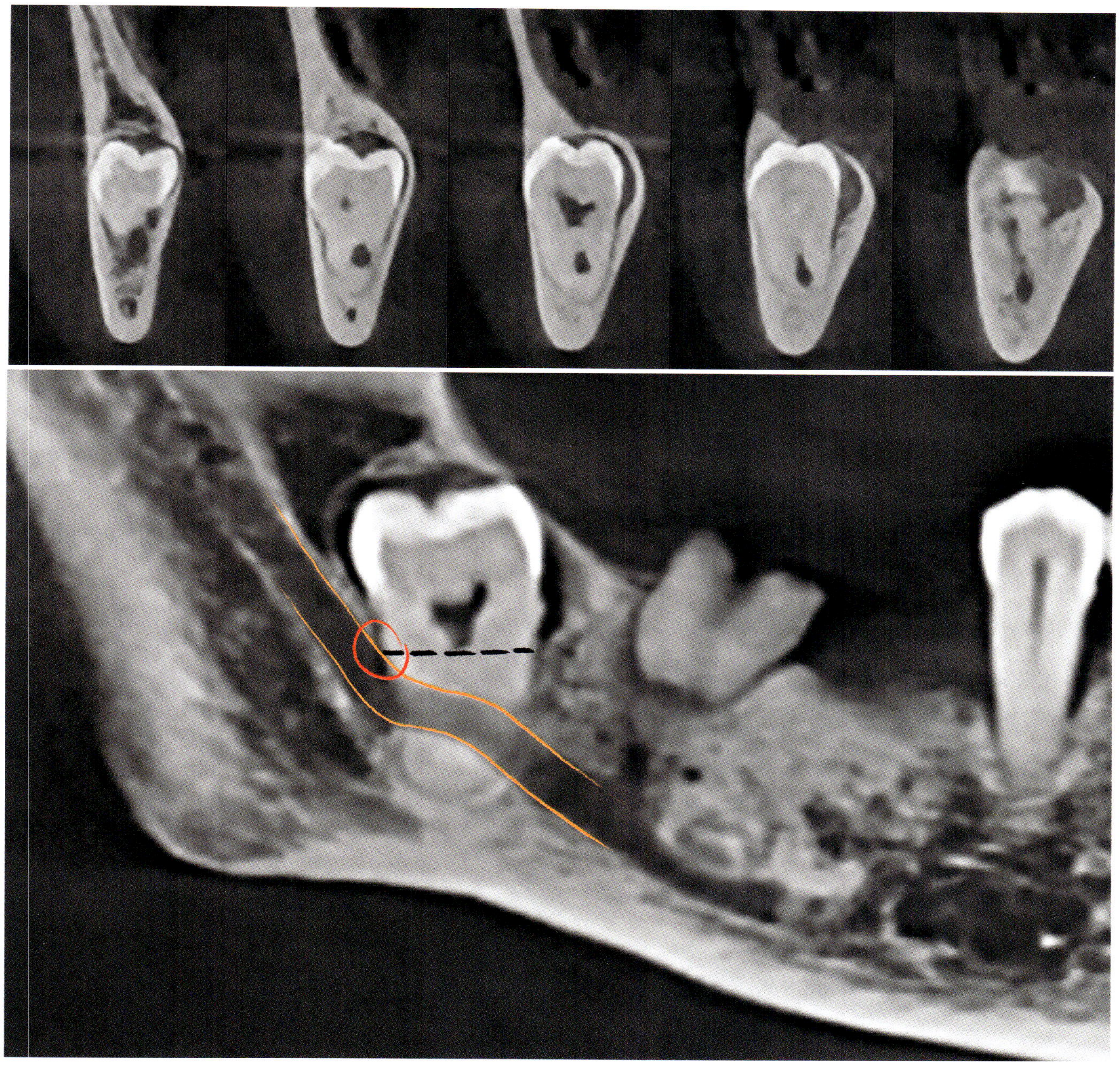

Figure 5-71 This tooth has developed entirely around the inferior alveolar nerve. Coronectomy significantly reduces the chances of nerve damage compared to extraction in this case. But look at how close the distal crown approximates the nerve. Pay close attention to that distal area to avoid nerve damage from the drill. Our goal is to reduce the tooth below the pulp chamber if possible. Less retained root structure is better.

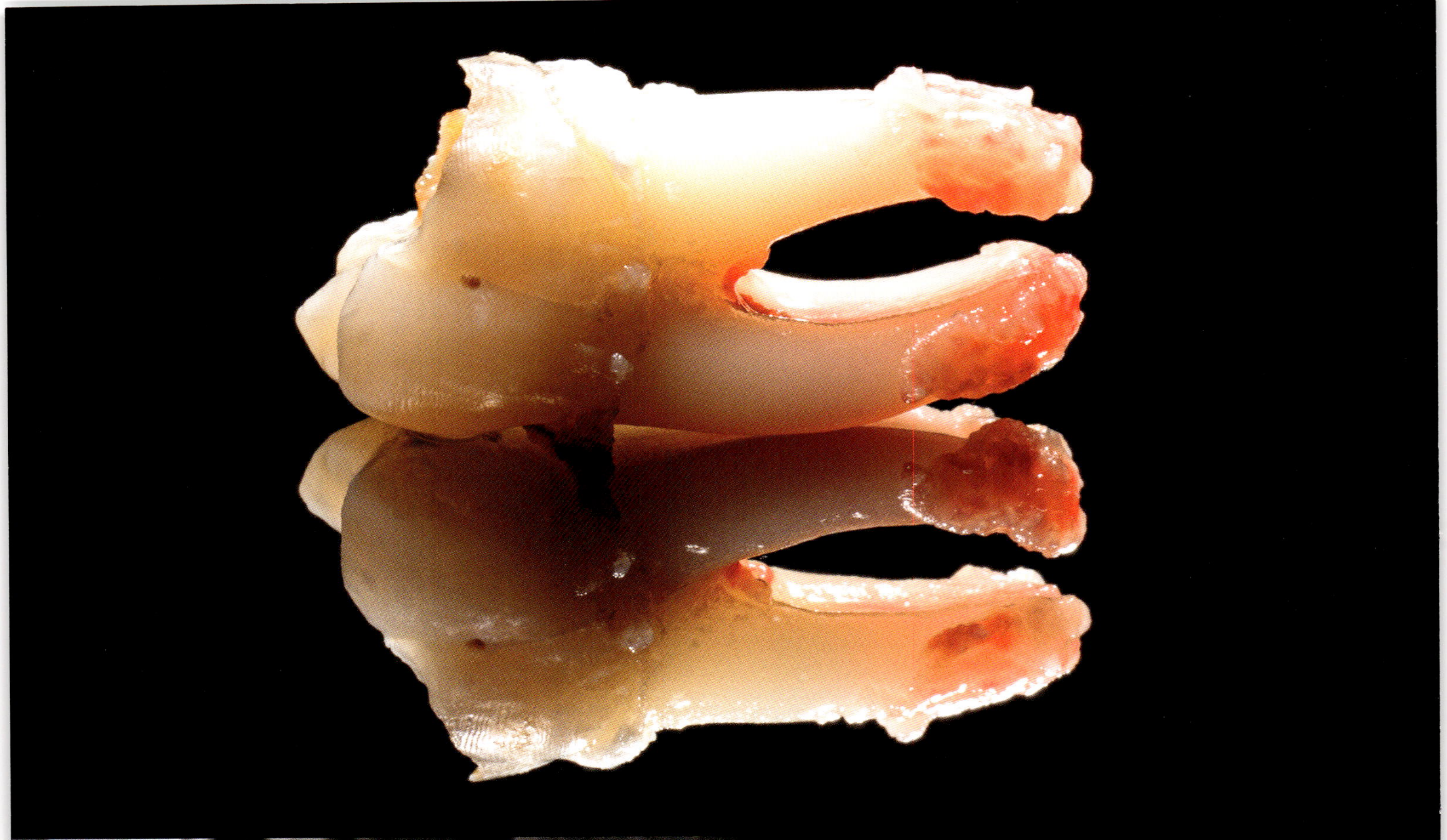

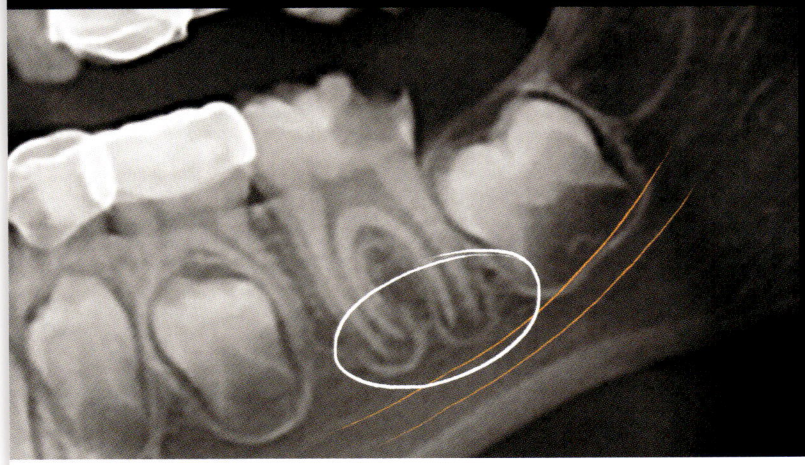

Figure 5-72 The apex of an incompletely developed tooth poses very little risk to a nearby nerve. Look at the radiographic root development. If this were overlying the nerve, it would still be unlikely to cause permanent nerve damage. (Coronectomy was not even considered in this case. These pictures help visualize root development radiographically with clinical anatomy.)

Root development

Undeveloped roots are a relative contraindication for coronectomy. Permanent nerve injury is less likely with an incompletely developed root. The soft tissue at the apex acts like a bumper protecting the nerve from damage by the root. And it is very difficult to maintain stability of the retained portion of an incompletely developed root. They are much more prone to migrate.

I find it helpful to begin evaluating the development of third molars in patients in their early to mid-teens. I would much rather have the option to wait rather than wish we could have done surgery sooner. In the context of this discussion regarding nerve injury, it is safer to remove impacted wisdom teeth before they become intimately involved with the nerve. However, many of our patients are not afforded that luxury. We often need to manage high risk impacted third molars after complete root development when there is a very intimate relationship between the entwined root and nerve.

While it is impossible to know if a patient truly understands, we want them to understand as well as possible. I like to use the following language in my documentation: *"Reviewed risks, benefits and alternatives to the proposed treatment. Patient indicated understanding and elects to proceed with treatment."* This is just a simple phrase I include after much more significant documentation of the findings and the conversation.

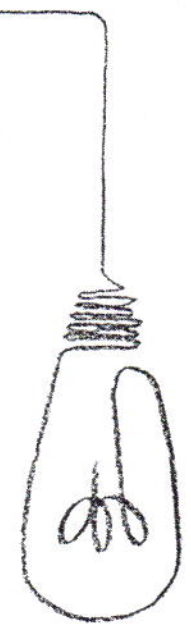

Age

Regenerative potential decreases with age. A similar injury is more likely to cause permanent changes in older patients[15]. Therefore, it may be more beneficial to consider coronectomy on an adult patient. Sometimes age is the determining factor even if the anatomy is similar. An identical tooth that may be safe for an extraction in an 18-year-old may be best as a coronectomy in a 60-year-old.

Treatment options

It is usually easy to identify high risk situations. It is obvious that a nerve running directly through a tooth has a high risk of injury. Planning becomes more challenging when the nerve is close but not obviously intwined with the roots. In these cases, clinical and radiographic judgment informs your conversation with the patient. Not all patients will make the same choice, even with identical findings and the same discussion. Patients must be informed of the risks, benefits and alternatives to the proposed treatment. They need to be involved in the decision. And their involvement must be documented in their chart. As surgeons, we investigate the situation, apply what

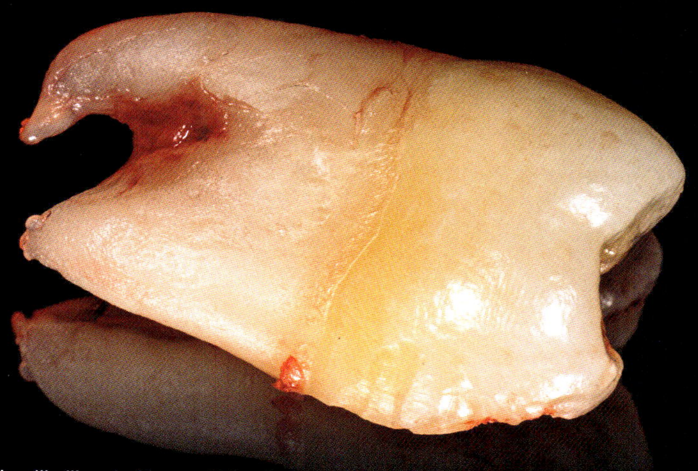

Figure 5-73 This tooth had a higher likelihood of traumatizing the nerve. You can see the path of the nerve at the apex. Thankfully, this patient had no resulting paresthesia.

we know, and do what we think is best. This is how we guide the planning for our patients.

When a tooth is near the nerve, there are three main options: retain the tooth, remove the tooth or resect the coronal portion of the tooth, which is called coronectomy. The patient must always be informed of the option and risks of doing nothing. That is a key component of a proper medicolegal informed consent.

Retain

In the absence of acute pathology, retention may be a reasonable and prudent option. But retaining a tooth with a hopeless prognosis and impending infection may result in higher risk and increased morbidity later. Patients tend to heal better when they are younger; every one of our patients is getting older.

Remove

Sometimes the infection is too bad or too much tooth structure is compromised to either retain the tooth or perform coronectomy. Despite close relationship to the nerve, the tooth may need to be removed. Protecting the nerve in these cases starts with knowing the anatomy where the nerve and root meet. Construct a mental image of the roots, bone and canal. See the relationship on the computer screen and in your mind. Envision what it would take to protect the nerve while removing the tooth. It can be helpful to section the tooth parallel to the mandibular canal. Envision using forces that move the tooth away from the canal. It is conceivable that enough tooth structure and bone could be removed to allow the root to be elevated away from the nerve without significant risk of harm. While this technique is conceivable, it may be unrealistic. The level of precision drilling, splitting and elevating without causing sharp or blunt injury to the nerve may not be practical or possible. We want to do the very best we can with the resources we have. In these cases, it is helpful to create adequate access and work efficiently. You also may consider referring to someone with more experience or better surgical resources.

Resect (Coronectomy)

The race is on. When a root tip is retained, either intentionally or unintentionally, a race begins between the root and the surrounding bone. The root is trying to erupt, and the bone is trying to heal over it. If the root wins by erupting into the mouth, it will likely need to be removed in a secondary surgery. Thankfully, the risk of nerve injury is then very low as the root has migrated away from the nerve. If the bone wins the race and completely covers the root, further surgery is not likely necessary as the root will likely remain in the bone for the long term. That is the goal. We want the bone to heal over to avoid additional procedures and potential complications. The vast majority of the time the bone wins and further surgery is not necessary.

Coronectomy procedure

How do we help the bone win the race to heal? By minimizing the size and mobility of the retained segment and maintaining as much bone in the site as possible. The smaller the root fragment, the more quickly the bone can heal over it. A stable root will erupt slower than a mobilized root. And a smaller defect in the bone will heal over faster. These outcomes are best achieved through precise drilling and a favorable split.

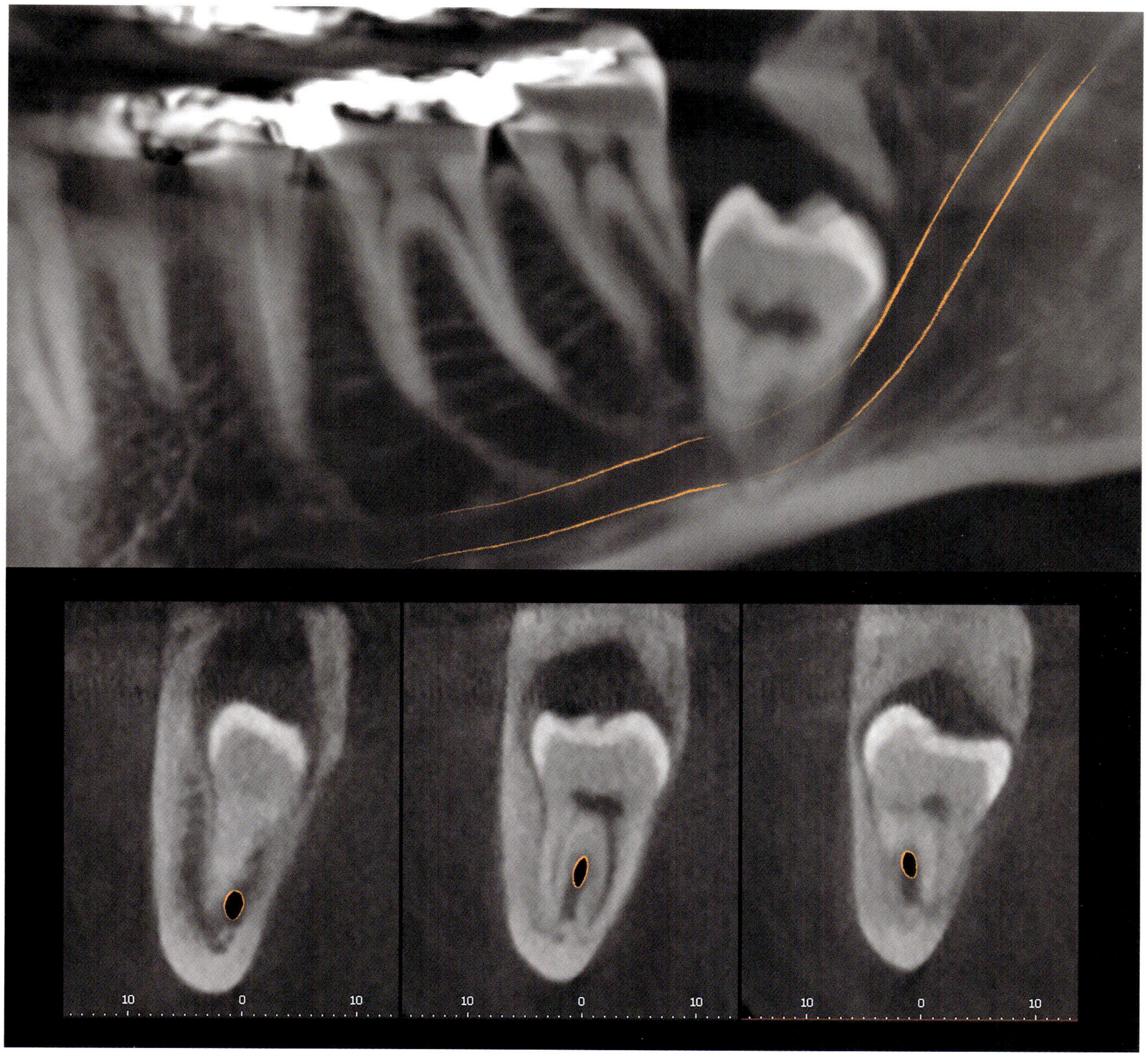

Figure 5-74 The path of the inferior alveolar nerve appears to go through the center of the roots of this lower third molar.

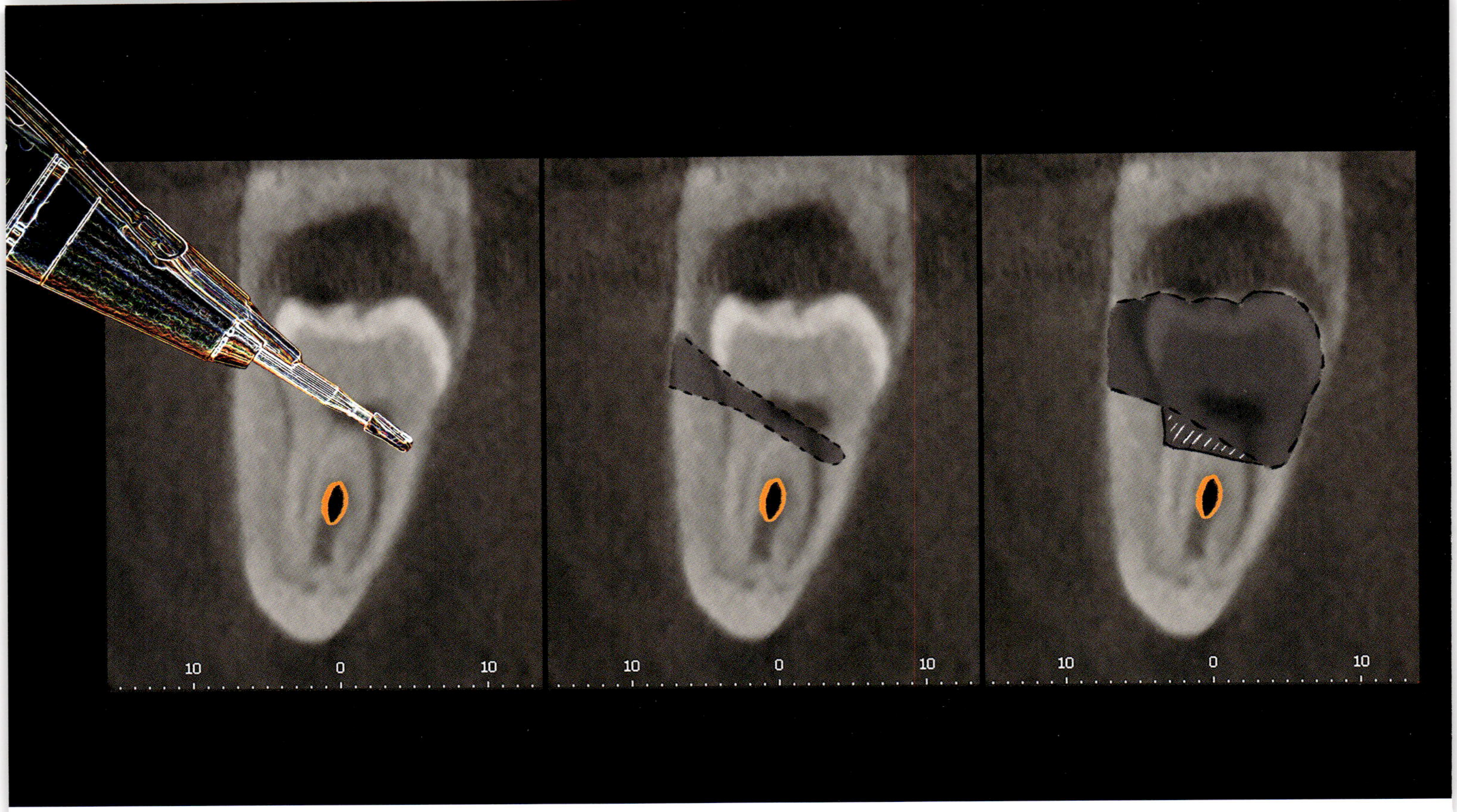

Figure 5-75 The angle of the drill extends more inferiorly on the lingual than buccal. After the coronal segment is fractured and removed, further root reduction is performed with a round bur favoring the buccal portion. The goal is to reduce the root below the pulp chamber, leaving as little root as possible while protecting the nerve. You know you are in the zone when you see two separate roots in the site.

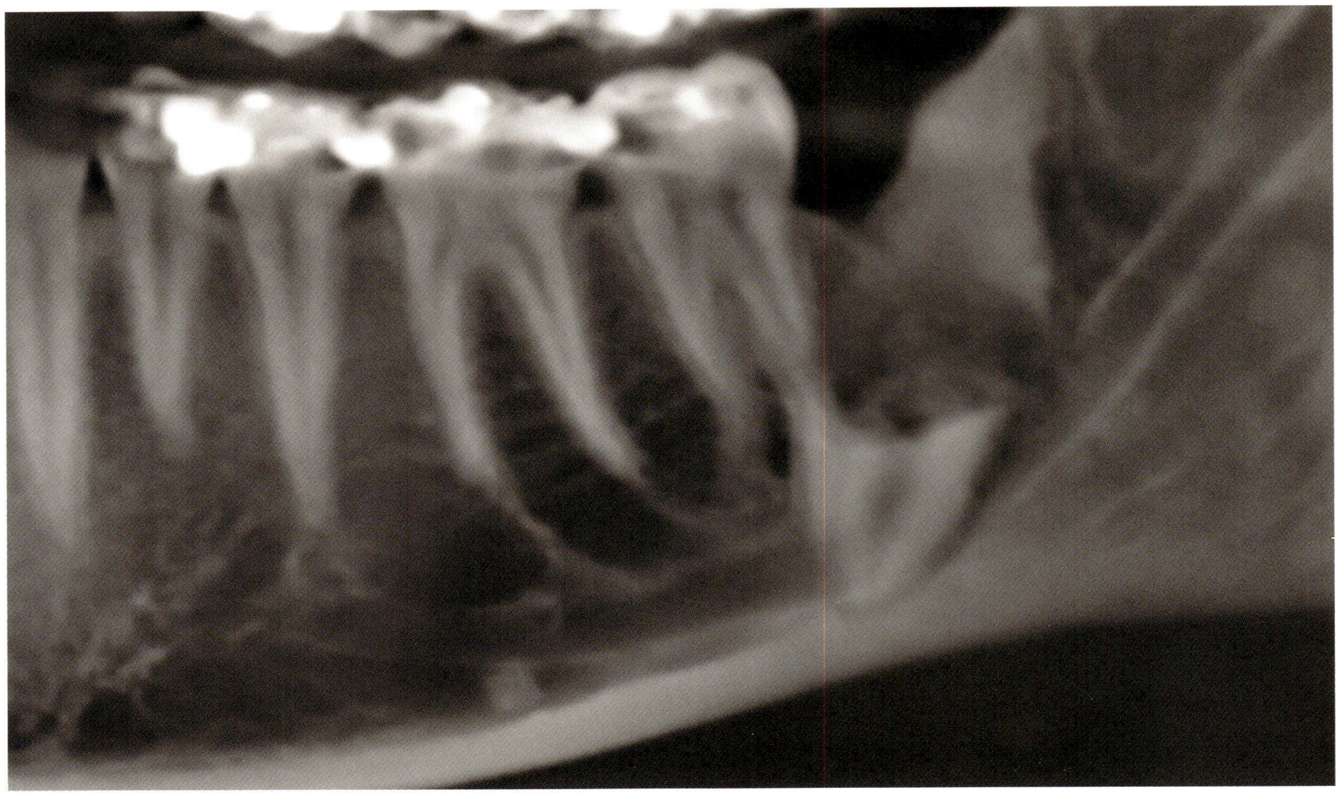

Figure 5-76 One year later, the bone has healed completely over the retained roots. The second molar is stable and the periodontal condition is healthy.

The typical technique for a coronectomy starts with a broad buccal access through bone. With the best visualization possible, the tooth is sectioned most of the way through the crown. This cut should be as apical as possible without compromising the nerve. A wide elevator or luxator is then placed into the deepest part of the cut and torqued to finish the split. The trick is to split the tooth without mobilizing the roots. They must remain stable.

The area of highest risk for a bad split occurs where the tooth remains most intact. Because of the limited access and visualization, this is often at the mesiolingual, distolingual or distobuccal aspects. Sectioning in these areas can be difficult due to the anatomy and angles of the bur. When completing the split, position the elevator all the way into the cut and rotate it in such a way as to propagate the fracture through the most intact portion of the tooth. Try not to lift the tooth out. Just complete the split.

You can usually hear or feel the tooth crack, but it can be difficult to know where it split. As a measure of caution, it is good to visualize the split before attempting to remove the coronal segment. If only one of the roots separated from the coronal segment with the split, the attached root will elevate out with the crown. I can tell you it doesn't feel good to see the crown come out with one root still attached.

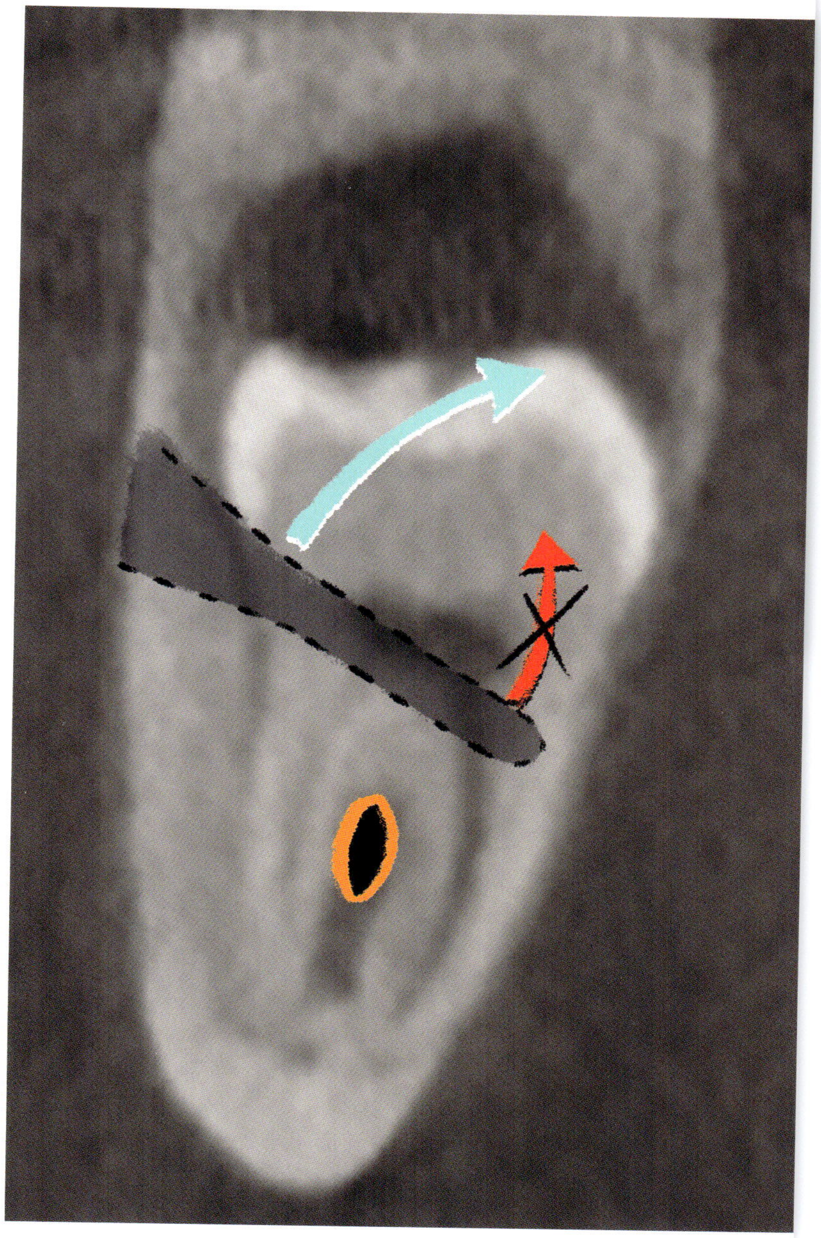

Figure 5-77 The leverage used to complete the split should propagate the fracture through the most intact portion of the tooth. A little force in the wrong direction can mobilize the tooth instead of completing the fracture.

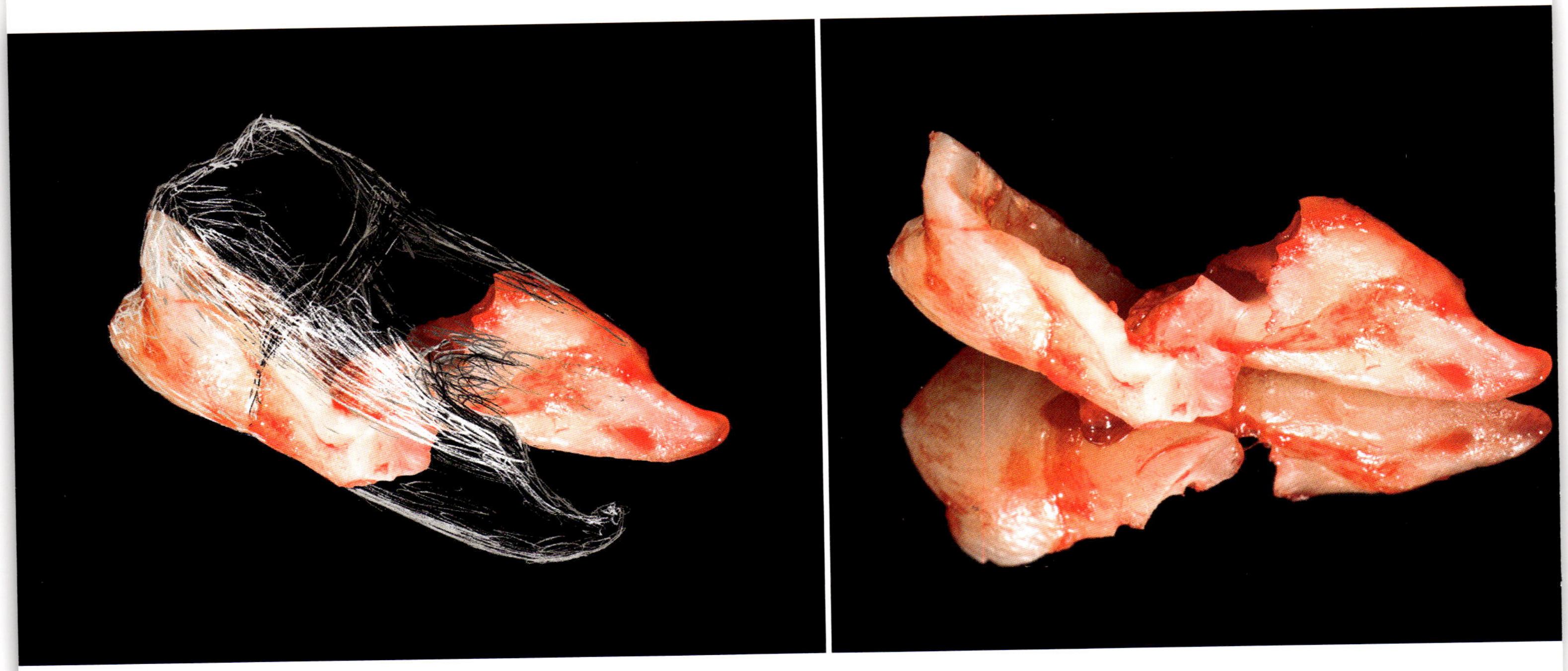

Figure 5-78 This cut went well over 2/3 through the crown. There was just enough structure remaining on the distobuccal that it didn't cleave the distal root when the crown fractured. Thankfully, this patient has recovered most of her sensation. After a few months, she reports the small amount of residual paresthesia on her chin is negligible.

Complete removal of the enamel is critical for coronectomy success. Inspecting the coronal segment when it is removed can help you visualize what portion of the crown has been removed and what remains. Due to the angle of the drill, the split is often sloped to include more lingual tooth structure than buccal. The coronal segment serves as a guidepost letting you know what structure still remains buried in the bone. Then you can go after the remaining enamel with a round bur. This is usually necessary on the buccal and mesial aspects. In addition to completely removing enamel, reducing the amount of retained root below the pulp chamber while maintaining its stability significantly improves outcomes. Less root structure leads to better bone healing and lower chances of spontaneous eruption or infection. My goal is to reduce the root at least beyond the pulp chamber and through the furcation. If possible, I like to see the separate roots. This gives me confidence I have reduced it adequately.

Key steps in coronectomy

- Adequate exposure
- Safe angle to protect the inferior alveolar nerve
- Depth of drill
  - Deep enough to fracture off the crown without mobilizing the roots: about ⅔ buccolingually.
  - Not too deep. Protect the lingual anatomy.
- Confirm the split
- Reduce the remaining root structure

Primary closure is referenced frequently in the literature as a component for success. In my practice, I have found the size and stability of the remaining root and the proper handling of the soft tissue are far more important.

Coronectomy surgery can be very stressful for the surgeon. You are working in the back of a small dark hole. You can't see your drill, but it needs to get at least ⅔ through the tooth for the roots to separate safely. If the drill goes in too far, it can perforate the lingual plate and sever the lingual nerve. If it is too coronal, the retained enamel causes failure. Too apical and the inferior alveolar nerve can be severed. And the longer surgery takes, the higher the risk of complications. I believe the challenges associated with successful coronectomy are the major reason for its lack of popularity. In my practice, I have found navigating the coronectomy procedure makes it much easier, less stressful, and far more predictable.

Changing Technology: Dynamic Navigation

Make it easier to do better. Then do better.

Navigated coronectomy

Coronectomy used to be one of the most stressful surgeries for me. As I have gained tremendous comfort and confidence in guided coronectomy, I now offer it as an option far more frequently. Sometimes, it makes me feel like Superman with his x-ray vision. I am able to drill at the optimal angle through a small opening, completely through the tooth. The risk of mobilizing the roots, retaining enamel, or damaging the nerve is dramatically reduced. As with any procedure, the easier and more predictable it is, the more likely an option it becomes. In my practice, navigating coronectomy procedures has become a routine option in high-risk situations.

Navigated procedure overview

1. The tags are applied and instruments calibrated per the Navident protocol.
2. A typical full thickness, distobuccal releasing incision is made, including the mesial papilla. Generous soft tissue exposure protects the flap and optimizes access.
3. Calibration accuracy is verified by placing the drill tip on nearby teeth or the overlying bone.
4. The surgery is visualized both by looking at the site and the computer monitor. Identify the path of the drill, mandibular canal, buccal access, vertical and horizontal position of entry, and position of second molar.
5. Remove buccal bone by fanning back and forth to allow the irrigation to remove bone debris and cool the site.
6. Angle the handpiece as perpendicular to the tooth as possible. Lower the Minnesota retractor to optimize the angle of the drill while keeping its tip firmly on bone. This helps protect the periosteum.
7. Drill to depth through the tooth fanning mesial and distal. Verify in the axial view that the cut extends most of the way through the mesial, distal and especially distobuccal portions of the tooth. It is easy to get focused on the lingual extent and retain a portion of the distobuccal tooth structure.
8. While clinically watching the coronal segment, apply a broad force at the depth of the cut with a wide instrument, like the spade elevator or wide luxator. Look to see if the coronal portion mobilizes when it fractures. If it looks like it is moving before feeling it fracture, the crown may have been completely cut off (this is fine) or you may be mobilizing the roots (not so good).
9. Deliver the coronal segment. With guided surgery the access is so small I often need to section the coronal segment. In contrast, when I did

non-guided coronectomy, a large buccal access was needed to adequately visualize the crown. This typically created space to remove it as a single coronal segment.

10. With the crown out, calibrate the round bur and further reduce the remaining root structure well below the crestal bone. Most often this is focused on the buccal aspect because of the angle of the drill. Direct vision seems to be most valuable at this stage while verifying the position and margin of safety with the navigation system.
11. Curette, irrigate, suture, place PRF, and administer Exparel as with routine impacted third molars.
12. Discharge with routine third molar instructions and prescriptions for steroid (Medrol Dosepak), mouth rinse, and a five-day course of antibiotics.

The risk of infection and nerve trauma is slightly higher than routine extractions. Post-operative prescriptions usually include a five-day course of amoxicillin or clindamycin, a five-day course of methylprednisolone (Medrol Dosepak), and chlorhexidine rinse. Patients are also instructed on over-the-counter pain management. A one year follow up appointment is scheduled for imaging and clinical evaluation. If there has been significant migration with no overlying bone, we may discuss removal. But most of the time no further intervention is needed.

Figure 5-79 Room setup for guided coronectomy. My attention moves between the surgical site and the wall monitor, which shows me the precise location of the drill.

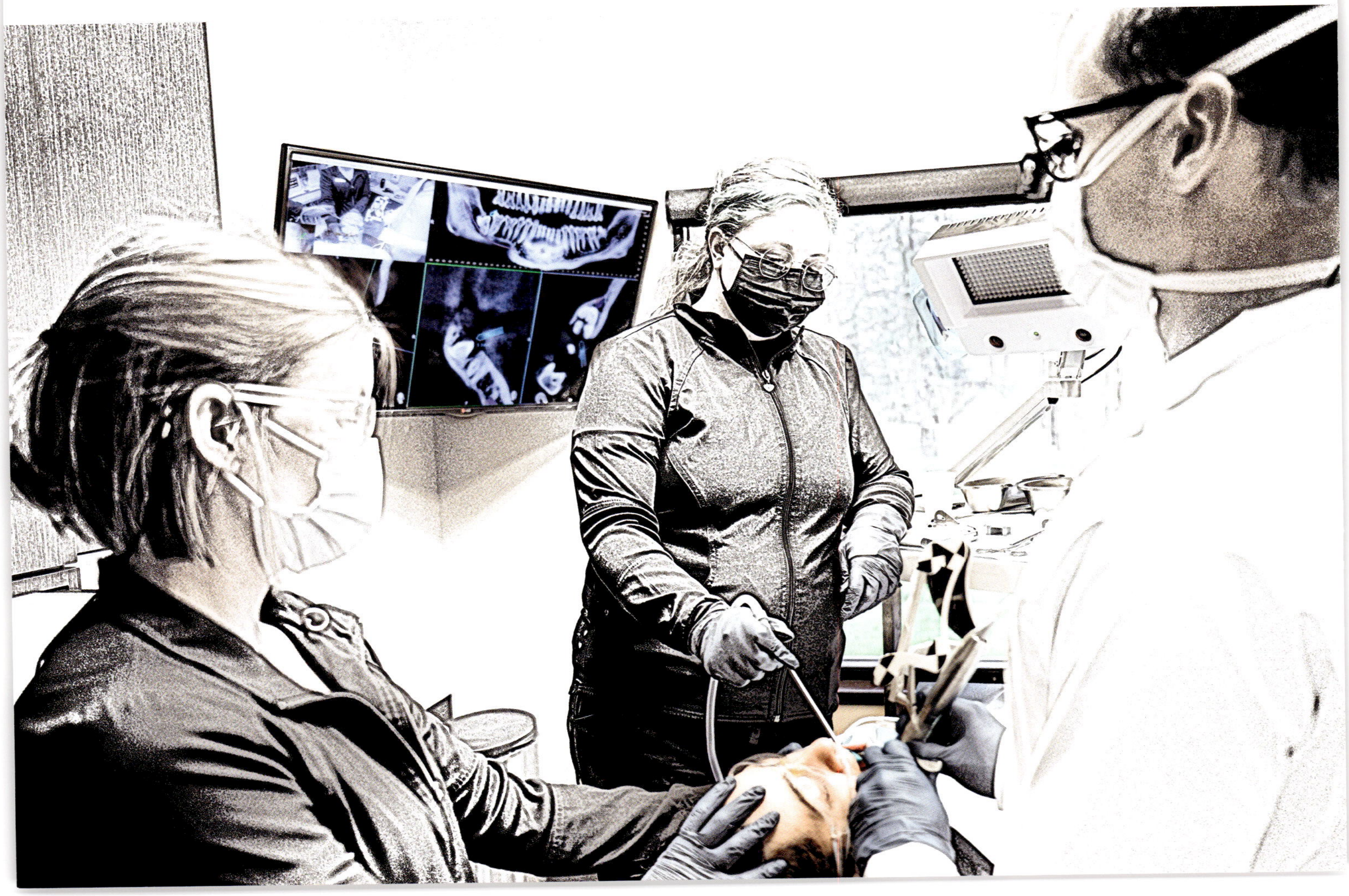

Guided biopsy

In this case, John's initial biopsy revealed an odontogenic keratocyst (OKC). He was followed closely due to the high chance of recurrence. With an OKC, any cells remaining will form daughter cysts. Therefore, complete removal of all cystic tissue is necessary. After two years, signs of recurrence were noted. Navigating treatment at this time allowed me to drill precisely into the small site of recurrence. It increased my confidence that this treatment would be definitive and it decreased morbidity of the surgery. And it also made my job more fun.

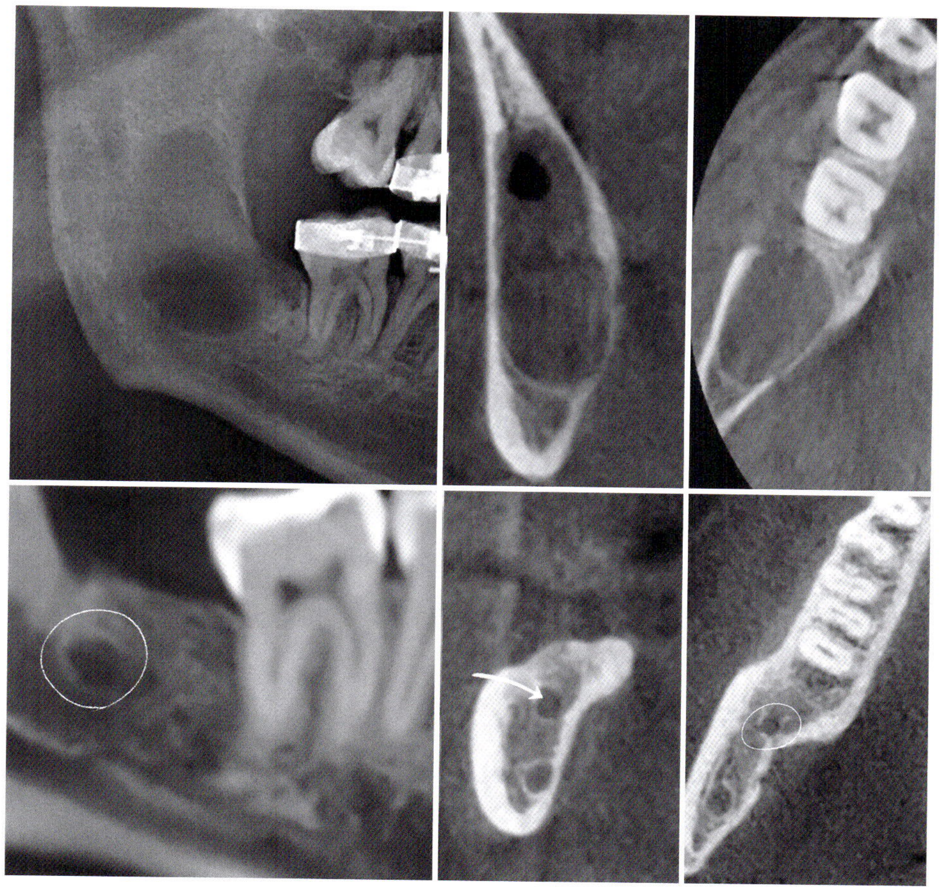

Figure 5-80 This lesion initially extended up the ramus. It recurred two years after the initial biopsy.

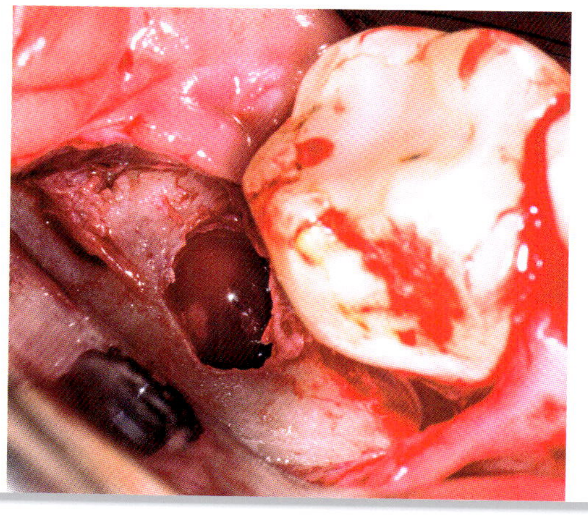

Figure 5-81 With dynamic navigation, the lesion was removed and the site was debrided through a small access. Watching on the monitor, I could direct my drill precisely to the area of recurrence.

Guided injection

The stakes were high for this lovely 17-year-old girl. Trisha's central giant cell granuloma had rapidly destroyed much of her anterior maxilla. Giant cells are the demolition crew in our bodies, employed to clean up cellular mess and debris. In this tumor, they are out of control, destroying everything around them. We can sometimes shut them down with serial steroid injections. To shut down this beast, I needed to make sure I canvased the entire lesion with the steroid. Attaching a navigation tag to a 10 cc syringe, I could see my position as I injected throughout the lesion. This technique also minimized the number of penetration sites. If there were multiple penetrations, the backpressure of injecting the steroid pushed the fluid back out the other holes, reducing the amount of steroid entering the lesion.

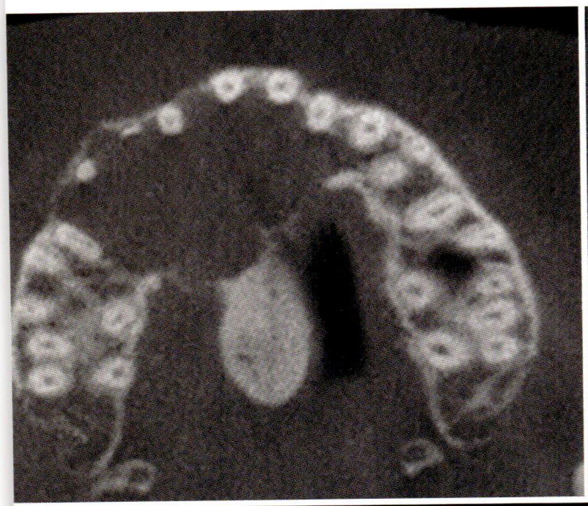

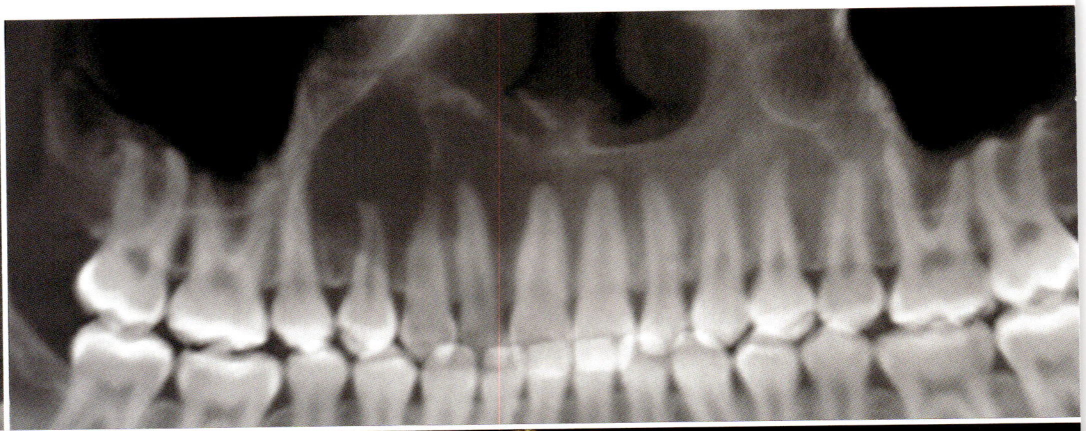

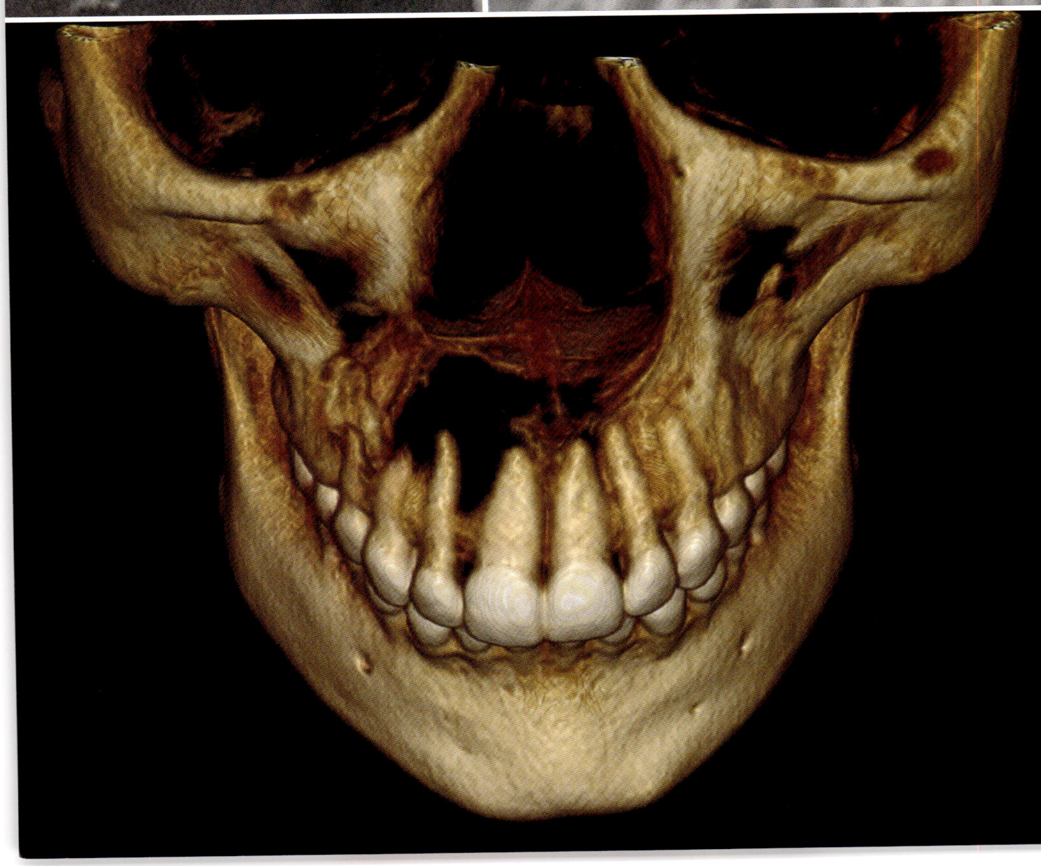

Figure 5-82 This central giant cell granuloma consumed the majority of the anterior maxilla. By attaching a tracking tag to the syringe, I was able to utilize navigation to optimize the injection throughout the lesion. I could see the position of the syringe in real-time on the monitor so I knew I was reaching the deepest margins.

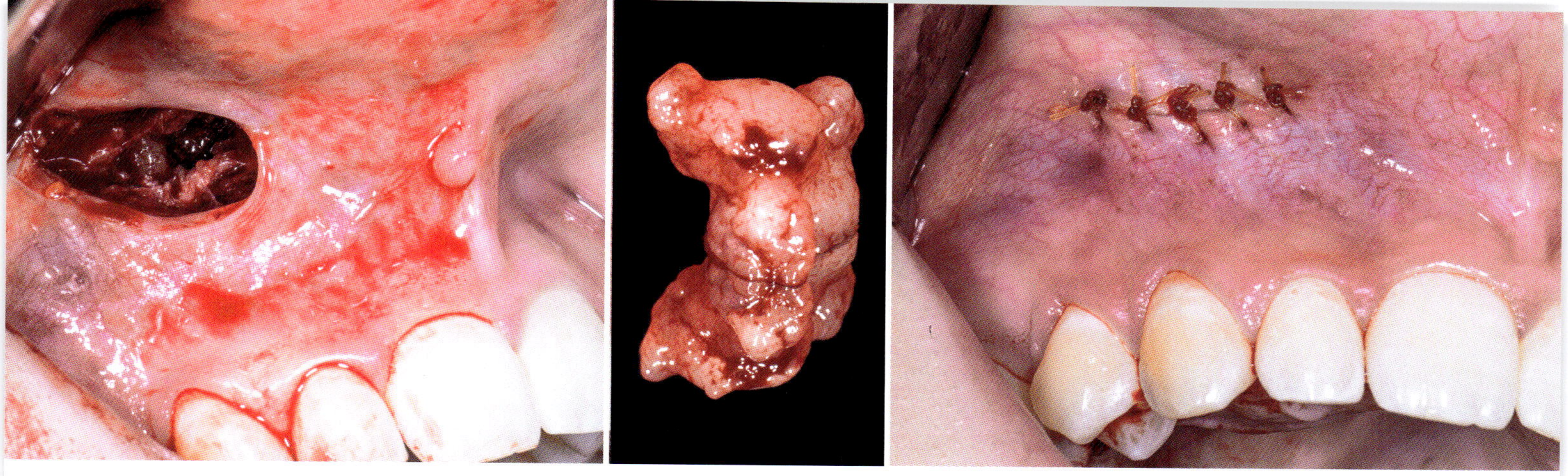

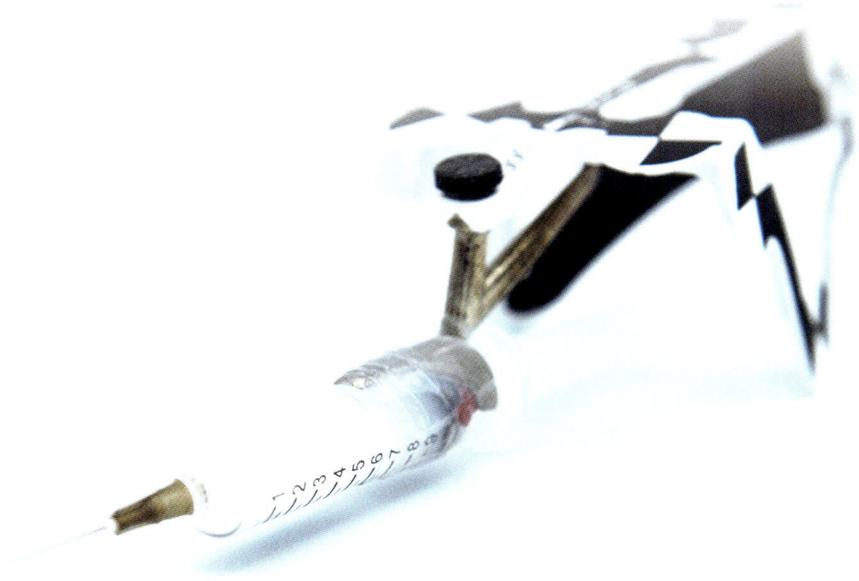

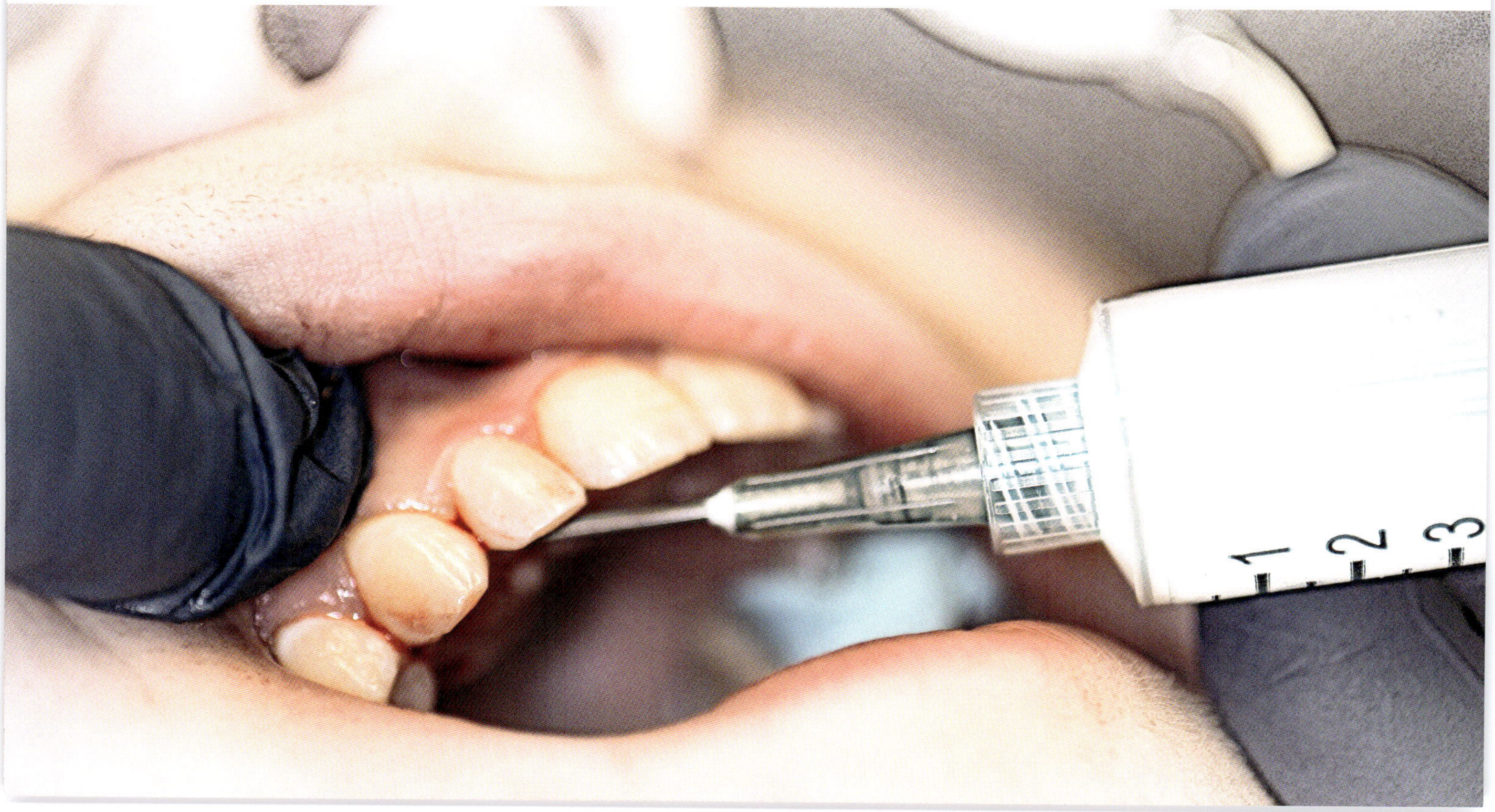

The Art of the Expose and Bond

There is not one right way to approach impacted canines, though there may be some ways that seem to work better. But when it comes to surgical exposure of impacted teeth, there are multiple effective philosophies on when and how they should be addressed. Some prefer to proactively go after a tooth early. Some allow time for it to declare what it is going to do. Others expose it to promote spontaneous eruption.

In treating impacted canines, the orthodontist is the overall "Master of Ceremonies"[16]. The orthodontist maintains the responsibility and privilege of formulating an overall treatment plan that will best achieve success for the patient's desired outcomes. Frequently, the surgeon and orthodontist work in concert to develop and execute a plan that best achieves the goals.

It is possible for any tooth to be impacted. The most common impacted tooth (apart from third molars) is the maxillary canine. The overall principles discussed here are geared toward impacted canines, but they can be applied to surgical management of any impacted teeth.

The classic "expose and bond" theory comes from a perspective that the impacted tooth can be managed best with three main steps: clearing the path of eruption, grabbing the tooth with a bracket and pulling it into place.

Three-dimensional imaging is critical for visualizing each step. It is also helpful in guiding treatment timelines, especially regarding adjacent teeth. It can reveal the ideal path of eruption and potential obstacles. When reviewing the image, check out the orientation, depth of impaction, adjacent structures, presence of periodontal ligament, and the overlying bone.

Try to envision the easiest path to reel the tooth into its final position in the arch. What bodily movement needs to happen? Will the tooth need to be translated laterally through the bone? If so, what bone can be reduced or removed to optimize this movement? Will the tooth need to rotate? Will there be adequate access to position the bracket well?

The angle of impaction and depth of impaction both influence the surgical and orthodontic plan. Horizontally impacted teeth will have two main vectors of movement, first correcting angulation and then erupting the tooth into the arch. At times, these moves are simultaneous. But often the orthodontist will need to address the orientation of the tooth prior to erupting it into the arch. This initial vector may seem counterintuitive, therefore communication and planning with the orthodontist will ensure optimal movements while protecting adjacent structures.

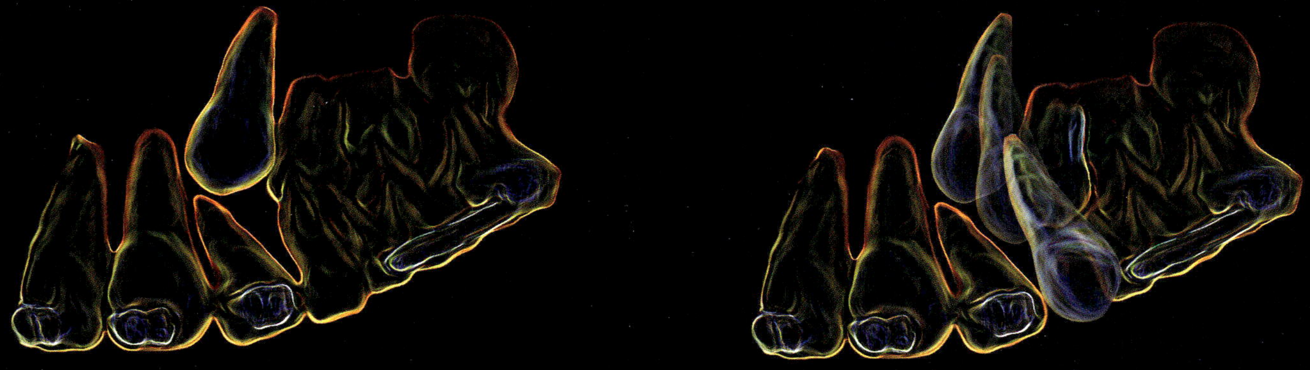

Figure 5-83 Three-dimensional imaging helps visualize the eruption path. In this case, the tooth needs to move distal, away from the lateral incisor to descend into position.

Clearing the path

Typically, the primary tooth is removed at the outset of the procedure. Attention to the relative position of the primary roots can be an effective guide or at least give some bearing on where to safely approach the impacted tooth. Visualizing the position of the primary extraction socket helps estimate the distance and orientation of the underlying tooth.

Judicious bone removal

Completely uncovering the crown of the impacted tooth down to the cementoenamel junction is critical in making an efficient path of eruption. If there is bone remaining coronal to the CEJ, there is more work that will need to be done by the body instead of by the surgeon. Minimize the work after surgery by optimizing surgical technique. The more space you create for the tooth to move, the less work it takes after surgery.

Limitations exist when adjacent teeth and roots are near or in the path of eruption. Extreme caution must be exercised to mitigate collateral damage and protect neighboring teeth. This requires visualizing both the current locations and anticipating the path of eruption. The enamel of a tooth being pulled through the bone can wreak havoc on the periodontal ligament and cementum of an erupted permanent tooth.

The Rapid Acceleratory Phenomenon (RAP) can facilitate this whole process[17]. Routine osteotomy or corticotomy can be performed where the root of the tooth needs to move. The metabolism of the injured bone increases the bone turnover, allowing teeth to move through the bone much faster and less traumatically.

Figure 5-84 Think like an excavator. The surgeon is the mighty machine. The surrounding tissue and remaining cells only have shovels. What can you do, as the surgeon, to help cells finish the work? The more effectively you utilize the power of surgery, the more efficiently the tissue will be able to complete the project.

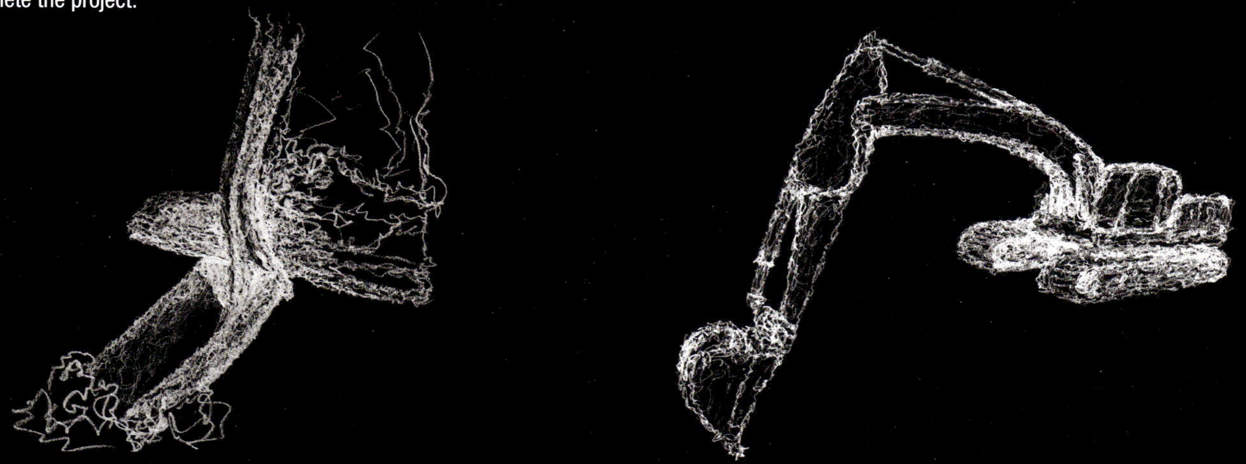

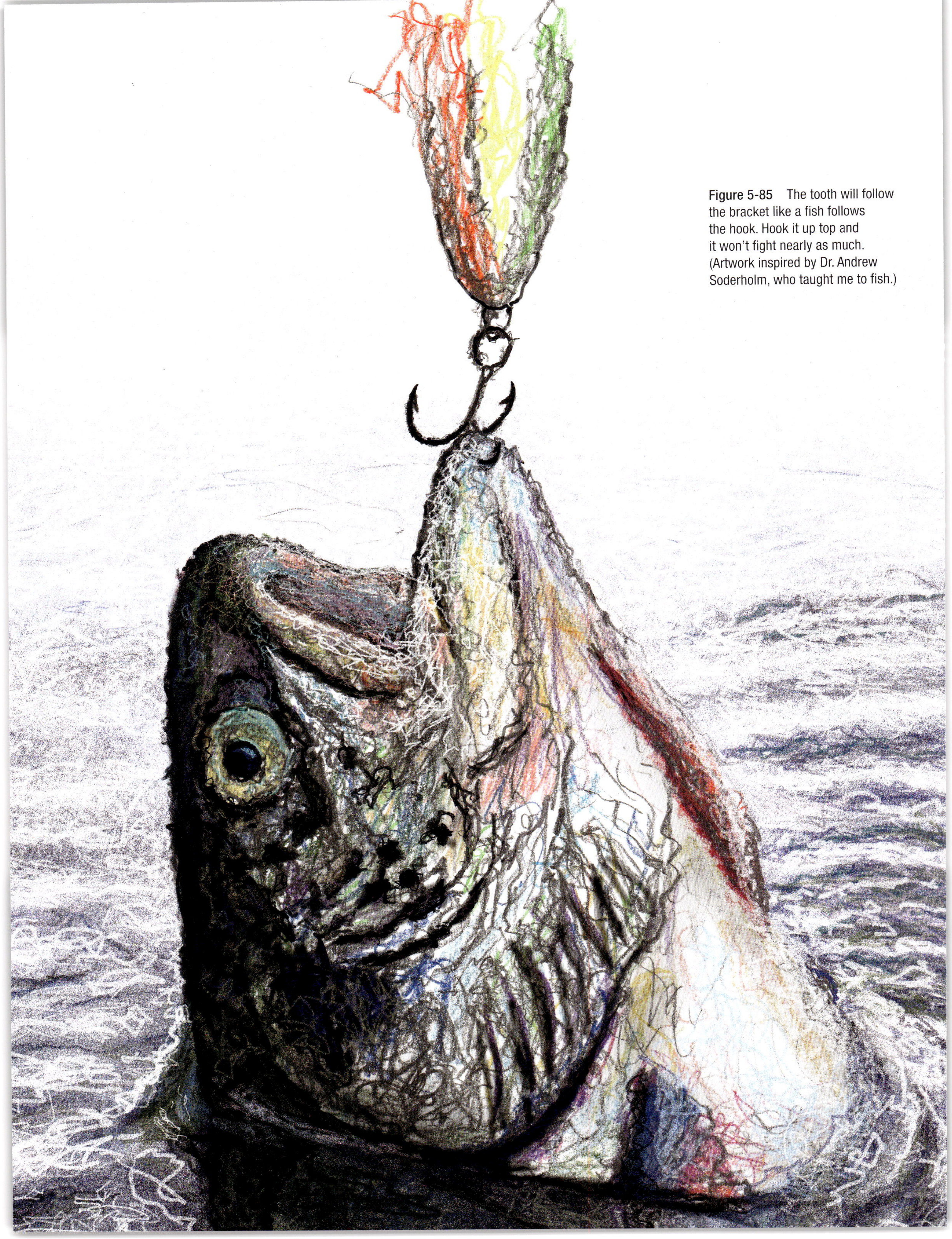

Figure 5-85 The tooth will follow the bracket like a fish follows the hook. Hook it up top and it won't fight nearly as much. (Artwork inspired by Dr. Andrew Soderholm, who taught me to fish.)

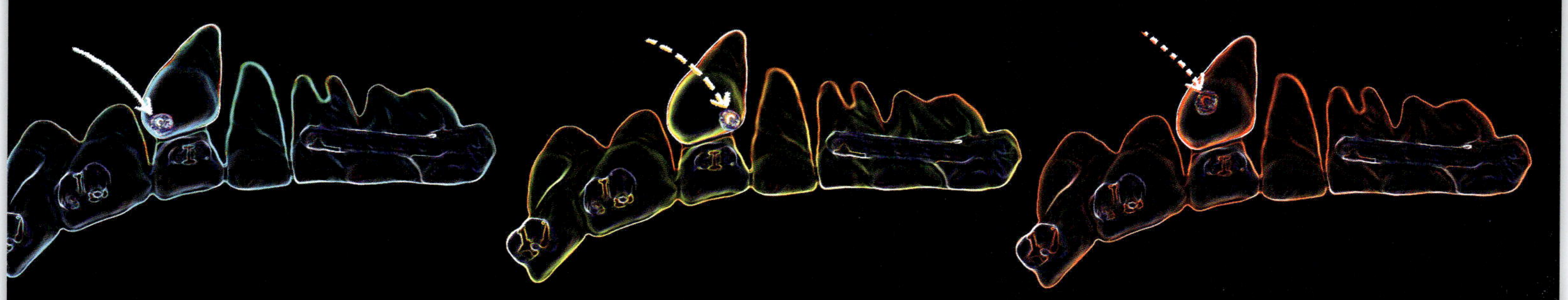

Figure 5-86 It is best to place the bracket on the incisal tip (*left*). It is often easier to place it on the distal, but this makes it more difficult for the orthodontist to manipulate the tooth (*middle*). Placing the bracket on the facial is the easiest surgically but sets the orthodontist up for the most difficulty (*right*).

Attaching a bracket

"Technique sensitive" is how I often explain this part of the procedure to a patient. The position of the bracket will determine how the forces are transferred to the tooth. A well-positioned bracket significantly improves the orthodontist's work as the tooth will more easily be guided as it moves. A good friend, Dr. Chad Harrington, gave me a visual that I always think of when determining bracket position. He said, "The tooth will follow the bracket like a fish follows a hook. Hook it in the cheek and it won't fight near as much." (The visual made perfect sense when I watched him flop a bit like a caught fish with his finger hooked in his cheek.)

The ideal position to "hook" the tooth is often nearest the incisal tip on the facial aspect. This guides the tooth right into position. It isn't a fight to translate the tooth laterally.

The actual bonding of the bracket is sometimes its own adventure. Isolation is key. The hard and soft tissue often bleed. Sometimes they bleed a lot. Any number of hemostatic methods may be used to dry the surgical site. The diode laser seems to work best to facilitate tissue removal and achieve adequate hemostasis. I say adequate because complete hemostasis is unnecessary. When the primary bleeders are stopped, a small amount of remaining oozing can be managed with a well-positioned suction cannula. The ideal position for the suction tip considers both the tissue and the planned bracket position. Blood will flow downhill. When a good suction position is determined, it should not move until the bracket is secured. Surrounding blood and fluid are eager to flow onto the etched tooth if the suction tip moves. Work with your assistant to find the best place and hold the position. If the position isn't working, adjust. Re-evaluate the site as blood

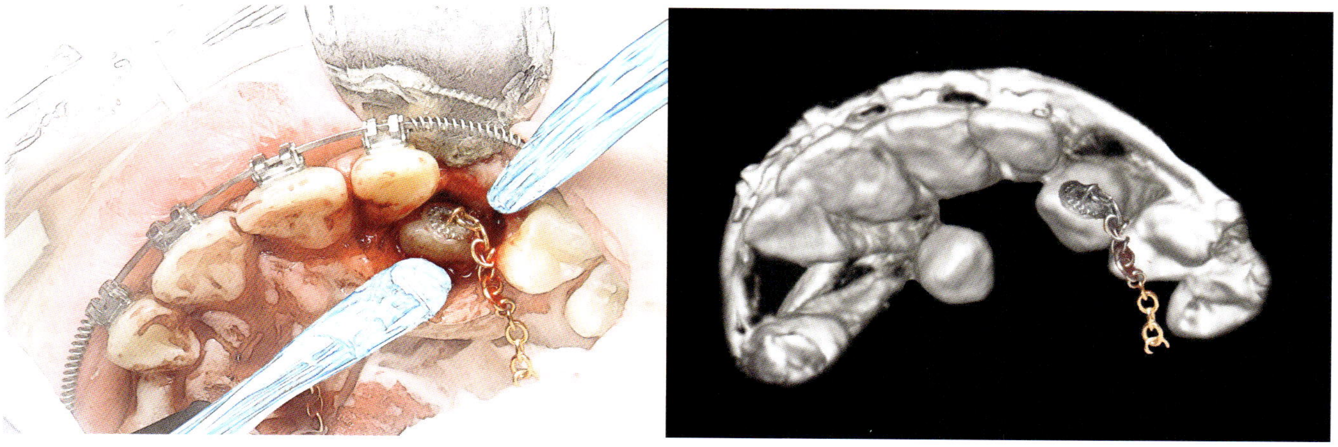

Figure 5-87 These pictures show surgical exposure and radiographic representation. Note bracket placement near the incisal tip.

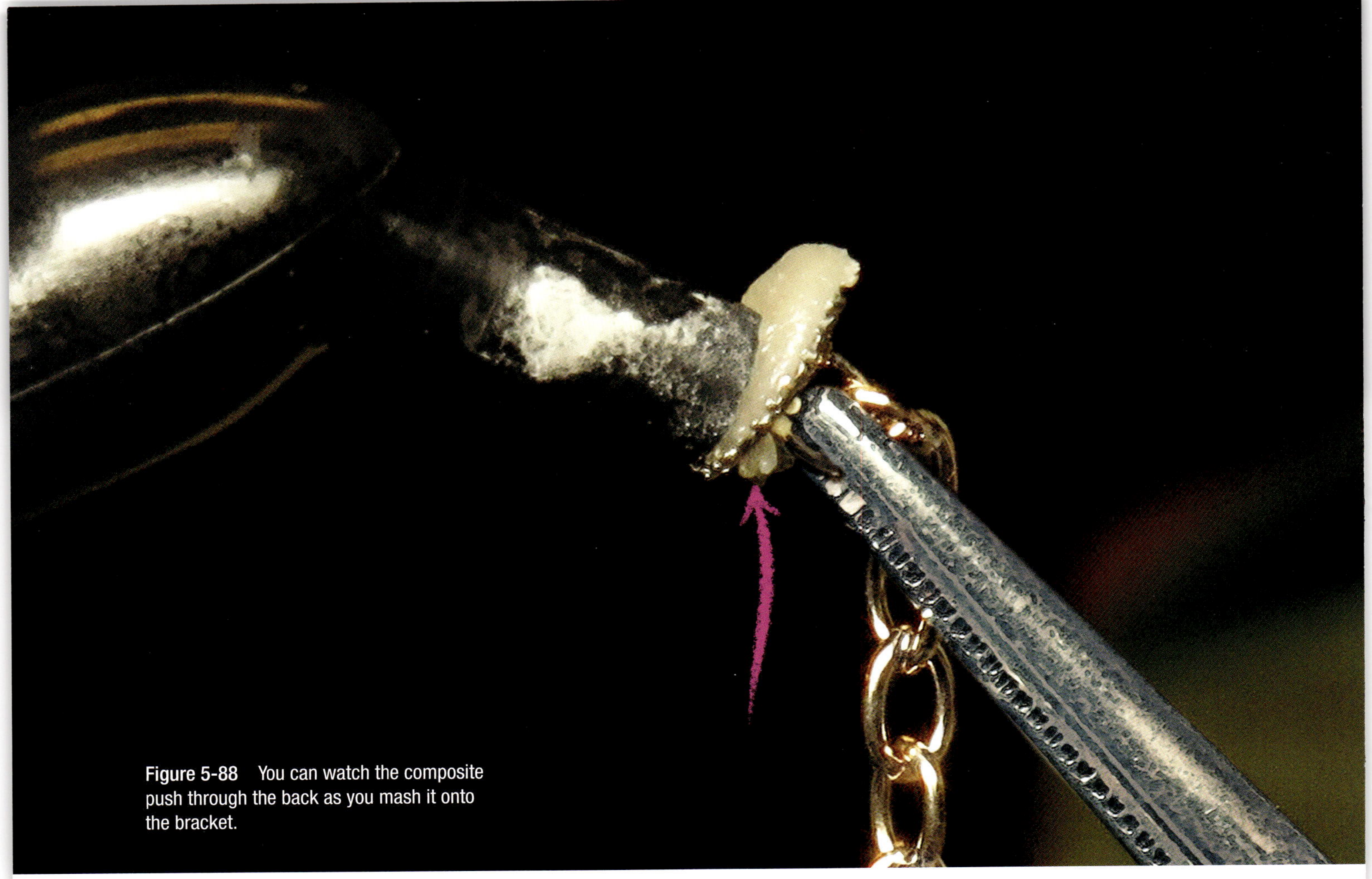

Figure 5-88 You can watch the composite push through the back as you mash it onto the bracket.

may have contaminated the bonding site. Even air turbulence from the suction can stir up the blood in the site, compromising the bond.

Following manufacturer's guidance, the tooth is etched, bonded and the bracket is luted to the enamel. Cotton forceps with moistened gauze are readily available and quite effective at cleaning the surface of the tooth prior to applying the etch. In my practice, I use 37% phosphoric acid for about 20 seconds. I then use a modified blow dryer to dry the tooth until it has a frosted appearance. I apply OptiBond, light cure, and then I mash the composite into the waffle matrix of the bracket, "like mashing in the butter," my friend says. While I press the composite coated bracket on the tooth, I am cautious to make sure the site hasn't been violated by blood or fluid. If there is any contamination apparent, I go back to short treatment with phosphoric acid. I find close attention to detail is a worthwhile challenge at these stages. When the site is contaminated, the bracket will not likely fulfill its duty. The responsibility to re-attach the bracket falls back on the surgeon.

Firm pressure between the bracket and tooth helps securely fasten the bracket. It is often difficult to get the curing light in close contact with the resin, so multiple curing rounds may be needed to adequately cure the resin. My routine is three 10 second cycles, adjusting the position each time.

Then comes the moment of truth. I grab the chain with a hemostat and give it a good tug. I want to see the patient's head move. I would much rather dislodge the bracket now and go through the steps to re-bond it while I have everything at my disposal. If it remains intact, it gets activated with elastic thread. If it pops off, I am thankful it happened now and not later.

Bonding: Self-etching primer may be convenient, but I favor a separate etch and primer. Because of their higher pH, self-etching primers demineralize less enamel, resulting in a lower shear bond strength of the resin attachment. Using a separate etch and primer gives me more confidence I will have a stable attachment until the tooth erupts. It is much more difficult to replace a bracket on a buried tooth in a surgical patient than a typical ortho patient.

Pulling on it: activation

Activating the tooth at the time of surgery gets a jump start on movement. Working with my orthodontists, I usually have a good idea of where they want me to pull. It may involve loops in an appliance, the arch wire, or an adjacent bracket. In any case, activating the tooth at the time of exposure maximizes the eruption potential and saves an appointment for the orthodontist.

Open exposure: palatal orientation

The main idea here is the tooth generally knows what to do and where to go, it just needs a little help getting unstuck. It is inhibited by the overlying bone and dense palatal tissue. When the overlying tissue is cleared away, the tooth may spontaneously erupt into a proper position, or at least erupt enough so the orthodontist can place a bracket.

References

1. Bali A, Bali D, Sharma A, et al. Is Pederson Index a True Predictive Difficulty Index for Impacted Mandibular Third Molar Surgery? A Meta-analysis. J Maxillofac Oral Surg. 2013 Sep;12(3):359-364.
2. MacGregor, A J. The impacted lower wisdom tooth [Internet]. Oxford ; New York : Oxford University Press, 1985.; 1985 [cited 2023 Jan 4]. Available from: https://www.ncbi.nlm.nih.gov/nlmcatalog/8700238
3. Indices of Difficulty [Internet]. Exodontia. [cited 2023 Jan 4]. Available from: https://exodontia.info/indices-of-difficulty/
4. Kautto A, Vehkalahti MM, Ventä I. Age of patient at the extraction of the third molar. Int J Oral Maxillofac Surg. 2018 Jul;47(7):947-951.
5. Kim JY. Third molar extraction in middle-aged and elderly patient. J Korean Assoc Oral Maxillofac Surg. 2021 Oct 31;47(5):407-408.
6. Xie Q, Wei S, Zhou N, et al. Modified envelope flap, a novel incision design, can relieve complications after extraction of fully horizontal impacted mandibular third molar. J Dent Sci. 2021 Mar 1;16(2):718-722.
7. Desai A, Patel R, Desai K, et al. Comparison of two incision designs for surgical removal of impacted mandibular third molar: A randomized comparative clinical study. Contemp Clin Dent. 2014;5(2):170-174.
8. Dwek JR. The periosteum: what is it, where is it, and what mimics it in its absence? Skeletal Radiol. 2010 Apr;39(4):319-323.
9. Mahajan A. Periosteum: A Highly Underrated Tool in Dentistry. Int J Dent. 2011 Sep 25;2012:e717816.
10. Behnia H, Kheradvar A, Shahrokhi M. An anatomic study of the lingual nerve in the third molar region. J Oral Maxillofac Surg. 2000 Jun;58(6):649-651; discussion 652-653.
11. Kiesselbach JE, Chamberlain JG. Clinical and anatomic observations on the relationship of the lingual nerve to the mandibular third molar region. J Oral Maxillofac Surg. 1984 Sep;42(9):565-567.
12. Miloro M, Halkias LE, Slone HW, et al. Assessment of the lingual nerve in the third molar region using magnetic resonance imaging. J Oral Maxillofac Surg. 1997 Feb;55(2):134-137.
13. Pasqualini D, Cocero N, Castella A, et al. Primary and secondary closure of the surgical wound after removal of impacted mandibular third molars: a comparative study. Int J Oral Maxillofac Surg. 2005 Jan 1;34(1):52-57.
14. Martin A, Perinetti G, Costantinides F, et al. Coronectomy as a surgical approach to impacted mandibular third molars: a systematic review. Head Face Med. 2015 Apr 10;11:9.
15. He L, Yadgarov A, Sharif S, et al. Aging profoundly delays functional recovery from gustatory nerve injury. Neuroscience. 2012 May 3;209:208-218.
16. Becker A, Chaushu S. Surgical Treatment of Impacted Canines: What the Orthodontist Would Like the Surgeon to Know. Oral Maxillofac Surg Clin North Am. 2015 Aug;27(3):449-458.
17. Wilcko MT, Wilcko WM, Pulver JJ, et al. Accelerated osteogenic orthodontics technique: a 1-stage surgically facilitated rapid orthodontic technique with alveolar augmentation. J Oral Maxillofac Surg. 2009 Oct;67(10):2149-2159.

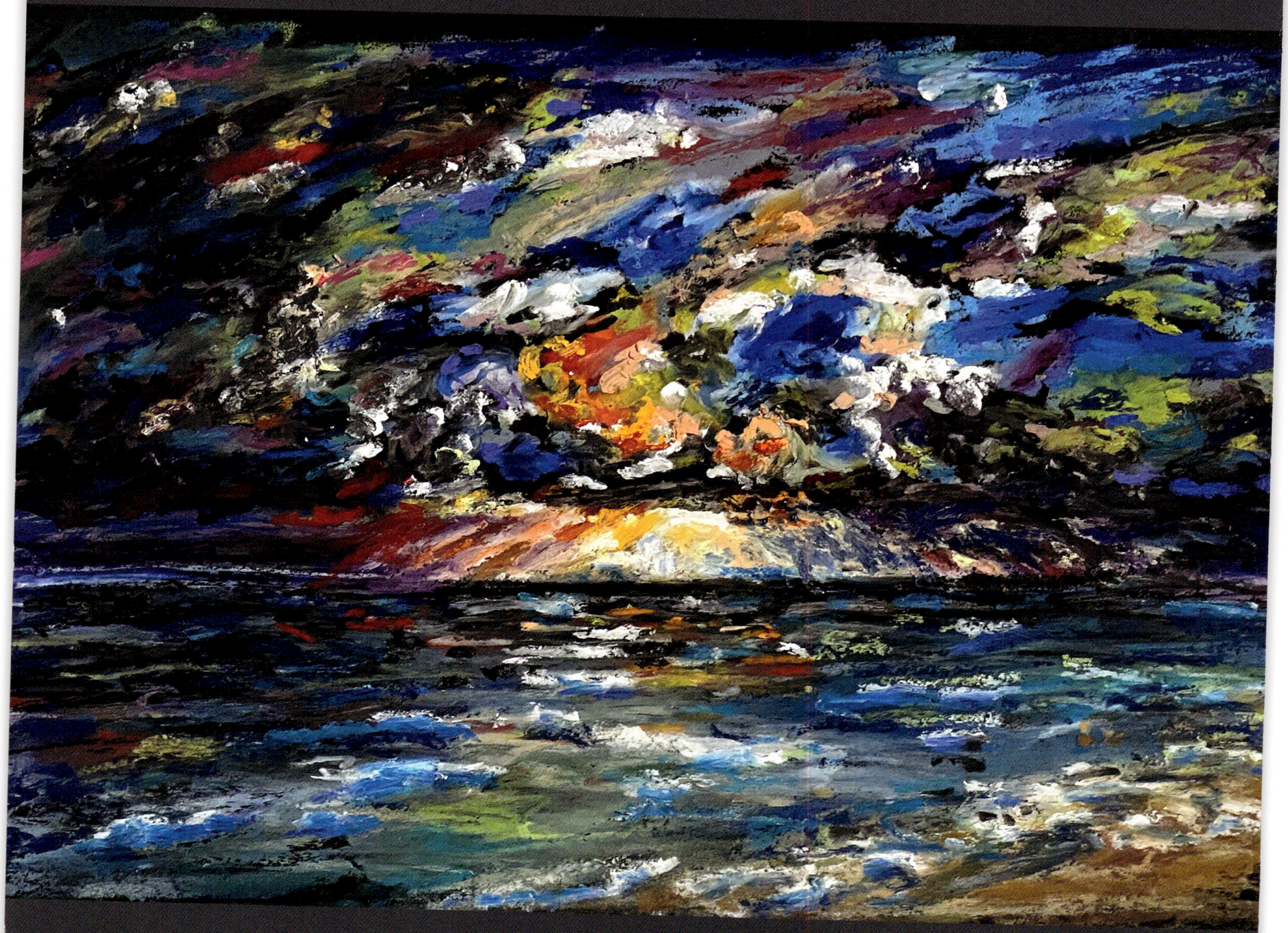

The Colors of Light. (Oil pastel)

CHAPTER 6

COMPLICATIONS OF EXODONTIA

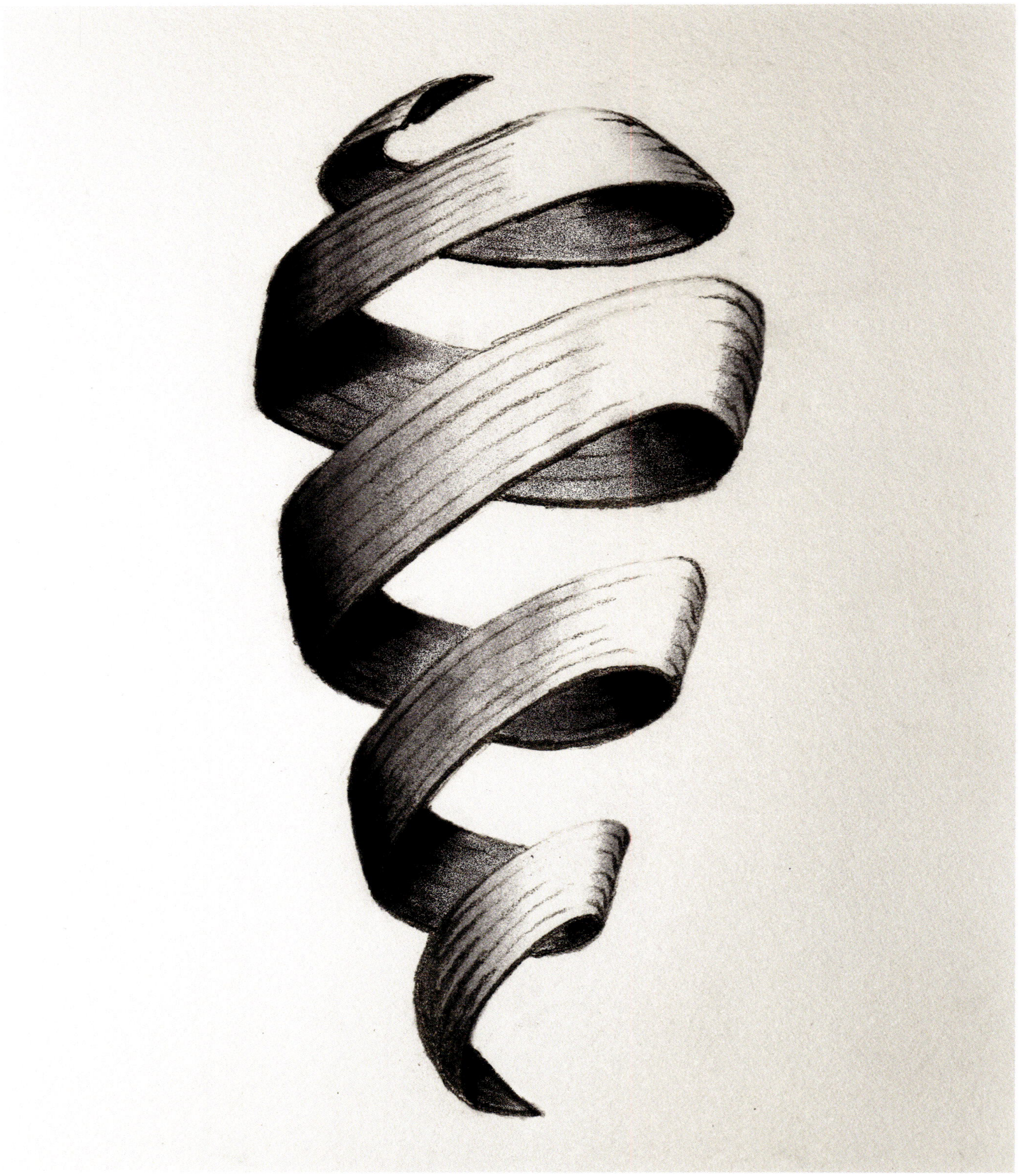

Figure 6-1 Unraveled (Artwork inspired by M.C. Escher.)

"The surgeon without complications is the one who doesn't operate."

Complications are an inherent risk of any given procedure. Thankfully, most complications can be avoided, or at least mitigated, through careful technique and a compliant patient. A flawless surgery performed on a non-compliant patient may not heal well. No surgeon is perfect. Let's talk about some common complications and how we can both avoid and manage them.

Displaced Teeth and Roots

The combination of thin bone and a bit of apical pressure can shove a root or whole tooth up into the maxillary sinus or out of the alveolus into the floor of the mouth, infratemporal fossa or into the adjacent tissue of the vestibule.

Displacement into the maxillary sinus is the most frequent of these and can cause chronic sinus infections if not managed well. The pre-op image is helpful in evaluating the location of the sinus floor as well as length and shape of the roots. When it looks high-risk, try sectioning the tooth into the separate roots, thus removing them individually. When the sinus floor is at the furcation and the roots are dilacerated, it is much safer to section the tooth when the majority of the crown remains intact. The biggest risk comes when there are small portions of root dangling into the maxillary sinus. There isn't much to get a hold of. And drilling way up there runs a high risk of pushing the drill into the sinus, perforating the membrane. Care must be taken to avoid sectioning too deep. If the roots don't section well and you end up with small portions of the root closely approximating the sinus, very gentle and intentional moves with a fine periotome or Micro Buser may mobilize and retrieve the piece. (Or it may disappear into a deep black hole.)

Think about the entire circumference of the retained fragment and try to visualize the safest place to execute your next move. Sometimes, there is a purchase point that is difficult to see without loupes, a mirror, irrigation and suction. Sometimes, a fine surgical bur can safely remove bone on the buccal or palatal plate, creating space for the tooth to be luxated or elevated. It is typically safer to remove bone on the buccal or palatal aspects when the sinus is close. These peripheral areas have a larger margin of safety than toward the center of the socket.

If a tooth or root becomes displaced through the lingual cortex, retrieval principles are similar to when an instrument breaks or a tooth is displaced into the sinus. Take a breath and focus. Try to retrieve it through the hole without further displacing it or losing sight of it. Place a finger on the lingual aspect of the soft tissue to feel where it is and possibly push it into a more accessible position or back through the hole. Consider enlarging the hole with hand instruments or possibly with a drill, using extreme caution. Attempt to retrieve it with slender curved hemostats, a curved curette, or possibly sinus lift curettes. (The angles of these instruments may do the trick.)

If it is not retrieved at the time of displacement due to patient factors or surgeon factors, the patient should be informed of the situation and placed on appropriate antibiotics. Follow-up must be established for definitive retrieval. Post-operative three-dimensional imaging can identify the location, guiding the retrieval. A CBCT may be sufficient in locating the tooth or fragment. At times, a medical

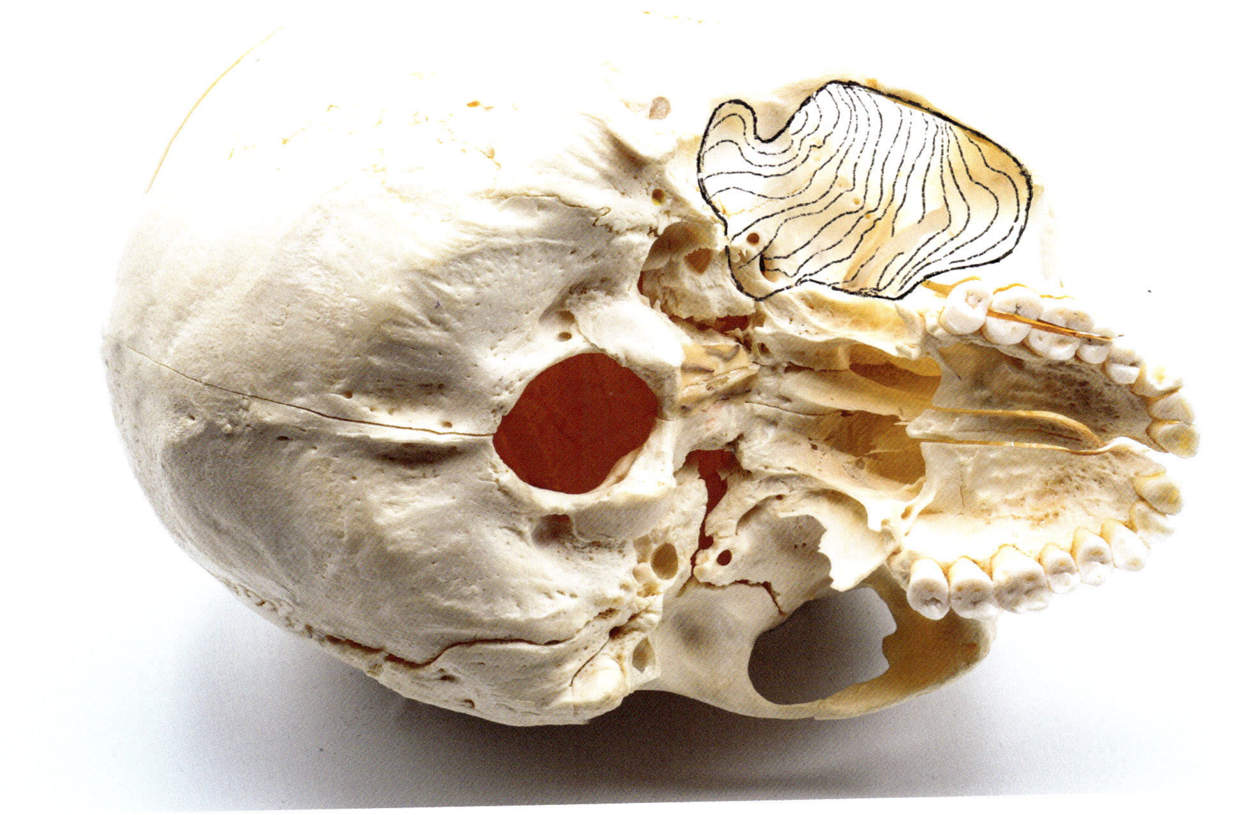

Figure 6-2 The infratemporal fossa is right behind the upper third molars. The tooth doesn't need to travel far to get in there. This space can swallow teeth. They can be removed, but it can be challenging. It is much easier to keep them out of the space by controlling the forces on the elevators, paying attention to how the tooth is moving, and using the tip of the Minnesota retractor to block the tooth from sliding up around the corner.

grade CT scan may be indicated as it can better identify the soft tissue anatomy. This may be useful to identify if a fragment is displaced above the mylohyoid into the sublingual space, below the mylohyoid into the submandibular space or more posteriorly into the pterygomandibular or lateral pharyngeal spaces. Finding a small root tip can feel like finding a needle in a haystack.

When a tooth gets displaced into the sinus, sometimes it hangs out just beyond the bone, held in place by the Schneiderian membrane. In this case, a little lateral pressure to gently outfracture the bone may improve the access and allow a curved hemostat or even a surgical suction tip to retrieve it. What a relief when that works. If it becomes more complicated, a few different techniques can be employed to safely remove the fragment and optimize the recovery.

First breathe. Slow down. Gather your thoughts. Evaluate the site. My team knows when I am in the sinus because I stop singing with the music, take a deep breath and get very focused.

If the hole is small, it is unlikely forceps or a hemostat will be able to grip the fragment without further displacing it into the sinus. A small, curved curette can sometimes sneak around the back side of the root and tease it out of a slightly enlarged hole. Keep in mind the hole the tooth just went through is the same size as the piece of tooth. The hole will probably need to be enlarged to get the piece of tooth back out. If the curette is unsuccessful, consider using a small instrument to enlarge the hole. Try to visualize how the tooth will come out so you can remove bone where it counts. Sometimes, more extensive bone removal is necessary to visualize or access the tooth. With an enlarged opening, try the suction, curette or hemostat again.

If that doesn't work, you may need to reflect a flap and perform either a Caldwell Luc approach to the sinus or remove more buccal bone to get adequate access. Before reflecting the flap, think about the closure. The tissue will need to be advanced over the site with passive primary closure (with or without buccal fat pad advancement) to promote healing. A vertical release one tooth distal to the site will protect the blood supply of the flap and optimize access to the buccal fat pad if needed. Another vertical release mesial to the site also can be quite beneficial. The better the flap, the better the tissue will heal. Continue to judiciously increase osseous access and work to tease it out until the tooth is retrieved. When the tooth is finally out, the remainder of the repair is similar to closing a sinus communication. Passive primary closure is key.

The floor of the mouth is another potential place for a tooth to go, and it can be intimidating. It can pop right through a dehiscence or thin bone in the lingual plate. The same general principles apply in this situation. First, avoid making it worse. Be incredibly cautious as the tooth can easily push farther into the tissue. Try using a surgical suction tip or teasing it out with a small angled curette. Try pushing it back through the hole with your finger on the lingual of the mandible. Having a finger in this position can also help hold the fragment in place while you try other maneuvers. It can feel like a mouth full to the patient, but it could keep the tooth from displacing farther out of sight.

If you need to increase access on the lingual, proceed with extreme caution. The lingual nerve is right on the other side of the lingual plate. Drilling the plate away will improve the chances of a successful root retrieval. But don't let your drill tip go past the plate. Most roots can be retrieved with these simple steps. If not, further dissection may be necessary by approaching the area through the lingual tissue or the floor of the mouth. The mylohyoid muscle will likely get torn a bit by this whole process. That's okay. It will heal.

Sinus Communication

Getting sinus communications to heal can be challenging, especially when they are greater than 5 mm. Why does size matter? All the blood supply and cellular growth come from the surrounding tissue. The cells must stretch themselves, suspending out over a void, to bridge the gap. A blood clot can cover a small communication of less than 2 mm. That clot undergoes transformation through the phases of healing, resulting in epithelialization. But it is quite fragile. A bit of air or fluid tearing it back open after the clot is stabilized can stop the steps toward healing and redirect the epithelium to line the opening instead of closing it. A compliant, low risk patient may heal spontaneously by simply avoiding positive or negative pressure in their nose or mouth. The chances of healing go down with smokers, diabetics, sleep apnea patients, or patients with dysfunctional sinuses. If a patient reports frequent sinus congestion or recurrent sinus infections, expect healing to take more time and effort. Plan for more involved procedures and longer antibiotic treatment.

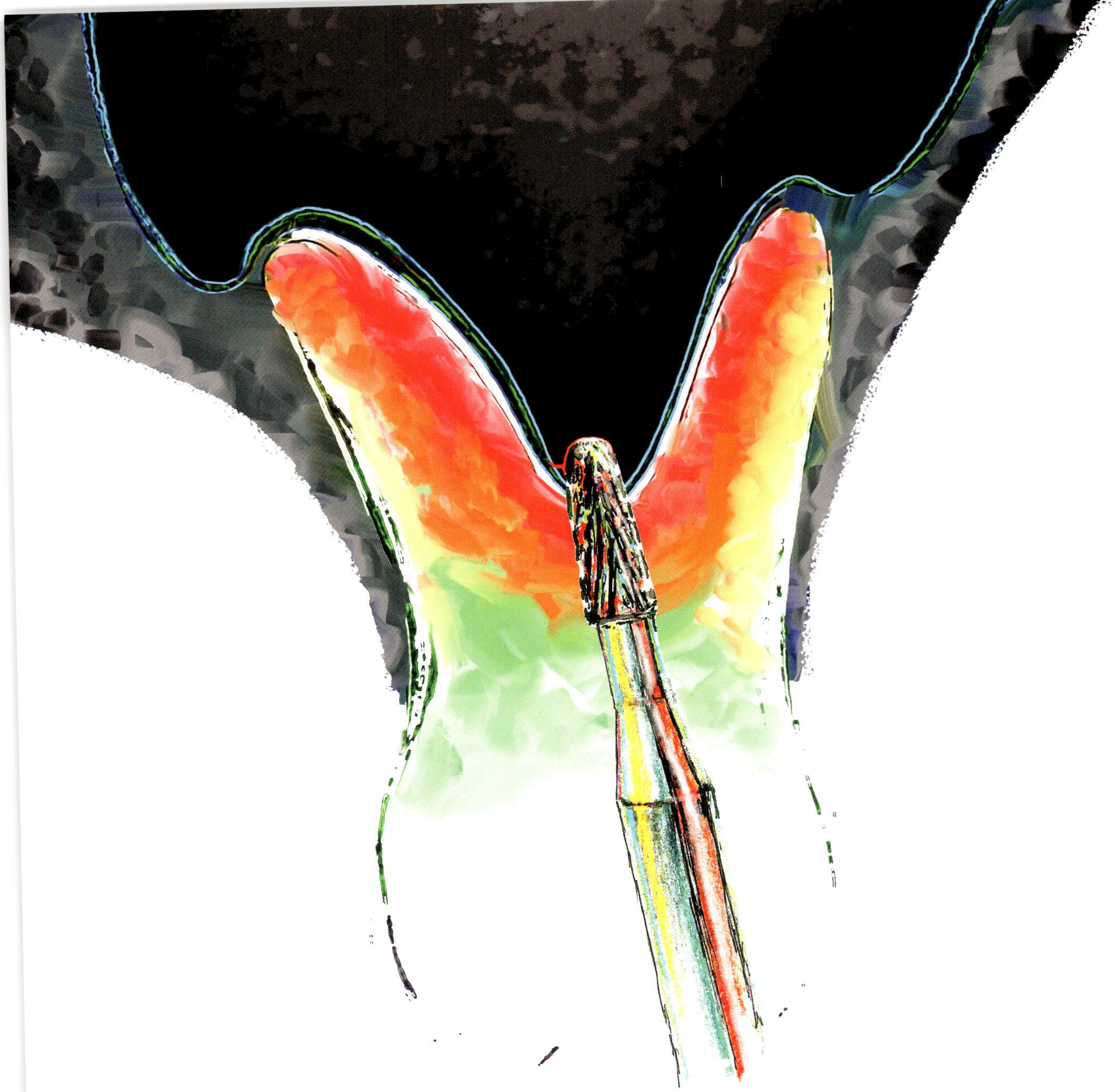

Figure 6-3 Safety zones in drilling for sectioning upper molars. Depending on the shape of the sinus and roots, there may be a high risk of perforating the sinus when sectioning in the middle of the tooth. It is also good to visualize the position and bone thickness around the apex, especially in the posterior maxilla and mandible.

If a sinus infection develops during the fragile early healing stages, it is much less likely to heal. The pressure, inflammation and biologic harm will unravel the body's attempts to close the hole. Antibiotic therapy can greatly reduce the bacterial load and help reduce the chances of secondary infection. When there is a hole between the mouth and the maxillary sinus, secretions become stagnant and contaminated with oral flora. The synchronous beating of the cilia is disrupted, and the fluid doesn't clear out the ostium. With these failures, the sinus becomes a cesspool, a perfect breeding ground for bacteria. Antibiotics are routinely prescribed prophylactically if any sinus communication is noted. (Relatively low risk patients in my current practice are prescribed seven days of amoxicillin 500 mg TID or a five-day course of azithromycin 500 mg day one and 250 mg days 2 to 5.)

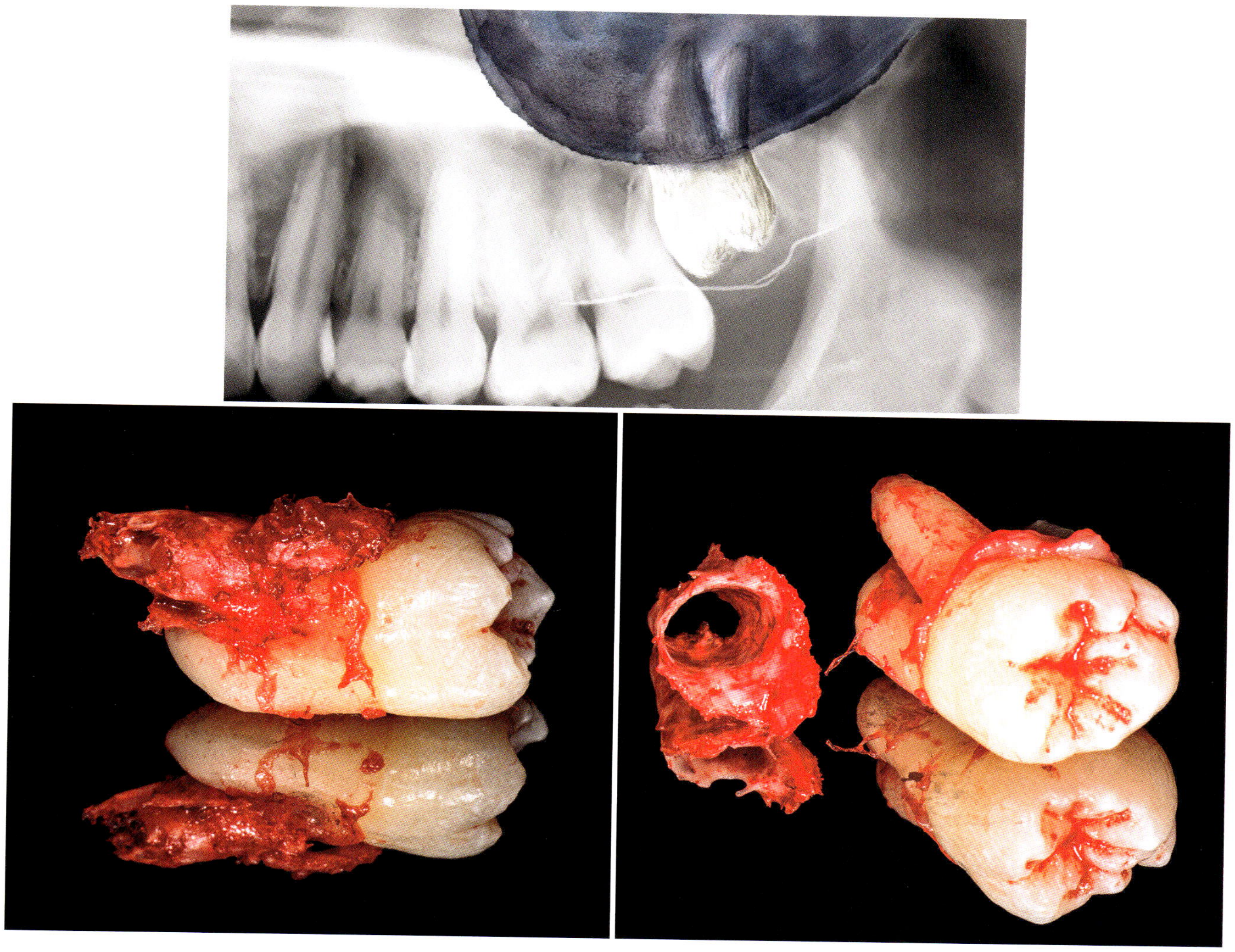

Figure 6-4 It can be difficult to assess sinus risk on a panoramic radiograph. There is often a very thin layer of bone covering the upper third molars. In this case, this sleeve of bone came out with this upper left third molar. Thankfully, the sinus lining remained intact.

When the defect is greater than 2 mm or the patient has elevated risk factors, the body is less likely to close the sinus on its own. Surgery is likely needed. Optimizing sinus health pre-operatively significantly improves the outcome. Antibiotic coverage (Augmentin 1000 mg BID or Clindamycin 300 mg TID for 10 days) and nasal decongestants (pseudoephedrine or phenylephrine) are recommended to optimize sinus function and decrease infection risk in these higher risk patients pre-operatively and post-operatively.

The most common surgical technique to successfully close a sinus communication is a buccal soft tissue flap advancement, with or without buccal fat pad advancement. To achieve passive primary closure, the flap must be adequately mobilized and advanced. This is typically done by elevating a full thickness crestal flap with mesial and distal vertical releases at least one tooth away from the site. A good subperiosteal dissection initially frees the tissue, and then a periosteal releasing incision significantly increases the mobility of the flap. It is important to confirm the periosteal release was complete by using an instrument to sweep laterally through the periosteal incision. If it gets hung up, work to further release the tissue that seems to be restricting the flap until it is fully mobilized. You know you've got it when the flap freely advances over the site, passively covering the defect.

Passive is the key word here. If there is any tension on the tissue when suturing, it has a substantially increased risk of dehiscing and prolonging the complication. It will likely require another surgery. Final soft tissue closure starts with two or three horizontal mattress sutures placed about 5 mm from the incision on each edge. These sling style sutures are primarily responsible for resisting any functional tension on the incision from eating or facial expressions. Next, the vertical releasing incisions are closed. The vertical releases need close attention to avoid future periodontal issues and recession. First, reapproximate the gingiva to avoid a gingival defect. The remainder of the release can then be closed with either interrupted or a running suture. After the releasing incisions are closed, a running-locking suture effectively reapproximates the incision with a watertight closure. Use caution when using a running locking suture technique. It provides better tensile strength between the edges but can easily strangle the tissue. This can reduce the blood supply and cause minor tissue necrosis. While the necrosis may not be obvious clinically, a resulting wound dehiscence sure is. My current routine is to use 3-0 PTFE sutures for the sling sutures and 4-0 chromic suture for the remaining stitches.

If the sinus defect is greater than 5 mm or the patient has higher risk factors, it can be helpful to mobilize the buccal fat pad and recruit its cells and blood supply to help. To access the fat pad, the periosteal releasing incision is extended. Sharp and blunt dissection gets you through the encapsulating fascia of the fat pad, allowing it to herniate through the opening. Once it starts peeking out, cautious blunt spreading dissection with a curved hemostat breaks up the adhesions and septae, allowing the tissue to advance quite freely. If you have ever inadvertently encountered the fat pad while removing upper third molars, you know how accessible this blob of tissue can become. The yellow, gelatinous fat seems to have an abnormally strong attraction to the suction. The fat pad's jelly-like properties are a liability in routine third molar extractions, but they are an asset in closure of sinus communications.

When the sinus opening isn't terribly large and the patient isn't high risk, sometimes advancing the buccal fat over the hole is enough without closing the overlying mucosa. Amazingly, when the pedicled fat flap is advanced and left exposed, a layer of epithelium grows over it. If I am going to do all the work to advance the fat pad, I usually take the extra steps to get passive primary closure as well. This is the proverbial "belt and suspenders," and I like it.

These three techniques all approach the site similarly. The defect gets covered. Either the soft tissue alone is closed, the fat is advanced and it alone is closed, or both the fat pad and the overlying mucosa are closed individually with passive primary closure. This two-layered closure approach has the highest success rate, but it can obliterate the vestibule. This may complicate future removable appliances or implant supported restorations[1].

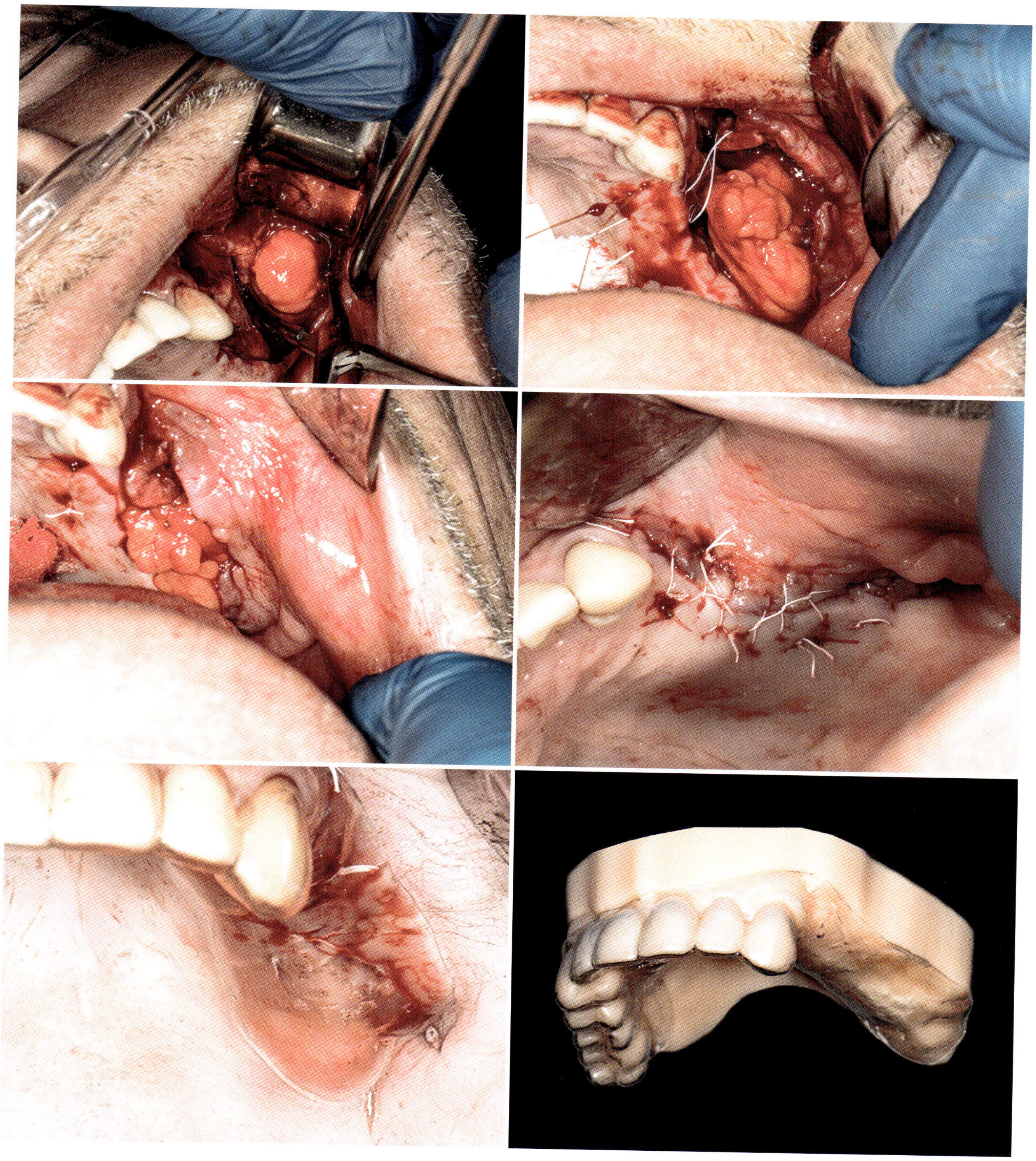

Figure 6-5 The buccal fat pad is approached through the periosteum beneath the flap. It is mobilized, sutured across the defect and layered closure is performed with resorbable and non-resorbable sutures. A "suck-down stent" is made and worn for two weeks post-operatively. Sinus precautions are given, and antibiotics prescribed.

Oral-Antral Fistula

The human body is always on defense. It must constantly protect itself from an onslaught of bacterial invasion. When the oral epithelium is compromised, resulting in an exposure to the sinus, the body attempts to close over the defect. If it cannot isolate the sinus from the oral cavity, it begins a process of epithelial ingrowth along the tract. This epithelialized tissue is much more resilient and protects the underlying bone and tissue. But these layers will not grow together to close the defect. They are each their own independent outer surface layer. Excise the fistula first and then develop the flaps, advance the tissue, and secure passive primary closure. The excision helps ensure success. It can also be helpful to treat with a few days of pre-operative antibiotics as well as 7 to 10 days post-operatively. This improves the sinus condition and optimizes the environment for healing.

Retained Roots

A necrotic canal is a safe harbor for bacteria. When the surrounding blood supply cannot adequately penetrate the space within the canal, the bacteria proliferate and can advance into the surrounding bone. If the body's immune system can access the space, an infection is much less likely to develop. Many of the teeth we remove are necrotic. If a root tip breaks off, the size of the remaining necrotic canal, not necessarily the fragment, seems to have the biggest impact on the outcome. Size isn't the only factor. It is also impacted by the condition of the tooth and surrounding bone, as well as the patient's overall condition. Generally, if the broken root tip is less than about 3 to 5 mm, the body can typically prevent an ongoing infection. I wish I could give an exact number, but the truth is the other factors play a big part in the decision as well. The smaller the better. Think about endodontics. If the fill is within 1 mm of the apex, it is likely to be successful. That means the terminal 1 mm of canal space is available for the bacteria to occupy. And the immune system only has access from one side. With retained roots there is access from both.

It isn't ideal to leave roots behind. An attempt at retrieval should be made or at least considered, but it is sometimes better to leave a portion of tooth. With the more than 2,500 teeth I remove each year, I knowingly choose to retain less than 20 fractured roots. When the risk of retrieval is high and the risk of retention is low, leave the root. If the root is larger than 5 mm or infected, the risk of retaining it goes up. How do you decide how hard to try? Apply this matrix to both sides of the equation. Here are some questions to ask:

How likely is the complication to occur? How big of an impact would the complication have on the patient?

Ask these questions for both retrieval and retention to help guide the decision. You can also have a conversation with your patient, if they are not sedated[2]. There is a nice risk reward benefit matrix described by Nayyar et al.[2].

Retaining a broken root should be the exception, not the rule.

For more discussion, see **Figure 4-21**.

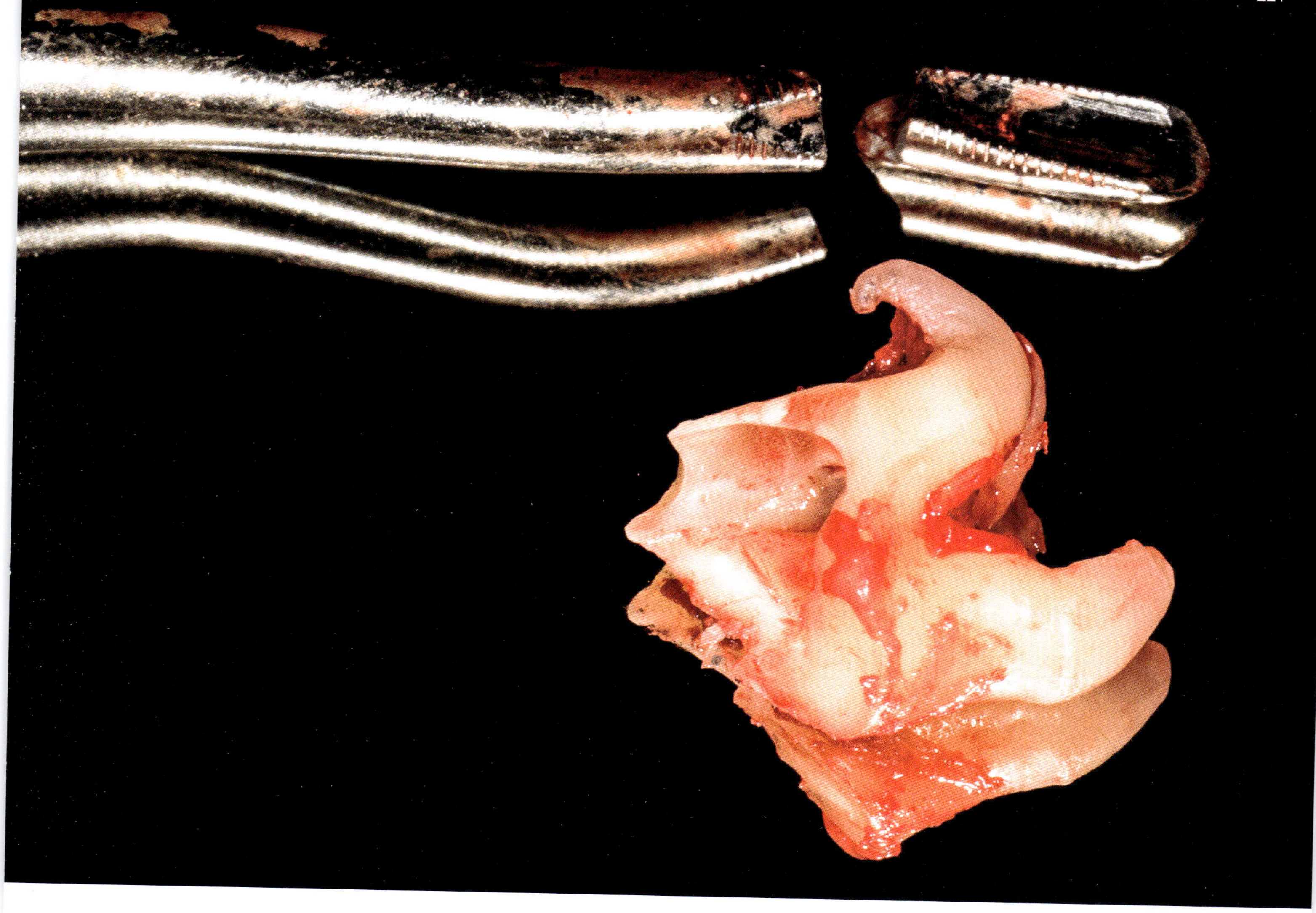

Figure 6-6 Slender instruments break easier, especially with mandibular teeth. Even a sturdy elevator can fracture when working on a tooth like this. You never know when it will break until it does.

Fractured Instruments

When an instrument fractures, things can get remarkably more complicated. The tooth is just as stuck as before. But now the fractured piece must also be retrieved. Now is the time to take a quick pause to regroup. Get yourself out of the cognitive tunnel that can limit your perspective. Stand up straight. Take a breath. The goal is still to create a healing extraction site, not just remove the tooth.

Keep a close eye on the broken piece. A pharyngeal curtain or throat pack is the standard of care in all our work. Now is a good time to verify it is adequately protecting the airway. If the piece cannot be accounted for and there is any chance it went down the patient's throat into their stomach or lungs, the patient must be sent for a lateral and PA (posterior-anterior) chest radiograph.

The fractured piece is typically wedged tightly between two objects, the tooth and either the bone or the adjacent tooth. Section the tooth in such a way as to mobilize it and remove the broken piece. Use great caution to avoid losing or displacing the broken piece. If the tooth came out but you didn't see the piece come with it, you must completely explore the site. Retained fragments can cause significant unnecessary harm to the patient and open the surgeon up to tremendous liability. For example, they can cause infection, migrate and cause erosive trauma to vessels and other anatomy, or heat up in an MRI. It is critical to ensure no broken pieces are left behind if possible.

Bleeding

The human body is programmed to stop bleeding. When bleeding occurs, an elaborate cascade of events transpires involving the vessel wall, platelets and various structural and signaling proteins. They coordinate to form the initial "platelet plug." This initial plug is relatively unstable and needs reinforcement. As the clotting cascade continues, the innate anticoagulant properties always at work to prevent aberrant clots are turned off. The myriad of clotting factors and associated enzymes are thrust into action. Thus, a clot develops.

Developing a stable clot requires a competent system and slow enough blood flow. If the body doesn't have adequate clotting resources, hemorrhage continues. If the blood is blasting out so fast it just flushes out everything the body throws at it, hemorrhage continues. But as they say, all bleeding stops … eventually. The two basic steps to controlling bleeding are: optimize the system and minimize the flow. Create an environment where the coagulation system can succeed. And then protect it so it will last. Promote clot formation and stabilization.

In medicine and science, we like order. We like to organize things like the coagulation cascade into a neat and tidy process. We define and arrange the various steps. We like it to be similar to the famous Dutch painter Piet Mondrian's work. Organized. Predictable. In reality, it is a lot more like Jackson Pollock's work: a flurry of coordinated chaos that results in an intricate tapestry, returning order and maintaining hemostasis.

Taking a thorough medical history helps identify systemic bleeding risks. The patient may have innate increased risk of bleeding such as low platelets (thrombocytopenia) or medication related risk from various anticoagulants. This must be evaluated and properly managed to attenuate the complications. Prevention is the best management.

A simple 4-0 chromic suture and some Gelfoam helps reduce post-operative bleeding. The suture slows the blood flow. The Gelfoam helps the clot get established by providing a framework for coagulation to take place. Platelet rich fibrin is even better. This isn't necessary for everyone. But for elderly patients or those with coagulopathy, a stitch may physically help reduce post-operative bleeding. It will also mentally help the patient, knowing that extra measures were taken to control blood loss. Little mental victories improve patient well-being and satisfaction. It also reduces post-op phone calls from worried patients.

Anticoagulation

Managing anticoagulated patients is all about weighing the risks and the benefits. These patients are anticoagulated because they have a condition that increases their risk of developing what could be a devastating clot. Is the risk of the patient having a thrombotic event greater than the risk of having major post-operative bleeding? Consideration must be given to both sides of the equation: thrombosis and bleeding. This risk stratification helps guide treatment. In evaluating the risk of a thrombotic event, consider the following factors: type of anticoagulant, reason for anticoagulation and history of thrombosis.

The ordering physician should be called upon to guide any changes in anticoagulant therapy. They know their patients and take seriously their responsibility for preventing a thrombotic event. For practical and medicolegal reasons, please consult the ordering physician and document their recommendations. Make sure patients understand their physician is involved and participating in the decision. I often tell my patients I would rather they bleed a bit more after surgery than throw a clot to their lungs or brain. Then we talk at length about steps they can take to help the bleeding stop. It is all a balance.

Type of anticoagulant

The type of anticoagulant medication the patient takes has a big impact on the risk of holding it. For example, discontinuing warfarin may result in a temporary rebound hypercoagulopathy, briefly putting patients at a potentially greater risk of thrombosis. Whereas holding a novel anticoagulant, such as Eliquis, the morning of surgery results in a temporary decrease in overall anticoagulation but does not result in a hypercoagulable state. The duration of action is also important to consider. Let's compare warfarin, Xarelto and aspirin.

Patients remain anticoagulated for several days after stopping warfarin. It blocks the formation of the reduced form of Vitamin K, which is a big player in the coagulation cascade. As this critical resource is used up in normal daily hemostasis, warfarin prevents it from being adequately replaced. This depletes the supply and thus decreases the efficacy of the coagulation cascade. It takes several days for the liver to restore the supply to a therapeutic level. Holding this medication for surgery can result in increased risk of clotting for up to 5 to7 days, but the big risk in holding warfarin may be the controversial rebound hypercoagulability. Their risk of a thrombotic event may be even higher than their baseline if they were never taking warfarin. Warfarin has the longest window of increased risk compared to the other types.

With a 12-hour half-life, Xarelto's effects only linger for one day before returning to near normal coagulation. It takes only a couple of hours to achieve peak effect again after restarting therapy. If the decision is made to hold Xarelto, the patient is at increased risk of thrombosis for only 24-36 hours.

The active component in aspirin, salicylic acid, is produced naturally by willow trees. Nature has been making it a lot longer than the modified version Bayer produces (acetylsalicylic acid). It is the most widely used medication in the world. When it enters a platelet, it irreversibly binds to the cyclooxygenase enzyme (COX-1). For the rest of the life of that platelet, it cannot form the protein thromboxane A2 (TxA2), which is responsible in part for platelet aggregation. The platelet inhibition happens very quickly, within 60 minutes of ingestion. These impotent platelets are replaced with functional platelets on their normal 8 to 10 day life cycle. At that time, platelet aggregation has returned to its baseline level. Therefore, aspirin must be held for 4 to 7 days before surgery to be of any benefit. When we hold aspirin, our patients are at a minimally increased risk of thrombosis for 4 to 7 days[3].

Some patients report aspirin makes them bruise and bleed easily and they have a difficult time getting it to stop. For these patients, it would be prudent to consider holding it. While holding aspirin may not make a huge difference in post-operative bleeding, it also doesn't usually pose a significant risk to the patient. The duration and significance of the risk when holding warfarin is much greater than Xarelto or aspirin.

It is important to know the reason your patient is anticoagulated and to be aware of the medication's mechanism and pharmacology. This is all changes constantly. I recommend checking the American Dental Association's current guidelines as they update them periodically on their website (https://www.ada.org/).

Reason for anticoagulation

Find out why the patient is anticoagulated. Some conditions requiring anticoagulation have very strict protocols. Patients with a mechanical prosthetic heart valve must remain anticoagulated. Otherwise, they have a significant risk of throwing a clot. If their procedure has a high risk of bleeding, perioperative management may include bridging their anticoagulation to decrease exposure and risk to a very short timeframe. Consulting with the cardiology or cardiothoracic team is imperative to the patient's wellbeing.

History of thrombosis

Recent history of a thrombotic event places the patient at high risk of having another event if anticoagulation is stopped. Proceed with extreme caution. That patient should probably continue the anticoagulant, even if it means a bit more blood loss from surgery. Local hemostatic measures are even more important in these cases.

Intraoperative bleeding

Bleeding can be high or low pressure (arterial or venous) and high or low flow (a large or small leak). Depending on the pressure and flow, intraoperative bleeding can range in severity from a nuisance of a trickle to an obstructive ooze to an unmanageable flood. And sometimes it is off the charts when an arterial bleed paints the patient's pulse through the air and onto the ceiling with a geyser of blood. Regardless of the cause, the goal is the same: control the bleeding.

With a nuisance of a trickle, the bleeding just gets in the way a bit. This can make it more difficult to see the details of the procedure. But the blood is easily evacuated with suction, allowing reasonable visualization again. Typically, intermittent suction is sufficient to manage this type of bleeding. At times, the flow is more obstructive. When the bleeding hampers the progress of the surgery, several steps can be taken to help control it and optimize the surgical field. When the bleeding seems like an unmanageable flood or a startling geyser, remain calm and work through these principles of hemostasis.

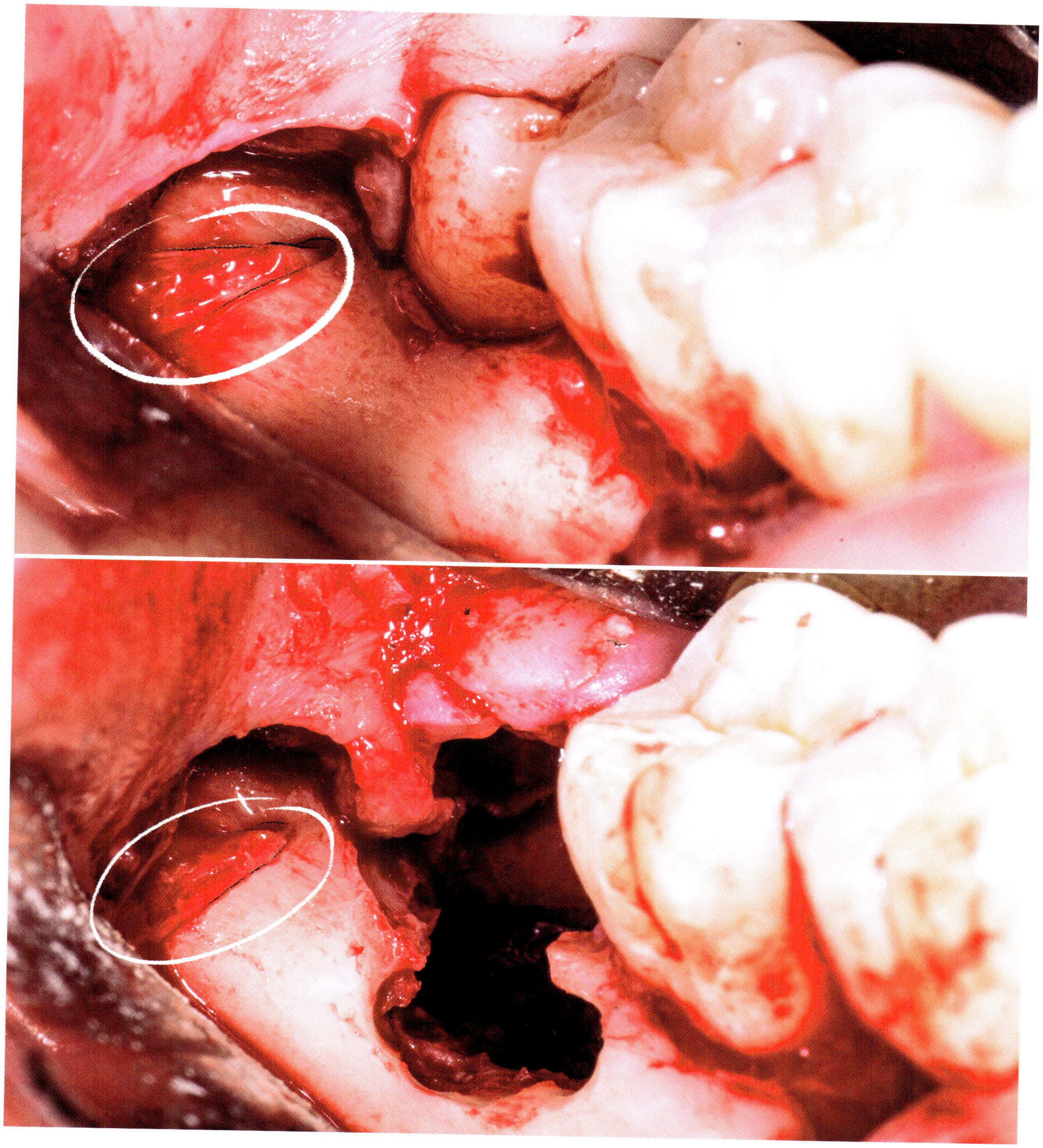

Figure 6-7 Vessels like this are often encountered when elevating a flap. Protect it by working around it if possible. It was relatively easy to preserve the vessel in this coronectomy. When you need to drill where a feeder vessel perforates the bone, expect increased bleeding. Consider compressing the overlying bone with a condenser or angled curette to obstruct the bleeding and improve hemostasis.

Principles of achieving hemostasis

There are many techniques to manage intraoperative bleeding. Thankfully, most bleeding encountered in routine oral surgery can be managed quite easily and quickly with a few simple and accessible techniques. Depending on the extent of the bleeding and the available resources, there are many other options available that we will discuss. But it all hinges on knowing where the bleeding is coming from.

1. Identify the source. Identifying the source is pivotal in managing intraoperative bleeding. If you can isolate the source, it is much easier to stop. Efforts can then be effectively focused where it counts. Some helpful tools to identify the source include a small tipped surgical suction, a small tissue elevator (Micro Buser), hemostats, gauze and irrigation. Blood flows downhill and pools in the lowest place. That may seem obvious as it is liquid, but keep this in mind while searching for the source. A small tipped surgical suction is a very handy tool. Use it to isolate the bleeding by following the blood to its source. When the suction is directly over the mark, that particular bleed appears to be gone. If there are multiple sites, isolate and manage them one at a time, starting with either the most obvious source or the one that is easiest to access. Packing the site with gauze and removing it slowly can also help locate the source.

When the source is challenging to find with suction and pressure alone, flush the site with saline. Clear away the blood so you can track where it seems to be coming from. This can help track down the leaking vessel. Take the time to precisely identify the source. If you don't deal with it at the source, you will spend considerable time mopping up the mess, which is time consuming and frustrating.

2. Apply pressure. The most basic and easy thing to do is apply pressure. The challenge is to maintain adequate pressure in a favorable spot long enough to promote a reasonable clot. Gauze can be very effective. If the bleeding seems to be coming from the soft tissue, roll some gauze and position it directly over the site of the bleeding and apply firm pressure. Depending on the site, this can be done by biting on the gauze or manually holding pressure. If there is considerable bleeding, apply pressure for at least 5 to10 minutes. That feels like a really long time during a procedure. It can be prohibitively long and other measures may achieve hemostasis quicker. But pressure is nearly free and quite effective. It takes some time for the initial plug to form. Make space for the body to do what it is designed to do. If the bleeding seems to be coming from deep within an extraction site or osteotomy, pack the site with moistened gauze. (It can be dry gauze, but some moisture will help prevent it from sticking to the site and later dislodging a clot.) Really pack it in there. The more pressure there is, the more stable the site, and the faster and more effectively the bleeding will be controlled. Use a hemostat or cotton forceps. Unfold a piece of gauze. Then layer it into the site, condensing it with each layer. If it is really bleeding, consider dousing local anesthetic with epinephrine on the gauze before packing it. The epinephrine can help with vasoconstriction. Then set a timer. Don't trust yourself to have the patience to wait long enough. You have things to do anyway. Proceed with another part of the surgery if possible, or even step out to do something else or just clear your head. (In full disclosure, I don't routinely set a timer anymore. This concept was ingrained in me when doing facelifts on my facial plastic surgery rotation. A little bleeding there can make a big difference to patient satisfaction. But the principles are wise, and I feel the need to pass them along.) If the gauze is soaking through with blood, make sure it is packed tightly and wait longer. Consider adjusting the gauze or replacing it only if you think the position can be improved. Otherwise, just reinforce it with more gauze if it becomes saturated. After the timer goes off, remove the gauze and evaluate. If the pressure was in the right spot long enough, the site is typically dry and the procedure can commence (with particular care taken to protect the delicate new clot).

Packing the site like this is most effective when the packing is directly pressing on the bleeding site. First, try to identify the source. If the source cannot be clearly located, blindly packing the site can be a Hail Mary attempt with relatively good outcomes and low risk. It often works as a sort of shotgun approach. This is particularly useful when apical granulation tissue is oozing. The combination of disorganized, fragile vasculature with localized inflammation is a recipe for bleeding deep within the socket. Ultimately, the granulation tissue should be excavated. This can be difficult and messy when it is actively hemorrhaging. A bit of pressure may do the trick to slow the bleeding enough to continue the operation effectively and efficiently.

3. Occlude the vessel. Directly occluding the bleeder can quickly and effectively stop the bleeding. This requires clear identification of the vessel to precisely obstruct its flow. If the bleeding is from within the bone, it may be possible to crush the bone. Any small instrument may work, but a small condenser or the tips of curved hemostats seem to be a good choice. Press firmly. Envision compressing the bone around the vessel. This doesn't work if the bone is too dense. But this is a slick trick when it works.

Bone wax can also obstruct a bleeding vessel. Mashing a dollop of wax right into the bleeding site can help stop the bleeding. Bone wax is cheap and a potentially effective aid.

Injecting local anesthetic with epinephrine causes vasoconstriction and can apply indirect pressure to the vessel to reduce bleeding. First, identify and isolate the bleeding. Then, inject right into the soft tissue where the bleeding is occurring and also around the site to help with pressure and vasoconstriction. This can help choke the vessel and reduce the outflow.

When ridge preservation is planned, if the extraction is completed and the site is adequately prepared, simply condensing the bone graft material into the site may occlude the vessel and help achieve hemostasis.

4. Introduce hemostatic agents. There is an entire bouquet of hemostatic agents available, each leveraging some part of the coagulation cascade. They can be passive or active. Passive agents generally create a matrix to promote clot formation and stability. Active agents trigger an event somewhere in the cascade to promote further coagulation. These can be very helpful, especially when used in combination with firm, constant pressure[4].

5. Cauterize. Electrosurgical or laser cauterization can dry up an oozing surgical site very well. There may be some collateral damage, so be judicious in applying these techniques. They can generate a good bit of heat, damaging cells beyond the local bleeding tissue. Electrosurgical cautery takes a bit of planning to set the patient up with a safe grounding pad. But it is also more effective at managing higher amounts of bleeding. A laser may be quicker to set up, but it may not have as much horsepower to deal with significant bleeding. Electrocautery can penetrate up the blood stream better as it is an electrical current. The laser is an optical transmission of energy that requires closer and more direct proximity to the bleeding vessel. These both require specialized equipment and training to be used safely and effectively. The settings are important. Too much energy can fry the site, further disrupting the vasculature. If the energy isn't high enough (or with the optimal frequency for lasers) it won't be effective.

6. Ligate, reverse anticoagulation, thrombose. If a soft tissue artery is cut, as in a biopsy or flap development, a ligature suture can be placed around the vessel as a little tourniquet. This may be a temporary measure, removed before finishing, or sometimes it is left in place to resorb over time. Consider the risk of post-operative bleeding before removing a ligature suture. If the established clot gives way, how will that impact the recovery?

Table 6-1 The most common things I use in my clinic

	Source	Mechanism	Use
Gelfoam	Absorbable gelatin sponge	Framework for clot formation and stabilization	Place in socket and may place suture to retain
Collaplug	Highly crosslinked collagen plug	Increases platelet adherence and promotes clot stabilization	Place in socket and can apply some pressure
Platelet rich fibrin	Autologous blood product	Fibrin matrix clot rich in platelets and cytokines that promotes coagulation	Place in socket and place suture
Surgical	Oxidized regenerated alpha cellulose woven into gauze	Stabilizes clot and promotes fibrin formation	I only use this in the hospital setting, emergency room or operating room
Tranexamic Acid (TXA)	Synthetic lysine analog	Inhibits fibrinolysis, thus stabilizing the clot	Orthognathic surgery. 10-15 mg/kg IV. Can also be used as topical oral rinse

In the hospital, I sometimes use 10 to 15 mg/kg of tranexamic acid infusion during the surgery, as in a maxillary down fracture.

Post-Operative Bleeding

Early and late post-operative bleeding can be unnerving for a patient. Some bleeding is normal after most oral surgery. Preparing patients to expect bleeding can do wonders for their anxiety if it persists. If they know it is common to bleed through today and into tomorrow, they will be much less anxious as the day goes on.

It is also very helpful to explain multiple times and in detail exactly how to manage bleeding: with good firm pressure right where the bleeding is coming from. If the gauze is placed between the teeth and not putting firm pressure on the wound, it is doing little more than absorbing the blood. Patients should be instructed on how and when to change the gauze as well. Instructing patients to maintain constant pressure on the site for 30 to 40 minutes at a time increases the likelihood of compliance (maybe getting the patient to at least apply pressure for 10 to15 minutes before checking it). The most common causes for prolonged bleeding are inadequate pressure either from not applying pressure long enough or improper tamponade. If a reasonable clot hasn't formed when the patient removes the gauze, the biological clock starts over with a new platelet plug. When this is explained, patients are more likely to comply and have a better recovery.

Excessive bleeding can occur from routine oral surgery, resulting in significant blood loss. It is rare to need a blood transfusion after oral surgery. But it must be at least entertained as a possibility in the surgeon's mind if a patient with compromised cardiovascular status is experiencing excessive bleeding.

When should surgeons intervene in post-operative bleeding? If the bleeding is pulsatile, surgical intervention is indicated. If the patient has already sustained significant blood loss and is showing signs of hypovolemia (weakness, fatigue, lightheaded, tachycardic, hypotensive) intervention is required. Otherwise, it is at the surgeon's discretion. The intervention itself may carry some risk of bleeding. If the plan is to open the site for exploration to control the bleeding, there is risk of destabilizing any clot that has formed. The art is in knowing what to do and when.

Liver clot/currant jelly clot

Venous hemorrhage can sometimes result in a liver clot or a currant jelly clot developing. These names describe an aberrant mass of clotting blood that can form at an intraoral surgical site. This seems to be a result of ectopic clotting beyond the vessel wall. The clot can't form at the injured vessel wall, possibly due to flow or disruption in the normal coagulation cascade. The vessel continues to hemorrhage blood into a developing fibrous capsule. The fibrin that is meant to stabilize the clot forms the barrier around the jelly-like mass. This type of clot can be very confusing for patients and can result in significant blood loss. The treatment for this odd problem is counterintuitive to patients. It would seem like disrupting this clot could further propagate the bleeding. Instead, treatment involves removing the clot and applying firm pressure directly to the site of bleeding.

Patients can often clear the clot and achieve hemostasis on their own with proper direction. Explain what caused the clot and that it needs to be completely removed. Have someone else help hold a light and retract the tissue so the clot can be visualized. Use a clean wash rag or gauze to completely remove the clot. It often comes out as a whole, but the site of the bleeding needs to be gently cleared as well a second time. Once all the clotted tissue is removed, apply firm, direct pressure to the site of the bleeding for 30 to 45 minutes at a time until the bleeding has resolved. If some of the liver clot remains or if it reforms, wipe the area clean and try again. If the patient is unsuccessful, it may require intervention under local anesthetic in an operatory to evacuate the site and apply additional hemostatic measures. Because of how the liver clot disrupts normal hemostasis, significant blood loss can be incurred. This must be taken seriously and properly managed.

Nerve Injury and Healing

Nerves send signals very quickly but supplies very slowly. They take a long time to heal.

I used to think electricity was something that actually flowed, like a garden hose of power. It turns out that when a current is generated, a chain reaction occurs in which the outer electrons in the atoms are excited just enough to bump the electrons of the neighboring atom out of its atomic orbit. That electron, in turn, bumps the next one out, and so the negative current travels down the line. In this way, it is more like Newton's pendulum, the mesmerizing toy my kids brought home from the Museum of Science and Industry in Chicago.

It is mind blowing to think about how a nerve transmits an electrical signal. Nerves function similarly to electrical wires, though they are far more complex and elegant. With nerves, the signal or current is not just an excited electron blasting another electron out of orbit. There is an elaborate flow of charged ions passing across a membrane that physically changes the shape of specialized protein channels. These different proteins function to passively allow and actively pump the charged ions in and out of the cell, generating a cascade that transfers the charge along the nerve axon to the cell body. When it arrives at the end of the nerve cell, it passes the signal across a synapse to the final destination or another nerve in the pathway.

In a nerve's resting state, a charge is generated and maintained by sodium-potassium pumps. These little protein pumps constantly ratchet back and forth, pushing three Na^+ ions out and two K^- ions into the cell. This creates a negative internal and positive external charge called the resting state or resting potential. The ions are desperately trying to neutralize the charge by flowing across the membrane.

▸
Figure 6-8 When the pendulum is loaded, the signal transmits almost instantly along the path. If one ball doesn't respond, the signal is broken.

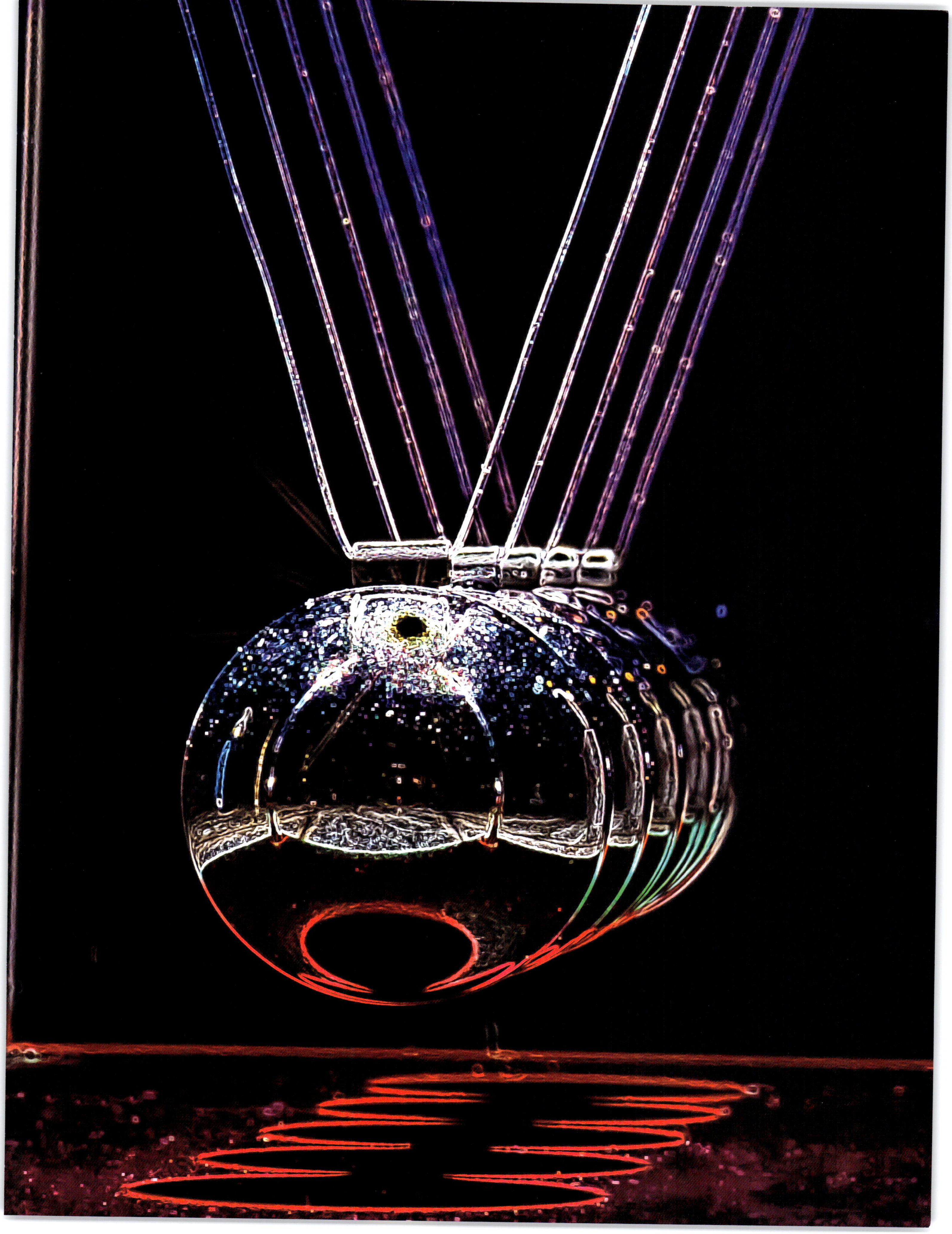

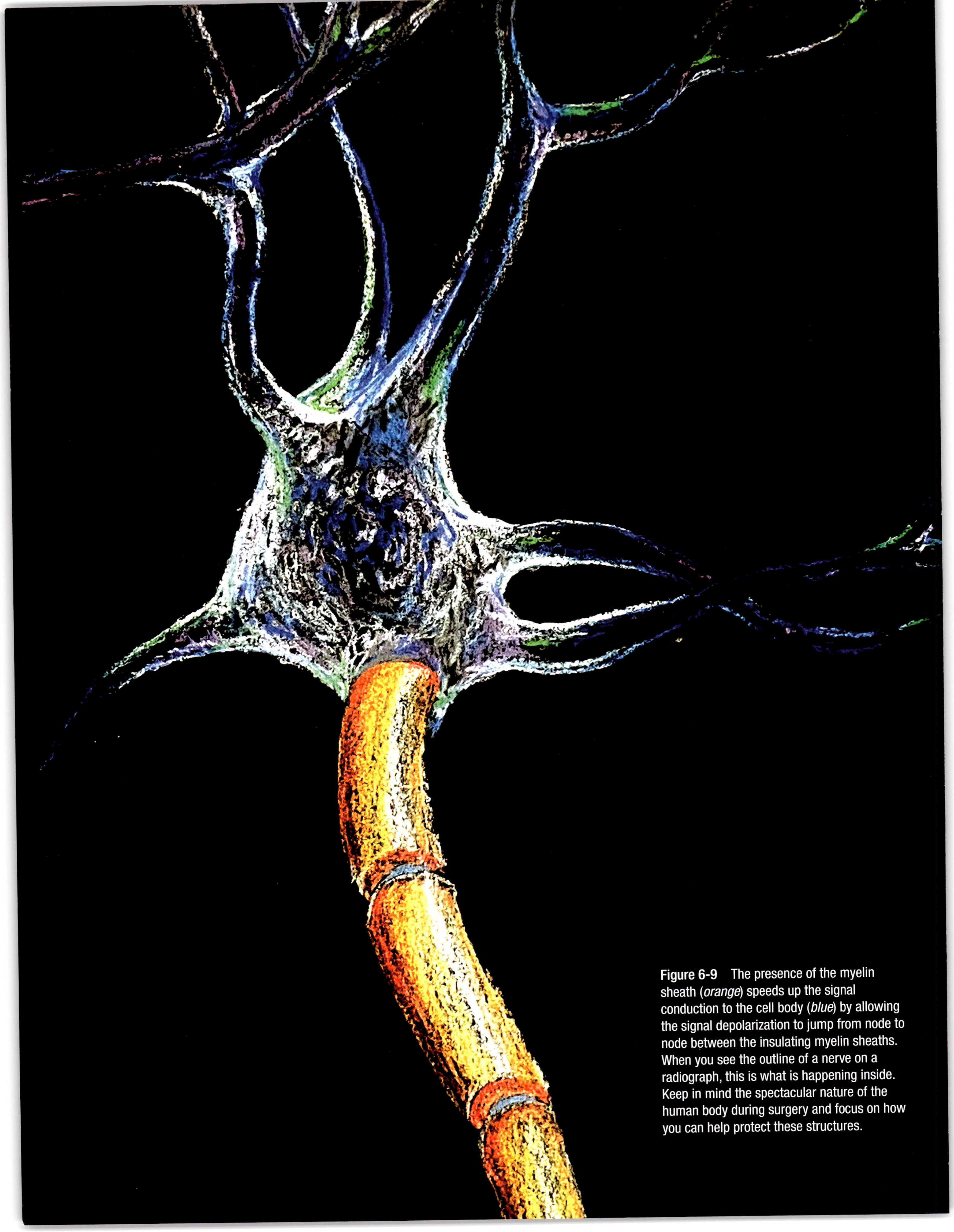

Figure 6-9 The presence of the myelin sheath (*orange*) speeds up the signal conduction to the cell body (*blue*) by allowing the signal depolarization to jump from node to node between the insulating myelin sheaths. When you see the outline of a nerve on a radiograph, this is what is happening inside. Keep in mind the spectacular nature of the human body during surgery and focus on how you can help protect these structures.

The difference between the positive external and negative internal charge is the voltage. When the voltage decreases, it triggers amazing little proteins called voltage-gated sodium channels to pop open, allowing the Na^+ ions to rush in across the membrane, thus decreasing the polarization or charge. As the Na^+ channels are wide open and the charge is neutralized, another protein channel opens, allowing the K^- ions to rush out of the cell. This results in a negative charge outside the cell. The outside of the cell instantly goes from positive to neutral and then to negative as it depolarizes. This flux triggers the adjacent voltage gated Na^+ channels along the nerve to pop open, depolarizing that portion of the membrane. Each one triggers the next one in line. And so, the signal is transduced down the axon toward the cell body. Nothing really flows along the axon except the changing current. There is a similarity with electrons moving a charge down a copper wire, but nerves are far more intricate and delicate. And way more amazing.

The signal journey

If you gently lick your lips right now, a specialized sensory cell at the base of the epidermis in your lower lip called a Merkel cell triggers depolarization at the end of a myelinated A-beta nerve fiber. The complex cascade of depolarization blazes at about 150 miles per hour (70,000 mm/second) along the axon through the deep tissue of the lip, past the mental foramen and shoots through the tunnel of the mandibular canal. It exits the mandibular foramen just behind the lingula and ascends through the infratemporal tissue, cruising past the skull walls through the foramen ovale into Meckel's cave. Here, the depolarization rips on through the trigeminal ganglion, which houses the cell body of this particular axon (as well as thousands of other trigeminal axons sending their own depolarization signals to and from the brain). The signal zooms into the nearby brainstem and heads to its second synapse on the journey in the Chief Sensory Nucleus. It takes about 0.5 milliseconds for the neurotransmitters to be released, diffuse across the gap, and trigger the postsynaptic receptor. The race is on again as the voltage gated channels fling open on the second order neuron and the action potential explodes up to the midbrain. The thalamus is the great relay station in the midbrain that ultimately sends the signal out to the pars oralis in the neocortex, letting you know something just touched your lip. That signal pathway has occurred thousands of times since you first noticed your lip a minute ago.

If you bite your lip, a similar process occurs. The free ending of an unmyelinated C-fiber axon follows the same pathway. But it only travels at about 5 miles per hour (2,000 millimeters per second) without insulation from the myelin sheath. These signals synapse in the Spinal Trigeminal Nucleus before proceeding up to the higher brain.

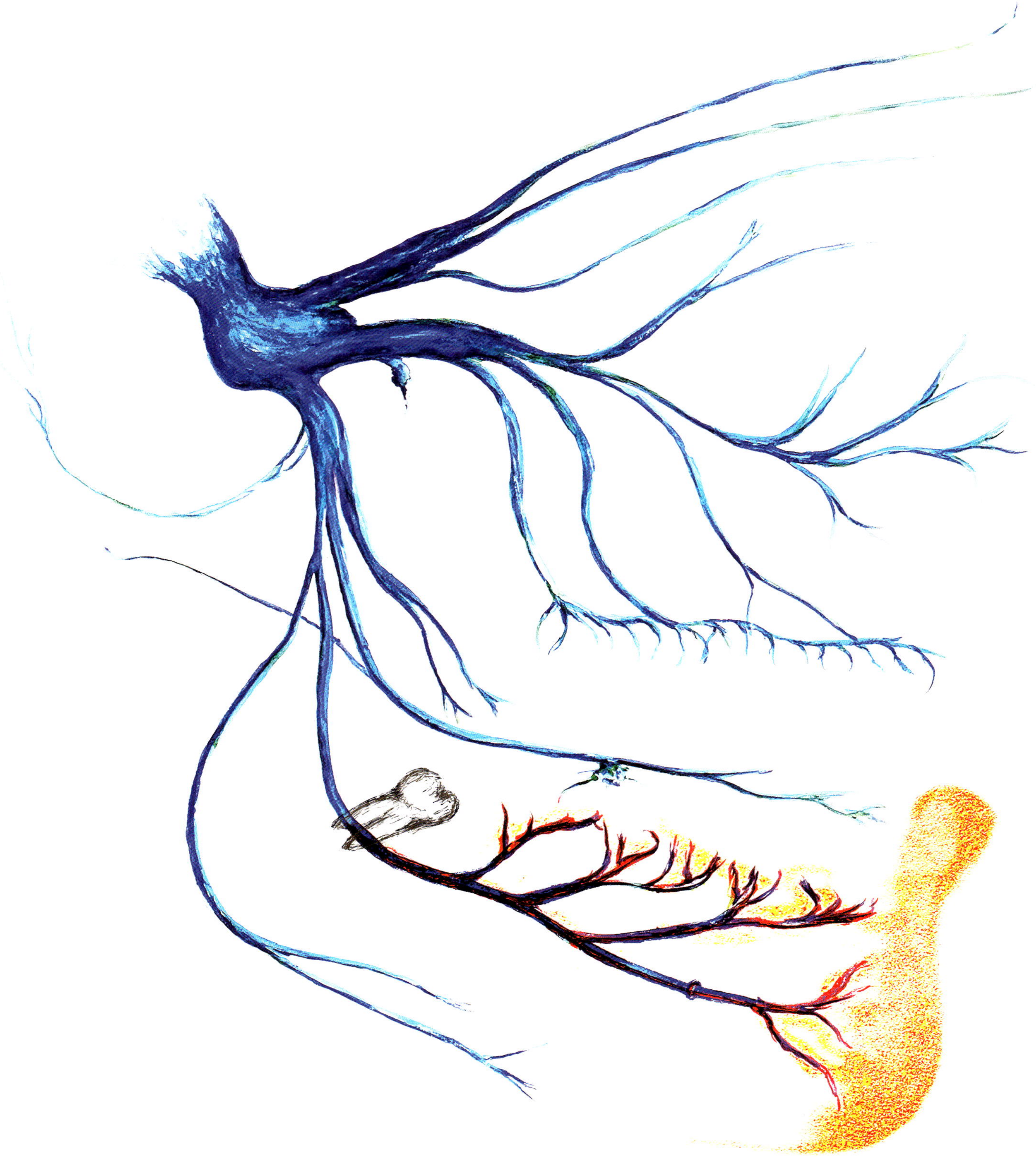

Figure 6-10 The trigeminal nerve has many branches. When it is damaged during a lower third molar extraction, sensation to the lower lip and chin is altered. At a minimum, this numbness can be obnoxious for patients, but it can also be downright debilitating in the case of anesthesia dolorosum. (Artwork inspired by Kaitlin Walsh.)

TYPES OF NERVE FIBERS

A-beta fibers: Touch and pressure. Myelinated. Merkel cell body in base layer of epithelium.

A-delta fibers: Pain and temperature. Myelinated. Merkel cell body in base layer of epithelium.

C fibers: Pain, temperature and itch. Unmyelinated. Free nerve endings in epidermis.

Nerve trauma

With all that complexity, it is no surprise nerve function can be easily disrupted. Nerves are fragile and fickle. They like to be protected and can be fussy when disrupted. Broadly speaking, the more layers of the nerve that are traumatized, and the worse the trauma, the lower the chances of quick and complete recovery. All a nerve's regenerative potential is mobilized from within the cell body. This is often far from a site of injury, contributing to the prolonged sensory recovery compared to other hard and soft tissue recovery.

A minor compression injury to a nerve can temporarily stop the signal from moving. Apraxia means without movement. When the nerve is "without movement," Sir Herbert Seddon labeled it "neurapraxia." In this type of injury, there is no significant structural damage, and the nerve can recover fairly quickly.

A more severe injury can cause axons to separate within the nerve bundle while the majority of the nerve remains intact. The suffix "tmesis" literally means the separation of parts, so Seddon called this type of injury "axonotmesis," or axon separation. These injuries require more time and effort from the nerve cell body to heal. They can have partial or complete recovery without surgical intervention, depending on how much damage was done.

The most severe nerve injury is a transection injury. When the nerve itself is separate, Seddon classified this as "neurotmesis," literally meaning nerve separation. Without surgical intervention, recovery is unlikely. The nerve needs a pathway to follow when healing. The ends of the severed nerve can be approximated or wrapped with a conduit type of graft. Without a track or guidance, it will simply form a bundle of scar tissue at the stump of the injury called a traumatic neuroma.

Seddon's classification is very practical using the following suffixes:
apraxia = without movement.
tmesis = separation of parts.

The longer and more numb a patient is, the higher the injury grade, and the lower the likelihood of complete recovery. Even in the absence of complete sensory recovery, the human brain has a marvelous ability to normalize and adapt to the changes in sensation.

Visualizing potential injury

What type of nerve injury is acceptable? Even neuropraxia can be alarming and concerning for a patient or their parents. And we don't really know the extent of the injury until it either recovers or doesn't. It can only be called temporary after it recovers.

If we can visualize the potential injury before it happens, we can hopefully mitigate the damage. Envision the path the root will take during extraction. Will it rub against the nerve or squeeze it? If a small portion of the root breaks off during extraction, how can it be retrieved while protecting the nerve? If the nerve gets bumped a little, it will likely recover its function completely. If it looks like the root curves around the nerve toward the apex, the injury will be more extensive and recovery more questionable. A few questions to ask when evaluating and considering removal could be:

- *How severe will the injury be?*
- *How much of the nerve will be compressed?*
- *How much room is there for the tooth to move?*

Envision the entire fascicle of the nerve and then think about each axon. They all carry valuable signals. No one wants to live without them.

Nerve injury management

What do we do when we have a patient with a nerve injury? Treat, track and refer.

Early treatment with supplements and steroids has been shown to improve the outcome. Neuroinflammatory processes can cause ongoing axonal damage. Immediately begin an anti-inflammatory medication, such as a Medrol Dosepak (tapered methylprednisolone regimen).

Support nerve healing with specific Neurotropic B vitamins for a few months[5]. These include:

- **B1**: Site-directed antioxidant. Facilitates energy production for nerve healing.
- **B6**: Balances nerve metabolism. Inhibits release of neurotoxic glutamate.
- **B12**: Maintains and regenerates myelin sheath. Helps the nerve cell survive the injury.

(These vitamins are available in a high dose combination prescription called Neurobion Forte. I don't know of any literature directly supporting its use in oral surgery related injuries, but it is worth considering.)

Identify and track the progression of the sensory defect. If it is not improving within a couple months, recommend referral to a specialist in micro neurosurgical repair. When the defect shrinks in size or shows signs of regeneration, surgery is not indicated. In the presence of complete prolonged anesthesia for 2 to 3 months or dysesthesia, surgical repair may be indicated. Refer the patient and let the specialist determine the next steps. The clearest indication for micro neurosurgical repair is a witnessed transection of the nerve. Thankfully, this is extremely rare, but it should be managed with prompt surgical repair.

Help your attorney defend you by providing clear, concise and contemporaneous documentation. Thoroughly documenting clinical findings as well as patient discussions is crucial if the case enters the legal system. If you have a patient with a nerve injury, spend a few minutes learning about neurosensory mapping with light touch, two point discrimination and pin prick discrimination[6].

Referred pain makes sense when you consider the incredible sequence of changes in polarity occurring within the epi and perineurium. The increased depolarizing activity of a few axons could potentially trigger some excitability in other adjacent axons. Additionally, the terminal receptor for the signal can also become excited with a high volume of impulses, resulting in a slightly broader area reception of the signal within the brain. A high-volume signal reverberates within the conduit of the nerve, confusing the final signal in the brain.

References

1. Hassani A, Shahmirzadi S, Saadat S, et al. Applications of the Buccal Fat Pad in Oral and Maxillofacial Surgery [Internet]. A Textbook of Advanced Oral and Maxillofacial Surgery Volume 3. IntechOpen; 2016 [cited 2022 Dec 24]. Available from: https://www.intechopen.com/state.item.id
2. Nayyar J, Clarke M, O'Sullivan M, et al. Fractured root tips during dental extractions and retained root fragments. A clinical dilemma? Br Dent J. 2015 Mar 13;218(5):285-290.
3. Ornelas A, Zacharias-Millward N, Menter DG, et al. Beyond COX-1: the effects of aspirin on platelet biology and potential mechanisms of chemoprevention. Cancer Metastasis Rev. 2017 Jun;36(2):289-303.
4. Moghadam HG, Caminiti MF. Life-Threatening Hemorrhage after Extraction of Third Molars: Case Report and Management Protocol. J Can Dent Assoc. 2002 Dec;68(11):670-674.
5. Baltrusch S. The Role of Neurotropic B Vitamins in Nerve Regeneration. Biomed Res Int. 2021;2021:9968228.
6. Ziccardi VB, Zuniga JR. Nerve Injuries After Third Molar Removal. Oral and Maxillofac Surg Clin North Am. 2007 Feb;19(1):105-115.

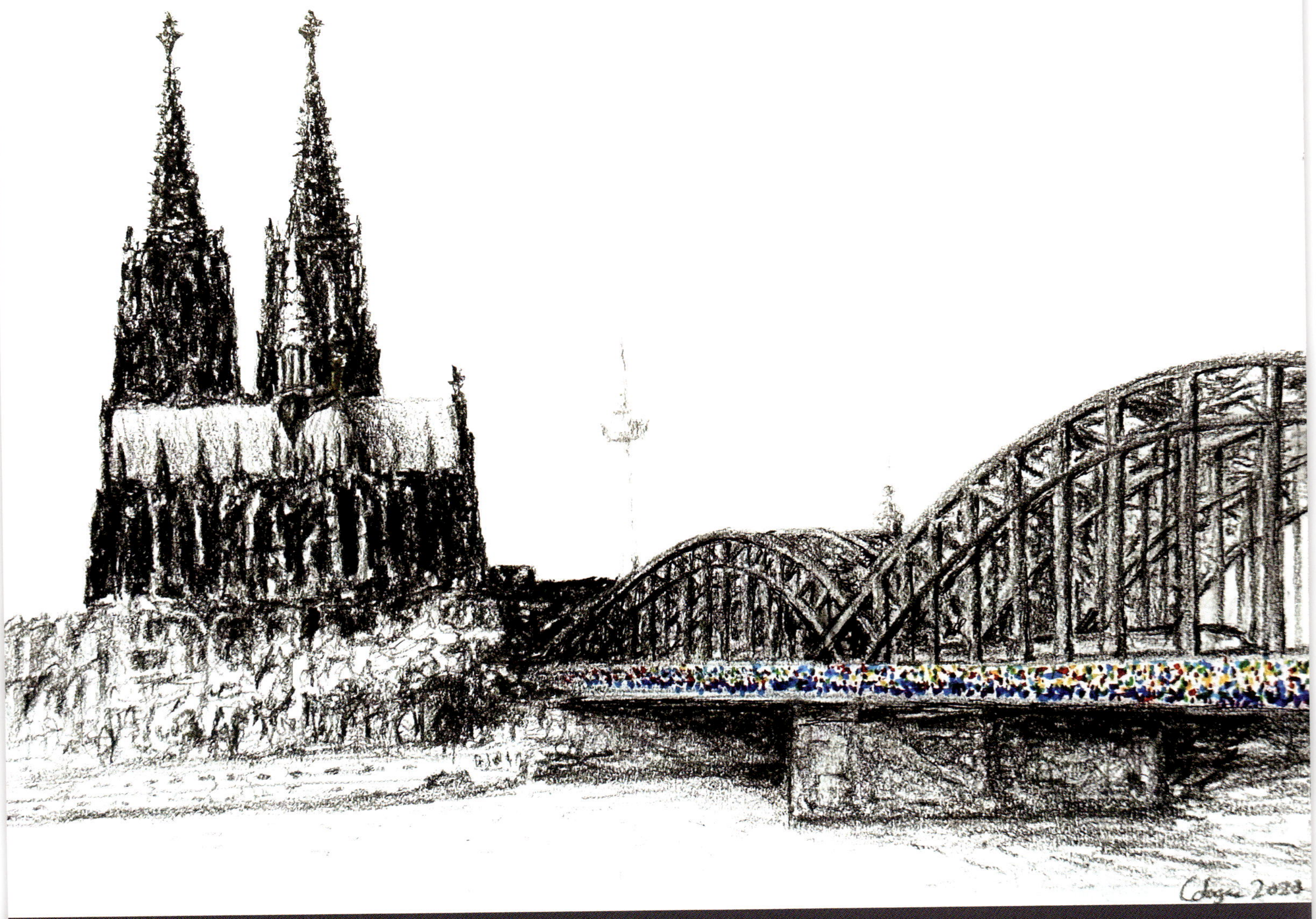

Color of Love. (Graphite and marker on paper)
My older brother, Jordan, taught me sketching engages the brain and locks in the memory. When traveling, I always make a little time to sketch. Looking at this picture instantly brings me back to my trip to IDS in Cologne, Germany. This bridge over the Rhine River was canvased with locks placed by people to symbolize their love.

CHAPTER 7

IMPLANT ARCHITECTURE

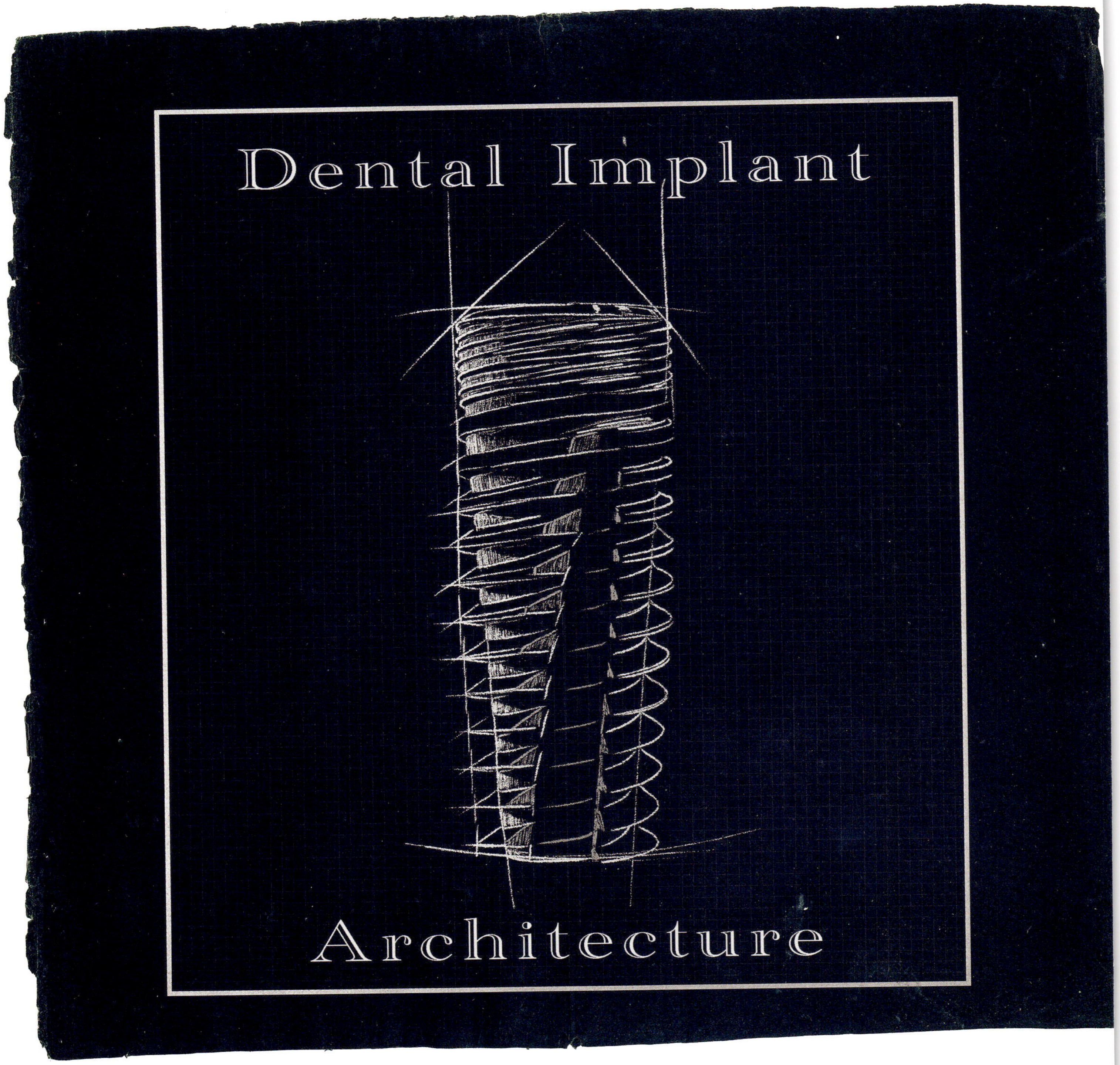

(Artwork inspired by Leonardo da Vinci.)

The best implant always begins with a surgeon who understands the principles of surgery and healing, and the design of the implant system.

We have a very high calling as architects of implant dentistry. Our ultimate goal is to provide a seamless transition by restoring esthetics and function so well patients are unaware they are missing a tooth. Essentially, we are to make them whole. Complete.

Architecture is a fascinating form of art. The artwork itself is inhabitable and functional. It is a blend between engineering and design. An excellent architect uses the resources available to create a beautiful structure that effortlessly serves its intended purpose. A well-designed building feels right to its occupants. This requires the architect to visualize the building's intended uses, possibly even more than the people who will be using it.

As an artist and architect in the first century, Vitruvius described three guiding principles that have stood the test of time: durability, utility and beauty (De architectura). These same principles guide our work in implantology today.

Durability

Teeth and implants take quite a beating. The physical and biological assault they sustain is incredible. We need to understand the burdens of the oral cavity to overcome them.

Utility

Mother Nature is very clever indeed. She has designed a system to harvest energy from glucose and oxygen by producing carbon dioxide and water. Chewing is a pretty important step in this whole process. To optimize function, we try to understand and replicate the natural occlusofacial complex. We want implants to work, to chew, as well as teeth. We all need to eat.

Beauty

We have moved far beyond simply accepting a screw in the jawbone as success. Our sophisticated materials and techniques allow us to design and construct a form of beauty nearly matching that of nature.

Implant architecture is the process of planning, designing and constructing replacement teeth. To do this well, we need to start with an overall plan. We gather and analyze data according to biological and mechanical principles. The design flows out from there, taking engineering, biomechanics and esthetics into consideration. Then comes the surgery, constructing a foundation to support the ideal restoration. The restoration should guide each step of the process. When the restoration is complete and the patient is again made whole, we become inspired. Inspired by the work of art. Inspired to continue to produce and expand our skills and understanding.

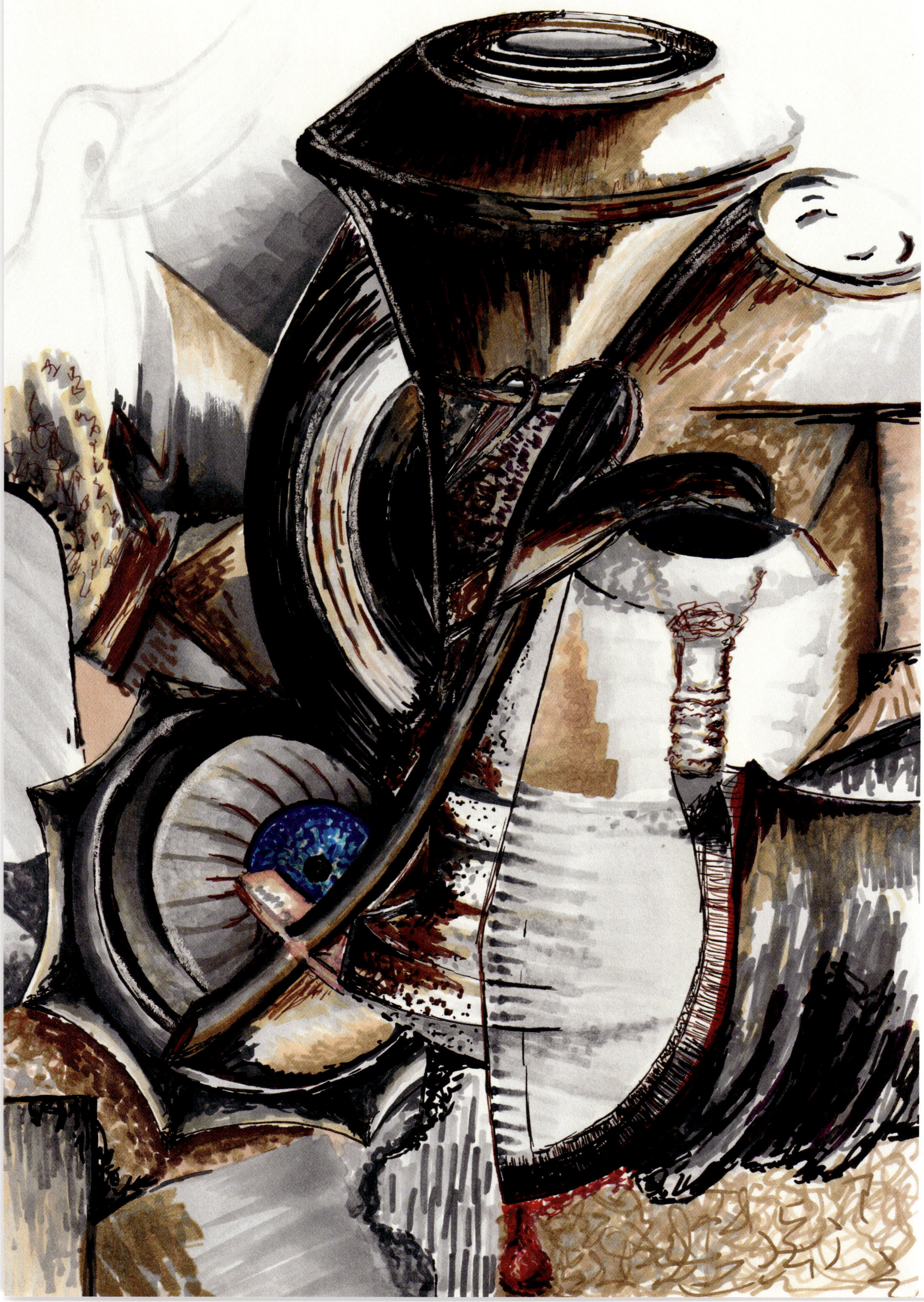

Evaluation

A great plan always begins with great questions. My mentor and friend Bryan Dodge taught me that if you want to change the outcome, you must ask the right questions. The questions we ask determine the conversation. The conversation reveals the wisdom. The wisdom informs the decisions. And all the decisions together ultimately determine the outcome. Therefore, if we want a great outcome, we must start with great questions.

What are the implant's esthetic needs? Ask patients about their hopes and expectations before looking at their teeth. This is your best chance at seeing it through their eyes. That way, you will get a much better feel for what it will take to make them happy. Find out what they want before planting ideas about what they should want or should be looking for. Don't dive into the gritty details of an esthetic assessment until you understand their preconceived desires and needs. Like an architect, we use our talent and skill to incorporate patient desires into a functional work of art. Patients need to be happy with the outcome. I think we need to be happy as well.

Work with what you have right in front of you.

Use patients' current teeth to lead them through an evaluation of their personal esthetic desires. Ask them open-ended questions. *Is there anything you would change about your smile right now? What changes would make you happier or more confident when you smile?* Starting with broad questions helps you understand their felt needs. These are what I think of as their personal esthetic desires. If they whip out their wedding picture, zoomed in on their bright, joyful smile, we can use that picture as a starting point to figure out what they like. We can guide them through the soft and hard tissue esthetics, evaluating the lip and smile line as well as the teeth and gingiva.

A picture is worth a thousand words and is a common language we share with our patients. It doesn't need to be fancy to be effective. Looking at a picture with patients is a point of reference that creates space to discuss what they see and what they want. We can then translate that into our language. If there is asymmetry in the gingival contours that show at high smile, point to it on the picture and ask if they would be happy with that as a final outcome.

◂
Figure 7-1 The Cubist movement has taught me a lot. Conceived by Pablo Picasso and Georges Braque, the artwork is a compilation of different angles and perspectives of a subject. You literally view the subject from different positions and add what you see to the canvas. Maybe this is how we should approach evaluation and learning. How helpful it is to see different perspectives. But it can get confusing. (Artwork inspired by Pablo Picasso.)

- Taking the picture. Don't let taking the photo get in the way. Make it easy. Find or develop a system that works for you, your team and your patients.
- Viewing the picture. Consider how you view the picture with your patients. This will certainly impact what they see and what they look for. Displaying a huge picture zoomed in on their teeth could show how detailed you are, impressing them. It could also make them think they too should be looking that closely at all the details. Sometimes, looking together at the picture on the viewfinder is more realistic and helpful.
- Documenting the picture. Include the picture in the chart and at least a brief overview of the conversation you had while looking at the picture. It can remind you and your patient what was discussed and the expectations. We all know expectations can change with time, so it is good to document the starting point.

Set realistic expectations according to the esthetic challenges. After we understand what they see and want, we can start to discuss what we see. This includes what we see in their current state, as well as what we want to see and expect to see in the final outcome. If there is a particular aspect I know will be challenging, I like to show that to patients and explain it. This gives them ownership of the problem and the process, and it gives me space to succeed. For example, when I am removing a failing central incisor implant with a big soft and hard tissue defect, I want patients to know how the tissue got to this state and how difficult it can be to restore it. I want them to know what we will be asking of their body, their own cells. We need the body to grow more bone and soft tissue than it currently has or thinks it needs. I personally am not growing the bone. I am merely setting the stage, to the best of my ability, for them to grow the bone. If the patient sees and understands growing bone and soft tissue is a big challenge for their cells in this situation, they will be more likely to accept a plan that includes multiple grafting procedures. It also creates space for them to be happy with an outcome that may not be perfect in their eyes. Either way, patients are more involved in the decision. They can see what they have to start with and what it may take to achieve different outcomes. They need to know the challenges so they can have realistic expectations. That way we all can win.

What are the functional needs of this implant? Picture it in use. Envision the motion and function of biting and chewing while examining the radiograph and oral cavity. How will this implant be used? What is the load moment? What does the rest of the occlusion look like? Is this going to bear a majority of the functional occlusal load? A second molar implant in a bruxer needs to accommodate significant vertical forces, whereas a maxillary incisor implant bears an almost entirely off-axis load. This can dramatically increase stress to the surrounding bone[1]. An implant retaining an overdenture ideally sustains only retentive forces, but with time and recession, it may sustain significant vertical and lateral forces if the denture is not relined. Keep the functional load in mind throughout the process and think beyond today. The anatomy and load will change as the patient ages. Think about the functional needs both now and later.

Inventory of resources

What resources are available?

Taking a systematic inventory of resources is critical to establishing realistic expectations. There may not be enough available to give them the result they want. A discrepancy between expectations and resources is an opportunity to adjust and set realistic expectations. If the resources available don't match expectations, diligently work to reset or recalibrate expectations. We all need to share the same expectations for success to be possible.

Bone volume and space

Implant success relies on the health of the surrounding bone. How much is enough? There needs to be enough bone to support both mechanical needs and biologic needs. The biologic needs depend on enough bone cells and blood supply to keep the bone alive and well under the load. For there to be enough bone, there first needs to be enough space for the bone around the implant[2]. Studies show that, on average, about 1.5 mm of bone around an implant is adequate to maintain long-term stability. Adjacent implants do well with about 1.5 mm each, or 3 mm total between them. These are statistical averages, not laws. Some patients have successful implants with much less bone volume. Failure is not guaranteed if these margins of safety are violated, but we want to stack the deck in favor of success.

In addition to adequate mesial-distal space for bone, there must also be adequate bucco-lingual and apico-coronal bone for the planned implant. General minimum dimensions are 1.5 to 2 mm buccolingually and 1 mm apically. Buccal bone is the most valuable for esthetics and the most frangible. The overall treatment plan is greatly simplified when there is adequate bone available. Most digital implant planning programs build these dimensions into the system. There is a natural rhythm guiding the safe distances we use to plan implant cases.

When there is inadequate bone volume for an implant, vertical or horizontal bone augmentation may be necessary. This is often necessary because implants need more surrounding bone than the teeth they are replacing. The periodontal ligament around a tooth provides collateral blood supply to the bone that is absent around implants. The blood supply to the bone around an implant comes only from the overlying periosteum and the adjacent medullary bone. Paper-thin facial or interdental bone may be stable for a tooth, but it is not predictably stable for an implant. The periodontal ligament also provides a mechanical advantage to the surrounding bone by absorbing some of the load. This reduces the load on the bone, protecting it from microfracture.

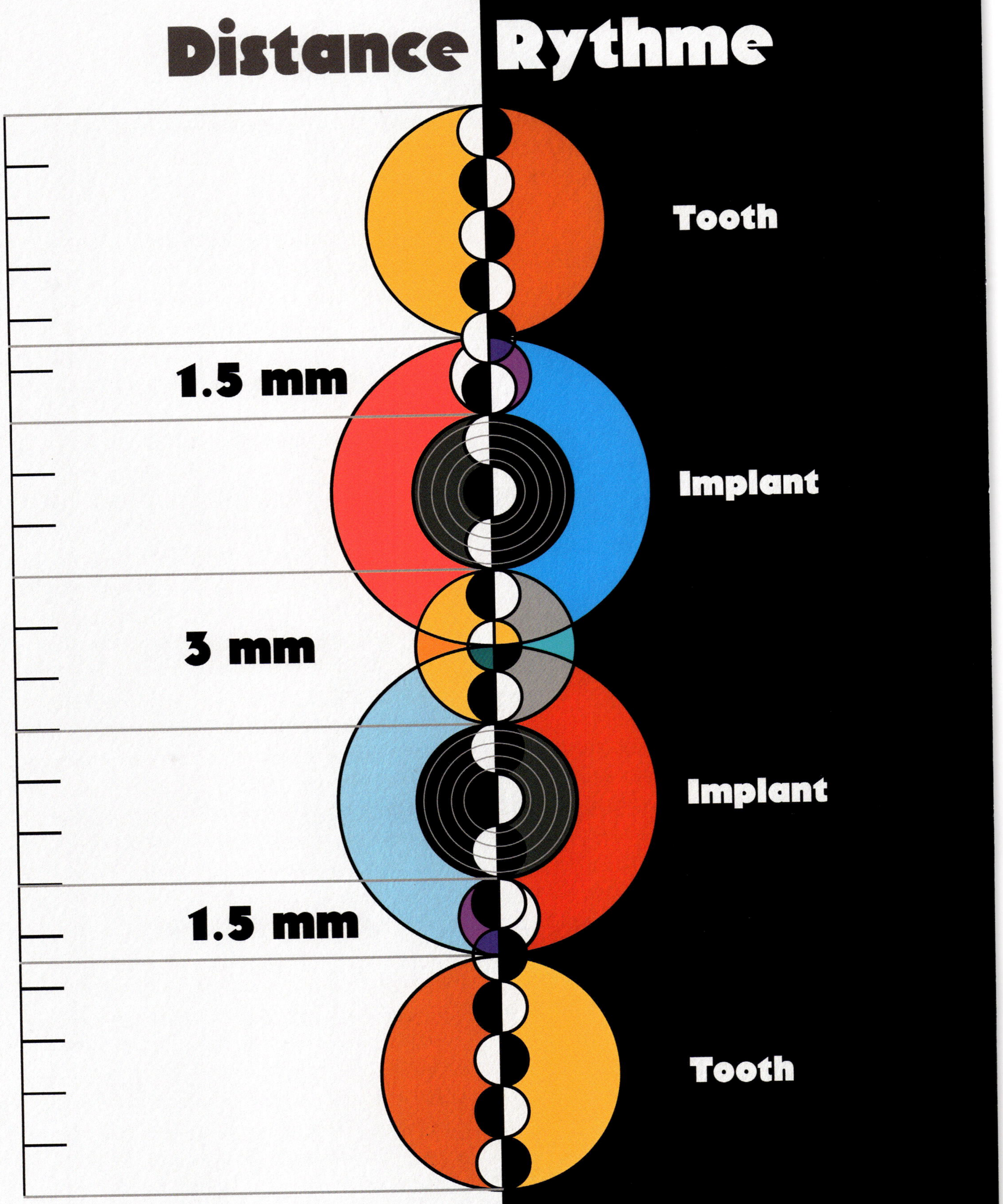

Figure 7-2 Minimum spacing between implants and teeth.
(Artwork inspired by Sonia Delaunay's Rythme series.)

Bone quality

An implant's durability also depends on the quality of the surrounding bone. This is the foundation upon which everything else is built. It is true there needs to be enough bone. But the bone also needs to be good enough for initial and sustained integration of the implant.

How do we know if the bone is good enough? Quality is more difficult to determine than quantity. Overall, quality is a gestalt of multiple desirable distinct qualities. The bone qualities that optimize implant success include density, cortical anatomy and blood supply. These qualities comprise the foundation upon which we base the architecture of implantology. They each impact aspects of the plan and surgery. A competent implant architect adapts the overall design according to the resources of the site.

Bone density

Adequate bone density is important[3], but density is not just a checkbox that is either adequate or inadequate. The density also varies within each site. This should be factored in when planning the implant's length and diameter. It also impacts surgical drilling and placement.

Every implant site has areas of bone with higher and lower density. Where the bone is denser, the implant may have increased stability. Plan the implant accordingly. Optimize the engagement of the dense bone. For example, in a recent extraction site or immediate implant site, the implant may need to be longer in order to engage the denser bone of the socket walls. In the posterior maxilla, where there is often very limited density, it may be beneficial to place a longer implant to engage the maxillary sinus floor by performing a minor sinus augmentation. In contrast, in cases of extremely dense mandibular bone, a long implant may introduce challenges that a slightly shorter implant may avoid. Longer implants in less vascular dense bone can suffer more from over-heating, over-torquing and over-compressing the limits of the bone.

In my mind, I make a mental image of the bone density in a site. I loosely refer to this as "density mapping." It can quickly and easily be done while evaluating the CBCT image. Just pay attention to where the bone appears most dense, then decide if you want to engage that area. Envision how the denser bone will push the drill and implant during surgery. A dense wall of bone can walk an implant laterally off course, sometimes right out of the alveolar bone. This density mapping isn't a formal diagnostic tool, but it provides tremendous insight into how to optimize the plan and procedure.

Density also has a huge impact on technical aspects of the surgery. For instance, in low-density bone you may make a smaller hole so the implant can engage more bone. This increases the initial stability of the implant. More elaborate techniques, such as osseodensification, further increase density by creating a controlled expanding and compacting force during drilling, pushing the bone outward rather than simply removing it. Every self-tapping implant inherently uses a form of osseodensification as the threads and implant body compress the surrounding bone upon insertion. This is how it achieves its primary stability. But the true osseodensification protocol does much more to preserve and control the density of the surrounding bone. This is a tool for controlling and adapting the implant site based on the available bone and its density.

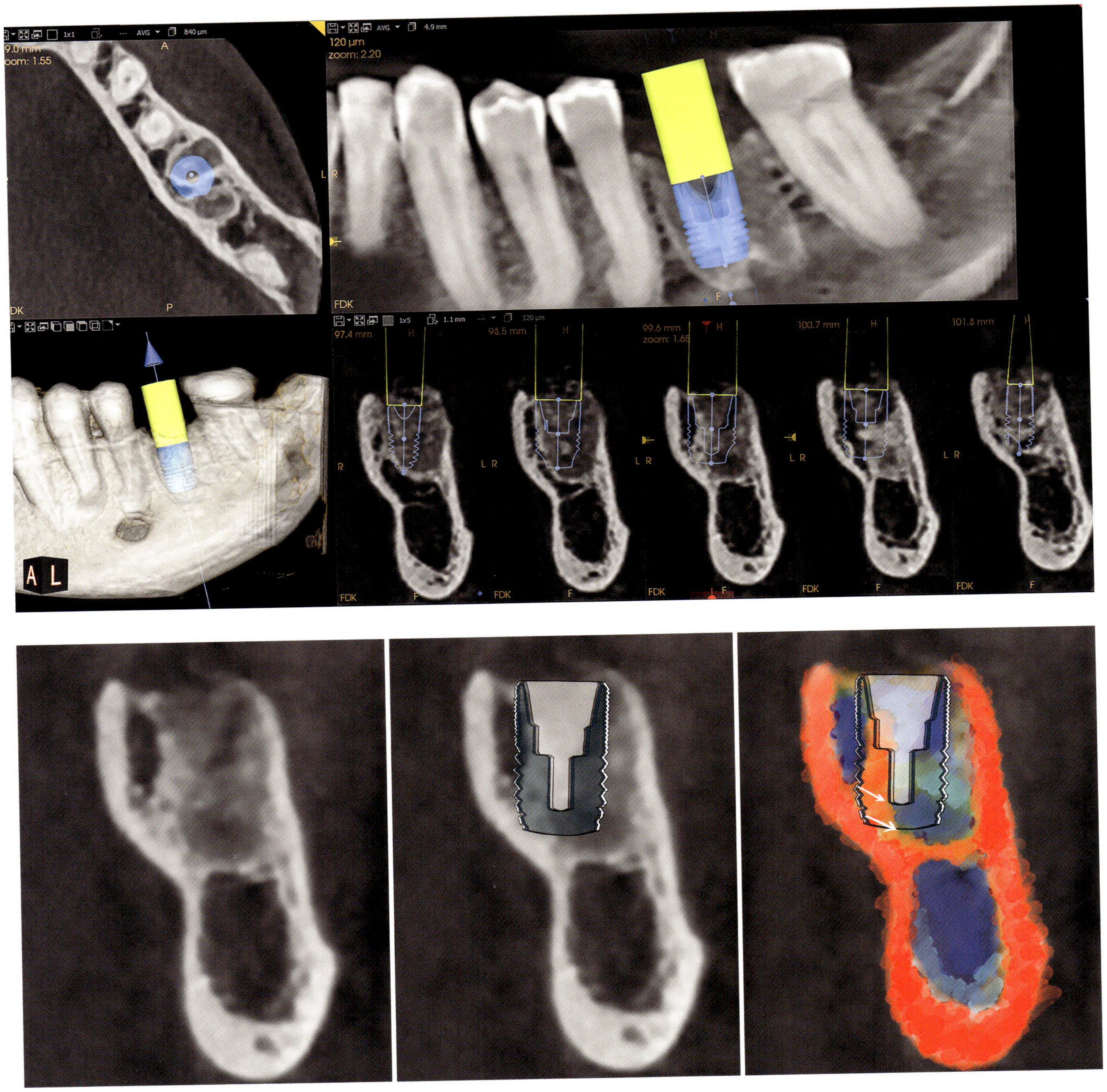

Figure 7-3 This implant will engage the dense lingual bone, pushing it lateral to the planned position. The variation in density visible on the radiograph can also be felt when drilling. Informally, I think of this as "density mapping." It is mental imagery of the bone density throughout the site and how that will impact surgery and integration. (The upper image shows the display I use during implant planning. The windows in this screen allow me to simultaneously visualize the implant and site in each of the three dimensions as well as in a three-dimensional reconstruction.)

In the case of high bone density, achieving initial stability is not the challenge. It can be all too easy to achieve very high torque, which can generate devastating heat and internal pressure leading to bone necrosis and painful implant failure. Dense bone drilling protocols can mitigate this risk by increasing irrigation, decreasing drilling speed (rpm, more drills, pausing), widening the osteotomy and creating thread space (tapping). Ultimately, these protocols safely create a larger osteotomy, decreasing the friction and pressure of the threads and implant body on the surrounding bone during insertion.

Increasing irrigation serves a few functions. It helps clear the dense bone collecting in the flutes of the drill, thus optimizing cutting efficiency. The flow of cool water absorbs the heat being generated. It also acts as a lubricant, decreasing the friction between the bone and the rotating drill[4].

Decreasing drilling speed can be done by slowing down the drill's revolutions per minute, using more drills to incrementally increase the osteotomy, and by advancing the drill more slowly. Reducing the rpm of the drill decreases the heat generated by drill friction on the adjacent dense bone. Drill kits for various implant systems often have optional dense bone drills that are otherwise unnecessary in normal bone, but are hugely valuable in very dense bone. For example, seven incremental drills may be used instead of four to achieve the same final osteotomy size. Advancing the drill slower through the dense bone decreases heat from the friction and effectively increases the irrigation's cooling capacity. Pumping the drill by backing it out slightly while advancing it flushes the flutes and allows the heat to dissipate more effectively.

Tapping creates a thread pattern within the bone, decreasing resistance and insertion pressure. It clears out a path that matches the implant's threads. They still engage the same amount of bone surface area, they just don't cut or compress the bone as much themselves upon insertion. The surrounding dense bone responds better when it is not compressed or heated as much. Additionally, lower torque is kinder to the implant's delicate internal components and the implant delivery system.

Density is not simply good or bad. It is a factor. A consideration. An opportunity for success. Inadequate stability in low density bone can contribute to failure, while excessive heat and pressure in high density bone can also ruin a perfectly good implant.

Cortical anatomy

The crestal cortical bone is the key. This is where the force is greatest between the implant and bone. In fact, there is very little force acting in the middle and apical portions of an implant during function. There are several elaborate finite element analysis studies that have shown this over and over. They look something like Figure 7-4. And it makes good sense mechanically. The greatest force is transferred right at the junction. As such, we want to engage good crestal bone and we must protect it during placement[5].

We are always worried about crestal bone loss. That is where bone loss occurs. We don't generally see apical bone loss on implants over time. The functional and biological stress is focused right at the crest. Having good crestal cortical bone is desirable and favorable throughout the life of an implant.

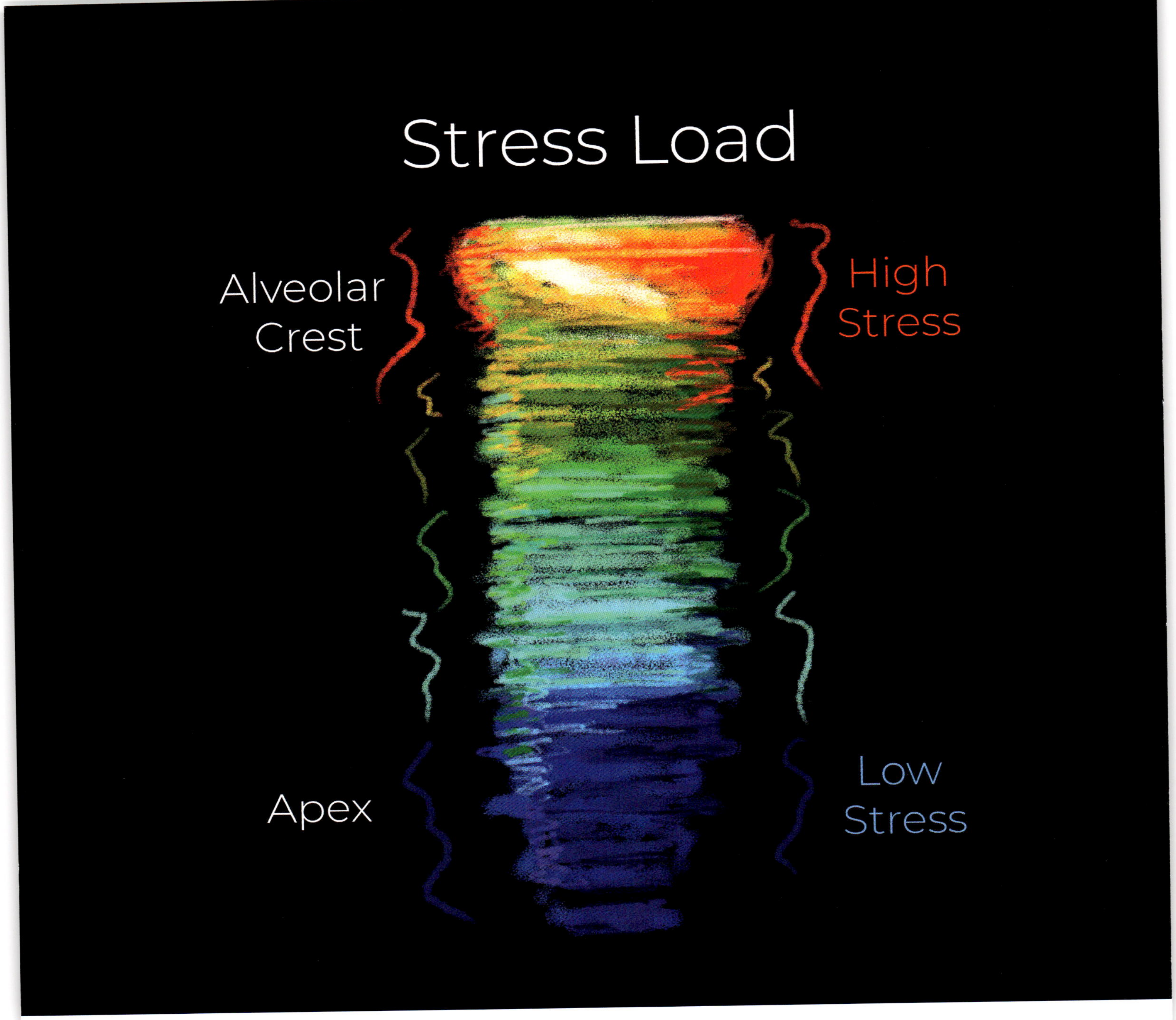

Figure 7-4 Finite element analysis reveals most of the implant's stress load is born at the crest. Progressively less stress is placed on the implant and surrounding bone toward the apex, with the majority of it right at the crest.

Blood supply

Bone receives blood supply internally through medullary perfusion and externally from the periosteum and the periodontal ligament. Healthy, robust periosteum supports the underlying bone, especially when it is protected during surgery. The periosteum becomes even more critical as bone density increases. There is much less internal blood supply in very dense bone. Envision how the bone around the implant will be nourished and perfused when planning an implant. We want to optimize each implant site by leveraging the benefit of stability from the densest bone with the perfusion of the less dense bone and the overlying periosteal blood supply.

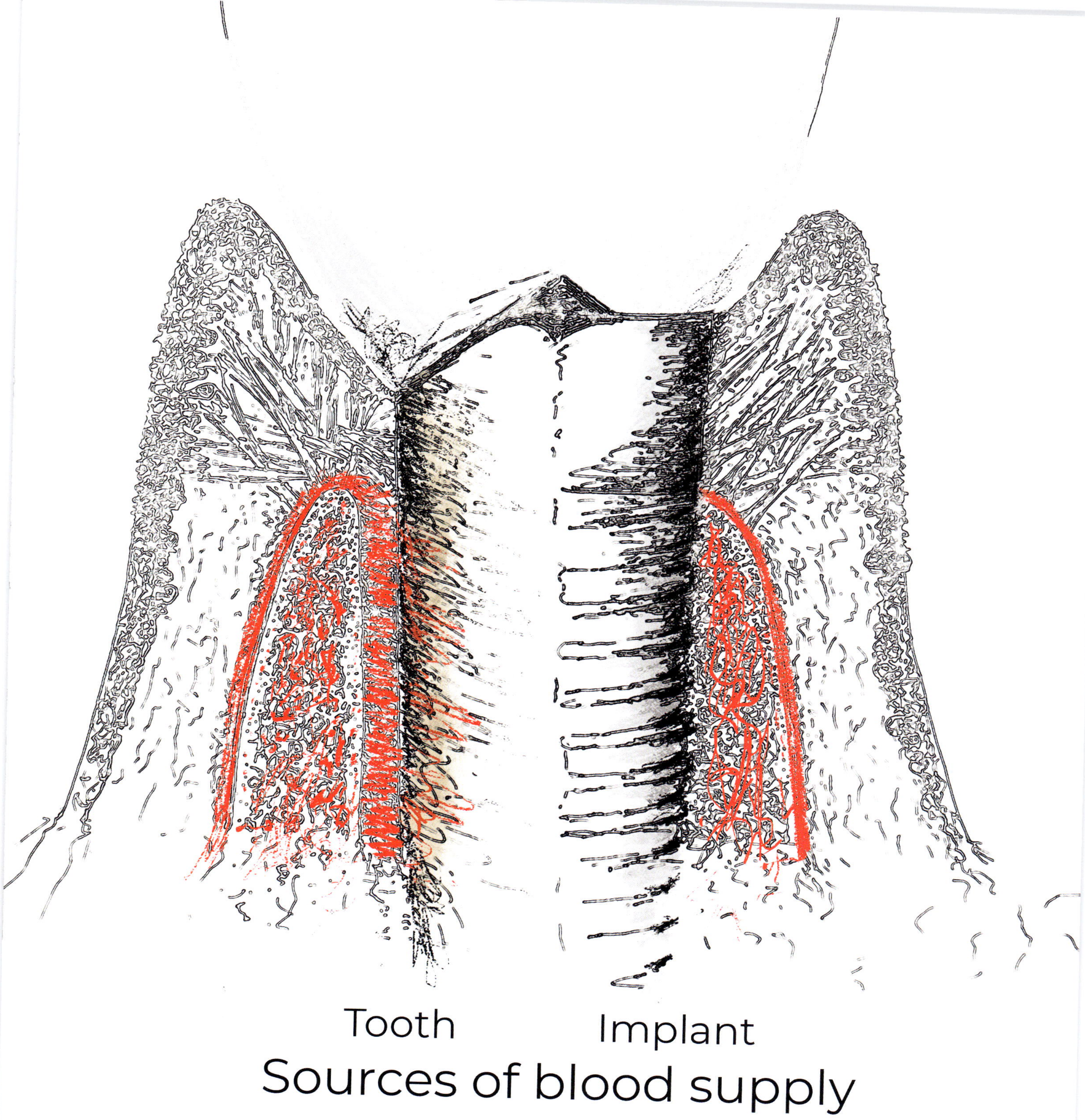

Figure 7-5 Bone surrounding a tooth receives blood supply from the periosteum, marrow, periodontal ligament and some collateral flow from the tooth. In contrast, the bone surrounding an implant only receives blood supply from the periosteum and the marrow space. To maintain adequate blood supply, the bone must be much more robust around implants.

Soft tissue quality

High quality soft tissue improves long term predictably and stability. It is one of the more important factors for success. While the controversy over the ultimate importance has yet to be fully resolved, it seems logical that optimizing keratinized gingiva is beneficial in implant dentistry[6]. As the first line of defense against mechanical and biological threats, the soft tissue around an implant takes tremendous abuse. The health of an implant is directly impacted by the health of the surrounding soft tissue. Evaluate the soft tissue as early in the process as you can. The radiographs only tell part of the story. It is wise to gather information early to avoid costly changes later.

If the tooth has not yet been removed, pay attention to tissue health: inflammation, recession, probing depths. These will all change when the tooth is removed, but it helps build the picture of what we have to work with. Diseased or compromised tissue may require more time to heal and may also benefit from additional grafting. It is also extremely valuable to pay attention to the adjacent tissue and overall periodontal health. A patient with severe generalized chronic periodontitis has a multitude of factors that are even more harmful for implants than teeth. If this complex disease process is not managed well, implants will likely fail.

Evaluating the soft tissue in an edentulous site is a bit more straightforward than a dentate site. The site has already shown how it will respond to initial extraction healing. Now, we can easily assess whether there is sufficient tissue to work with, or if we need to consider augmentation. It is still just as important to evaluate the adjacent teeth and mouth as a whole whether the tooth has been extracted or not.

The position of the implant must first be visualized to understand what we have to work with. Where it will emerge from the tissue provides key insight into how the tissue can be manipulated and optimized. There may be adequate volume of thick keratinized tissue, but it may need to be repositioned facially to effectively protect the implant. If there is inadequate tissue volume, grafting options can be incorporated into the overall plan and design.

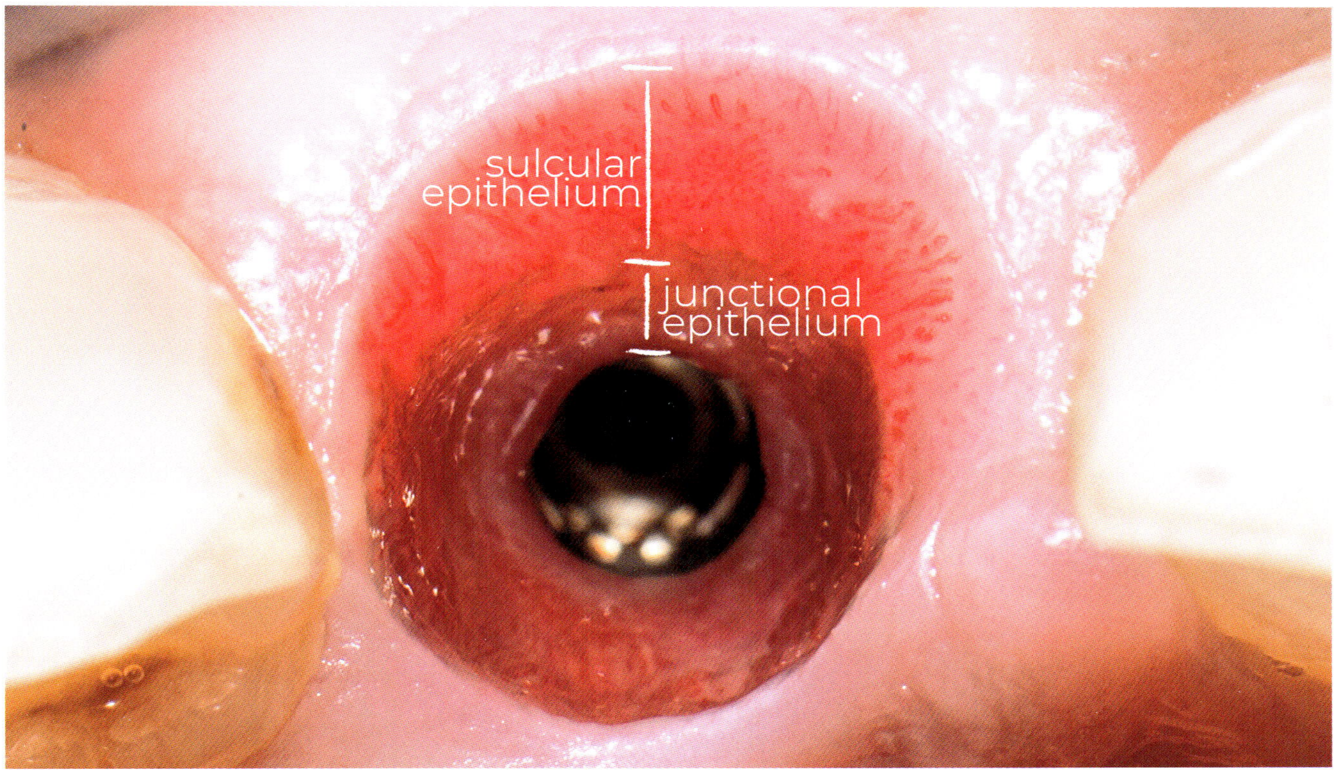

Figure 7-6 This is where it counts. We want healthy tissue surrounding the implant. This protects the underlying bone and implant. The microanatomy here shows the complexity of the sulcular and junctional epithelium.

Esthetic soft tissue evaluation

Soft tissue evaluation and management is such a broad, important topic that entire textbooks have been written on it alone. I simply cannot do it justice in this book. But there are a few things I would like to touch on related to this topic.

Develop a routine in your practice to evaluate and discuss esthetics with every implant evaluation. Routines promote consistency. Consistent evaluations will result in more consistent outcomes. We only see what we look for. We become better at seeing the soft tissue when we routinely look at it. As mentioned previously, our patient's expectations can surprise us. And their expectations are best addressed at the onset of treatment. Most patients don't care much about the soft tissue esthetics of an upper second molar implant, but some do. And they will care about your overall attention to detail. If they care, you better care. Either way, it makes you look a lot better when you care at least as much as they do about the results of your work.

The overall esthetic evaluation can go well beyond just the soft tissue[7]. It can include facial contours, smile line height and shape, tooth shape and inclination, and buccal corridor. And the upper lip! There is an entire industry built on upper lip esthetics and rejuvenation. There are certainly extreme expectations at times, but a simple and focused evaluation can set the stage for success in most cases. The lips are hugely dependent on the underlying dental and alveolar structure. How you proceed with this evaluation will depend on the goals and expectations of both you and your patient.

Have you noticed most famous old portraits don't have a smiling subject? Think about it; the great masters never really painted a portrait with a full smile. In classical art, it may not even be considered a portrait if there is a smile. Everything about the face changes with a smile, eyes and all. Can you imagine trying to sit for a portrait while holding a sincere smile for hours on end? A smirk, maybe. (What was she smirking about anyway?) But not a genuine smile. In the past, people didn't want to be remembered smiling. Smiling, especially showing teeth, was long regarded as beneath the aristocracy class. It was unfashionable, even vulgar. And so, the masters never painted a smiling portrait.

In our culture, smiles have become part of everyone's identity. It represents who people are (at least online). Much of dentistry exists in its present form because of the rising popularity of the smile. Nowadays, smiling is the cool thing to do. Everyone is doing it. People come to us desperately wanting to restore or improve their smile. It is their first impression out there in the world. As dentists, we get to meet people in that vulnerable space. So much is on the line when a smile is failing. Confidence. Self-esteem. Social acceptance. Patients feel psychological and emotional stress when they have a defective smile, especially if they are missing one or more front teeth. They feel anxious. Exposed. Ashamed. That is where we come in with our expertise to solve the problem and our creative energy to make something beautiful.

In visual art, the point where the brightest bright meets the darkest dark is the area of greatest interest. The eye is drawn immediately to that point. It is the focus of attention. This is one reason we are so captivated by a smile. The reflection of light from the pearly white enamel falls off the incisal edge below. And above, it meets the soft shadow and depth of the lip or gingiva. This is where our eyes naturally go. We are allured by this contrast of light and dark.

When the drape of the upper lip conceals the underlying gingiva, the gingival contours and esthetics are almost irrelevant. But when an elevated lip reveals the gingiva, everything about it matters. The dynamic of a patient's lip is constantly changing. The movement is far more pronounced with an unposed smile or laugh. That's where it counts. Many people don't show any gingiva, even with the most genuine high smile. But many do. And when they do, everyone sees it. We refer to this as smile type and gingival display. When the tissue shows at high smile, a few simple tools can help guide evaluation and treatment, whether you choose to manage the case or refer it out.

Esthetic evaluation tools

The "Pink Esthetic Score" and "Esthetic Risk Analysis" are two practical systems to evaluate and address soft tissue esthetics[8]. We can use tools like the pink esthetic score to quantify and systematically evaluate tissue. We also can use this concept to build a mental framework in our minds of what the tissue looks like. Consistently using a system like this trains our eyes what to look for and our brains what to evaluate, even if we don't employ the actual system in our charting.

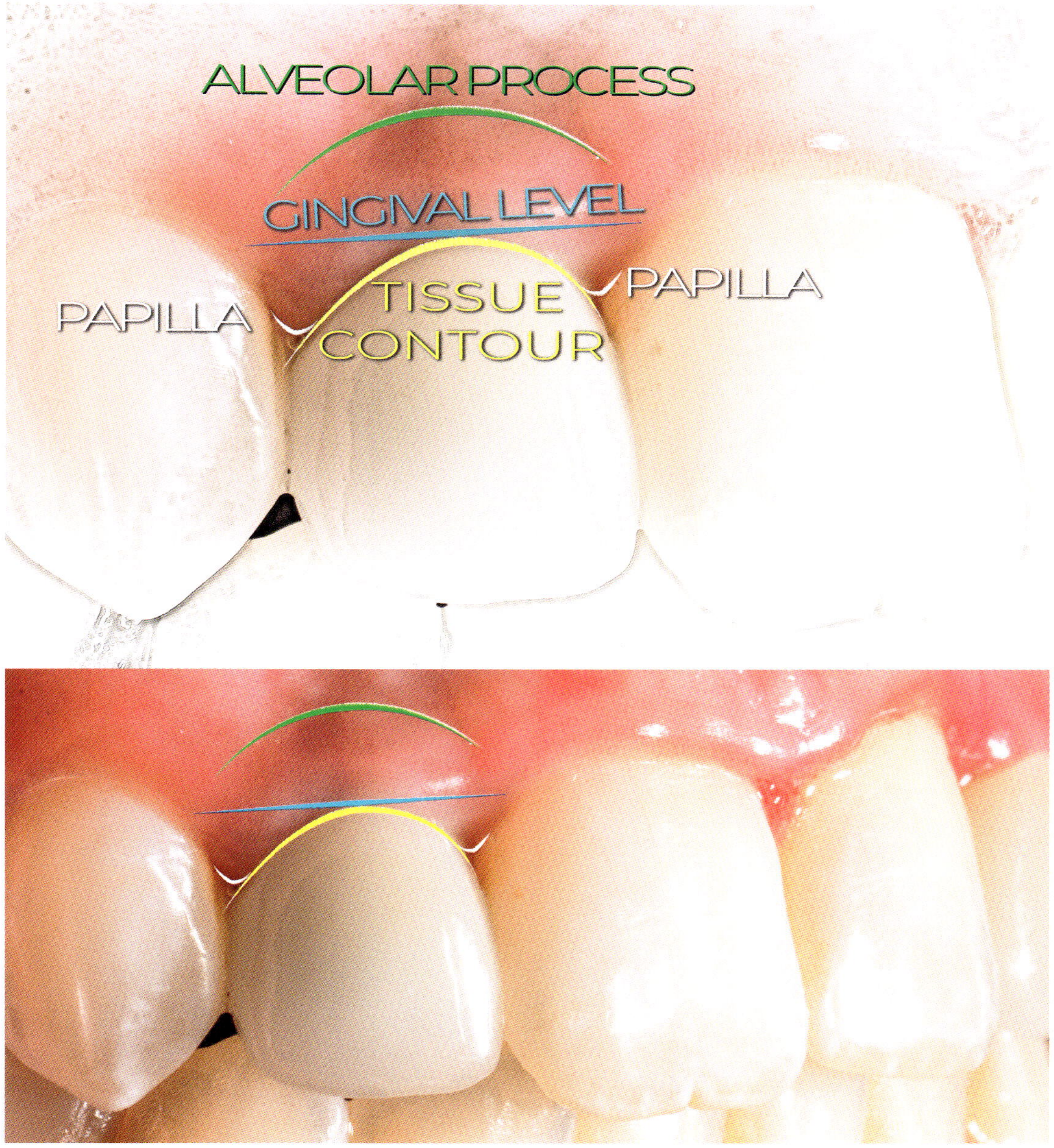

Figure 7-7 An evaluation of the mesial and distal papilla, gingival level, contour of the alveolar process, and tissue contour provides a good framework for esthetic evaluation.

Gingival contour

This is influenced by the fine-tuned positioning of an implant. An implant positioned to favor the height of contour or gingival zenith will make the crown and soft tissue look better.

Papilla

We want harmony and symmetry. Long, slender papillae are difficult to reproduce. The papilla height has been shown to correlate to underlying bone height[9]. And the papilla fills in overtime after an implant is restored. We need to be patient when evaluating the final papilla. And we need to counsel our patients likewise. Wait several months before finalizing a verdict on how the papilla will respond. Sometimes it is surprising.

Figure 7-8 Consider the desired gingival zenith when planning the implant position. The height of contour naturally forms along the midline of the implant. If this is slightly distal, consider placing the implant slightly distal, as long as there is adequate space. Implant position is not the only factor here, but it is one we can control when planning an implant.

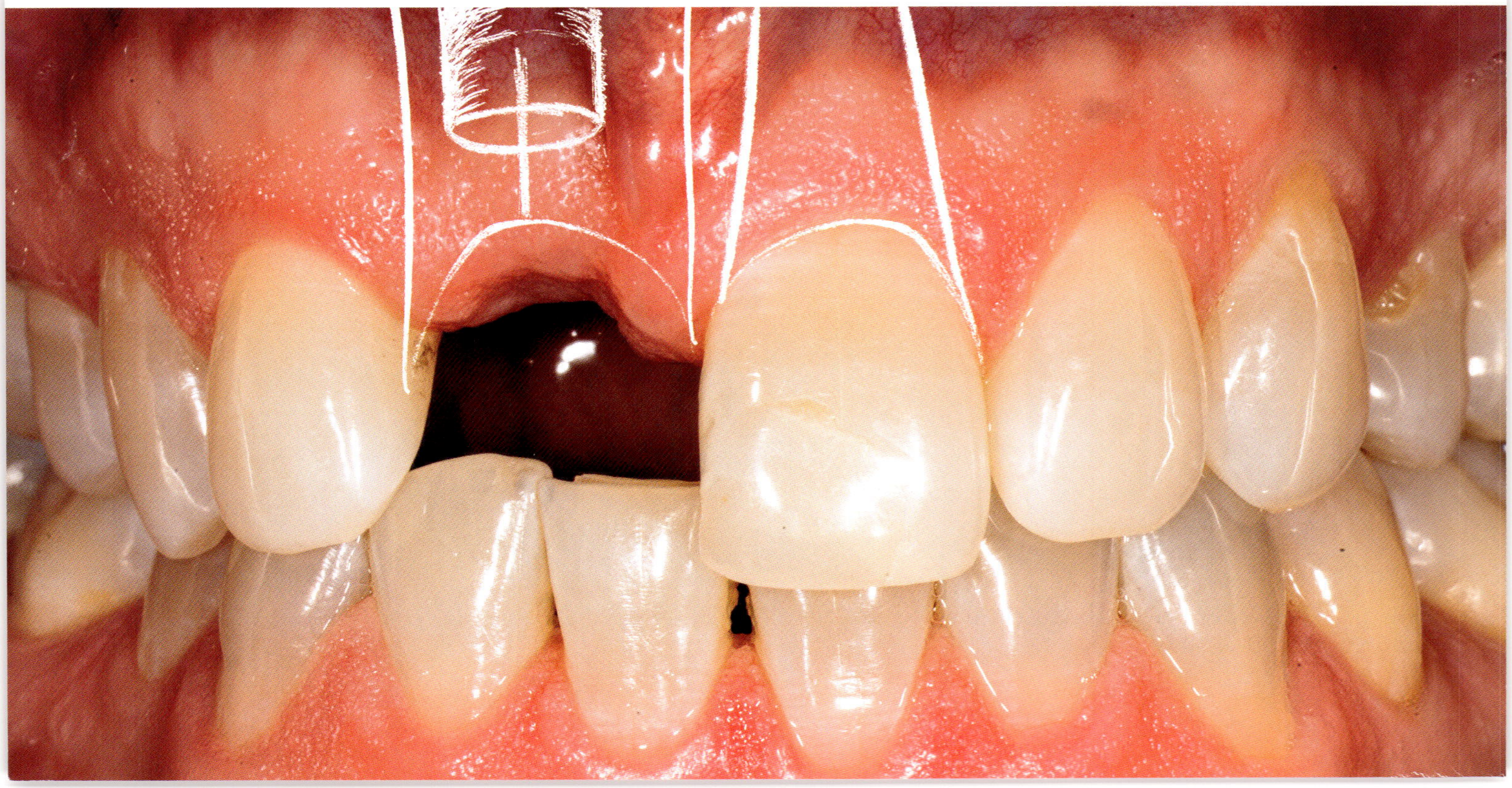

Gingival health

Gingival health is important for both esthetics and longevity. The shape and position of the tissue will change when it transitions between disease and health. Evaluating inflamed tissue gives an inaccurate baseline. The crown length can be impacted by gingivitis and periodontitis. In cases of periodontitis or recession, the tissue can undergo dramatic changes in shape and form at different stages of the process. Gingival health is also a function of the long-term predictability and anticipated tissue change over time[8]. Be aware of the impacts tissue health has on the implant.

Esthetic Risk Assessment

The Esthetic Risk Assessment (ERA) is a simple and elegant tool you can use to assess an esthetic case's overall risk and complexity[10]. It uses simple metrics to classify a case as low, moderate or high esthetic risk. Depending on your skill and confidence, you can use this to decide whether to begin treatment or recruit help from other specialists. These same metrics can also guide the smile design process.

The patient and the implant are the two most basic components of implant architecture. The principles of durability, utility and beauty apply to evaluation as well as implant design.

Figure 7-9 As a surgeon, I seldom use a scaler. But if there is significant calculus adjacent to my implant, I like to take a few seconds to scrape it off. It would be ideal to do this a few weeks before surgery to allow the tissue to respond with some healing.

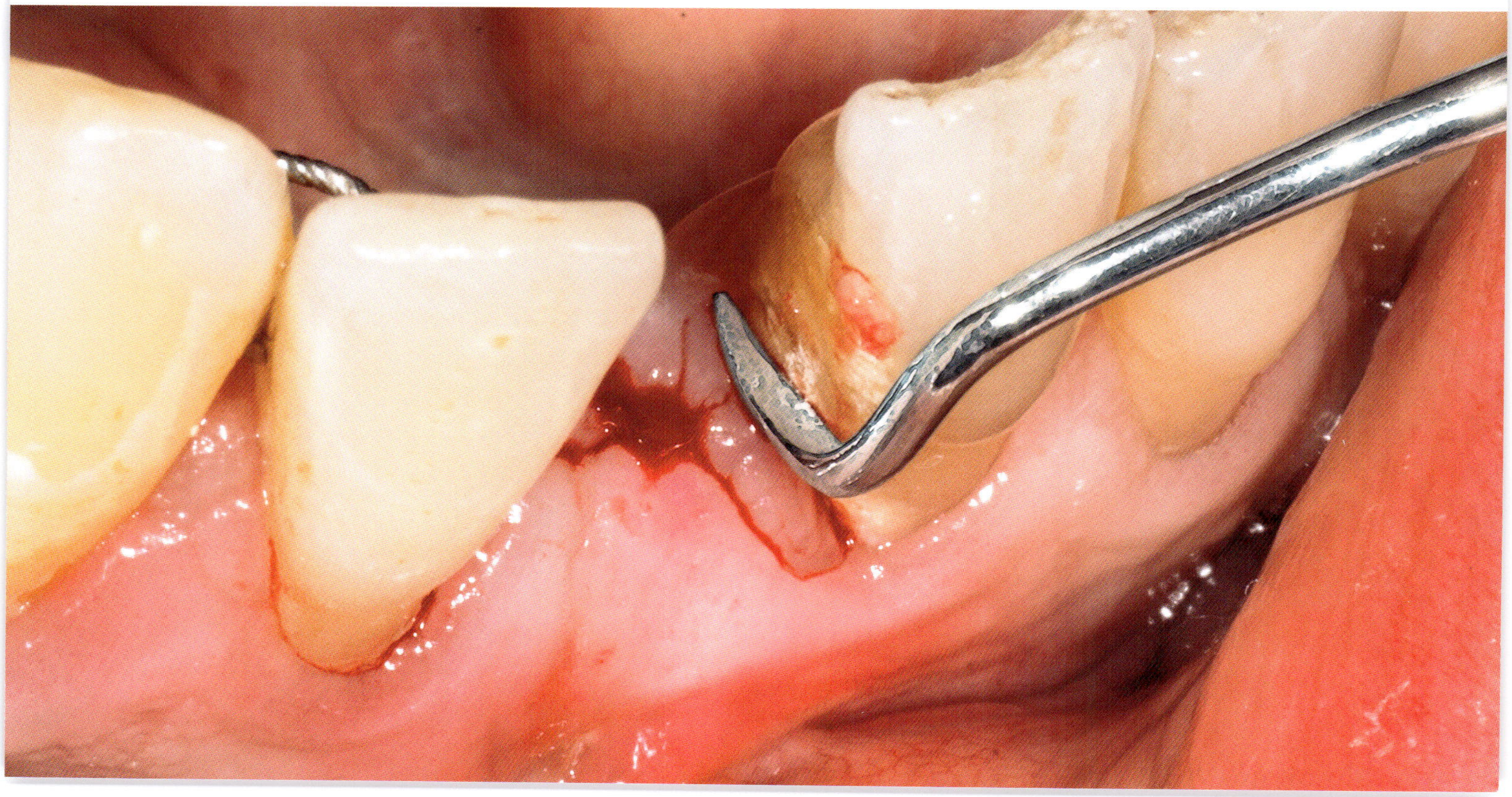

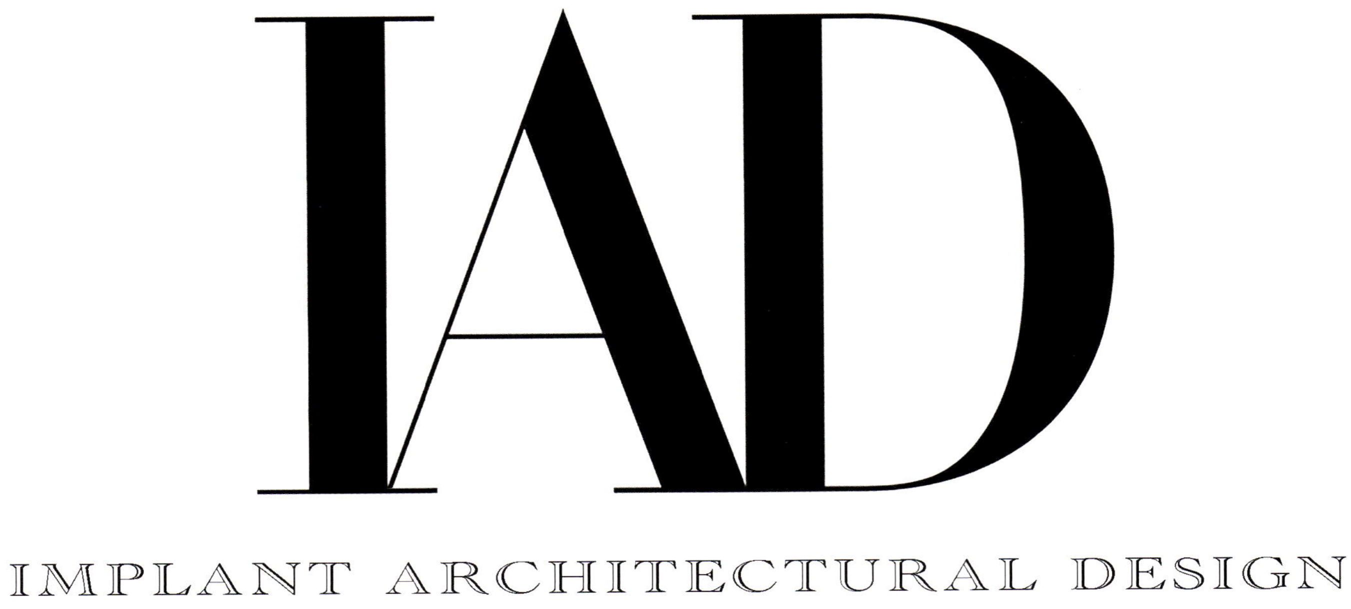

Figure 7-10 Designing the world's best implants. (Artwork inspired by Architectural Digest.)

Implant Design

The best implant is not a product you can buy. Nor can your patients buy it. As surgeons, we can set our patients up for success, but they alone bring healing to the equation. We just try to set them up for success as well as we possibly can.

The Goal: Stability

Implant stability is the most important factor for integration. The word stability can be described as being firm, solid or immovable. If an implant is not stable, the bone around it won't heal properly and integrate with the implant. If an implant is stable and integrated and it becomes unstable over time, it is said to have lost its integration and the implant fails. An implant must remain stable for the bone surrounding it to accept it and incorporate it into its daily function.

The life of a dental implant has two main phases: the early healing phase (surgery and actively integrating) and long-term maintenance phase (functional and maintaining integration). It needs to integrate and then maintain integration. The initial phase includes surgical treatment (site preparation, development and insertion) and healing (process of integrating). The second phase is the implant's functional life. It is the state of being integrated and maintaining integration.

There is a window of vulnerability in implant healing when the primary stability decreases and the secondary stability has not yet increased significantly. During this time, the risk of exceeding the micromovement threshold is elevated. Too much movement now and the implant will not integrate. We want to decrease the risk during this time. Soft diet and good hygiene are helpful, but the technological improvements in implant systems seem to be shortening this window and increasing the margin of safety. The less time our patients spend in this critical time between primary and secondary stability, the less likely they are to stimulate fibroblasts instead of osteoblasts.

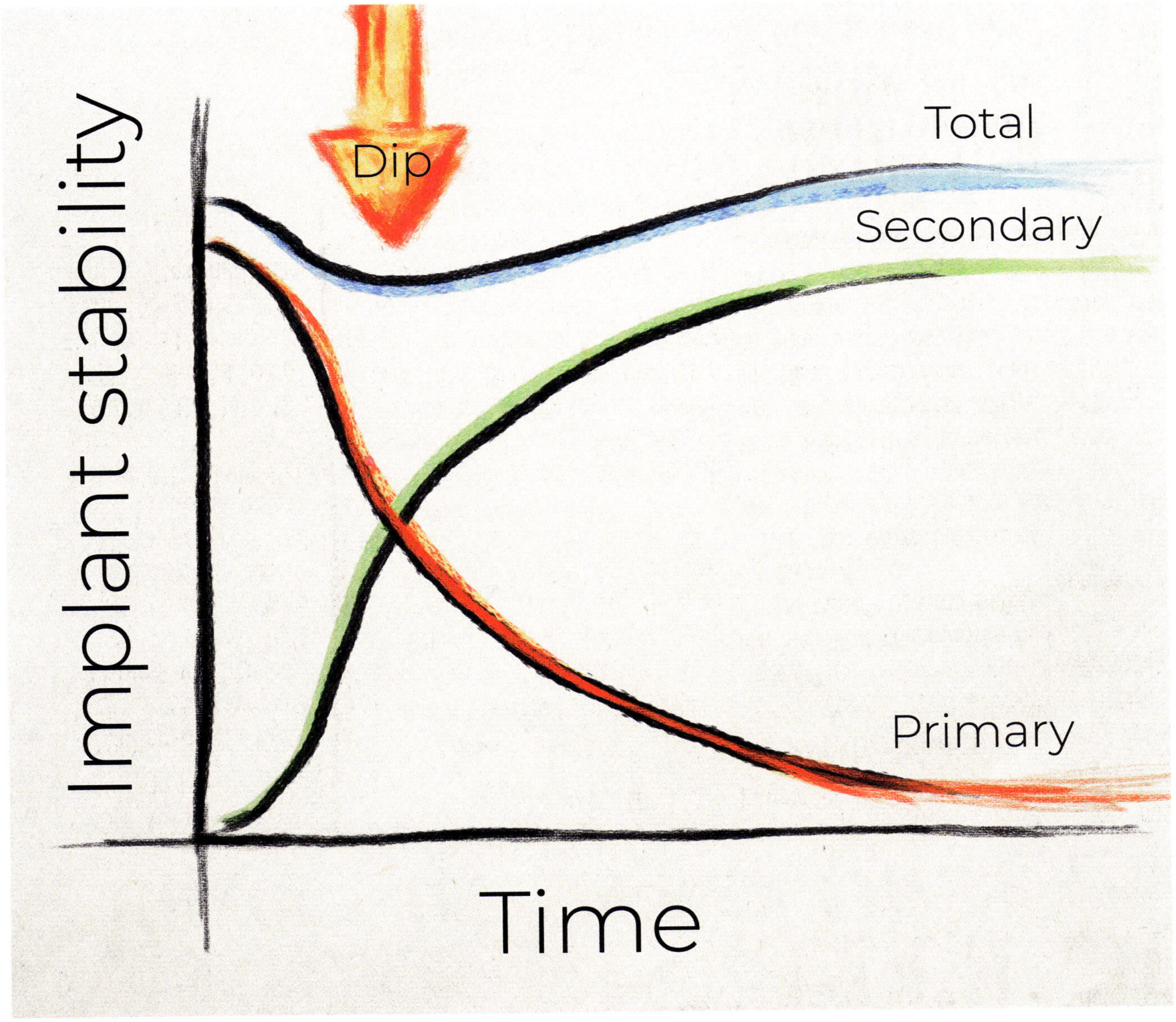

Figure 7-11 Time of greatest risk of implant failure. The mechanical stability (*red*) is decreasing, and the biological stability (*green*) is not high yet. This results in a temporary dip in the total stability (*blue*) of the implant.

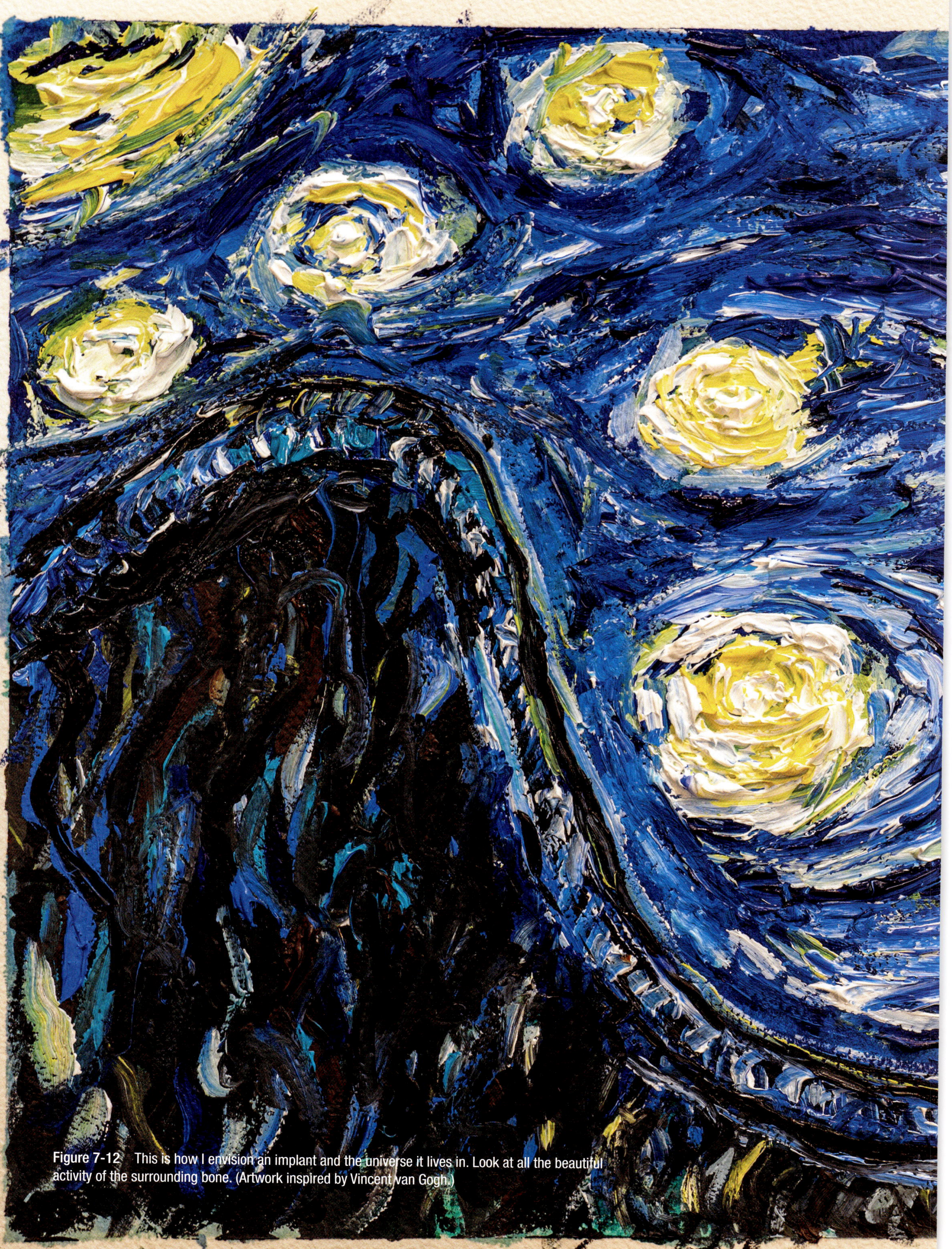

Figure 7-12 This is how I envision an implant and the universe it lives in. Look at all the beautiful activity of the surrounding bone. (Artwork inspired by Vincent van Gogh.)

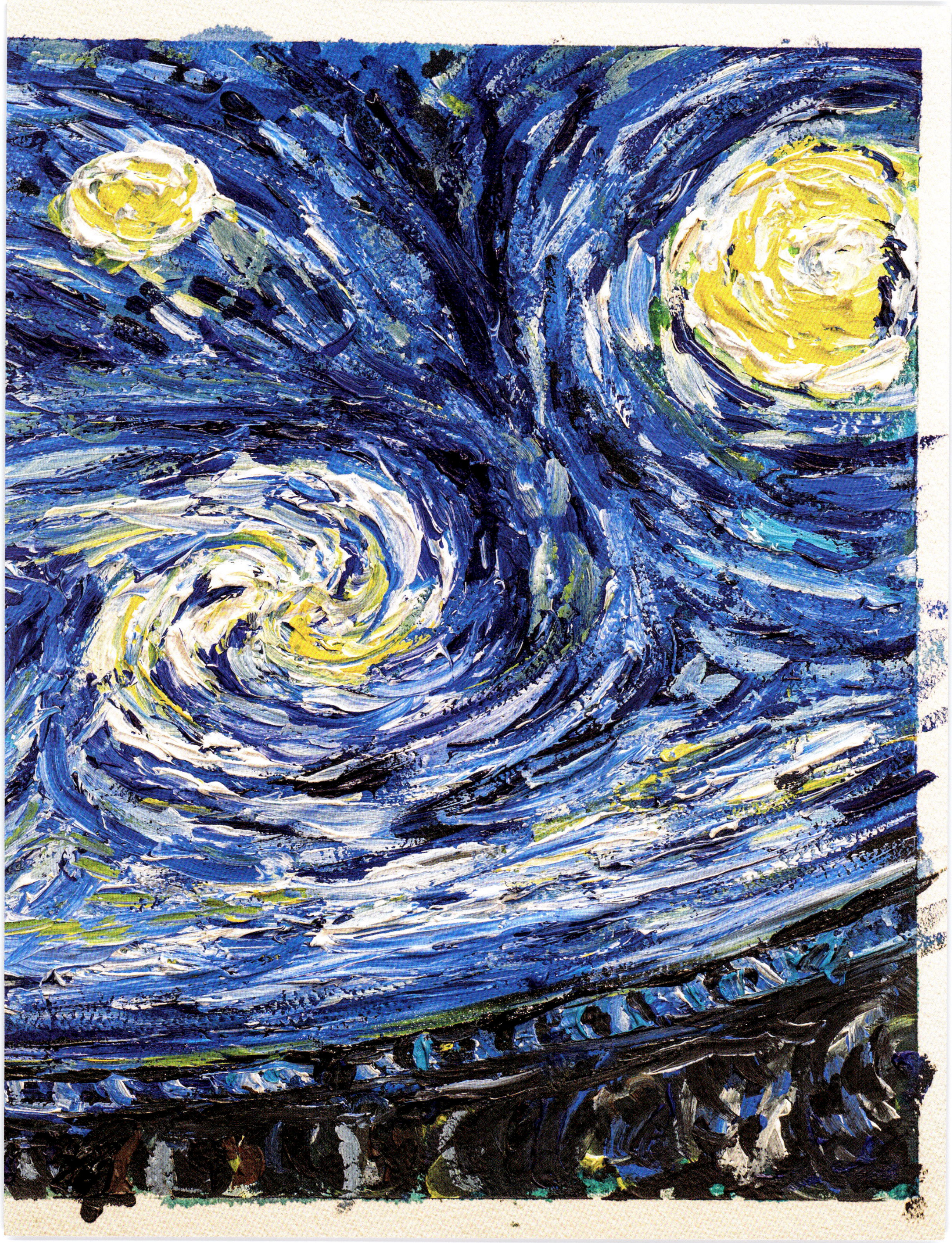

Osseointegration is the key. It is the foundation for a healthy implant. Without integration, an implant fails. There are other factors that can lead to implant failure (soft tissue health, restorative function, esthetics). But the most important piece of the equation is osseointegration.

Integration is the process or status of being made whole. This is the goal of implant dentistry, to restore and maintain the optimal overall health of the patients who are entrusted to our care. To make them whole. It is pretty much like an extraction reversal. We want to undo tooth loss.

As the industry continually improves and changes, there are countless products and systems that all claim to have an edge on success. This can get a bit confusing. My hope is to explore some basic elements of a dental implant and how they can be leveraged for success. In full disclosure, some of this information will be limited by what's available as I am sitting here writing this. Thankfully, this field continues to evolve and improve.

Several methods of testing stability have been described and studied with more continuing to emerge. The most basic and rudimentary methods include insertion torque, percussion testing, and the surgeon's perception. These are important and helpful, but they are limited in how well they predict the ultimate success of an implant[11]. More advanced testing methods have been developed that improve the accuracy and predictive value for success.

The more common advanced techniques for implant stability testing are simply based on one thing: motion. More specifically, the microscopic movement of an implant within the bone under a specific load. This information provides insight into the surrounding bone architecture as well as the interface between the implant surface and the bone. If the bone is very dense around an implant and is holding it very tightly, it moves very little under a load. It is stable. If the bone is not very dense or the surrounding bone has a loose grip on the implant, it moves a little more. It is less stable. The movement we are talking about is so tiny it can't be seen. But it can be heard. And it can be measured. Think about a guitar string. As it tightens, the string vibrates faster with a shorter distance between waves. We hear the pitch go up. Pitch is measured in hertz or frequency: the number of vibrations per second. The shorter the wavelength when it is plucked, the higher the frequency. Now, let's apply that principle to implant stability.

The less an implant moves, the more stable it is. If we could "pluck" an implant like a guitar string and measure its vibration, we would have insight into how much it moves within the bone. The advanced techniques testing implant stability are basically different ways to "pluck" the implant and measure the pitch. It is like we are making a form of music in implant surgery.

A simple tap on an abutment with the back of a mirror handle can give a sense of implant stability. A stable implant has been described as having a high pitch ring or a clear "crystal" sound. It doesn't move much at all. It resonates with a high pitch. An unstable implant will move more when percussed. This absorbs more of the force and produces a dull or low pitch sound.

The most widely used and well-studied advanced stability test uses the Resonance Frequency Analysis (RFA) method. Osstell™ combines magnetic and electronic technology to measure the vibration of an implant. A small aluminum peg (SmartPeg™) with a magnetic tip is screwed into the implant. The tip

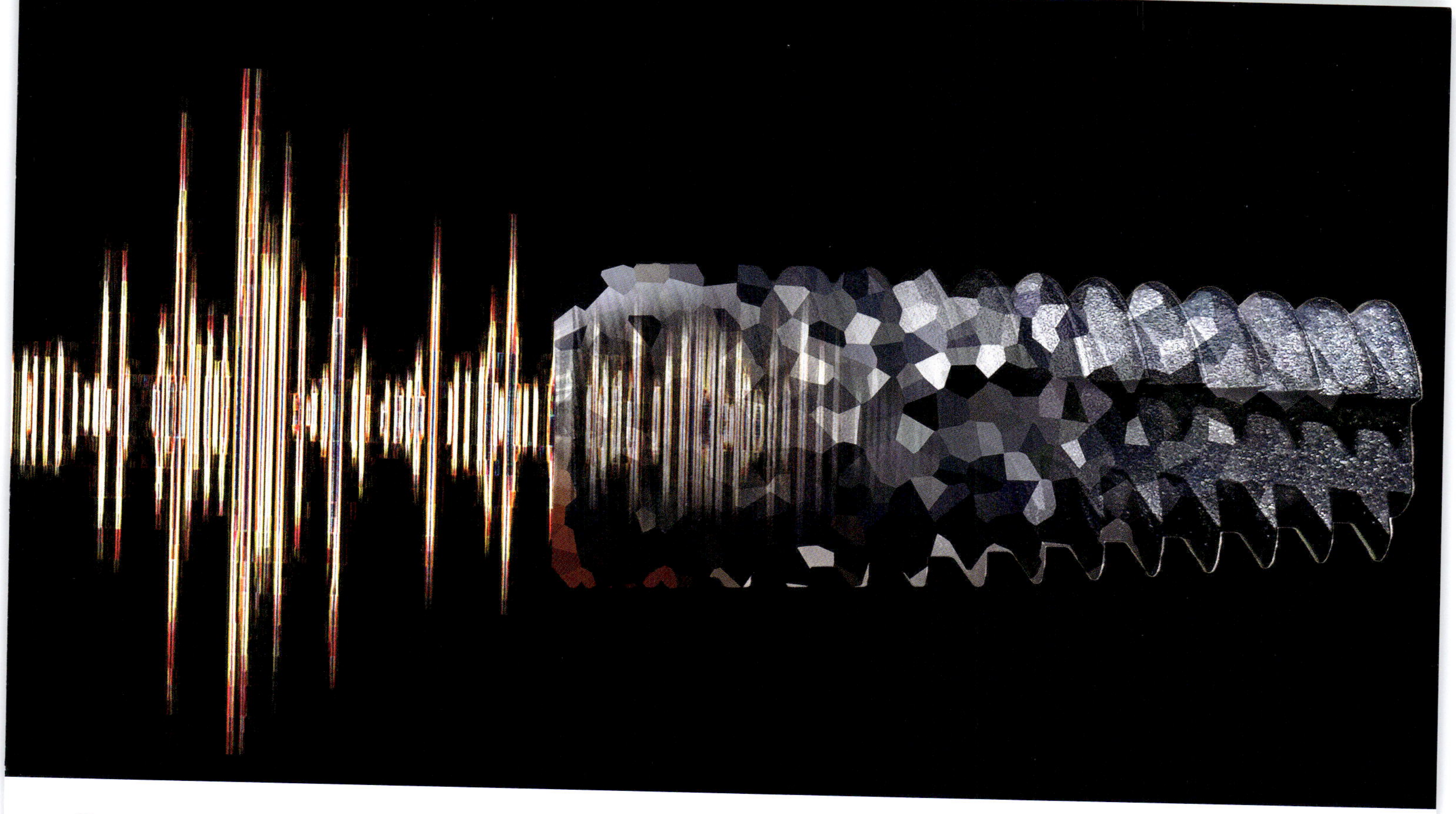

Figure 7-13 Resonance Frequency Analysis (RFA) measures the vibrations or the sound of the implant.

is magnetically "plucked" or "pinged" with a special wand unit that reads the waveforms and applies a calculation to provide a specific unitless measurement called the Implant Stability Quotient (ISQ). The higher the number, the more stable the implant. This information can be used to determine stability at placement and to track it over time. It is an objective measurement that can help guide decisions about when to restore the implant or even whether the implant has failed and needs to be removed.

A high ISQ at the time of implant placement has been associated with increased success in immediate loading. A steady or increasing ISQ over time indicates successful osseointegration. A low or decreasing ISQ may indicate the implant does not have stable surrounding bone or that the implant is not integrating. Many factors influence the ISQ, and it is not a perfect system. It is a tool. Another useful piece of information that, when used wisely, can help optimize outcomes.

I like that the Implant Stability Quotient (ISQ) is a unitless measurement. Usually, we have to measure things in a specific unit. Not this, though. There is no unit. Units are fascinating. One meter was originally defined as one ten-millionth of the distance between the North Pole and the equator through the observatory in Paris. One unit of Botox is the median lethal intraperitoneal dose of the toxin as measured in Swiss-webster mice. The unit of resonance frequency is hertz. But the ISQ is a scale developed specifically to track the resonance of dental implants based on their micromobility[12].

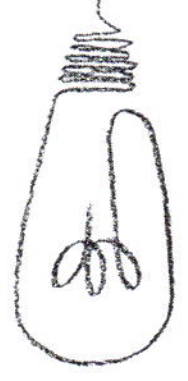

Implant stability can be differentiated as primary and secondary stability. Primary stability describes how firm or strong the implant is retained within the bone when it is screwed into place, how well it grips the bone after the last twist of the implant driver. This is a function of the implant's mechanical engagement with the old bone that is already there involving the surrounding bone as well as the implant design. The surrounding bone's quality is the biggest factor in achieving primary stability. Site preparation and osteotomy formation has the second biggest impact on potential primary stability. Implant elements such as shape, thread and surface design also contribute, but they may not be as influential as bone quality and osteotomy design[13].

Secondary stability describes how the bone heals to and around the implant. This is how it remodels and regenerates. It is the new bone. Secondary stability denotes the osseointegrated implant. This is heavily dependent on the surrounding bone. But it too is impacted by design elements of the implant[11].

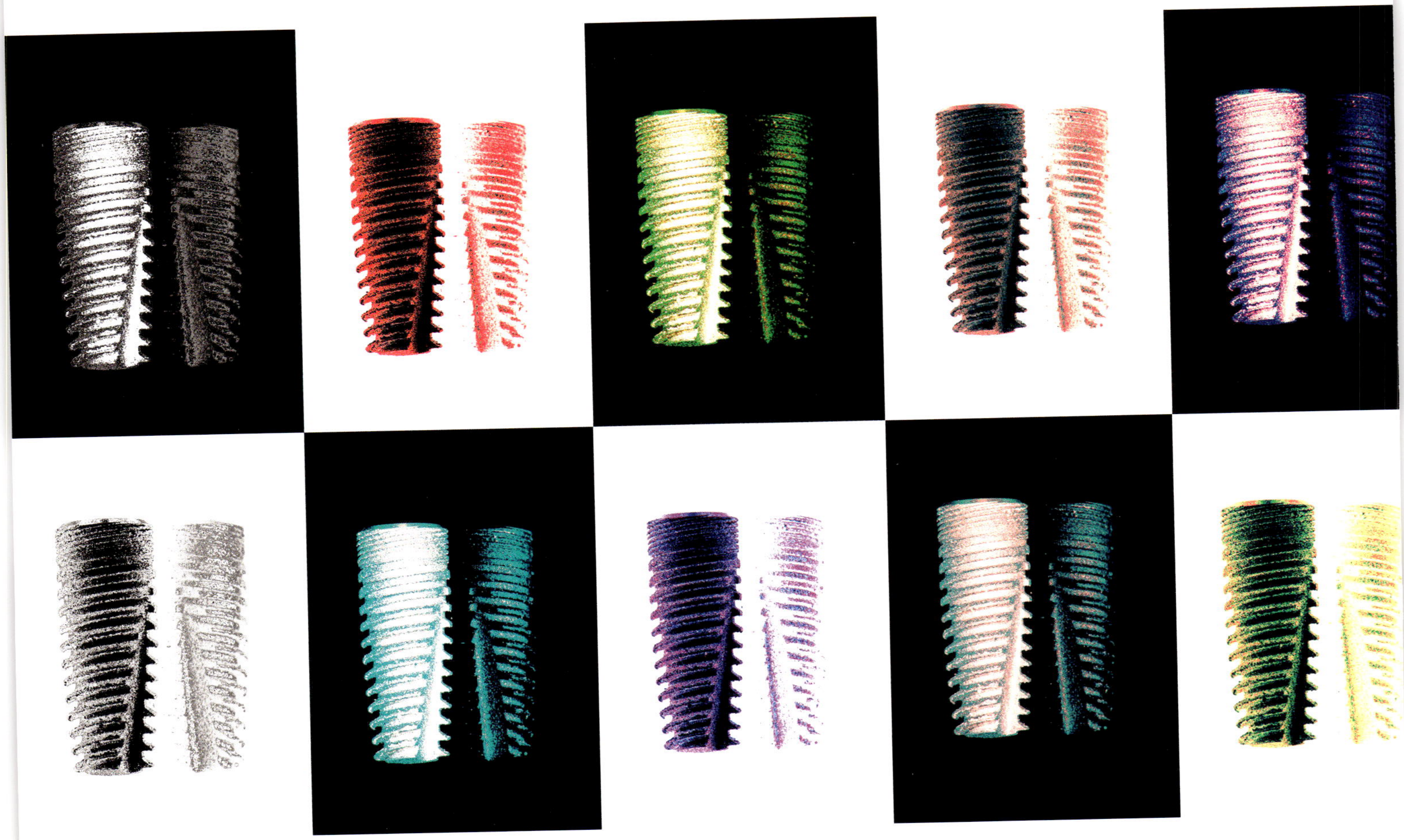

Figure 7-14 (Artwork inspired by Andy Warhol.)

The designers

Today, all major implant companies are producing implants with an inherent capacity to integrate. Bone can heal around them. Implant design is all about tipping the scales in favor of healing. We want to leverage our understanding of the science to increase the bone's ability and likelihood of integrating with this foreign body we are inserting.

Implant success is on a continuum. It is not dualistic. Black or white. Yea or nay. Integrated or not. If you have placed many implants, you likely have stared down an implant or two that has "the look" that says it is stable for now, but don't push your luck, buddy. It may not be bad enough to remove it or even open the site and graft it. But it sure won't stand up to very much abuse, either mechanical or biological. Determining what to do clinically is difficult in these cases. Our goal is to use well-designed implants in well-designed sites to decrease the need for these challenging decisions.

The work of implant companies is to improve implant design to make it as close to a natural tooth as possible. We are looking for incremental improvements in the quality, speed and predictability of the integration. We want the best possible relationship between the implant and the surrounding hard and soft tissue. Until our technology exceeds Mother Nature's success rate (which I cannot fathom happening), there will continue to be a drive for improvement. This expensive and tremendously valuable competition between the many implant companies is fascinating. It seems to me like some of the small gains implant companies achieve get over promoted, claiming more progress than may be due. But with relentless effort, the many small steps add up to great gains for dental implants over time.

When it all comes down to it, should we really be asking which implant is best? Best is relative, after all. It must be excellent. It must be innovative. It must have strong scientific support for its claims. It must support your goals and needs surgically and restoratively. How significant is the difference between the leading systems? The answer to that question will always be changing.

Dental implant companies study success and design implants to be successful both in the initial phase and in the long-term phase. They are constantly researching and developing materials, designs and protocols to make their product the best on the market. And that is what we all want: the best. Consider this a shout-out to all the people at dental implant companies investing their lives in improving our patients' lives; cheers to you.

The design

Basic features in the design of an implant include surface, shape, size, threads, platform (connection) and restorative components. Each one impacts different aspects of implant stability, osseointegration, soft tissue health and restorative outcomes.

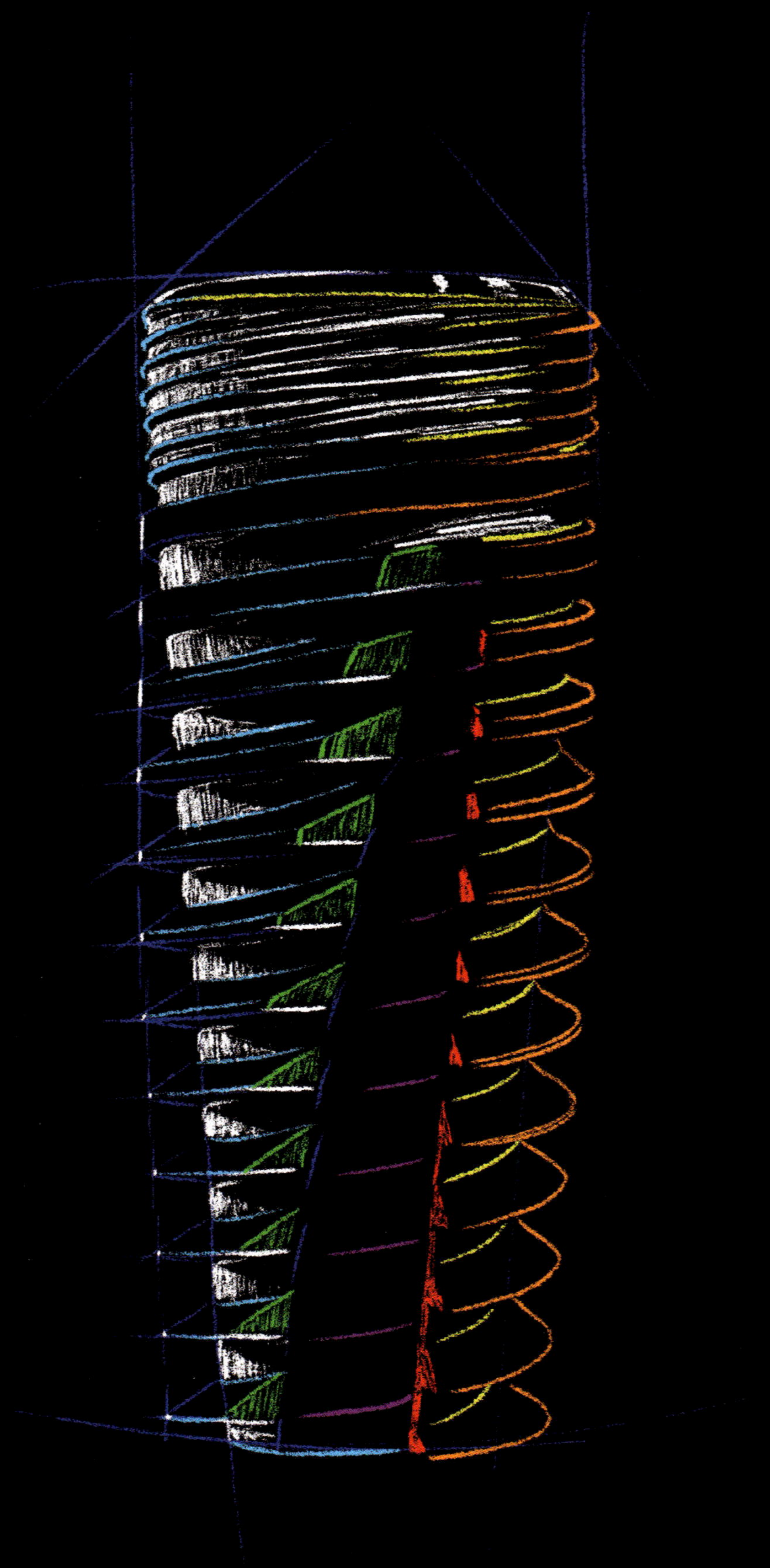

Figure 7-15 Implant design has a few main considerations. The leading edge of the threads (*red*) in this type of implant progresses from cutting to compressing. You can see how the threads are sharp toward the apex and become flat toward the platform (*blue* and *orange*). The channel (*purple*) collects the cut bone fragments at the leading edge of the threads. The implant body (*white*) is tapered more than the threads. Each of these design features becomes a tool we can use to optimize success and leverage our resources. Implant design is its own functional artform. It complements all the other various aspects in the art of oral surgery (for example, the stress load seen previously in this chapter). The better we understand how the body responds, the better we can leverage our efforts for short and long-term success.

Surface

Dental implants are great replacements for missing teeth. But like most replacement parts, they are never quite as good as the original. A healthy periodontal complex is far more sophisticated and durable than any dental implant surface could ever be. Tremendous research is being poured into understanding and improving the union between the mechanical (implant) and the biological (tissue). And it keeps on changing.

These days, most implants are made of surgical grade titanium. Titanium is strong as steel but 45% lighter. It is heavier than aluminum, but twice as strong. And the beauty is biology likes it. Well, it doesn't really like raw titanium.

Like all other metals, titanium corrodes. Biology generally doesn't like corrosion. But when titanium oxidizes, it becomes very biocompatible.

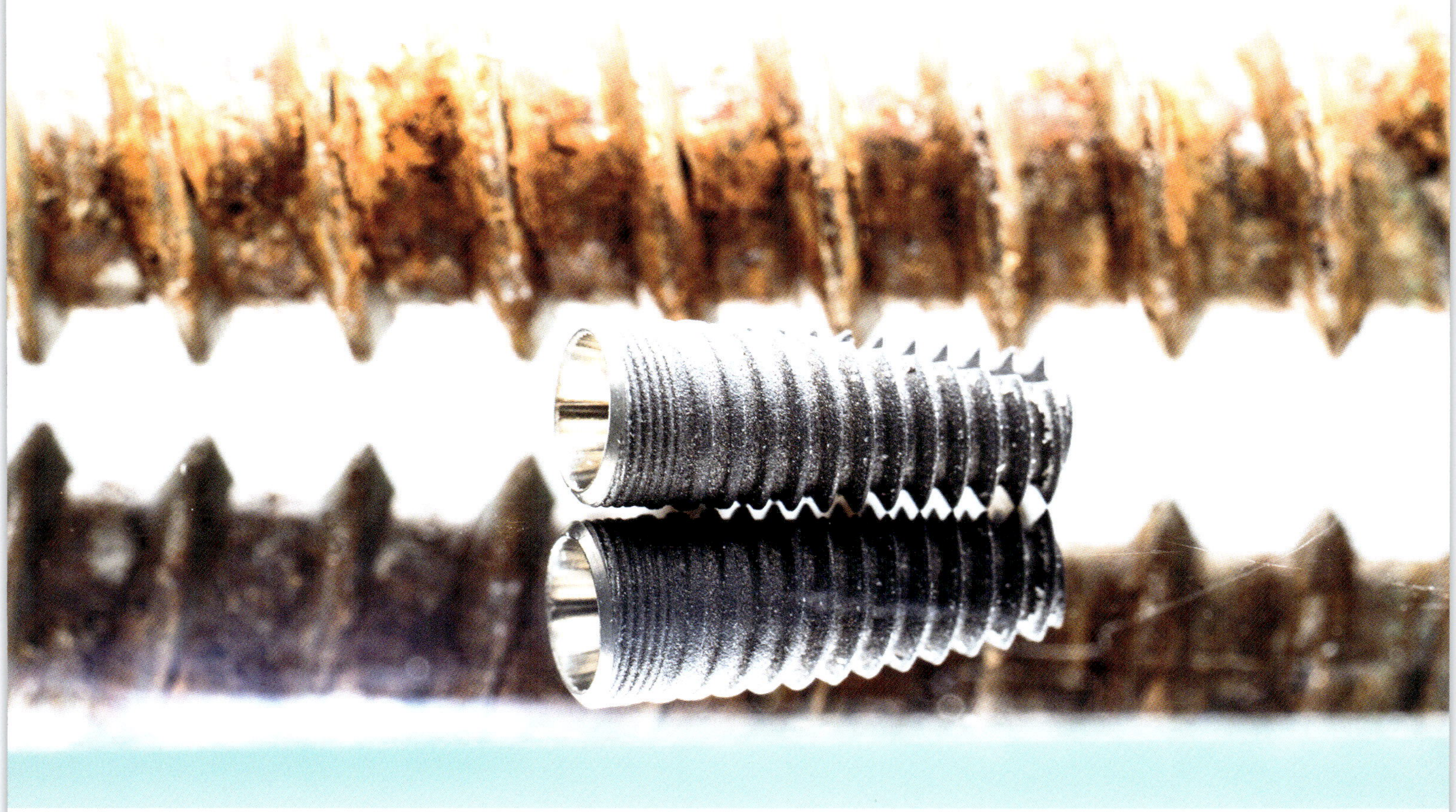

Figure 7-16 While corrosion, or oxidation, typically degrades the properties of metal, the properties of titanium that we rely on for implant success depend on it.

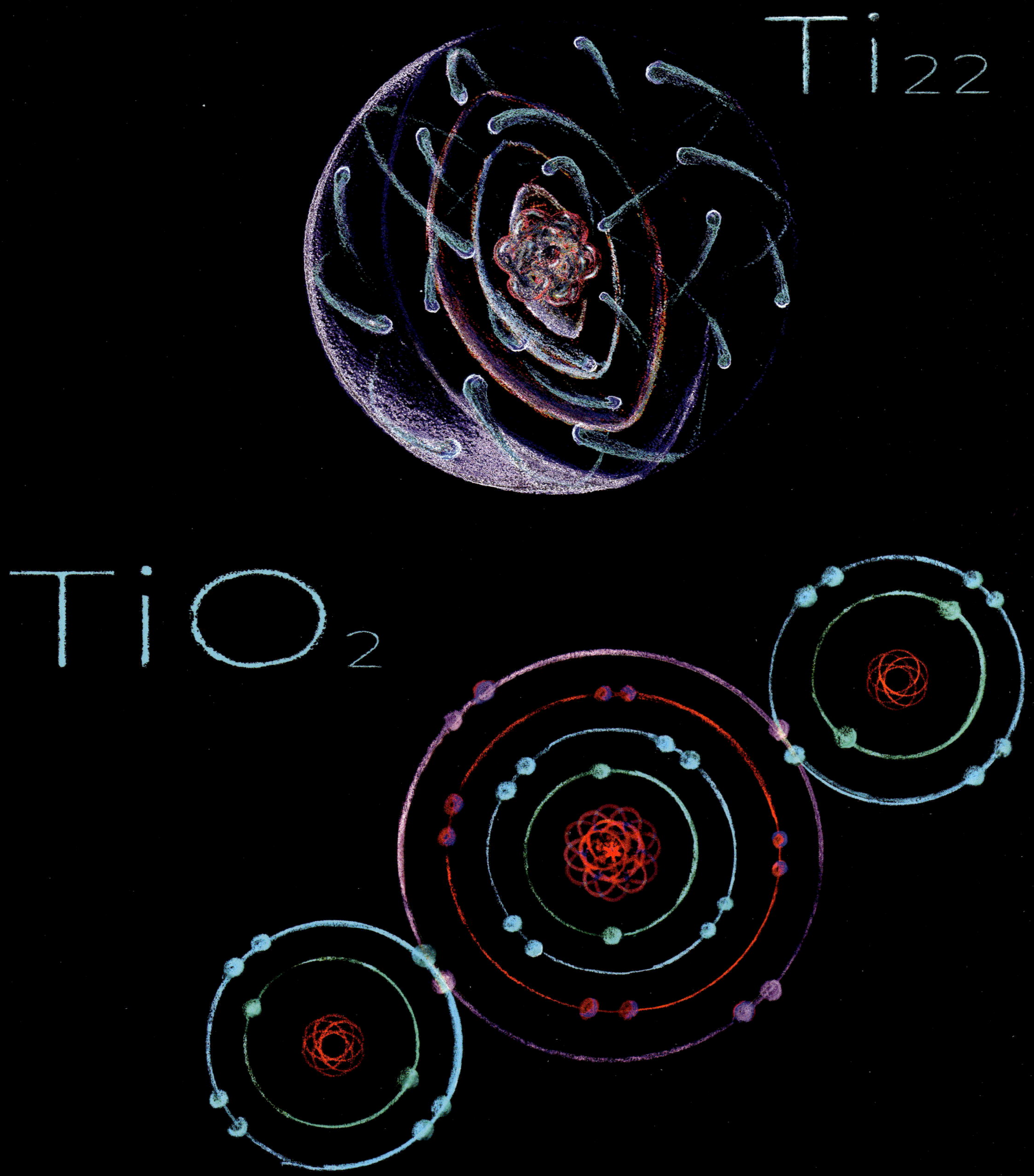

Figure 7-17 Let's look closer at titanium. Titanium has 22 electrons buzzing around its nucleus. Electrons like to be balanced, especially in the outer, valence layer. In titanium, the outer few electrons are not well balanced. They are unstable.

The instant raw or elemental titanium is exposed to the air, it oxidizes. A couple oxygen atoms help stabilize titanium's outer electrons by pairing up with them. Two electrons from each oxygen atom hang out with the outer electrons in the titanium atom, making a stable eight in the outer layer. That makes everyone happy. Titanium dioxide is very stable and corrosion resistant. And biology really likes that. Refined metals corrode. The surface atoms of metals, like titanium, naturally have an unstable charge. When exposed to air, oxygen binds to the titanium, forming a stable atomic layer of titanium dioxide (TiO_2). This oxidization is corrosion that actually protects underlying metal from further corrosion. Iron is different than titanium. When iron corrodes it forms rust, and its physical properties are degraded. This causes further corrosion that progressively penetrates deeper into the metal. Commercially pure titanium, on the other hand, has improved biological properties when it forms titanium oxide. Nature likes stability. Our bodies naturally prefer stability. They don't get along well with unstable or reactive things.

Treating the surface of a titanium implant can dramatically reduce undesirable reactivity and make the bone like it a lot more[14]. Every implant company has its own way of improving the biocompatibility of the surface of the implant. They study protein adsorption, fibrin adhesion and ultimately long term osseointegration. And they all have sophisticated studies with great data supporting their edge on the market. Together as a whole, implant dentistry is becoming better at knowing what the bone likes. Maybe someday we will find something as good as a vital periodontal ligament. Until then, it is important to know at least a bit about the science of it all.

Titanium dioxide is well accepted by bone. But we want to improve this relationship. The relationship inherently has two parties: the bone and the implant surface. To improve this relationship, any modifications must consider both the bone and the implant. One such modification is adding fluoride ions to the titanium dioxide surface (Dentsply Sirona DS Prime Taper). While fluoride is not essential for cellular growth or maintenance, it has been shown to improve bone mechanics and biology[15].

If we want the bone to accept and embrace the implant, we must first understand how to optimize the relationship between the bone and implant.

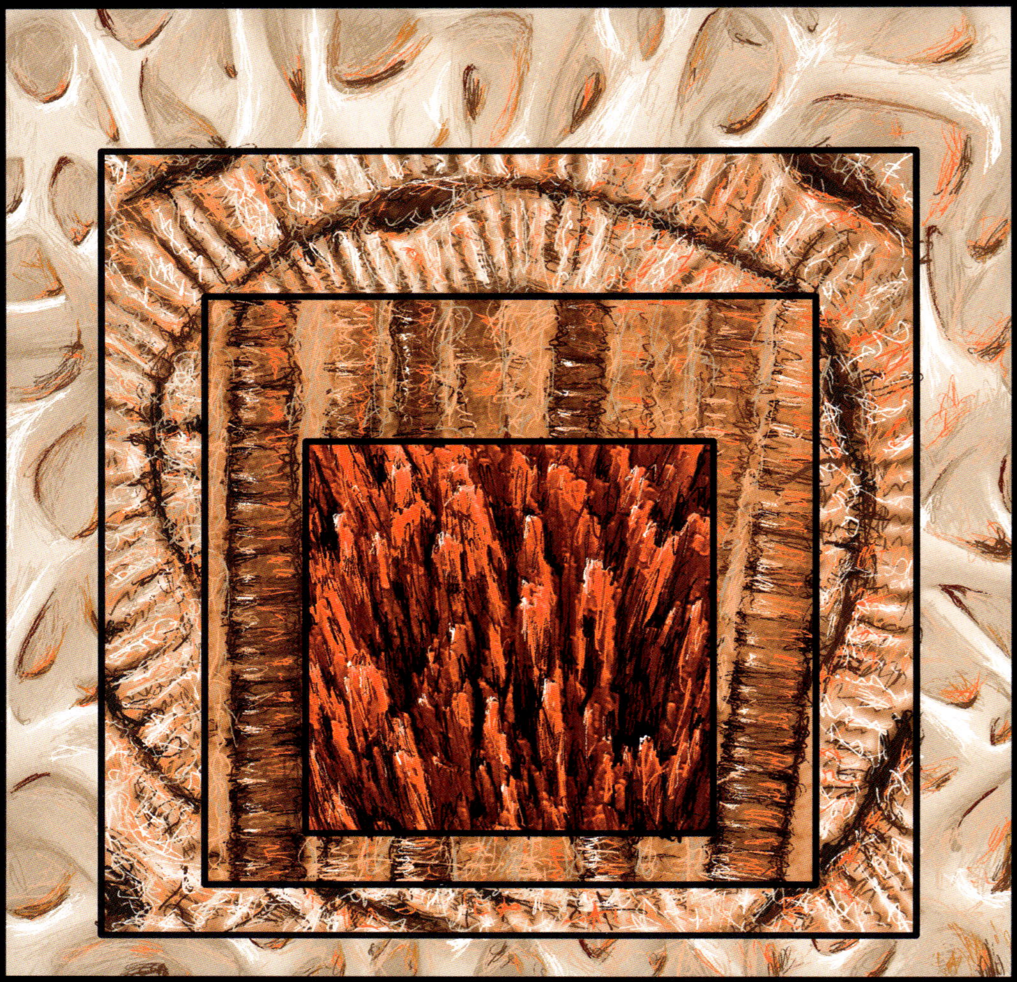

Figure 7-18
(Artwork inspired by Josef Albers.)

The more we understand about bone at every level, the better we can adapt to its needs.
We need to understand and respect the trabeculae at the macro level, osteoid at the micro level, collagen fibers at the nano level and hydroxyapatite crystals at the atomic level.

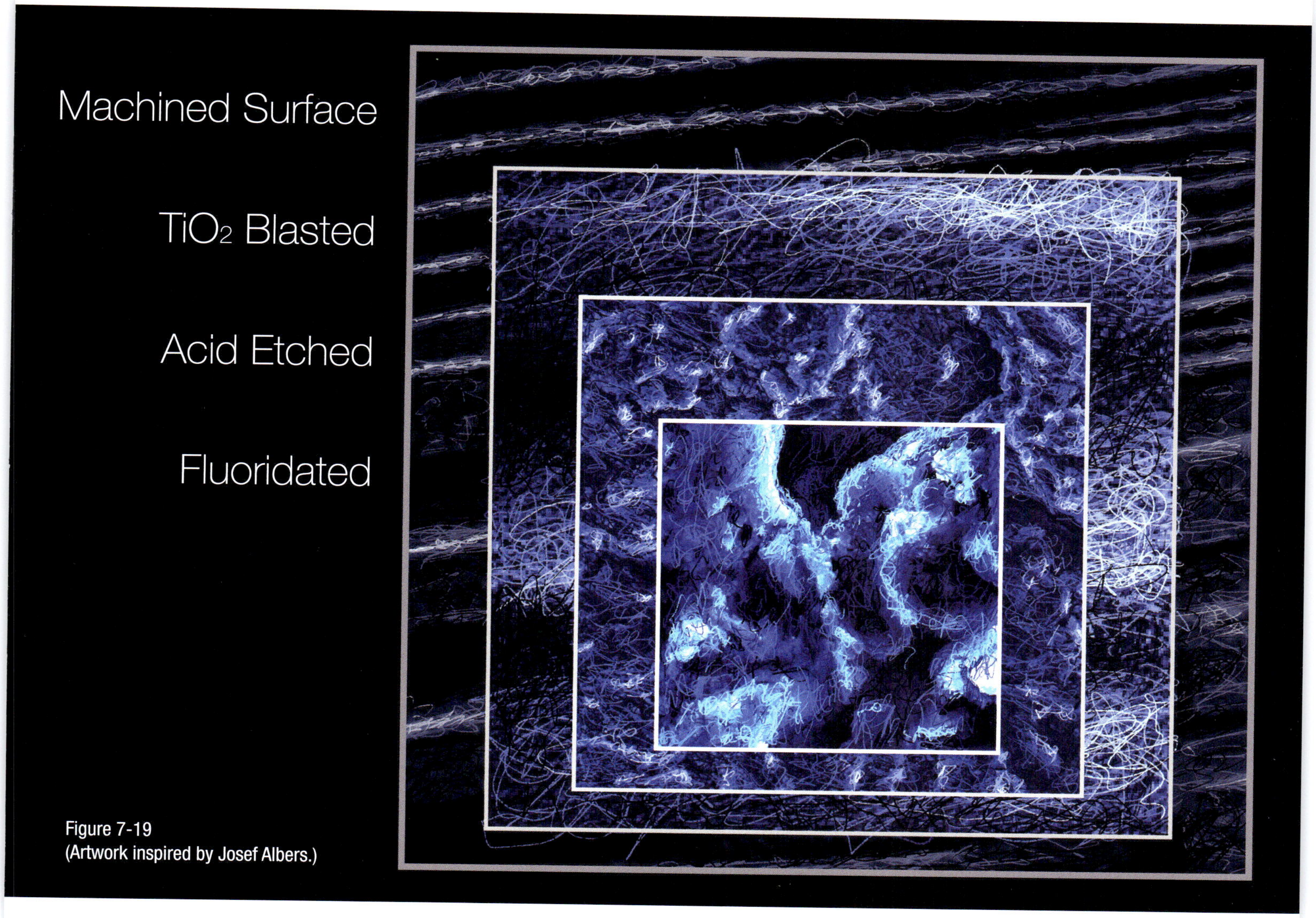

Figure 7-19
(Artwork inspired by Josef Albers.)

A machined implant is blasted with oxidized titanium particles to roughen the surface without contaminating it.

It is then treated with hydrofluoric acid, etching the surface and increasing the nano roughness. The composition of the hydrofluoric acid further modifies the nano roughness by evenly depositing fluoride ions on the surface and rounding off some of the nano-roughness. About 5% of the titanium dioxide surface has fluoride ions replacing a previous hydroxyl group.

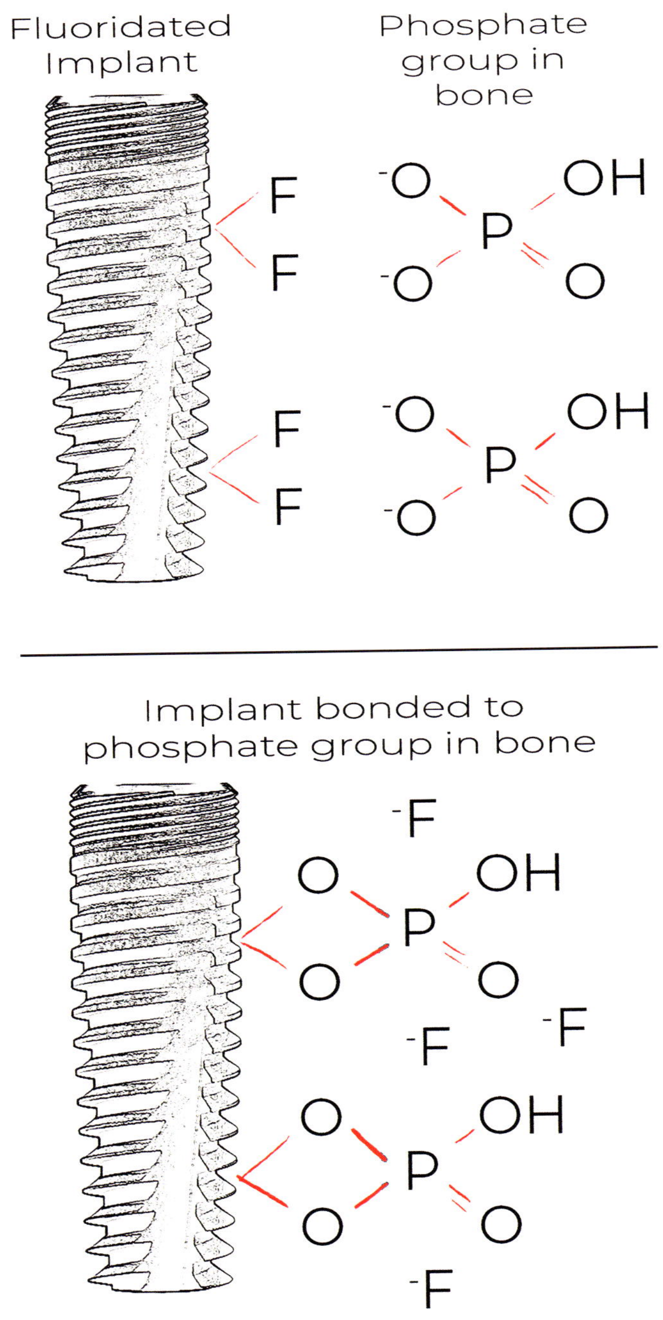

Figure 7-20 The fluoride ions on the implant surface promote the chemical bond formation between the titanium dioxide and the phosphate groups of the surrounding bone.

As the bone heals, it has been proposed that the fluoride ions on the implant are replaced by the phosphate groups of the surrounding bone. This liberates the fluoride and bonds the implant surface to the mineral structure of the bone.

Fluoride ions play well with the implant surface and the bone. By improving properties on both sides of this equation, adding fluoride ions on the implant surface serves to:

- Increase the trabecular density and calcification, improving the functional strength of the bone surrounding the implant.
- Increase the number of osteoblasts and improve their production of collagen and mineralized hydroxyapatite. This also speeds up the osseointegration process.
- Attract calcium and phosphate to the implant surface. This increases mineral density at the bone-implant interface.

It is good for the implant. And it is very good for the bone.

The late Per-Ingvar (P-I) Brånemark described osseointegration as "direct structural and functional connection between ordered living bone and the surface of a load-carrying implant."[17]

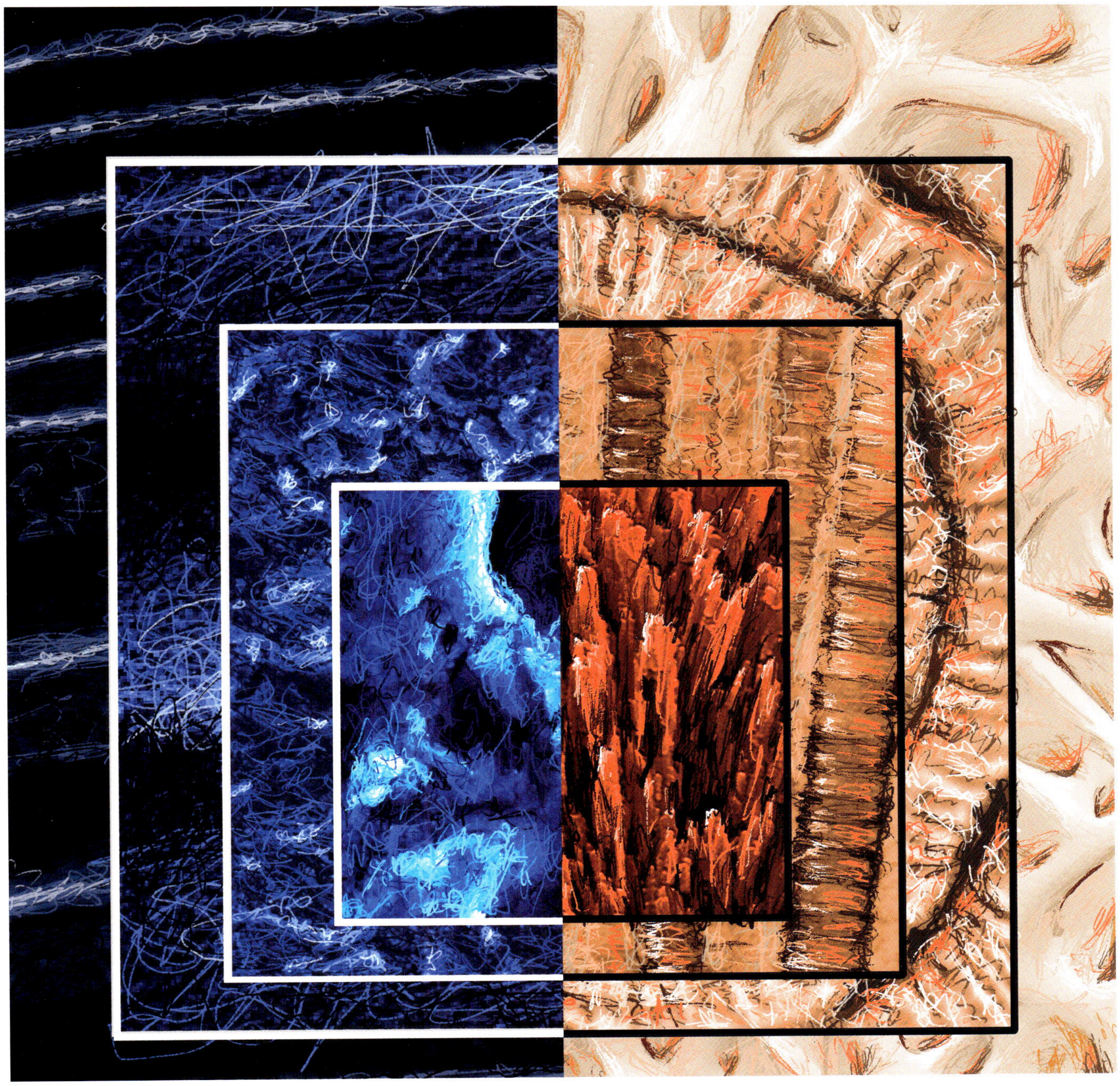

Figure 7-21 (Artwork inspired by Josef Albers.)

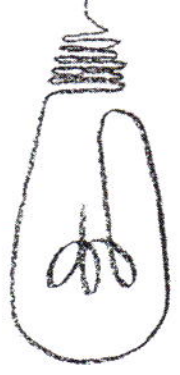

Desirable qualities of implant-bone interaction:

- Strong trabecular pattern from healthy, functional bone (implant shape)[16].
- Robust osteoid formation by recruiting osteoblasts to form from osteoprogenitor cells. (Fluoride promotes osteoblast differentiation.)
- Increased collagen production by stimulated osteoblasts. (Fluoride increases collagen production.)
- An atomic interaction between the hydroxyapatite and the implant surface. (Fluoride stimulates HA production by osteoblasts.)

Shape

Tapered (conical) and parallel (straight) are the two most basic implant shapes. Tapered implants are narrower at apex, resulting in a more active engagement with the bone as the implant is inserted. They are like a wedge: the outward pressure increases the deeper they are placed. Because of this, they may achieve higher levels of primary stability. But they can also cause increased pressure on the surrounding bone[13]. The narrow tip of a tapered implant is beneficial when there is limited apical bone available. Parallel wall implants maintain a relatively consistent width through the body of the implant. They are designed to engage the surrounding bone more uniformly as the implant is placed. In contemporary implant dentistry, there are no truly parallel wall implants. All implants taper to some degree toward the apex. It is more of a spectrum going from more parallel to more tapered.

Implant shape seems to be a matter of individual surgeon preference and is often site-specific. Each shape has its own distinct feel and response, both when drilling and when placing the implant. This is discussed further in *Chapter 8: Implant Surgical Principles*.

Threads

Implant threads actively engage bone during insertion. They are mainly responsible for primary stability. As the bone heals, the threads no longer actively engage the bone and become passive within the remodeled bone. The action of the thread no longer holds the implant in place. Secondary stability comes from the bone-implant interface and has less to do with thread design. Threads pull the implant into the site as it is screwed into place. And like so many simple machines, the force is greatly multiplied. A little more torque on the wrench can translate into a lot more force inside the bone. Therefore, it is important to know and follow the implant manufacturers' maximum recommended torque. Respecting this will protect the bone from excessive force, which can cause devastating necrosis of surrounding bone.

Threads engage bone by compressing and cutting into it. The friction of the threads during placement makes the implant functionally "self-locking." As bone density increases, the friction and resulting heat does as well. The friction and pressure provide increased primary stability, but they can also contribute to complications if they are not handled well. Most implant systems have protocols in place for soft or regular bone as well as dense bone. This may include tapping the osteotomy to decrease the pressure and friction the threads generate. Tapping addresses the space for the threads but not necessarily the body of the implant. The cutting action that happens when the threads cut into the bone generates bone debris. These bone fragments or chips get displaced between the implant and bone. There is a channel at the cutting edge of the threads that creates space for this bone debris. Every implant system has its own variation. It is important to understand the overall principles common to all systems to apply them skillfully in each individual surgery.

It is not only the thread that engages the bone. The body of the implant also engages the bone, impacting the torque and surrounding pressure. When the implant body is wider than the osteotomy, engagement increases significantly. While the threading both cuts and compresses the bone, the implant body only compresses it. The drill shape and size are designed for each implant to optimize bone engagement of the implant body and threads. They both need to be factored into the equation. Visualizing and understanding the relationship between the drill, implant design and bone density empowers you to leverage these factors for the success of every implant.

There are some implant systems with a more aggressive shape and surface intended to increase primary stability. These are often marketed for immediate placement and immediate loading, especially in low density bone. If this same aggressive type of low-density system and drilling protocol was used in high density bone, it would be more than frustrating surgically and would have devastating outcomes post-operatively. It all boils down to knowing your implant and the bone.

The stress transferred to the bone surrounding an implant is increased at the angles and junctions of the threads. This is a basic principle in mechanical engineering. The angle amplifies the functional stress on the system. While the primary stability is the main consideration for thread design, implant companies also factor in these and other long-term impacts on the implant-bone interface.

Wettability

An impressive microscopic flood takes place when an implant contacts fresh blood. The red tidal wave rushes over the vast network of crevices and pores, carrying with it a host of cells and biological products for healing. In many ways, blood directs and delivers the components needed for the initial phase of osseointegration. This is such a critical part of healing. Manipulating this wetting of blood on the implant surface influences the outcome. Wettability is impacted by many factors, including surface topography and chemistry.

Anodization is an interesting phenomenon. Titanium naturally forms an oxidized outer layer that can be manipulated with electricity. When the titanium is set up as the anode (positive charge that attracts the negatively charged electrons) this flow of electrons significantly alters the surface oxide layer (Nobel TiUltra™). It becomes thicker and rougher. This changes the microstructure of the surface layer[18].

In another system, the oxidized surface is blasted and acid etched (Straumann SLActive). The surface is then covered with hydrogen atoms, forming a hydroxylated layer that is uniquely hydrophilic. This attracts blood to the surface, increasing its penetration throughout the porous, roughened surface. It is as though the surface layer is activated by the hydroxylation. This treatment has been shown to improve early osseointegration.

The many different surface treatment methods are each quite unique, but they share common goals and outcomes: faster and better biomechanical connection with the bone.

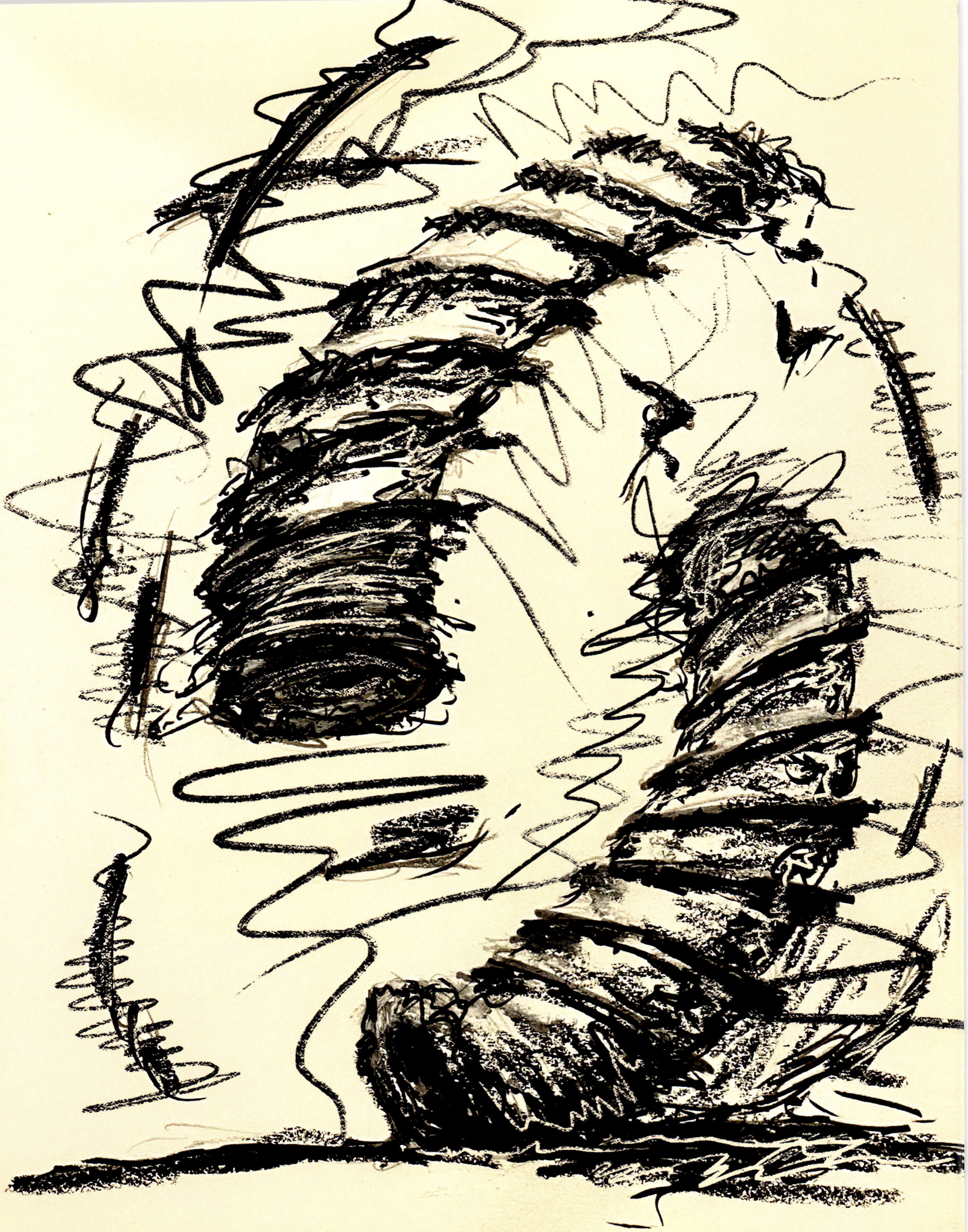

Figure 7-22 Implants must be resilient. Their environment is relentless and unforgiving. (Artwork inspired by Claes Oldenburg.)

Size: The balancing act

Size matters. But bigger isn't always better. It seems natural that a longer and wider implant would be stronger and last longer. This logic is true to a certain degree. An implant absorbs chewing forces and transfers that force from the biting surface down through its components and disperses the force from the implant surface to the surrounding bone. If the components are too small, they break. If there isn't enough implant surface area contacting the bone, the force can overload that bond and break it. If there isn't enough bone around the implant or the bone isn't strong enough, it can create microfractures triggering bone resorption. This whole system needs to be strong enough to last[19].

How much is enough? That is the question of the research. Failure anywhere the force is transferred is failure of the whole thing. Each of these areas is being studied and improved. As we improve our techniques and materials, we can push the limits of shorter and narrower implants with increasing success. The implant-bone interface is the most complex and difficult to study. Understanding how and where the force transfers to the bone is critical to solving this puzzle.

Implant success is far more dependent on recipient bone quality than implant length[20].

Frost's law states that bone reacts to functional load by improving its architecture[21].

The crestal bone matters the most. This is where the load is primarily transferred. Very little force is present in the middle or apical portions of an implant. Because most of the load is absorbed at the crest, the length of the implant beneath doesn't matter nearly as much. The diameter of the implant at the crest has a significant impact on the load transfer, reducing the forces as the diameter increases. Wider implants transfer the load better. But wider implants take up more space and may limit the amount of surrounding bone. Optimizing the width of the implant and the width of the bone is critical. A big fat implant without sufficient bone is worse than a narrower implant with stable bone. The restorative plan directs the final design. The implant platform diameter is the starting point for the emergence profile of the crown. Make it easy to restore and easy for the patient to maintain.

Small implant or bone graft?

It is a balancing act when the bone is limited. Short implants work. Narrow implants work. This has been proven time and again[22, 23]. Our job as implant architects is to know when longer or wider is better. As much as short and narrow implants have been studied and improved, bone grafting to improve height and width has also been researched and developed. Simpler is generally better. If we can avoid grafting by placing a shorter or narrower implant without compromising the final outcome, the answer is clear. Even if there is enough bone, grafting may improve the position of the implant, which can improve esthetics and hygiene.

When there is a shorter implant with longer restoration, the increased mechanical strain increases risk of prosthetic complications (screw loosening, decementation, ceramic chipping and ceramic failure)[23]. Consider splinting adjacent short implants. This decreases the stress concentration at the implant platform, leading to decreased load at the alveolar crest[24]. One of the main challenges with shorter implants relates to the engagement of the bone. They can be more technically challenging to place with adequate stability. Underpreparing the osteotomy can improve this success.

The following is my current decision-making protocol in my private practice. This is what I have found to be most predictable for me with my current implant system (DS Prime Taper):

POSTERIOR MAXILLA

- ***Implant length:*** 8 to 11 mm ideally. Prefer sinus augmentation to place an 8 mm implant but will consider 6 mm implant if higher risk for sinus augmentation.
- ***Implant width:*** 4.8 to 5.4 mm ideally. Prefer guided bone regeneration to place at least 4.2 mm implant but could consider 3.0 to 3.6 mm if higher risk for grafting.

POSTERIOR MANDIBLE

- ***Implant length:*** 8 to 11 mm ideally. Consider a 6 mm implant to avoid vertical grafting. Guided bone regeneration if needed.
- ***Implant width:*** 4.8 to 5.4 mm ideally. Prefer guided bone regeneration to place at least 4.2 mm but could consider 3.0 to 3.6 mm if higher risk for grafting.

ANTERIOR MAXILLA

- ***Implant length:*** 8 to 11 mm ideally. Limited bone height here often results in compromised platform position. Typically, if I cannot place an 8 mm long implant, guided bone regeneration is needed to optimize the restorative outcome.
- ***Implant width:*** 3.0 to 4.2 mm ideally. Interdental space and restorative driven needs are often the determining factor in implant width. Frequently perform bone augmentation to optimize the restorative outcome and maximize the critical facial bone volume.

ANTERIOR MANDIBLE

- ***Implant length:*** 9 to 11 mm ideally. A vertical defect here often results in compromised platform position. The total height of the mandible is not the issue. The platform of the implant may be more apical than ideal, making the restoration and hygiene challenging. Guided bone regeneration may be needed to optimize the restorative outcome.
- ***Implant width:*** 3.0 to 3.6 mm ideally. Interdental space and restorative driven needs are often the determining factor in implant width. Frequently perform facial bone augmentation to optimize the restorative outcome and maximize the critical facial bone volume. This can be challenging with the mentalis and typically very thin soft tissue.

Platform switching

Like microwave cooking and post-it notes, the idea for platform switching was an incidental finding that spawned a brilliant invention. As wider diameter implants were hitting the market in the 1980s, there was a shortage of wider abutments. As a result, regular diameter abutments (4.1 mm) were placed on wide diameter platforms (5.0 to 6.0 mm). They had switched the platform diameter. Hence the term "platform switching" came about. While this seemed to be a compromise at the time, the bone and tissue around these implants was better and more stable. This concept was published in 2006. This encourages me to pay attention to everything around me. The best inventions may be sitting right in front of us[3].

Platform switching moves the mechanical stress favorably toward the center of the implant, improving the implant-bone force transfer. More importantly, it improves the biologic response by shifting the interface farther from the bone, resulting in a more stable bone level. The interface at the microgap retains bacteria causing localized inflammation. Bone doesn't like inflammation and it distances itself. Ground zero in the assault on the bone is at the abutment-implant junction. Moving that junction helps protect the bone.

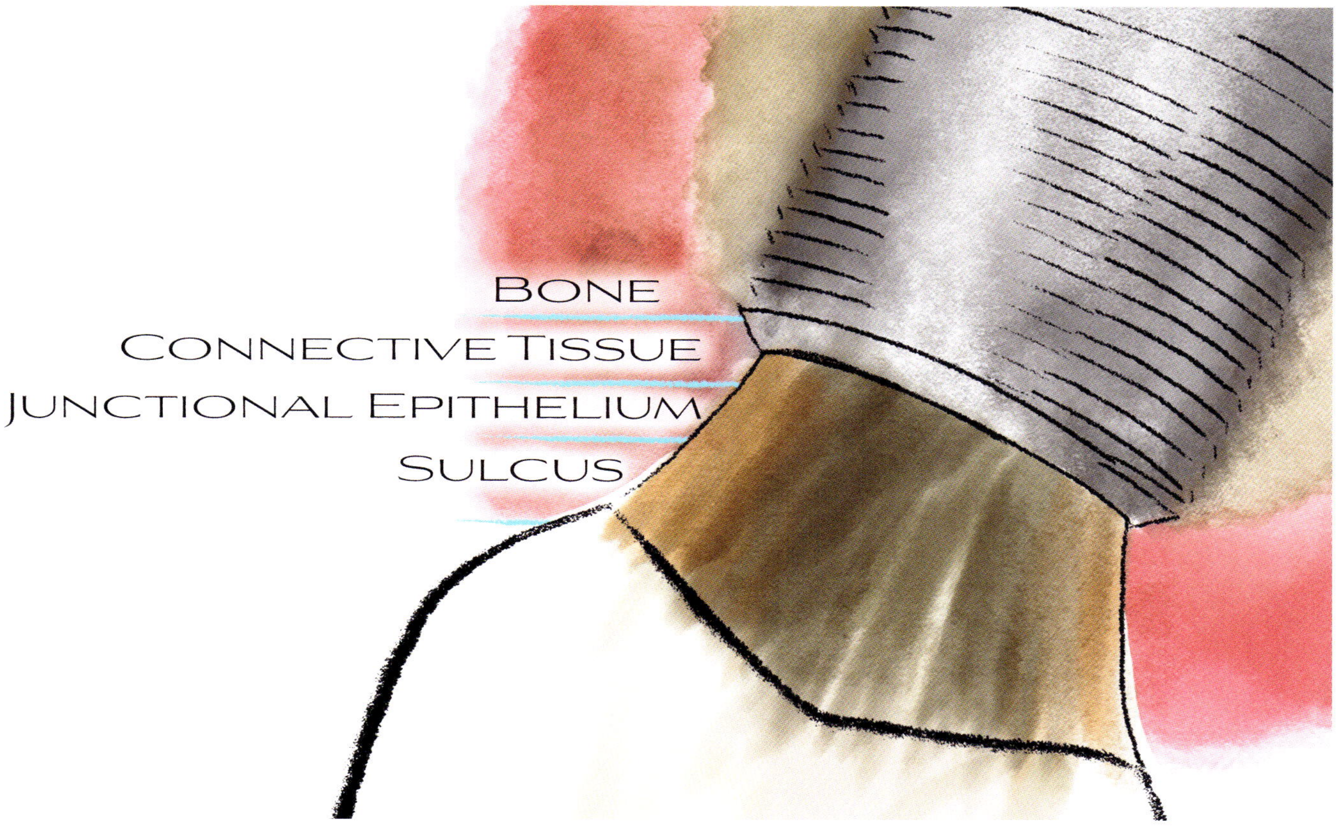

Figure 7-23 Moving the microgap farther from the bone by platform switching improves the thickness of overlying soft tissue and optimizes bone levels. The distance begins at the abutment-implant interface. When that is moved inward, there is more running room for the soft tissue.

Bone needs protection. Most implanted medical devices are buried within the tissue. The confluence of titanium, soft tissue and bone around dental implants is a unique environment. The bone around implants requires about 3 mm of overlying soft tissue for its protection and nourishment. This distance is referred to as “biologic width” in both periodontal and periimplant situations. This tissue is composed of junctional epithelium and connective tissue. The junctional epithelium is the initial line of defense, forming hemidesmosomal attachments to the abutment or implant surface. Below that, there is a layer of connective tissue, and then crestal bone. The attachment of the junctional epithelium is not stable above the microgap. Therefore, the best-case scenario for bone height would be measured from the implant-abutment junction. Platform switching moves this junction farther from the bone, creating more space for the overlying tissue. For further discussion, refer to the abutment section in *Chapter 8, Implant Surgical Principles*.

Platform level

Supracrestal, crestal and subcrestal.
Bone and soft tissue have different requirements for successful integration and long-term stability. Features that improve osseous stability, such as increased surface roughness, may compromise long-term soft tissue stability. Bacterial biofilm loves a rough surface. If a roughened portion of an implant is exposed to the soft tissue, there is a substantially increased risk of peri-implant mucositis and peri-implantitis. Substantial research is presently identifying the optimal properties for hard and soft tissue. The ultimate goal is to develop properties that optimize both hard and soft tissue integration. Then, the implant would better adapt to some bone loss, and the platform level would not be as significant.

The implant design relative to its soft and hard tissue compatibility defines the planned platform level. Many contemporary implants are designed for the platform of the implant to be level with the alveolar crest. These are typically referred to as “crestal” or “bone level” implants. The design of some implants favors deeper placement with the platform below bone level. These are “subcrestal implants.” And others thrive with the platform at the soft tissue level, raising the platform far above the bone. These are called “supracrestal” or “tissue level” implants. Each of these has specific advantages and drawbacks for different situations. Following the defined protocols and using the various types of implants properly is critical. Placing a tissue level implant subcrestally will compromise the outcome, as would placing a subcrestal implant at the soft tissue level.

If the crestal bone was perfectly flat, a truly "crestal" implant would be possible. In reality, the shape is usually curved or sloped. A single implant could actually be placed crestal, supracrestal, and subcrestal at different areas around the platform. Attention to these subtle nuances embodies the essence of the art of oral surgery.

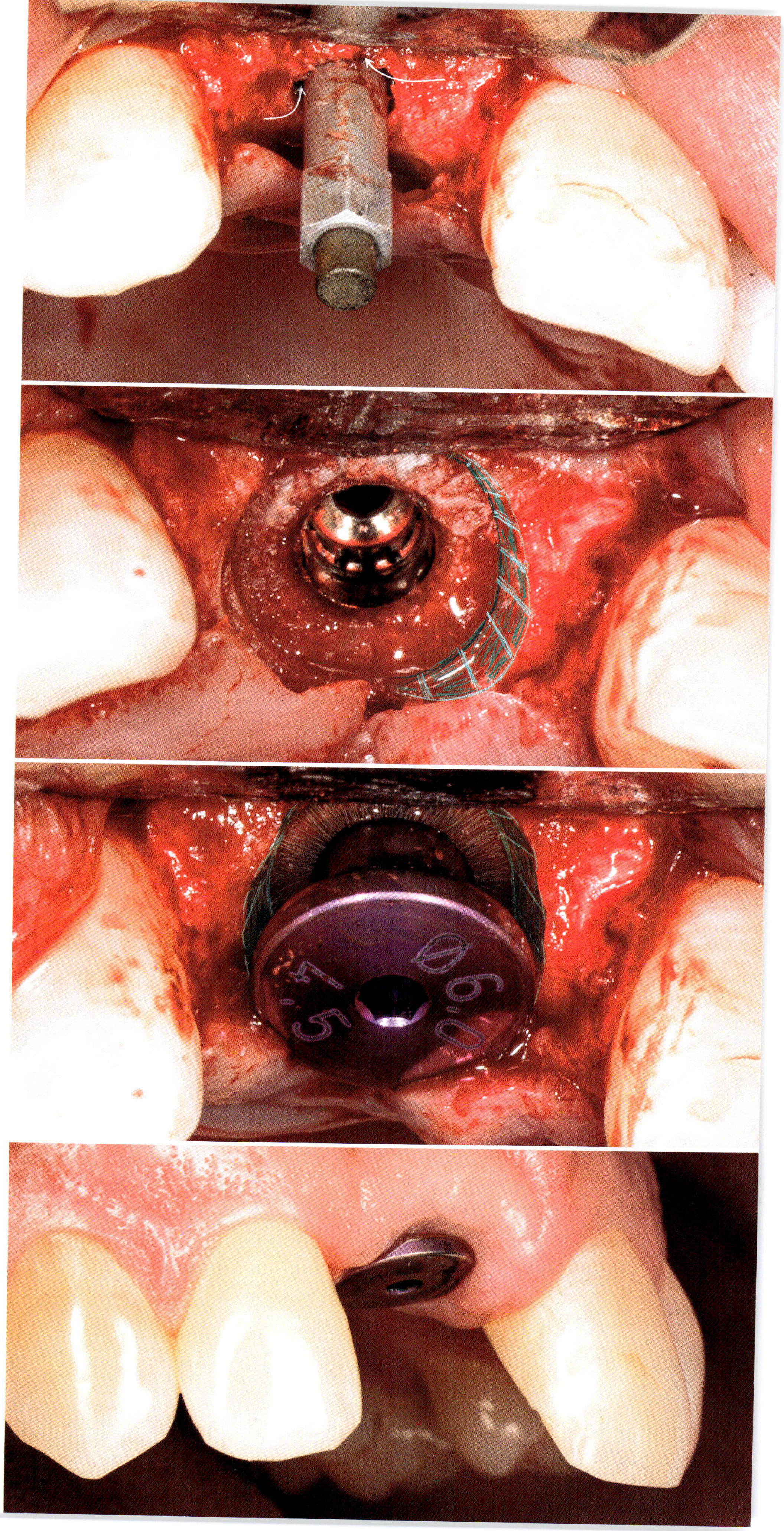

Figure 7-24 The platform of this implant is mostly subcrestal, but at the facial it is flush with the crest. Profiling the bone created uniform space for the abutment, soft tissue and bone. This implant could be classified as "crestal" on the facial and "subcrestal" everywhere else. Profiling makes the entire implant "crestal." Most cases are like this variable bone height.

Restorative components

Restorative driven implant dentistry is the industry standard. The goal is not merely a stable screw in the jawbone. It is the confluence of function and esthetics, with long term stability and maintenance as the foundation. A dental implant is useless without a restoration. The various interchangeable components involved in the surgery, impression and final restoration must all support the higher goals of durability, function and esthetics. They also have to work well in the provider's hands.

As with all things implants these days, there continues to be significant development in the efficiency and predictability of the restorative components. The main restorative components include the healing abutment (develops soft tissue contours), impression coping (captures emergence profile), final abutment (fixed or removable), prosthetic screw (engagement of threads) and the functional crown (fixed or removable, single or multiple). Implant surgery cannot be separated from the restorative process. A basic understanding of the restorative components and needs is fundamental in the art of oral surgery.

Internal conical connection

Simple physics.

The design of the implant-abutment connection impacts the stability of the restoration and the size of the microgap, two areas of potential compromise in implants. When the connection flexes, a microgap forms between the abutment and the implant[25]. The greater this gap, the more bacterial contamination and biofilm smear can develop. There is also evidence that using manufacturer specific components provides a much better fit[26]. We want this junction to be as snug as possible. The current data seems overwhelming that an internal conical connection (internal morse taper) is best.

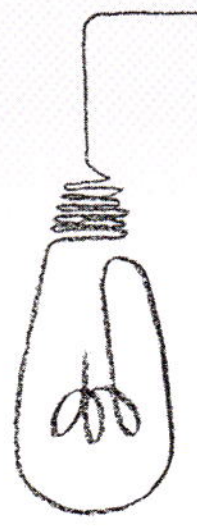

Know your implant. Understand the design and features. They are your biggest ally. Or they can be your worst enemy if they are misunderstood or misapplied.

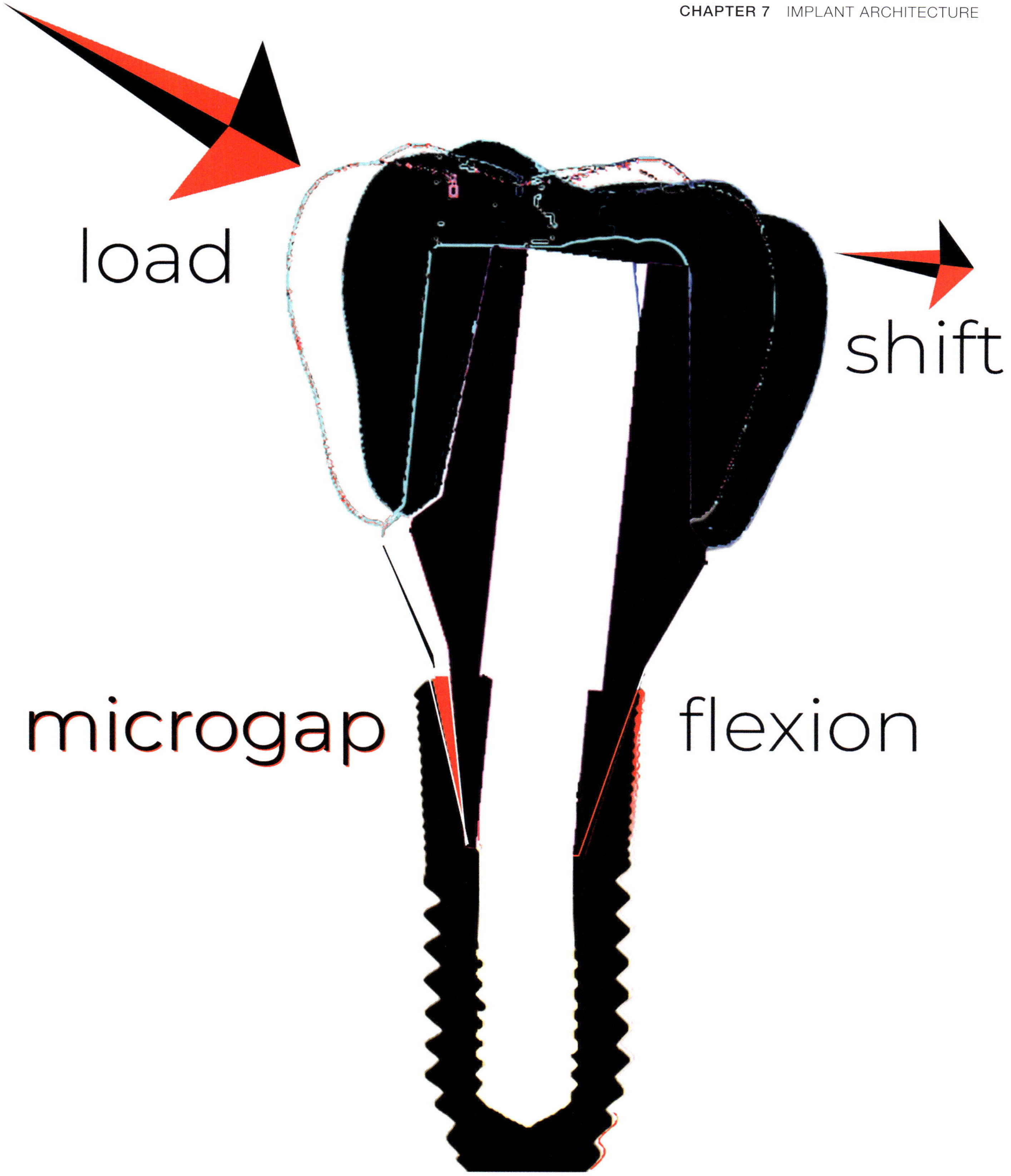

Figure 7-25 When the restoration is loaded off axis, the abutment and crown move slightly. As the metal components flex microscopically, a microgap (*red*) forms between the implant and the abutment. This causes wear and fragmentation of the titanium and creates space for problematic biofilm formation. (Artwork inspired by Andy Warhol.)

Prosthetic screw

The definitive prosthetic screw fascinates me. This tiny little screw holds it all together. It is solely responsible for maintaining the union between the implant and abutment. As the screw reaches final torque, friction builds under the head of the screw and between the threads. The screw also bends slightly at the shank and in the threads as it elongates slightly. This is called preload. This preload is engineered by the manufacturer matching the implant threads, screw threads, and the implant and screw material. The marriage of implant and screw is not only in diameter and thread pitch but in material properties. Each implant manufacturer has created a unique mighty little screw to fit their specifications. This is worth respecting by using both the manufacturer's components and torque specifications. Third party components are different in their shape and material properties. These suboptimal choices may save a few bucks now, but the increased chance of complications of screw loosening and fracture may not be worth it in the long run. Just ask your patients.

Tighter isn't better. In an attempt to improve retention, it seems natural to just tighten the screw a little more than recommended. But this additional torque decreases the true retention of the screw by exceeding the tolerance of its metal. It is also more likely to weaken or strip the head of the screw.

The best practice is to use original equipment manufacturer (OEM) parts and to follow recommended specs throughout the process. This also protects the warranty with most companies[27].

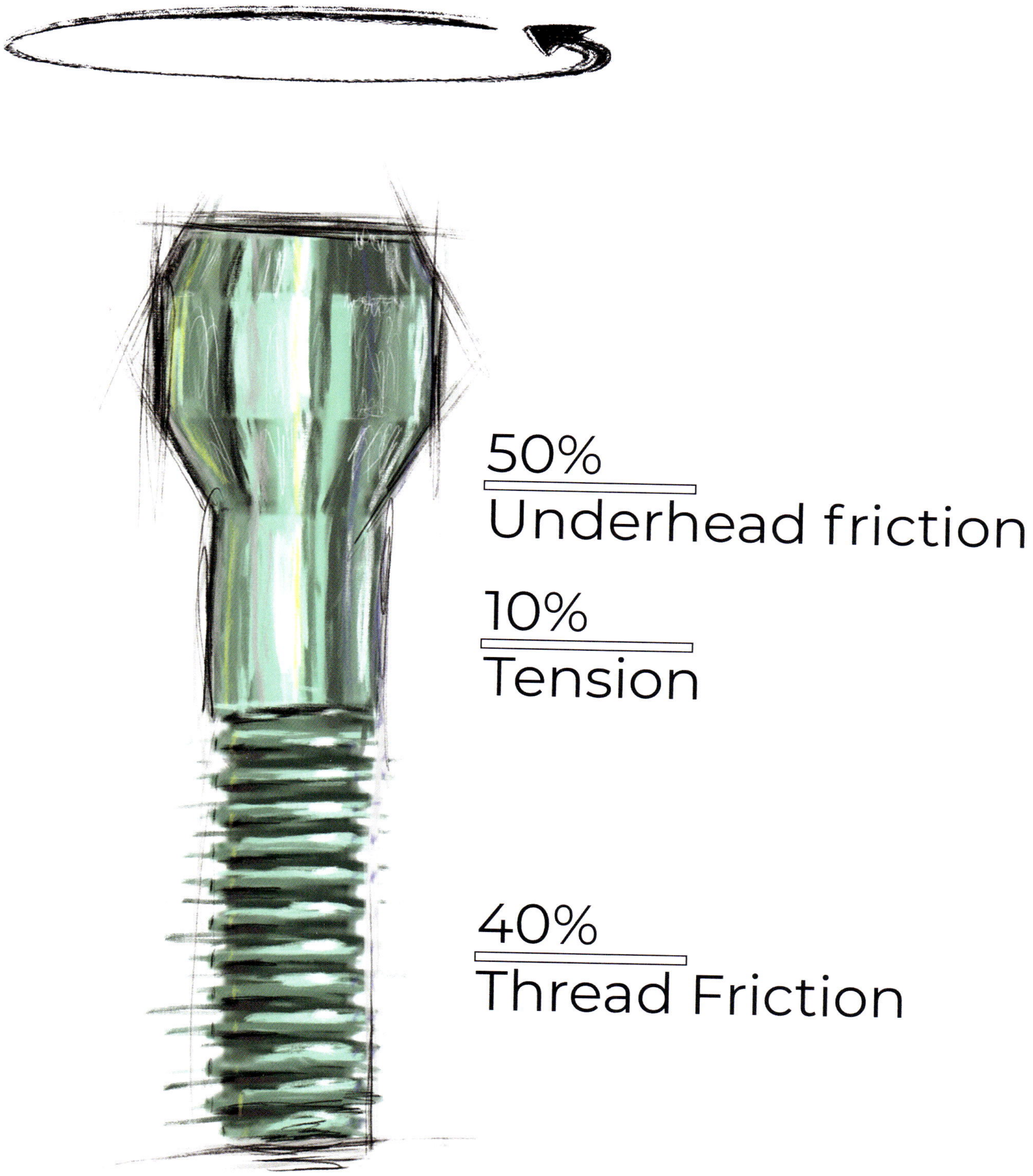

Figure 7-26 Torque is distributed between the head and the platform (underhead friction), between the threads (thread friction), and some is loaded as tension in the shank of the screw. These estimated percentages vary considerably depending on the design and materials.

BROKEN SCREW

Prosthetic screws break sometimes, and their retrieval can be intimidating. Simplify retrieval by figuring out why it broke, where it broke, and what is holding it in. The main issues I have found are stripped head, cross threading and fracture of the shank. The head will strip if the driver is not fully engaged or if it is over torqued. Make sure the driver is in line with the axis of the screw and follow manufacturer's instructions on final torque. If the screw is cross-threaded, it will never fully seat and it can permanently damage the internal threading of the implant. If it doesn't feel totally passive when the screw is engaging, and for the first few twists, it may be cross threading. Make sure everything is lined up straight and that the access through the crown or abutment is adequate.

Screws most often fracture from excessive lateral forces fatiguing the metal over time. When this happens, there is usually a part of the screw retained within the implant. Thankfully, this piece is usually somewhat loose in there. The majority of the retention of the screw was between the underhead friction and thread friction. When it breaks, the retained piece doesn't have much retention. Using an explorer tip and a lot of patience, think of drawing counterclockwise circles on the retained piece. An ultrasonic tip may also be beneficial. After working at it for a while, consider taking a PA to determine the progress. A slow spinning end cutting bur could also loosen it up. If this doesn't work, several companies offer kits specifically designed for screw retrieval. Follow their instructions carefully to avoid damaging the implant. In my experience, my implant rep has been quite helpful in these situations.

References

1. Misch CE, Bidez MW. Implant-protected occlusion: a biomechanical rationale. Compendium. 1994 Nov;15(11):1330, 1332, 1334 passim; quiz 1344.
2. Tarnow DP, Cho SC, Wallace SS. The effect of inter-implant distance on the height of inter-implant bone crest. J Periodontol. 2000 Apr;71(4):546-549.
3. Monje A, Chan HL, Galindo-Moreno P, et al. Alveolar Bone Architecture: A Systematic Review and Meta-Analysis. J Periodontol. 2015 Nov;86(11):1231-1248.
4. Strbac GD, Giannis K, Unger E, Mittlböck M, Vasak C, Watzek G, et al. Drilling- and withdrawing-related thermal changes during implant site osteotomies. Clin Implant Dent Relat Res. 2015 Feb;17(1):32-43.
5. Arsalanloo Z, Telchi R, Osgouie KG. Optimum Selection of the Dental Implants according to Length and Diameter Parameters by FE Method in the Anterior Position. Int J Biosci Biochem Bioinforma. 2014;4(4):265-269.
6. Tavelli L, Barootchi S, Avila-Ortiz G, et al. Peri-implant soft tissue phenotype modification and its impact on peri-implant health: A systematic review and network meta-analysis. J Periodontol. 2021 Jan;92(1):21-44.
7. Hulsey CM. An esthetic evaluation of lip-teeth relationships present in the smile. Am J Orthod. 1970 Feb;57(2):132-144.
8. Fürhauser R, Florescu D, Benesch T, et al. Evaluation of soft tissue around single-tooth implant crowns: the pink esthetic score. Clin Oral Implants Res. 2005 Dec;16(6):639-644.
9. Tarnow DP, Magner AW, Fletcher P. The effect of the distance from the contact point to the crest of bone on the presence or absence of the interproximal dental papilla. J Periodontol. 1992 Dec;63(12):995-996.
10. MS AC By Robert Levine, DDS, William Martin, DMD. Esthetic Risk Assessment in Implant Dentistry | Inside Dentistry [Internet]. [cited 2022 Dec 17]. Available from: https://www.aegisdentalnetwork.com/id/2012/08/esthetic-risk-assessment-in-implant-dentistry
11. Swami V, Vijayaraghavan V, Swami V. Current trends to measure implant stability. J Indian Prosthodont Soc. 2016;16(2):124-130.
12. Resonance Frequency Analysis in Implant Dentistry [Internet]. Decisions in Dentistry. 2017 [cited 2023 Apr 19]. Available from: https://decisionsindentistry.com/article/resonance-frequency-analysis-implant-dentistry/
13. Jokstad A, Ganeles J. Systematic review of clinical and patient-reported outcomes following oral rehabilitation on dental implants with a tapered compared to a non-tapered implant design. Clin Oral Implants Res. 2018 Oct;29 Suppl 16:41-54.
14. Jemat A, Ghazali MJ, Razali M, et al. Surface Modifications and Their Effects on Titanium Dental Implants. Biomed Res Int. 2015;2015:791725.
15. Norton MR, Åström M. The Influence of Implant Surface on Maintenance of Marginal Bone Levels for Three Premium Implant Brands: A Systematic Review and Meta-analysis. Int J Oral Maxillofac Implants. 2020;35(6):1099-1111.
16. Zhang H, Shan J, Zhang P, et al. Trabeculae microstructure parameters serve as effective predictors for marginal bone loss of dental implant in the mandible. Sci Rep. 2020 Oct 28;10(1):18437.
17. Brånemark PI. Introduction to osseointegration. In: Brånemark PI, Zarb G, Albrektsson T, editors. Tissue-integrated prostheses. Osseointegration in clinical dentistry. Chicago and Tokyo: Quintessence; 1985.
18. Rupp F, Liang L, Geis-Gerstorfer J, et al. Surface characteristics of dental implants: A review. Dent Mater. 2018 Jan;34(1):40-57.
19. Himmlová L, Dostálová T, Kácovský A, et al. Influence of implant length and diameter on stress distribution: a finite element analysis. J Prosthet Dent. 2004 Jan;91(1):20-25.
20. Li T, Hu K, Cheng L, Ding Y, Ding Y, Shao J, et al. Optimum selection of the dental implant diameter and length in the posterior mandible with poor bone quality – A 3D finite element analysis. Applied Mathematical Modelling. 2011 Jan 1;35(1):446-456.
21. Frost HM. Skeletal structural adaptations to mechanical usage (SATMU): 1. Redefining Wolff's law: the bone modeling problem. Anat Rec. 1990 Apr;226(4):403-413.
22. Petrie CS, Williams JL. Comparative evaluation of implant designs: influence of diameter, length, and taper on strains in the alveolar crest. Clin Oral Implants Res. 2005;16(4):486-494.
23. Rameh S, Menhall A, Younes R. Key factors influencing short implant success. Oral Maxillofac Surg. 2020 Sep;24(3):263-275.
24. Toniollo MB, Macedo AP, Pupim D, et al. Three-Dimensional Finite Element Analysis Surface Stress Distribution on Regular and Short Morse Taper Implants Generated by Splinted and Nonsplinted Prostheses in the Rehabilitation of Various Bony Ridges. J Craniofac Surg. 2016 May;27(3):e276-280.
25. Fokas G, Ma L, Chronopoulos V, et al. Differences in micromorphology of the implant–abutment junction for original and third-party abutments on a representative dental implant. J Prosthet Dent. 2019 Jan 1;121(1):143-150.
26. Gigandet M, Bigolin G, Faoro F, et al. Implants with original and non-original abutment connections. Clin Implant Dent Relat Res. 2014 Apr;16(2):303-311.
27. Ebadian B, Fathi A, Khodadad S. Comparison of the Effect of Four Different Abutment Screw Torques on Screw Loosening in Single Implant-Supported Prosthesis after the Application of Mechanical Loading. Int J Dent. 2021 Jul 19;2021:3595064.

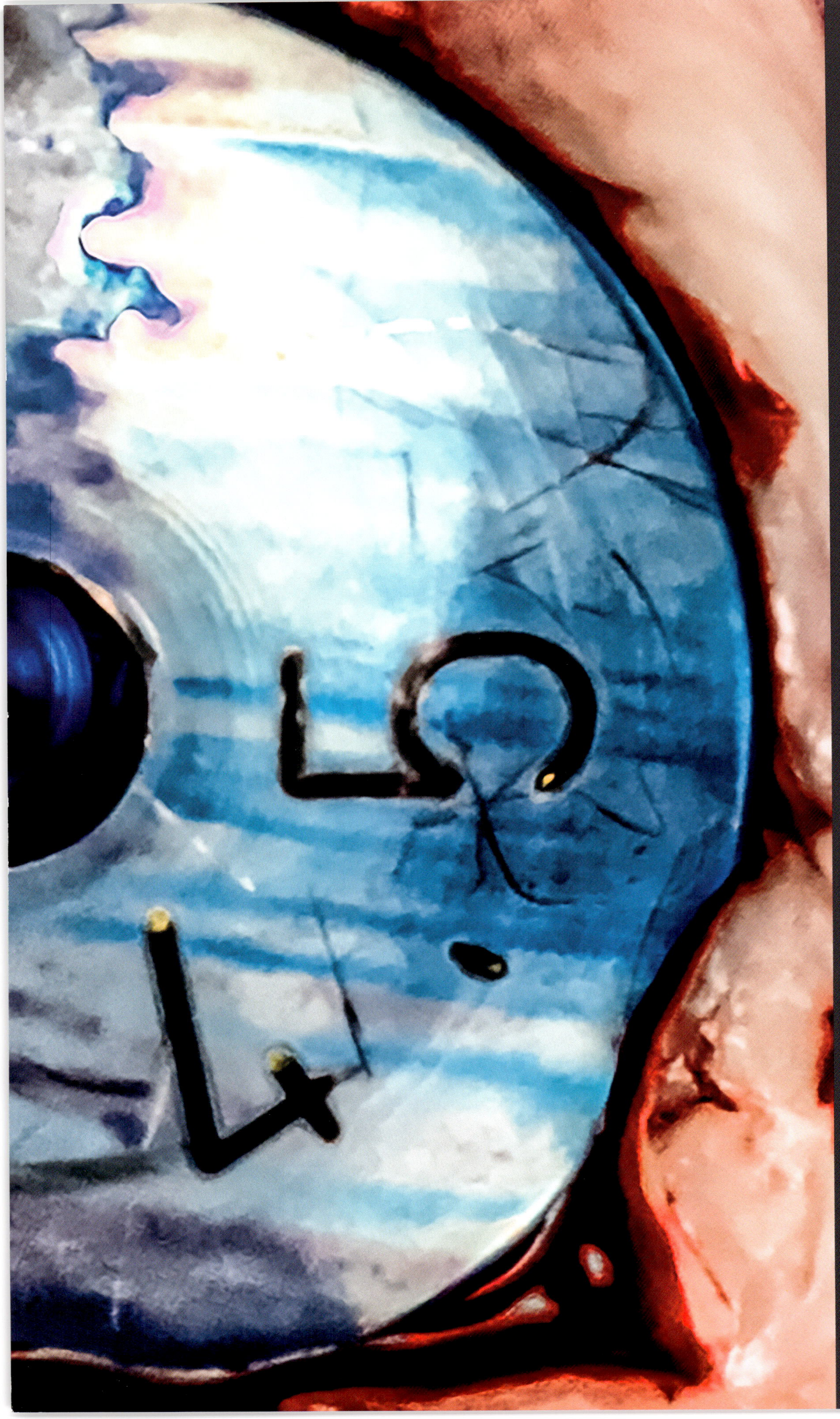

Titanium Record.

CHAPTER 8

IMPLANT SURGICAL PRINCIPLES: THE MOVEMENT OF IMPLANT SURGERY

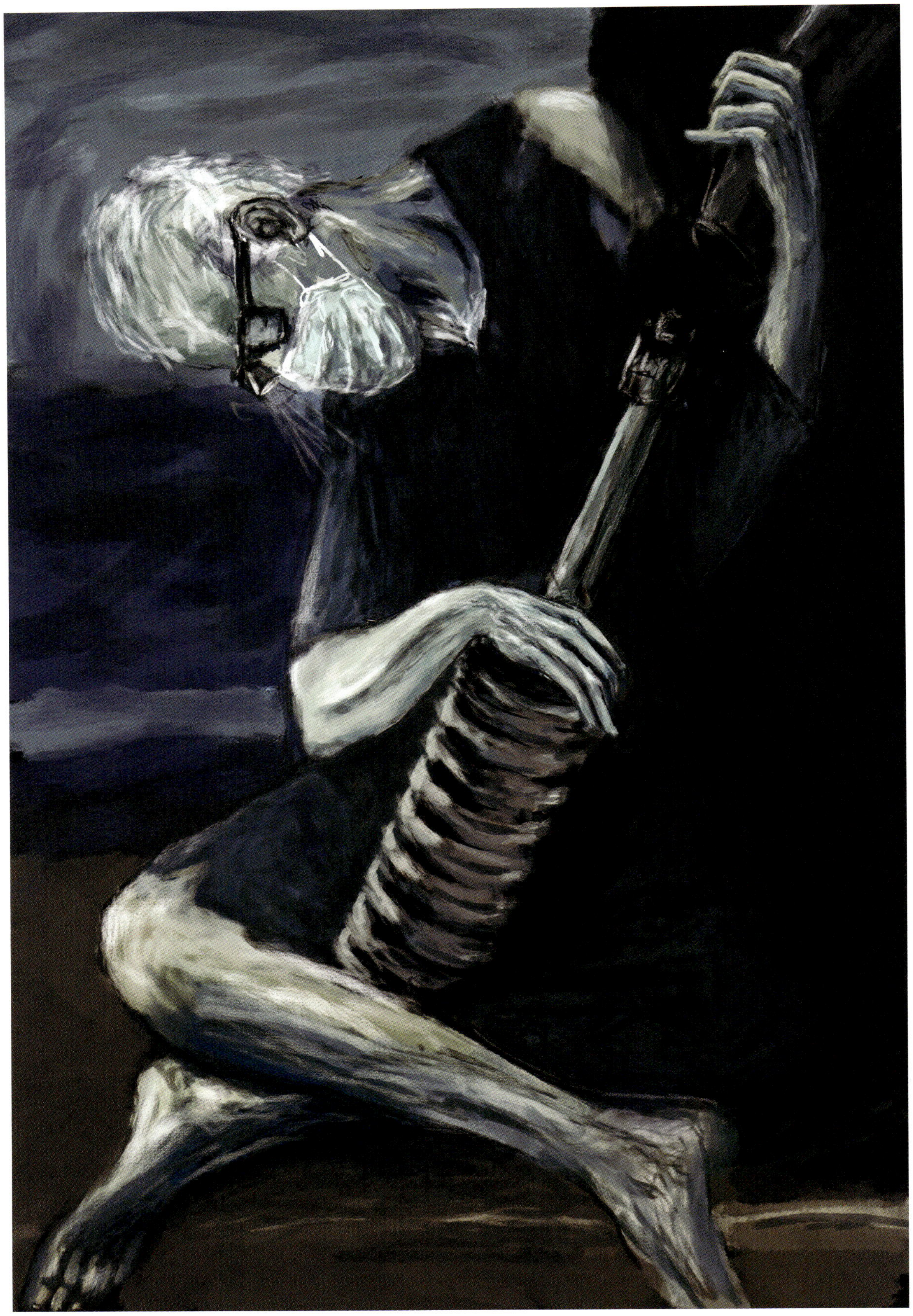

"The Old Implantologist." This painting says so much. (Artwork inspired by Pablo Picasso.)

In the movement of implant surgery, there are some consistent core surgical principles that play out as general themes as well as countless variations playing on those general themes. When I think about it, the idea of "theme and variations" keeps coming to mind. It is like some of the piano pieces I played growing up: There is a core melody that is the theme, and the variations are the melodic and rhythmic changes that make the music what it is. The many different successful techniques in implant surgery are all variations on a theme. These procedural variations all retain specific elements or themes fundamental to successful surgery. Let's explore some of the core themes and variations in the movement of implant surgery.

Theme 1: Implant Position

Surgery starts with the incision. This is when planning transforms into reality. A perfectly planned implant must be translated from a radiographic image and mental concept to flesh and blood. The incision is where the rubber first meets the road. It is the first commitment in implant surgery. The incision frames the implant. Take the time to acclimate and orient yourself to the anatomy and the plan just before cutting. It helps ensure the implant ends up exactly where it was planned to be.

Variations

Freehand or guided

The ideal position of an implant depends on the restoration as well as the available bone and soft tissue. But ultimately, an implant is no good if it can't be restored. There are three main techniques to control the position of an implant during surgery: freehand, static guide and dynamic navigation. Depending on the circumstances and surgeon, an argument can be made for each technique. Accuracy and precision are better with static or dynamic guided surgery than with freehand surgery[1]. Static guidance uses a prefabricated jig to direct the instruments. Dynamic guidance is like a GPS system for the instruments, showing your position in relation to the anatomy in real time. It uses cameras and markers that provide live feedback through a computer system showing the position of the instruments on the CBCT. Dynamic navigation is more fluid and adaptable during surgery. The plan can be adjusted intraoperatively, allowing the surgeon to accommodate nuances and variations as they develop.

Both static and dynamic guidance rely on accurate planning and execution. If planning and preparation are not accurately executed, they can guide an implant right through a nerve. A level of competence and awareness is critical regardless of the system you use. Trust but verify.

Regardless of whether the implant is guided or placed freehand (some call this brain guided), it is tremendously beneficial to orient yourself to the site before making the incision. Line up the starter drill in the planned position. Observe the angulation of the axis and lateral position from multiple angles. Even with dynamic navigation, it is quite beneficial to use a mirror to confirm the implant will be as close to dead-center as possible. The mirror allows you to view the implant from palatal, buccal and occlusal perspectives that you can't see with direct vision. A centered implant optimizes the emergence profile. It also looks good on an x-ray for the rest of the patient's life. It takes only a few seconds to confirm the position. It is worth it.

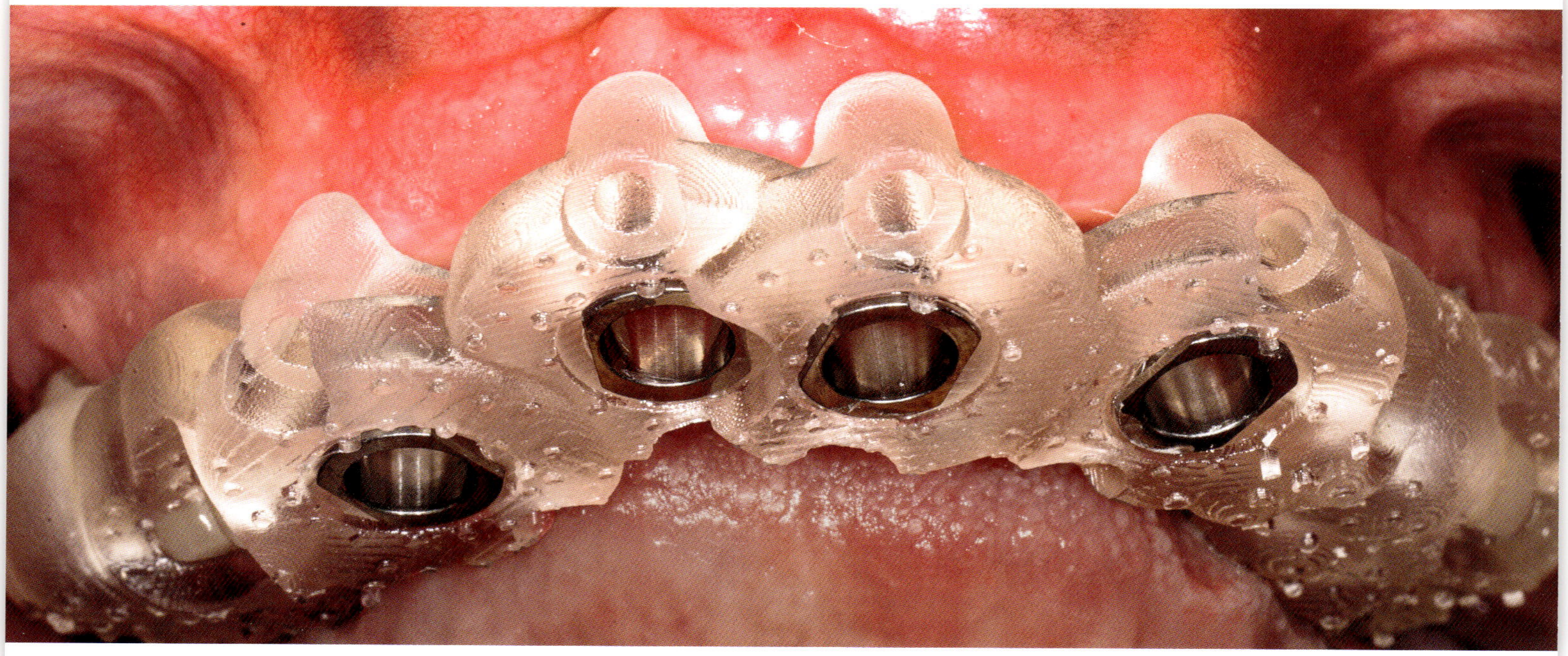

Figure 8-1 Static printed guides rely on pre-operative planning, so there is less flexibility during surgery. There are a few key factors that help when using these guides. Irrigation channels on the buccal and lingual optimize access. Generous cutouts verify complete seating if it is a tooth-born guide. The entire process relies on the guide being fully seated. Clearance around the crowns must be adequate so the guide doesn't engage undercuts. I always prefer my guides to have less coverage. I would prefer this guide to have larger cutouts around the teeth, less crown coverage, and more clearance in the entire anterior portion for the flap. When I elevated the flap for surgery, it was difficult to reflect it and maintain adequate seating of the guide.

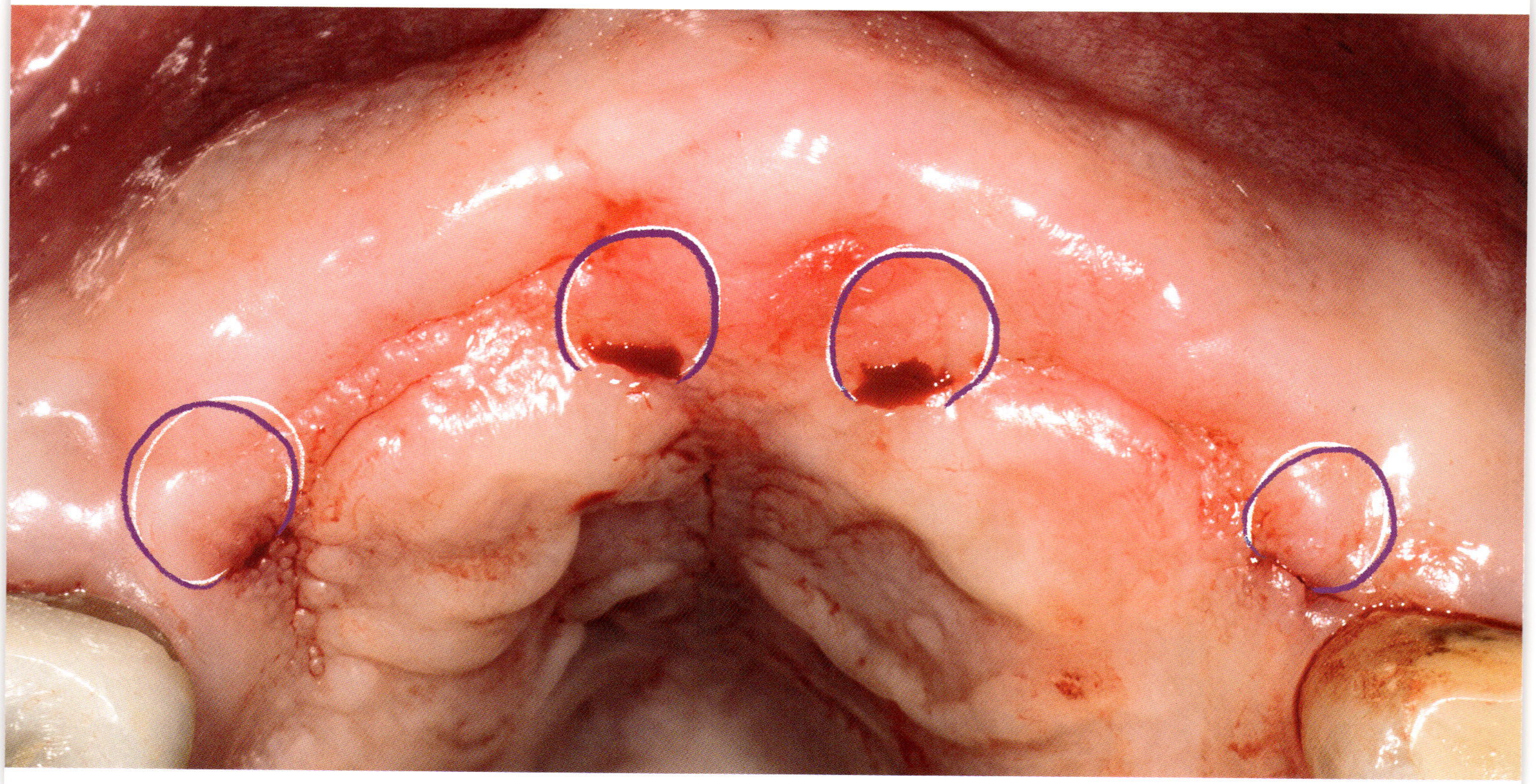

Figure 8-2 The outlines of the anticipated implants are drawn here. The palatal aspect of the implant position is marked through the guide. The incision usually follows these marks, reflecting the thick keratinized gingiva facially.

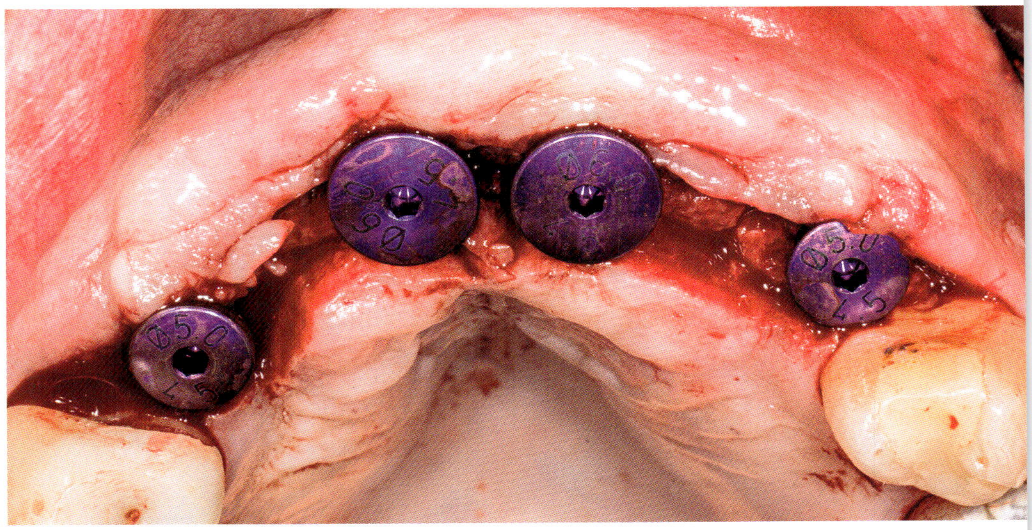

Figure 8-3 Guiding surgery allows implants to be ideally positioned for the restorations. It also helps with soft tissue management. There is no guessing where the implant will emerge. This provides tremendous confidence when planning the incision.

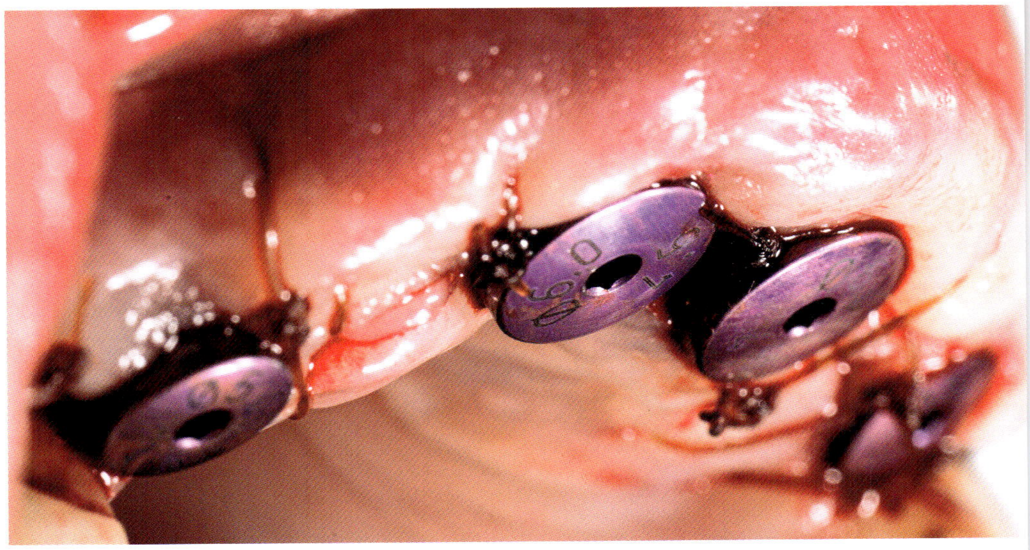

Figure 8-4 Multiple interrupted 4-0 chromic sutures stabilized the tissue. It was left to heal in by secondary intention between the implants.

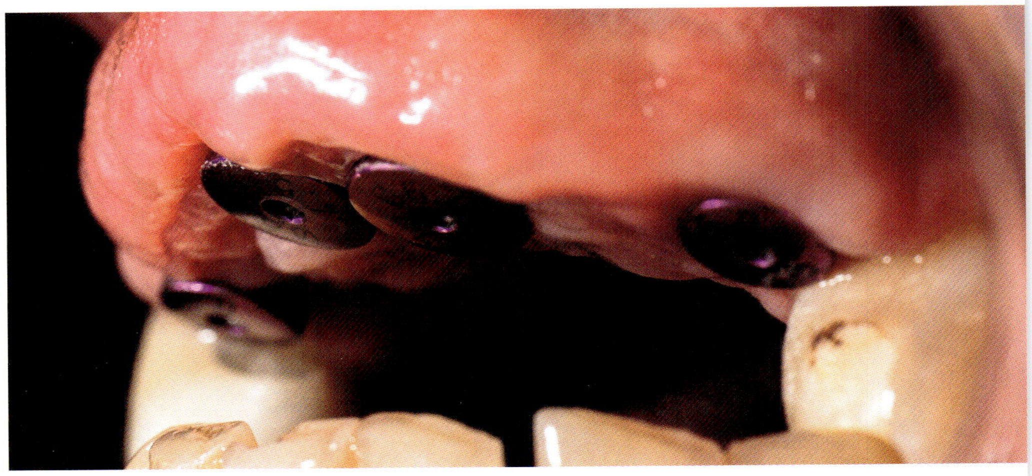

Figure 8-5 After 2 weeks of healing, the gingiva is filling in nicely.

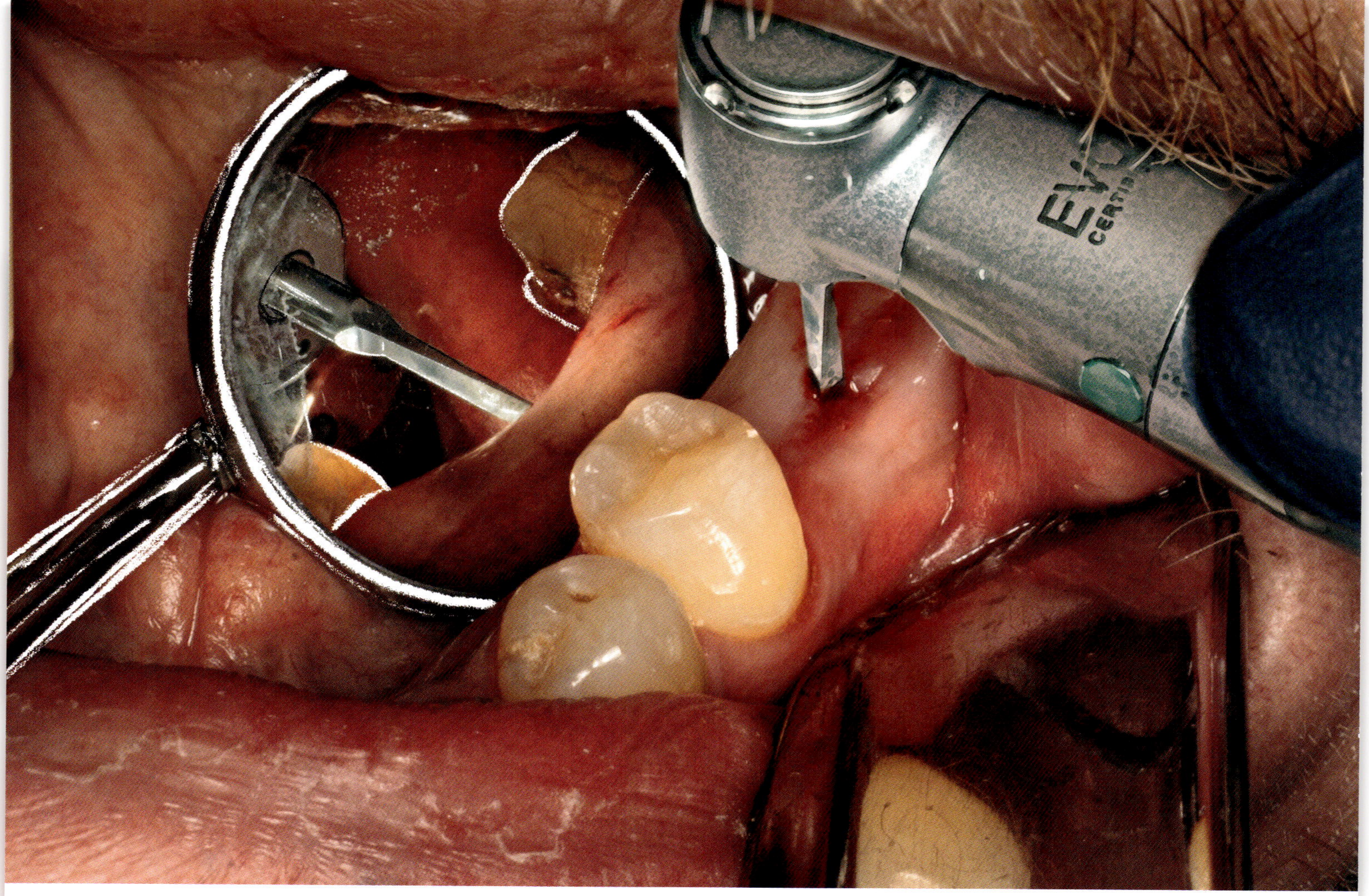

Figure 8-6 Even with dynamic navigation, the mirror can be used to verify optimal mesial-distal position. If it doesn't appear perfect, the plan can be tweaked to ensure ideal position.

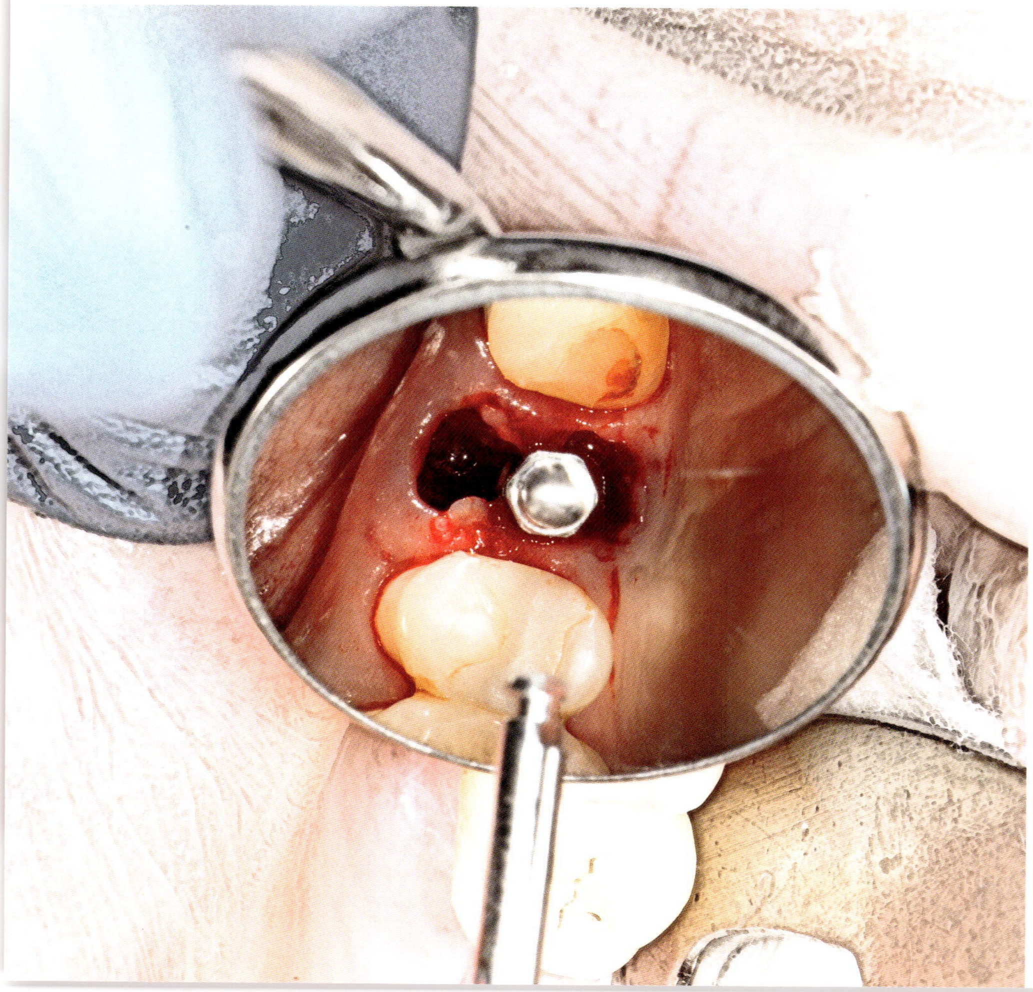

Figure 8-7 Verify the position throughout the implant process. An implant drill can simply be placed into the osteotomy after it is used to confirm the angulation clinically. A radiograph can also be taken with the drill in the site.

Most starter drills have a sharp enough point to mark the tissue in the center of the planned implant position. The small red dot created by gently pressing the tip into the tissue provides great perspective on where to make the incision. (This is further discussed in Chapter 9: Implant Site Development.) In an edentulous site, there is typically some hard or soft tissue atrophy. A lingually or palatally favored incision develops a small flap that can be translated buccally to improve the tissue thickness and overall tissue contours. If the incision is placed directly over the middle of the planned implant, half of the crestal soft tissue will be mobilized to the lingual and only half to the buccal. At times, this is ideal. More commonly, though, the buccal tissue has suffered from atrophy and needs increased thickness. I find it rare that a site is best served by simply excising a plug with a tissue punch. It may be slightly quicker or easier, but preserving and manipulating the tissue with a well-placed incision is low hanging fruit. It also sets up the site if you want to reflect a slightly larger flap to confirm the position and the overlying bone. The incision can also be extended to include the papilla, raising a conservative envelope flap for tissue manipulation or minor augmentation. The slight bit of increased discomfort a patient may experience from broadening the exposure is far less than the lifelong challenges that come with a poorly positioned implant.

Technology is an adjunct to skill and experience, not a replacement. Plan the implant to optimize the outcome. When guiding surgery, it always pays off to confirm the accuracy by looking at the angulation of the drills or even taking a quick intraoperative PA radiograph.

Theme 2: Protect the Bone

My grandfather used to tell me a sharp knife is safer than a dull one. (He had a small side business sharpening knives and scissors in his shop for about 60 years.) The same is true with drills. A sharp cutting edge on a drill reduces heat and improves control. It is important to replace drills on a schedule. This advice can be a bit tough to swallow when it comes from an implant rep who makes money on each drill. I will admit I previously used drills until they felt like they needed to be replaced. That was early in my solo practice career. I have learned over the years the cost of compromising is not worth it.

One of the most common surgical causes of implant failure is thermal injury to the surrounding bone[2]. It is the very bone contacting the implant that is responsible for the process of osseointegration. Drilling an implant osteotomy and placing the implant pose a tremendous threat to the health of the bone. Thermal injury triggers a cascade of events leading to necrosis of the bone and expulsion of the implant as a foreign object rather than integration and long-term stability. When bone reaches an excess of 47 degrees Celsius, proteins become denatured, which ultimately leads to necrosis. Two ways to protect the bone from thermal injury are to reduce heat generation and cool the bone with irrigation.

Friction is a force opposing motion between two touching objects. When two objects (like a drill and bone) are forced to move against each other, some of the kinetic energy is transformed to heat. The molecules on the surface of a drill and the bone cells it is rubbing against move faster when they rub together. The faster the molecules move, the more heat is generated. Reducing friction reduces this heat.

There are a few ways to reduce friction. If the objects are rubbing together slower, they generate less heat. Lower speed drilling may take a bit more time or be a bit more difficult to control, but it will decrease the potential for thermal injury to the bone.

A sharp cutting edge on a drill reduces friction by cutting the bone more efficiently. There is less rubbing of the molecules and more cutting. When a drill bit is dull, there is a tendency to press harder to get it to cut through the bone, further increasing the heat. Maintaining fresh, quality drills will improve success by protecting the bone. Irrigation decreases friction through lubrication, and it helps dissipate the heat. Copious irrigation can clear bone debris from the flutes of certain drill designs, improving cutting efficiency.

Figure 8-8 Typical implant drills cut bone as they drill. When the flutes fill with bone, the efficiency of the cutting-edge decreases. There is nowhere for the cut bone to go. This decreases effectiveness and increases friction. Pay attention to the efficiency of the drill. If it gets clogged with bone, consider clearing it before advancing it further. Increasing irrigation and pumping the drill in and out while advancing it can also improve the bone clearing.

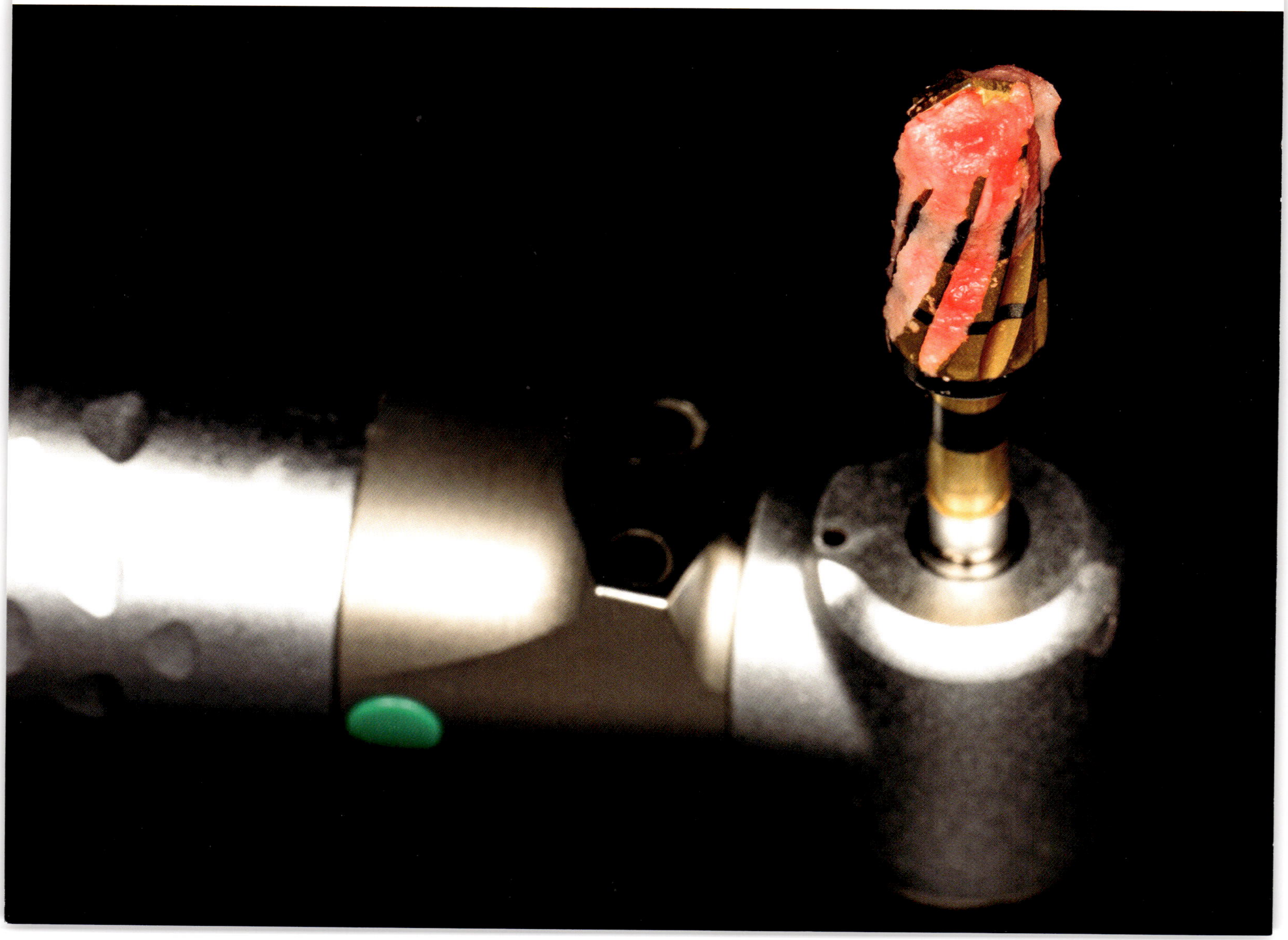

Variations

Drilling speed

Implant systems have their own recommended rpm settings for drilling and implant placement. There may even be different recommendations for different drills within the kit or different bone density situations. The unique design of each drill changes how it engages the bone, thus influencing the ideal drilling speed. If the drill is spinning too slow, cutting efficiency declines, and it takes more pressure to make progress. This can have a deleterious effect on the bone as well[3]. It is wise to set the drill speed at or slightly below the recommended speed and work within that range.

Pauses

Intermittent breaks from advancing the drill also allow heat to dissipate. Consider releasing the pressure for short, 2 to 3 second breaks while continuing to irrigate. Backing the drill up a few millimeters briefly will accomplish this as well and potentially clear some of the bone from the flutes of the drill. Be careful to maintain a precise drilling axis. This pumping action can ream out the osteotomy, making it slightly wider if the drill axis shifts.

Self-irrigating handpiece

Automating the irrigation process through the handpiece has pros and cons. It gives up some control of where the irrigation goes. A great assistant, at times, may be able to irrigate better than a self-irrigating handpiece. But self-irrigation is like giving your assistant a third hand that doesn't ever get in your way. They are still able to retract and suction with their other two hands while the drill irrigates the site. Keep an eye on the irrigation. It may easily be deflected without notice. When drilling through a CT guide, for instance, great attention must be given to ensure adequate irrigation reaches the surgical site. A guide can deflect most of the irrigation away from the site. When using a static guide, consider that an irrigating syringe can most effectively cool the site when there are properly designed irrigation holes in the guide. In these cases, turn off the self-irrigating function to prevent drowning the patient.

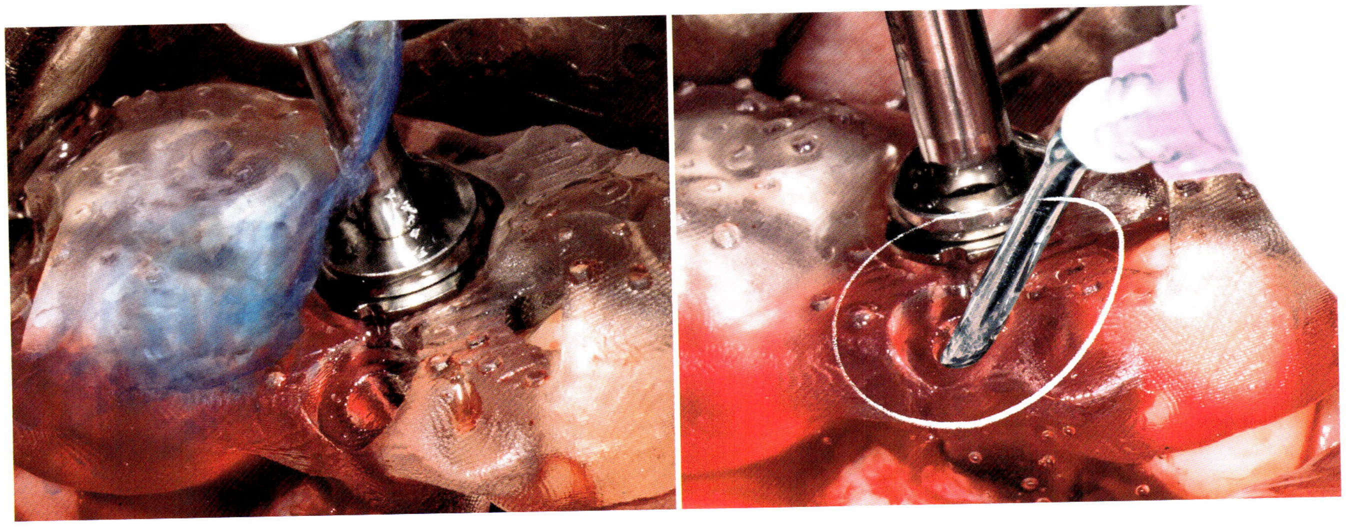

Figure 8-9 The water from a self-irrigating drill can easily get deflected from the osteotomy with potentially devastating results. A hole in the guide is designed to direct irrigation into the osteotomy, optimizing cooling and clearing of the water.

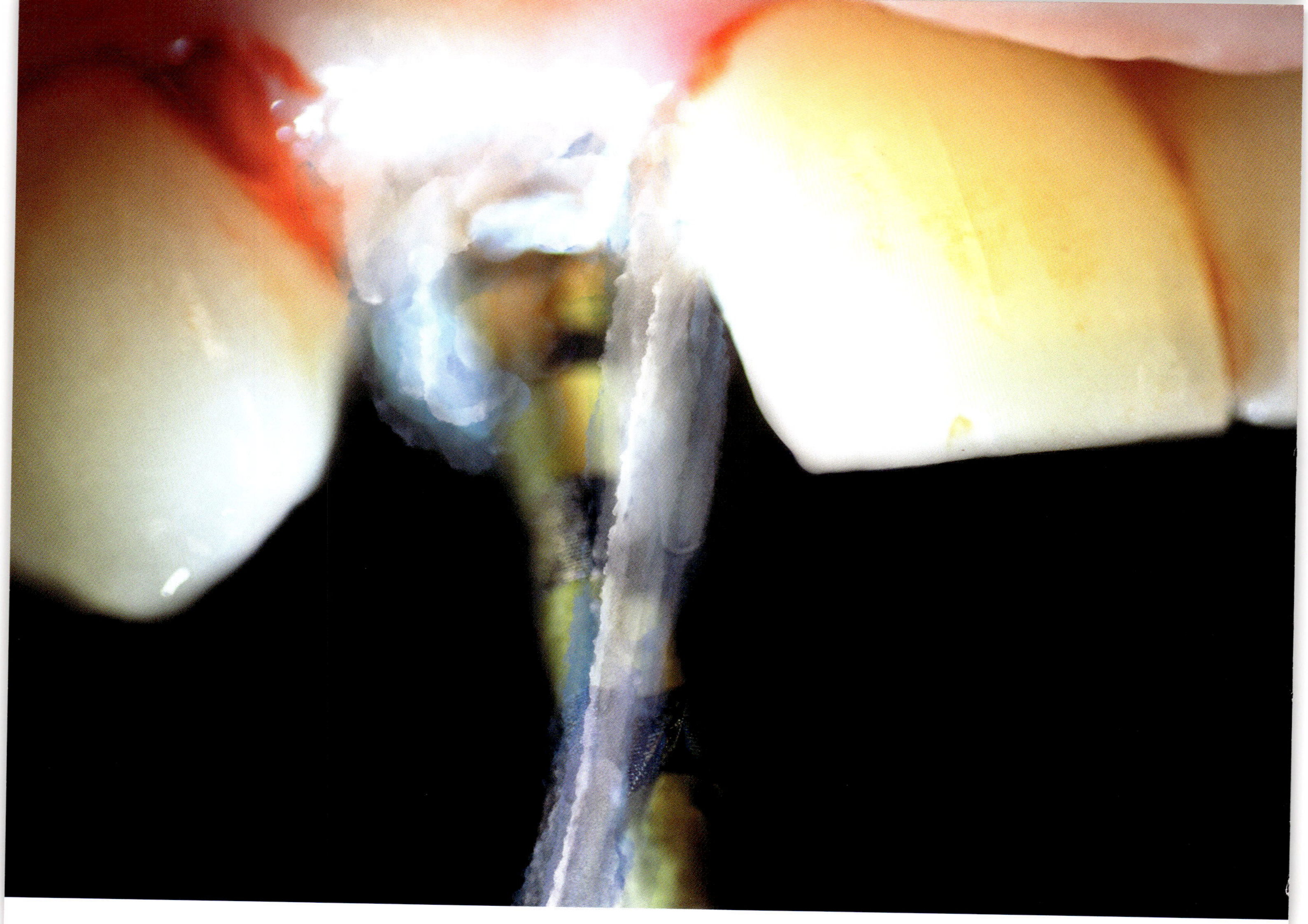

Figure 8-10 Water from self-irrigating drills hits the drill part way up the shank. Keep a close eye to ensure irrigation reaches the bur and is adequately cooling and clearing the drill.

Osseodensification

This clever variation in drill design is intended to retain the majority of the bone in the implant preparation site. Instead of removing it with a cutting edge, the bone is displaced laterally in incremental steps. This increases the density of the bone lining the implant site and potentially increases the bone width surrounding the implant. This system follows the core theme of protecting the bone by promoting copious irrigation and caution to avoid overheating the bone. But there are some key distinctions with this system that seem to contradict conventional protocols. Its design can be used in a clockwise or counterclockwise rotation. The flutes are beveled to cut in clockwise rotation to remove bone in situations where it is too dense to apply the densification technique. In the counterclockwise rotation, they are specifically designed to safely spread and condense the bone outward. This relies on the elasticity and plasticity of the bone in a technique sensitive preparation protocol described as "pumping the bur with haptic feedback." The advantage of moving instead of removing the patient's bone to optimize the site is attractive and can overcome the limitations of soft bone better than if you just under prepare the osteotomy. This technique has established its place in my practice. I especially like it for sinus augmentations and low-density, maxillary situations.

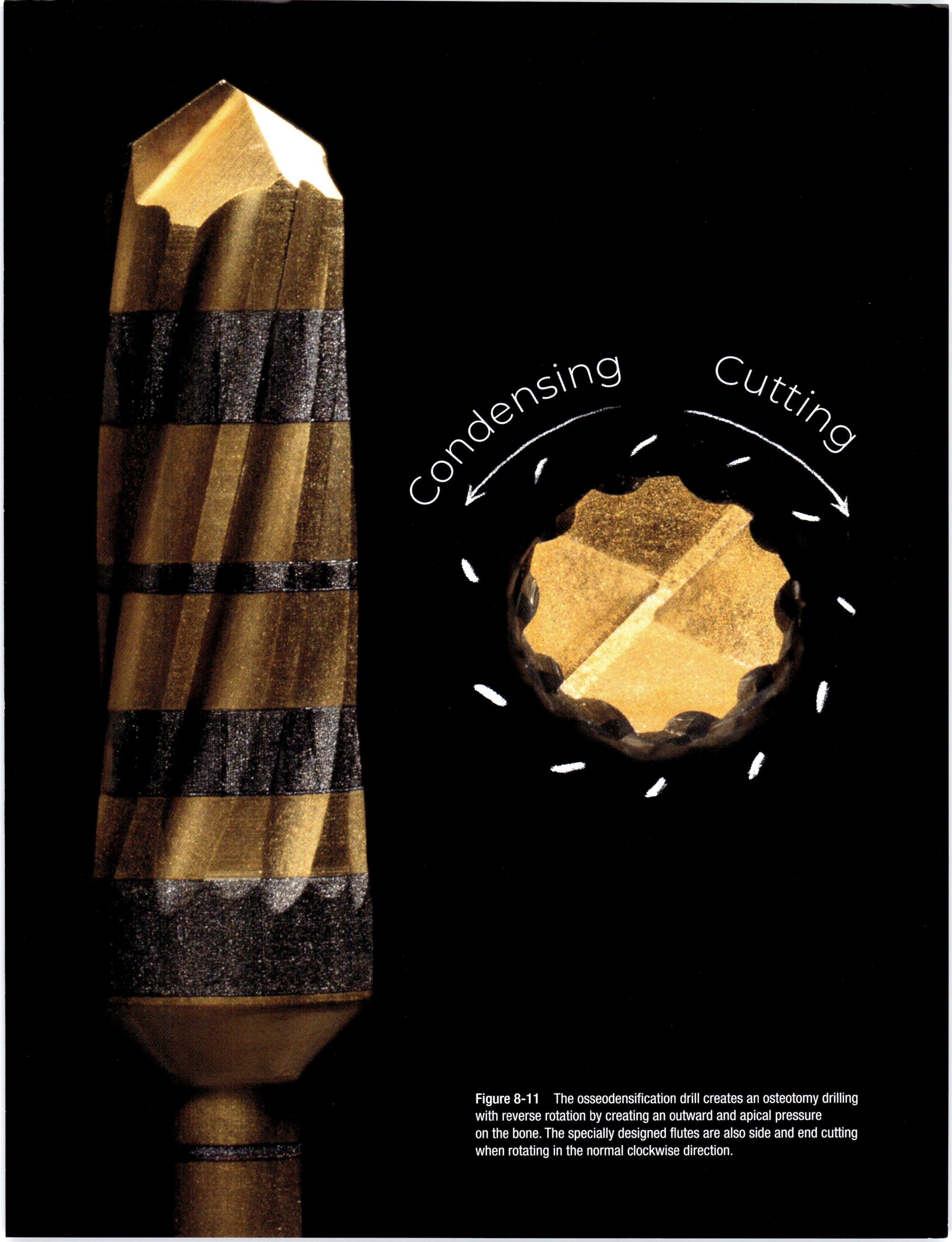

Figure 8-11 The osseodensification drill creates an osteotomy drilling with reverse rotation by creating an outward and apical pressure on the bone. The specially designed flutes are also side and end cutting when rotating in the normal clockwise direction.

Theme 3: Stability

An implant must be relatively immobile for the bone to heal properly around it. Implant threads engage the bone, stabilizing it upon insertion (Refer to the discussion in Chapter 7: Implant Architecture). Insertion torque is the most obvious and immediate indication of stability. There is a general range, or sweet spot, for insertion torque for each implant system as indicated by the manufacturer. Too much torque and the bone or implant can be damaged. Too little torque and the potential micromotion stimulates fibrous healing instead of osseous healing.

Preparation of each individual implant site is unique. You can't just use drills 1 through 5 for every type of bone. Feedback from the instruments while drilling helps guide the preparation and achieve ideal stability. High density bone requires preparing a larger osteotomy, very near the size of the implant fixture. This reduces friction and excessive insertion torque. Low density bone requires a much narrower osteotomy to increase the bone contact and torque, optimizing stability. Even when using the protocols recommended for the specific bone density, there are times when the implant insertion torque either exceeds or fails to hit the sweet spot.

Variations

Sweet spot

Each system has its own recommended torque range, typically between 15 to 70 Ncm. Some systems claim success with torque values in the single digits. Others recommend a maximum torque of 45 Ncm while others may allow exceeding 70 Ncm. It should be our goal to understand the limits and requirements of the systems we are using. In addition to reading the manual, it may be beneficial to talk with the implant rep. Good reps often have insight on how to optimize their implant for success. However, this must not be confused with the value of clinical judgment and surgical experience.

High torque

There is typically a progressive increase in torque as an implant is inserted to its final position. Several different techniques can be employed when the maximum torque is achieved before the implant is fully seated. If an implant is almost to the ideal position when max torque is hit, it is tempting to leave it slightly high or just crank on the wrench and over torque the implant into the final position. But that may compromise the outcome.

When torque is too high, the osteotomy may be too narrow, too short or both. The nuances of determining this and accommodating for it depend on the design of the individual implant. Tapered implants will behave differently than straight walled implants. But in general, if the implant torques out just before final seating, it may be because there are bone chips in the apical portion of the osteotomy, the osteotomy is not deep enough, or the apical portion is not wide enough. Clearing the apical portion or deepening the osteotomy should help. If high resistance is met when the implant is seated only halfway or less, the whole osteotomy likely needs to be widened.

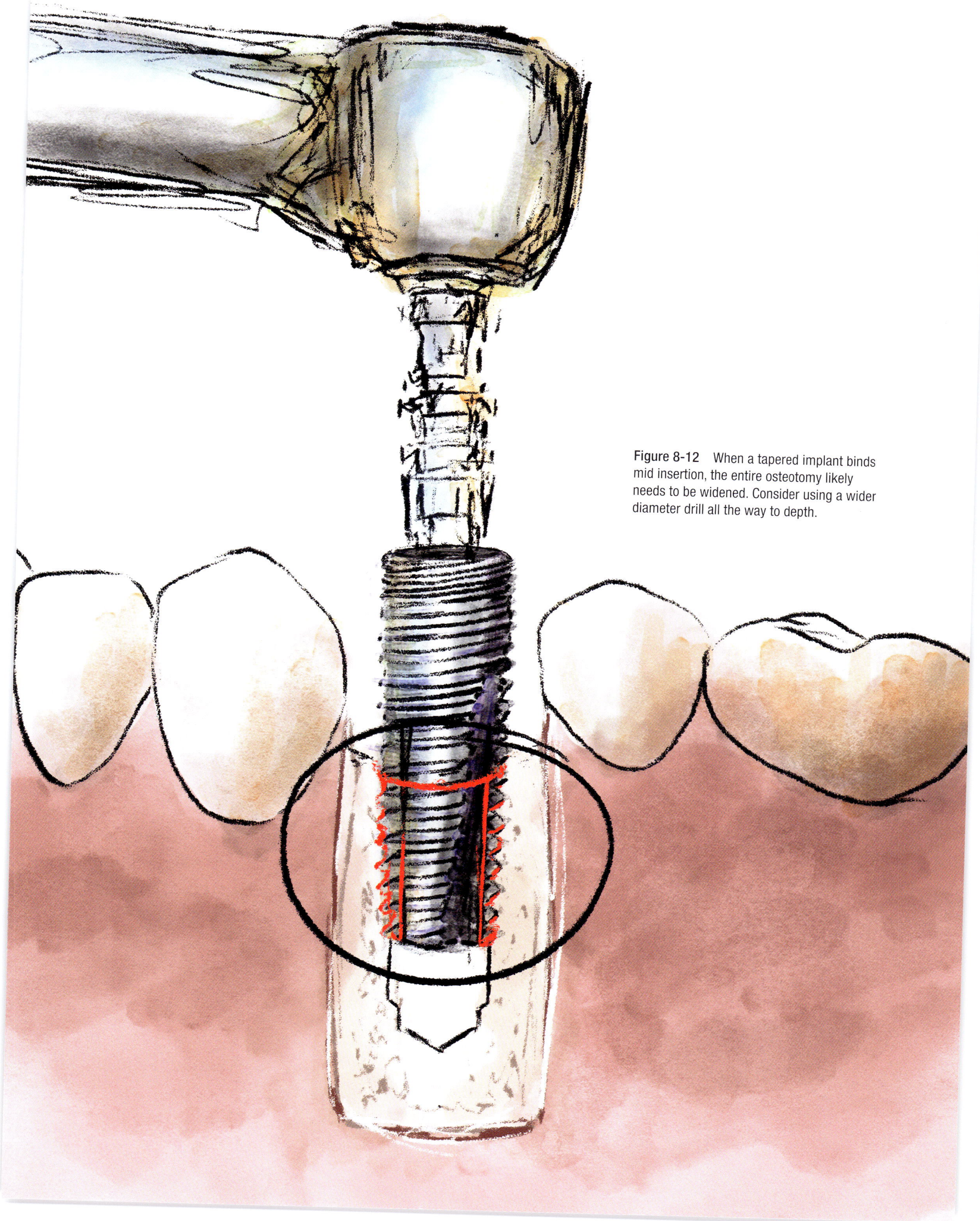

Figure 8-12 When a tapered implant binds mid insertion, the entire osteotomy likely needs to be widened. Consider using a wider diameter drill all the way to depth.

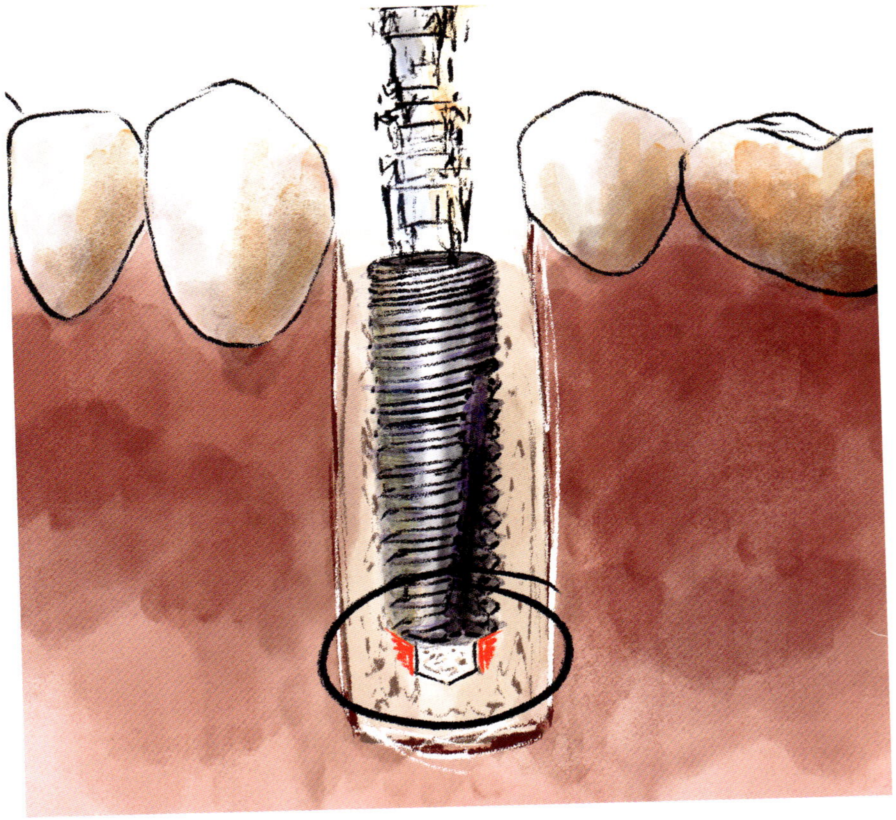

Figure 8-13 When the implant binds near its final depth, the apical portion may need to be cleared out, or the osteotomy may need to be deepened. In these cases, you may consider using the initial "final drill" and just go deeper to clear out the apex.

Drill more

Ensure the osteotomy is completely to depth or the implant will certainly not seat adequately. If the initial osteotomy was slightly short, pass the final drill a bit deeper to make space for the implant to seat fully in the bone. It may also be beneficial to go slightly beyond the planned depth with the final drill if there is adequate apical clearance. Flushing the site to remove debris can clear out the most apical portion of the osteotomy, making room for the implant.

Drill feedback is priceless. Pay attention to it. Notice where and how the drill engages bone. It may feel like the apical extent of the site is a solid wall of bone resisting the drill. The radiograph will usually corroborate the surgical feel. In this situation, it may be necessary to revert back to some of the initial end-cutting drills and work your way back up to the final diameter to safely deepen it without too much heat. Significant heat can be generated if a side cutting or shaping drill is used as an end-cutting drill to increase the depth. If it feels like the apical portion was easily cleared with additional drilling, it may be time to try placing the implant again. Sometimes, you can feel the drill engage bone at about the depth the implant had previously stopped. In these instances, it is relatively easy to know how much more drilling is needed to fully seat the implant. Be a bit cautious to avoid removing too much bone. It can be frustrating to go from excessive torque to no torque if the site gets over prepped.

If the implant torques out, binding halfway down, the width and possibly length of the osteotomy may need to be increased. If the implant system has a dense bone protocol, this may be the time to use it. In rare cases, the dense bone protocol used to the proper depth still results in excessive torque. In such cases, consider further increasing osteotomy depth or possibly placing a shorter implant. But beware. If the bone is that dense, it likely has very poor blood supply and limited cellular availability, increasing the potential for failure. These high torque situations can also generate more heat. And this extremely dense bone is the least tolerant of heat. Proceed with caution. It may seem counterintuitive, but these are the situations that benefit from slightly lower insertion torque. With high density bone, aim for the low end of the recommended insertion torque. This is less taxing on bone that is already less cellular and less vascular.

Tapping

Implants are self-tapping by design. They cut their own thread pattern in the bone. Tapping bone creates a path for the implant threads to advance. Implant systems often have specific instrumentation for tapping dense bone. The implant itself may be able to effectively tap the site. But specific tapping drills are safer, more effective and more efficient at creating an internal thread pattern in high density bone. When a site has been tapped, the implant will abruptly meet high resistance when the implant threads encounter the un-tapped bone. Therefore, when using a tapping drill, make sure it is tapped deep enough to ensure the best final implant position.

Another technique to optimize torque in a high-density situation is to insert the implant slightly beyond the desired position, back the implant out a turn or two, and then reseat the implant to the desired depth. This effectively taps the bone and reduces the final torque to a safer level.

This is how I like to do it in my practice. My implant drill system has four presets:

1. 1500 rpm, full irrigation
2. 25 Ncm, 25 rpm, no irrigation
3. 45 Ncm, 25 rpm, no irrigation
4. 70 Ncm, 15 rpm, no irrigation

The first preset is for drilling. Normally, I don't go full speed for drilling. It depends on bone density and feedback from the drill. I often hover around 300 to 800 rpm. Preset two is for implant placement. I love it when the implant fully seats right at 25 Ncm. That just feels good. If it hits 25 Ncm very early, I go back to drilling. If it is almost completely seated, I use the third preset at 45 Ncm. With the current system I am using (Dentsply DS Prime Taper) I don't want to exceed 45 Ncm and would prefer to be around 25 Ncm. If the final turn hits 45, I may leave it. If I am concerned about bone vitality or the patient's healing potential, I may back it out a smidge and then re-insert it, stopping short of 45 Ncm.

If the torque exceeds 45 Ncm on the third preset, there are times I will advance to the fourth preset to get past that initial binding. At this higher torque, I slow the rotations down to 15 rpm to decrease the heat of friction and increase my control. I often turn irrigation on to further reduce the heat. At this point, the implant surface has been wetted by the blood and is covered by tissue, so the irrigation will not impact surface wetting. It may be beneficial to position the implant slightly beyond the final depth at this higher torque temporarily in order to back it out and then advance it to the final depth. When used judiciously, this often achieves an optimal torque. This technique of temporarily advancing the implant beyond the final depth to effectively "tap" the bone can be better than backing the implant out and drilling the site again for a few other reasons. It decreases the potential of contaminating the implant surface when removing it. The initial blood and implant surface wetting may be compromised by drying outside of the site. It is much quicker. And sometimes, the initial stability or position can be compromised if the site is over-prepared.

There are distinct risks with this technique as well. There is potential to cause pressure or thermal damage to the bone or harm the implant. Using the implant to tap dense bone in this way also runs the risk of damaging the implant's internal components. An implant driver is designed to engage the implant during insertion under normal load. Excessive force may damage or strip the anti-rotational components of the implant or driver. Over time, implant drivers can wear out and increase the chance of stripping or damaging internal components. If the driver is not fully seated, the risk of damaging internal components skyrockets.

If an implant is irreparably damaged or stripped due to high insertion torque, it may be extremely challenging to remove. The driver may no longer adequately engage the implant to back it out. This can be a big problem. You don't want to let a compromised implant integrate. If a guided implant kit is available with a driver that screws into the implant, it may be possible to adequately engage a damaged implant to remove it. Commercially available implant removal kits function in a similar way. They engage and stabilize the driver, the internal thread of the implant to engage the anti-rotational components. This significantly increases the amount of torque you can use to back the implant out. If all else fails in a situation like this, you may need to remove some of the precious surrounding alveolar bone to retrieve a damaged implant that is stuck due to high insertion torque. Afterall, the damaged fixture cannot be retained and would be even more difficult to remove if it integrates.

Damage to the precision internal components can also be a nightmare when delivering the restoration. It can make it impossible to fully seat the abutment or thread in the screw. If there is any suspicion of damage to the internal components, it must be thoroughly evaluated prior to proceeding. Removing and replacing a damaged implant during placement is so much easier than dealing with a damaged integrated implant. Visually inspecting the inside of the implant may reveal damage. Consider trying on a restorative component that engages the internal connection if you have one available. If there is any resistance or difficulty seating it, the implant should be replaced during surgery.

At the far end of the spectrum, extremely high torque may even fracture an implant. This is very uncommon upon insertion of normal diameter implants. It is more often encountered when attempting to remove a failing implant that is already osseointegrated. An integrated implant can also fracture if it sustains excessive functional load over a period of time. Similar to a fractured tooth, bacteria populate the internal fracture line of the implant and bone resorption occurs. A fractured implant is not only non-functional, but it is a liability to the surrounding bone and structures. It must be removed.

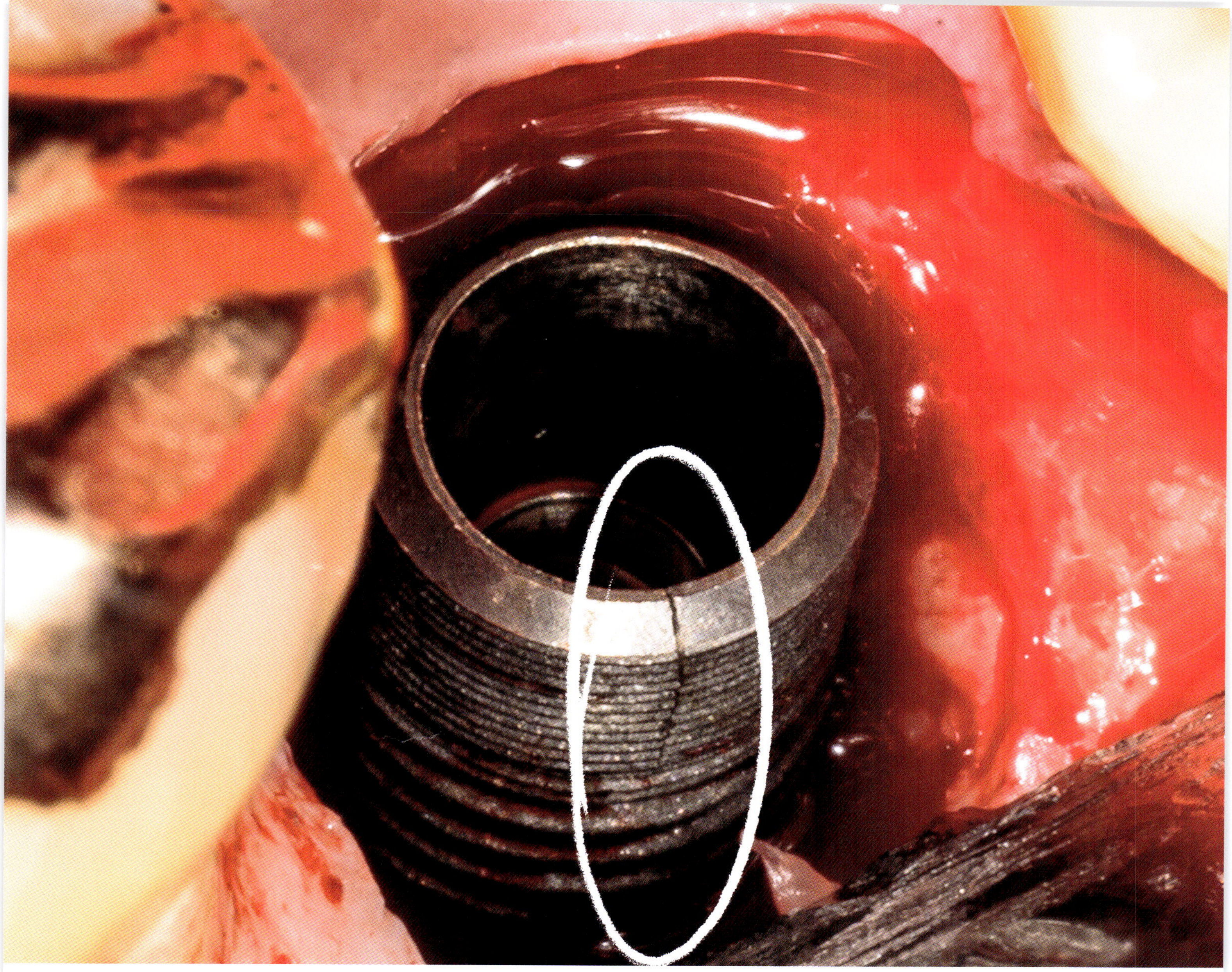

Figure 8-14 Bone responds to a fractured implant like it does a fractured tooth. It retreats away from the inflammatory response to the bacteria. The only solution is to remove the implant. This implant fractured within a couple of years due to traumatic occlusion and had to be removed.

Understanding the anatomy of the implant site is important to knowing what to expect and how to interpret the feedback when drilling and placing the implant. Depending on where the binding occurs and what the internal bone looks like, I may anticipate an early high torque and then a lower torque as the implant advances. This happens when the cortical bone is dense, and the marrow is not. As the tapered portion of the implant engages the cortical bone, the cutting edge of the threads meets increased resistance. Once it has tapped this bone, the resistance decreases as the tapered part of the implant is now engaging the less dense medullary bone. Sometimes, the torque temporarily exceeds the upper limit and then settles into a good range at the final position. In these cases, if you were to back the implant out and drill the cortical bone more, you may end up with inadequate torque. In contrast, when the deeper bone is denser, that same early high torque indicates the osteotomy needs to be enlarged.

It is all an art, with science and physics to back it up.

Binding

There is a notable binding that takes place between the implant and the bone when you stop advancing it on insertion. It feels almost like it locks into place. If you stop advancing at 25 Ncm, it may take 35 Ncm to get it moving again. But then the torque may drop back down to the mid-20s after it breaks that initial frictional binding. It will usually increase again as it is further advanced in the site. The same can be true when reversing the implant. If you hit 45 Ncm and want to back the implant out to drill more, it may take much more than 45 Ncm to initially break the implant free to remove it. It is helpful to know this both when advancing and removing an implant.

Low torque

The final turn when placing an implant can be disappointing sometimes. The torque seemed good as you were inserting it, but all of a sudden, it drops to nothing at the very end. You no longer have the solid implant you wanted and expected. This situation can sometimes be avoided by preparing the site with a low-density protocol, under sizing the osteotomy. Simply decreasing the osteotomy size allows the implant threads and implant body to engage more bone. This is the premise behind the typical low density bone protocol in most implant systems. But sometimes the stability seems to fall off a cliff right at the end anyway. Take a minute to figure out why this happened and then consider either increasing the length or diameter of the implant or burying the implant. In some situations, it is best to remove the implant.

Paying attention to the radiograph and the feedback from the instruments can help solve this problem. Imaging will indicate bone density. If there is dense crestal bone, the stability and torque of insertion may dissipate as the implant traverses or extends beyond it. If a wider diameter implant is possible, it may be inserted right into the same osteotomy. This will engage the bone better, improving stability.

If there is dense apical bone, the implant may have stripped the walls of the site. When the implant bottoms out at the apical extent of the osteotomy, any further rotation can force the threads to strip the bone, compromising stability. In this case, if you can't place a wider implant, consider a longer one to engage that dense apical bone. Don't count on the walls or crest to engage as they have already been stripped. Any increased stability will come from the apical bone. When you increase the osteotomy depth, be cautious to create enough space for the apex of the implant but not so much that you don't get adequate torque. This is a delicate balance.

At times, the torque may be so low when the implant is fully inserted that the implant spins in the site. We call this a "spinner." While this is not ideal, it is not necessarily a complete loss. Some implant designs fare better with spinners than others. Consider burying the implant or just removing it and grafting the site for future placement. If an implant is not stable within the bone, fibrous tissue may form instead of osseous integration. I view this process as though the body is responding to what the implant is doing. If the implant is moving in the bone, the body will surround it with tissue that is mobile: fibrous tissue. If the implant is not moving, the body interacts with tissue that is immobile: bone. This may not be scientifically perfect, but it helps me picture what is going on.

It is possible to unintentionally back the implant out with the Ostell peg if the torque is too low. If the final torque is less than 10 Ncm, you may consider postponing stability testing until after the implant has been uncovered to avoid accidentally removing the implant.

Every implant system has its own sweet spot, but there are options on either side of that ideal torque to achieve predictable outcomes. Pay attention to the site and know your implant system.

Theme 4: Aseptic Implant

The micro roughened titanium surface that most implants have does an incredible job of integrating with surrounding bone. But it is also a fertile environment for contamination and the formation of harmful bacterial biofilm. Great care should be taken to avoid contaminating the implant surface. All attempts must be made to ensure the implant itself is aseptic upon final positioning. Pre-operative antiseptic mouth rinse, such as 0.12% chlorhexidine gluconate, is a common way to reduce bacterial load in the oral cavity, but it does not achieve complete asepsis. We never achieve a truly sterile surgical field in the oral cavity. The instruments and tray are sterile when they are opened, but the oral cavity is not. As we discuss asepsis, let's assume proper universal precautions are employed, and the surgical site is generally clean.

The most critical time for asepsis is the moment of implant insertion. The instant it leaves its sterile packaging cocoon, it is exposed and vulnerable to contamination. It must be diligently protected as it travels from the packaging to the oral cavity, passes by the lips, dodges the tongue, sneaks past the retractor reflecting the flap, and spirals its way into the bone until the entire implant is safely protected by the surrounding tissue. Contact with anything on this journey is a potential threat. This can be a tricky route to navigate with the implant, depending on the environment of the oral cavity. Once the implant is fully seated, it is safe again. Or, at least, it should be safe.

If the final osteotomy gets contaminated, the implant also will be contaminated. For instance, if the sinus membrane is checked with a blunt probe for an indirect sinus lift, it could contaminate the site. If you want to verify that the apex didn't penetrate the lingual plate, examine with a clean instrument. If bone graft is added to an indirect sinus augmentation, a contaminated condenser could taint the tissue. Pay attention to ensure the final drill and any instruments or materials immediately preceding implant placement maintain sterility. And make sure it has a clean pass from the tray into the osteotomy site.

Variations

Sterile field

A truly sterile operating field is not achievable in most oral surgery procedures. The mouth cannot be sterile. All oral surgery should be carried out with sterile instruments and a clean work environment. That is a clear standard of care. Some providers practice "sterile technique" with a full sterile prep, drape, gown and gloves for certain procedures. This adds significant cost and time to the procedure. There is no inherent harm in operating under strict sterile protocols. This may theoretically decrease the chance of contaminating the implant surface if the implant unintentionally contacts something in the surgical field. Though, even in a sterile field, it is not recommended to place an implant that contacts something other than the surgical site. It would be far less risky to simply place a different, fresh implant. And the literature doesn't seem to indicate any real benefit from this added precaution[4]. It is the responsibility of the surgeon and the surgical team to minimize potential surgical site contamination during surgery. The literature supports clean non-sterile gloves and an overall clean procedural environment, much of which is sterile by means of autoclave. A disciplined and well controlled surgical technique, guarding the implant from any contact, is essential in mitigating risk of implant contamination[4].

Pre-operative hygiene

Consider the patient's oral hygiene. Some patients develop an incredible amount of plaque and others may not remove it very well. In these cases, it would be worthwhile to have a prophy before implant placement. These patients should also receive thorough instructions on home hygiene. Some providers require a professional cleaning prior to implant placement, which is wonderful. Other providers may find it more realistic to selectively recommend or require some patients with high risk factors or particularly high plaque scores to see their hygienist before implant surgery. A clean mouth heals better. Removing plaque and calculus adjacent to an implant site can easily be done with a scaler and some gauze at the time of implant placement.

Theme 5: Abutment Selection

Healing abutment selection is a surgical matter. Whether it is a one or two stage implant, the surgeon places the healing abutment. And the abutment matters. This theme has many variations because the healing abutment sets the stage for the soft tissue emergence profile. The emergence profile is the blossoming of the crown from the underlying implant. The transition from titanium to tooth. Molding and sculpting the soft tissue before taking the final impression dramatically impacts the restoration's design. It is the proverbial "alley-oop" for the slam dunk of the final result. This may seem a little exaggerated, but it is easy to overlook, and it deserves attention. If the tissue is not properly developed leading up to the final impression, the lab cannot possibly deliver the best results.

The healing abutment defines and develops the transition from the implant platform, through the tissue, into the oral cavity. Thankfully, tissue can be further developed after the healing abutment. It adapts to the restoration, whether pressure is applied to push the tissue back or space is created for the tissue to fill in. But when the tissue is developed with the final profile in mind, the lab technician, who has never seen your patient, can more predictably design and fabricate an esthetic and functional prosthesis.

Proper healing relies on proper hygiene. The occlusal surface of the abutment must be accessible to be hygienic. A flap of soft tissue overlying an abutment is a protected little nook for biofilm to develop and irritate the tissue (similar to pericoronitis). The abutment should emerge completely from the tissue. When selecting an abutment, measure the tissue height at the highest area, which is often interproximal. Don't just measure the facial tissue height. This will often result in the interproximal tissue crowding the space. If you measure and pick the best abutment the first time, you don't have to decide whether to take the time to remove the abutment, open a new one and place it. The fewer of these types of decisions you need to make, the better your outcome.

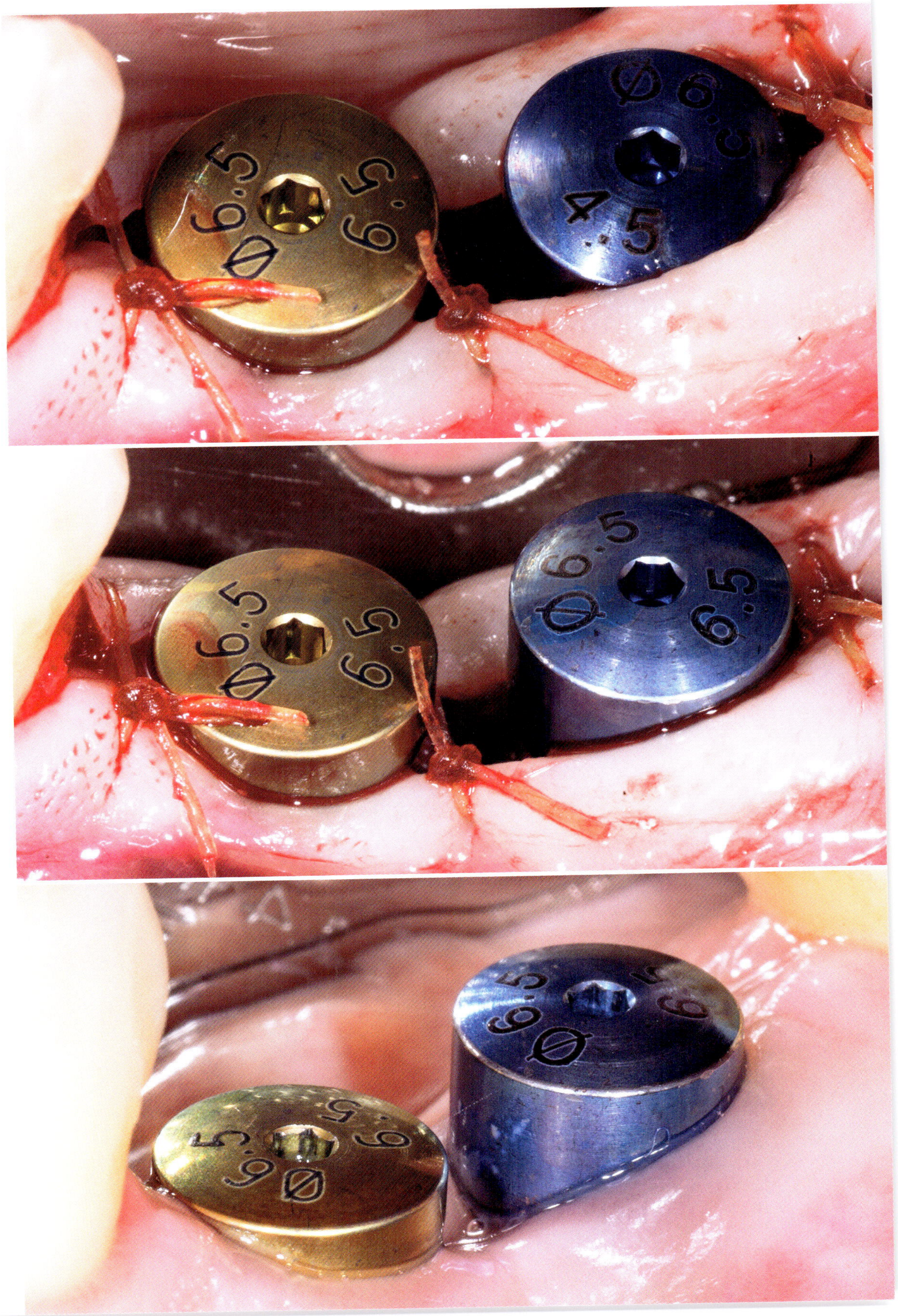

Figure 8-15 Tissue covering the abutment makes the area inaccessible to routine hygiene (*top*). Placing a taller abutment (*middle*) improves tissue health and makes it easier for the patient to clean the abutment (*bottom*). There are times when a temporary appliance or the patient's occlusion limits abutment height and tissue extends over the top of the abutment. Emphasize hygiene instructions in these cases.

The final restoration may displace the tissue, which can be quite uncomfortable. Optimize the emergence of the healing abutment and ensure there is no tissue over the occlusal of the abutment. The better the tissue is developed with the healing abutment, the better the final emergence profile, and the more comfortable it is for your patient[5, 6].

Variations

Bone profile

The abutment should not contact the bone directly. If there is no space for the soft tissue between the abutment and the bone, the bone will have to remodel to accommodate the space for the peri-implant soft tissue. This is also known as recession. And it can increase discomfort during healing. Relieving the surrounding crestal bone can be accomplished with the implant manufacturer's system (typically called a bone profiler) to ensure full abutment seating and adequate space for healthy peri-implant tissue. Profiling the bone may also allow a more flared abutment, further optimizing the development of the emergence profile.

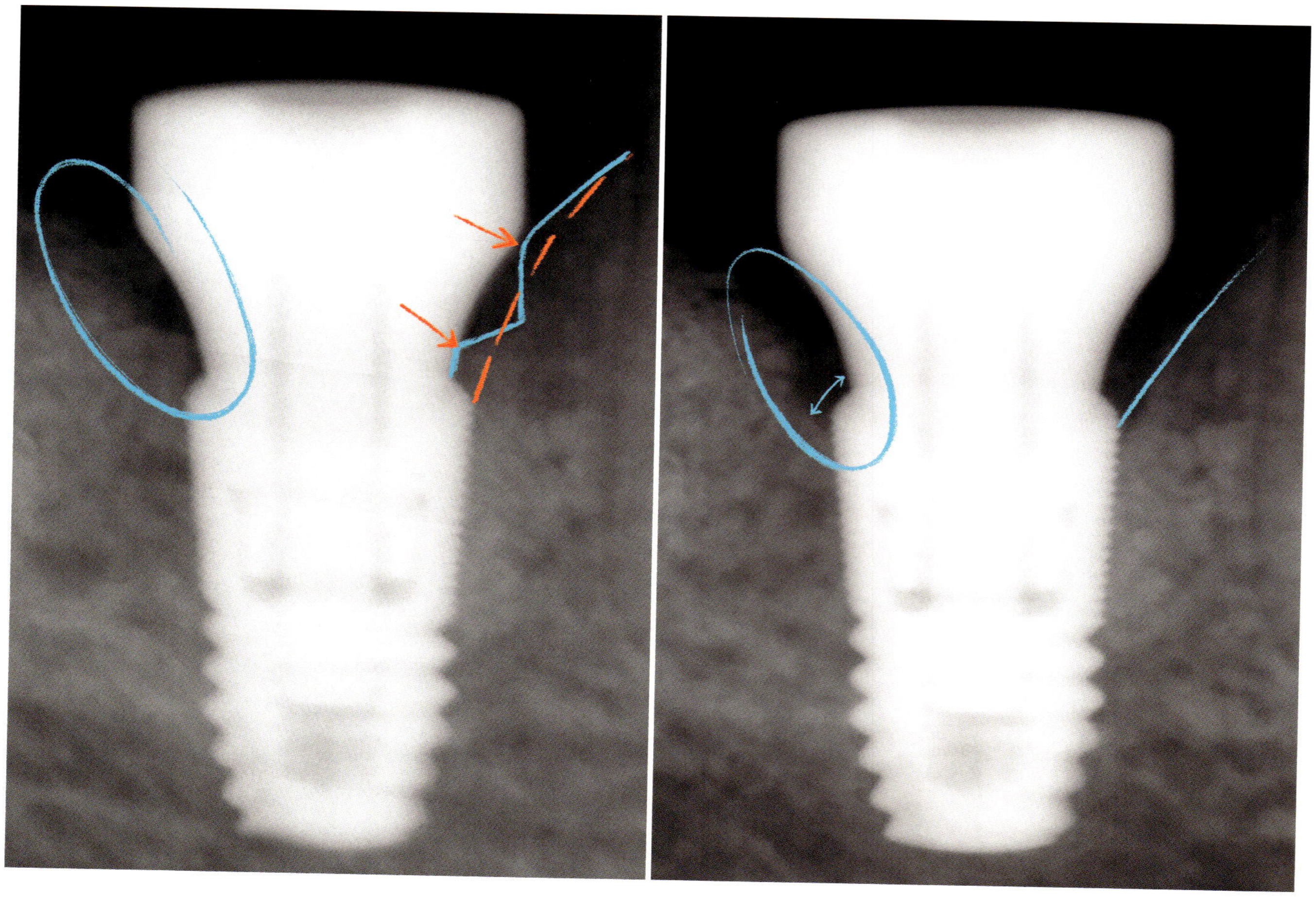

Figure 8-16 The body creates biologic width. We can help it by profiling the implant site so it doesn't need to resorb excess bone. These images were taken at placement (*left*) and at clearance three months later (*right*). Note the bone resorption that took place to create space for the soft tissue.

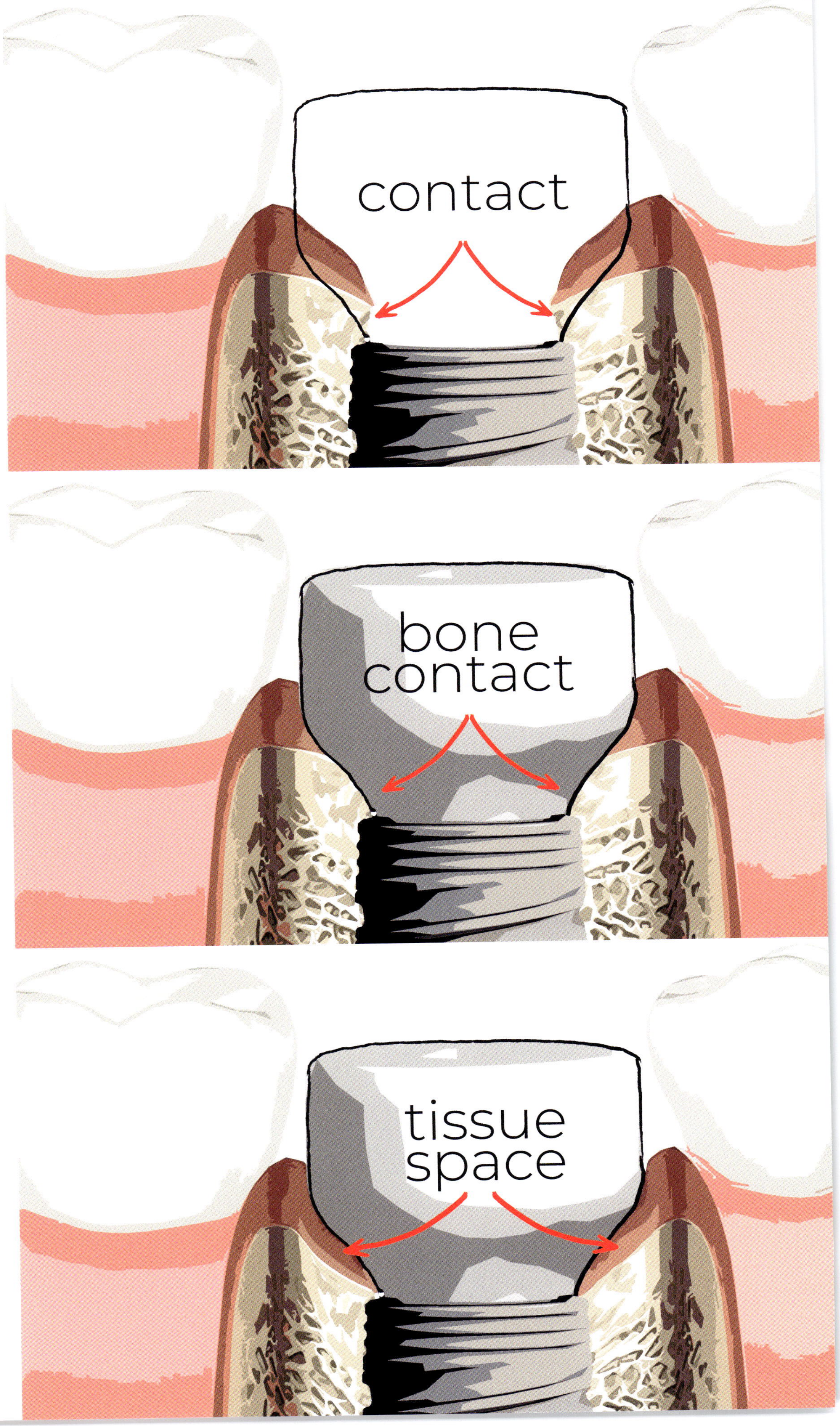

Figure 8-17 A flared healing abutment will often contact bone and soft tissue in a crestal or subcrestal implant. If it is profiled to allow the abutment to fully seat but is still contacting bone, there is no space for the soft tissue. Space must be made for the bone and soft tissue.

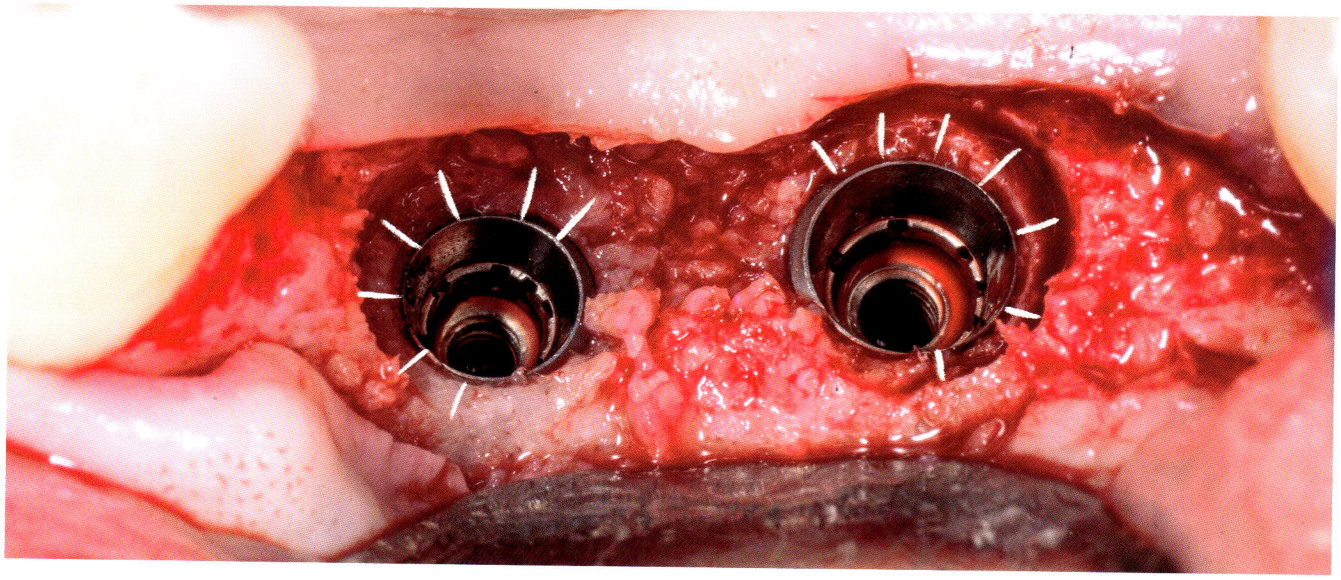

Figure 8-18 Creating space for the abutment by profiling the bone improves tissue health and emergence profile.

Figure 8-19 The crestal bone is the most critical and it can heat up, so use plenty of irrigation when profiling or countersinking.

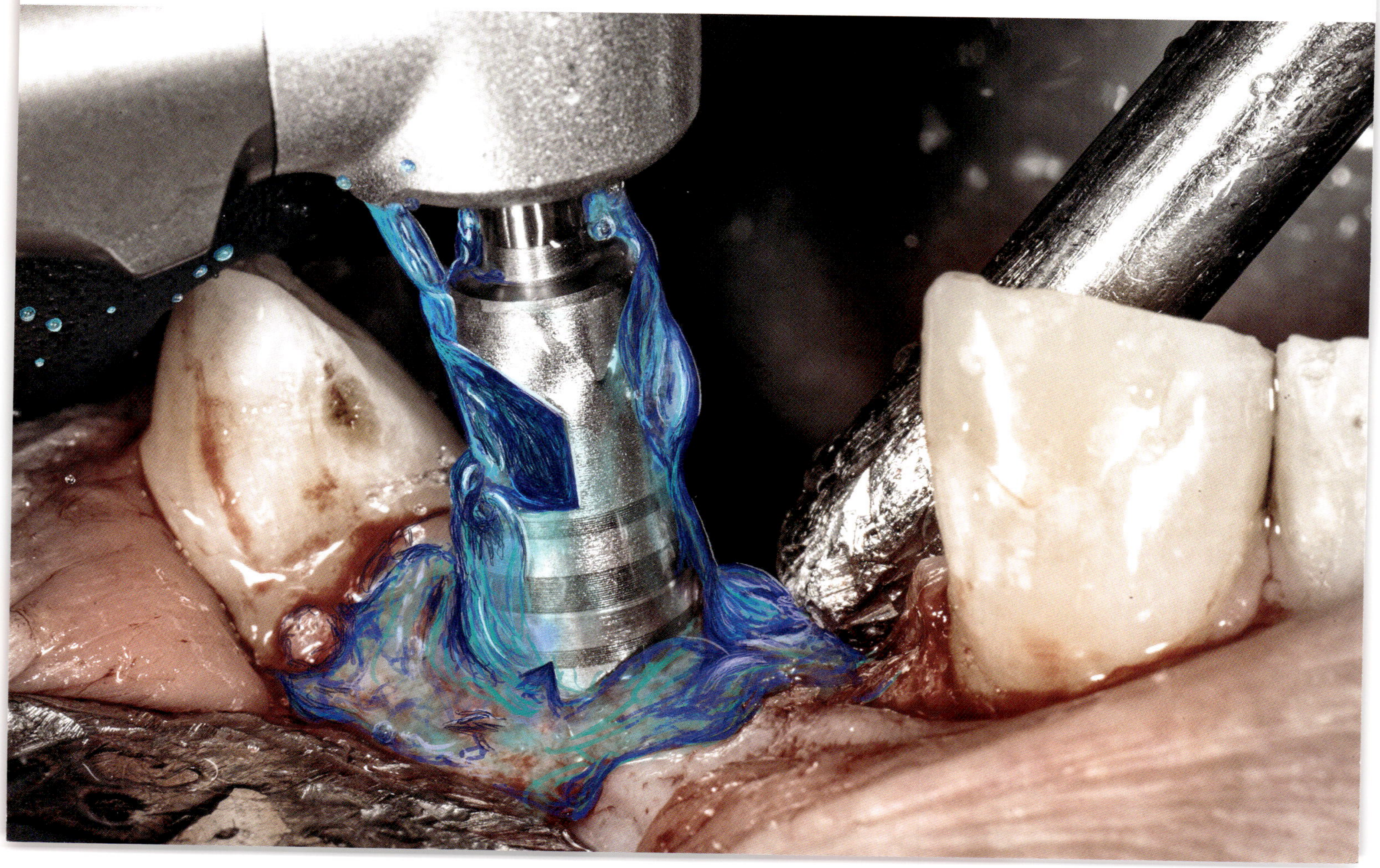

Definitive healing abutment

"One abutment—one time" is a concept that capitalizes on the soft tissue's healing properties. The hemidesmosomal attachment that has been shown to form between the soft tissue and the abutment is compromised each time an abutment is removed. The ideal technique would allow the definitive healing abutment to be placed during surgery to protect the fragile attachments and enhance the peri-implant soft tissue seal. There are several ways to accomplish this, and they all require a bit of pre-surgical planning. The planning takes into consideration the angulation and position of the planned implant. It also takes in the depth of the implant platform and the timing, or rotational position. When these are all accounted for and used to plan the case from the crown down, this concept has great value to soft tissue stability and underlying bone stability. Abutment material also has a significant impact on the soft tissue. This is being studied extensively and I hope will be an area of significant advancement in implant dentistry.

Anatomic abutment

This is the old "square peg in a round hole" dilemma. If the peg is square, you may as well make the hole square too. Stock healing abutments are typically round. Custom healing abutments take into consideration the complex transition from a cylindrical implant platform to an oblong or more square shaped restoration. Custom healing abutments deserve custom definitive abutments. If the tissue has been custom developed, a stock abutment wastes the gain.

Custom healing abutments, or anatomical healing abutments, factor in each individual tooth's dental anatomy. Implants are all cylindrical and teeth are never cylindrical. It makes sense that a custom or anatomical abutment will help transition the bionic limitations of the round implant shape seamlessly to the custom restoration.

The vast majority of implants have stock healing abutments. Overall, they are quite successful. It is important to know when it is worth the added cost of a custom healing abutment. While it can be beneficial for any implant, custom abutments are primarily placed in the esthetic zone where soft tissue is showing. A flared stock abutment may develop the tissue emergence better than a straight abutment. Some exceptions to this are when there is limited interdental space for a flared augment or if a locator attachment will be used for an implant retained overdenture. In general, pick the abutment that will best prepare the tissue for the final restoration.

Theme 6: Operative Imaging

Operative imaging is any radiograph taken during an operation used to guide the surgeon to optimal outcomes. In my mind, this includes intraoperative and immediate post-operative images. Intraoperative images are commonly taken to confirm the angulation and position of the initial osteotomy and to guide subsequent drilling. Immediate post-operative images are often used to document the final position and confirm seating of the abutment. But the immediate post-op image can be as valuable for guiding the procedure as the intraoperative images. Surgery is not necessarily completed when the immediate post-op image is taken. Don't get stuck seeing the immediate post-op image as the final answer. It may just be a rough draft. If you don't like the angle of the implant, change it. There must be room in the surgeon's mind to at least consider revision when viewing the immediate post-op image. It is only "post-operative" when the surgeon approves and sends the patient off to heal and integrate the implant into that final position.

Variations

Intraoperative periapical image

Early in my private practice, I took an intraoperative PA on every implant case after the pilot drill. As I was learning and establishing my practice, I needed that information and confidence. It was worth it, even though it added at least five minutes to the procedure to develop the film. (I did not have digital radiography when I first started my practice. My, how things have changed.) With time and experience, I have become selective on taking intraoperative images. The evolution of guided implant surgery has significantly improved predictability, decreasing, but not eliminating, the value of the intraoperative image. Guidance is not perfection. If there ever is concern or doubt about the position, the 20 seconds it takes for a digital PA is well worth the information and peace of mind. (I dare say, it would still be worth the five minutes to develop film to ensure ideal positioning.)

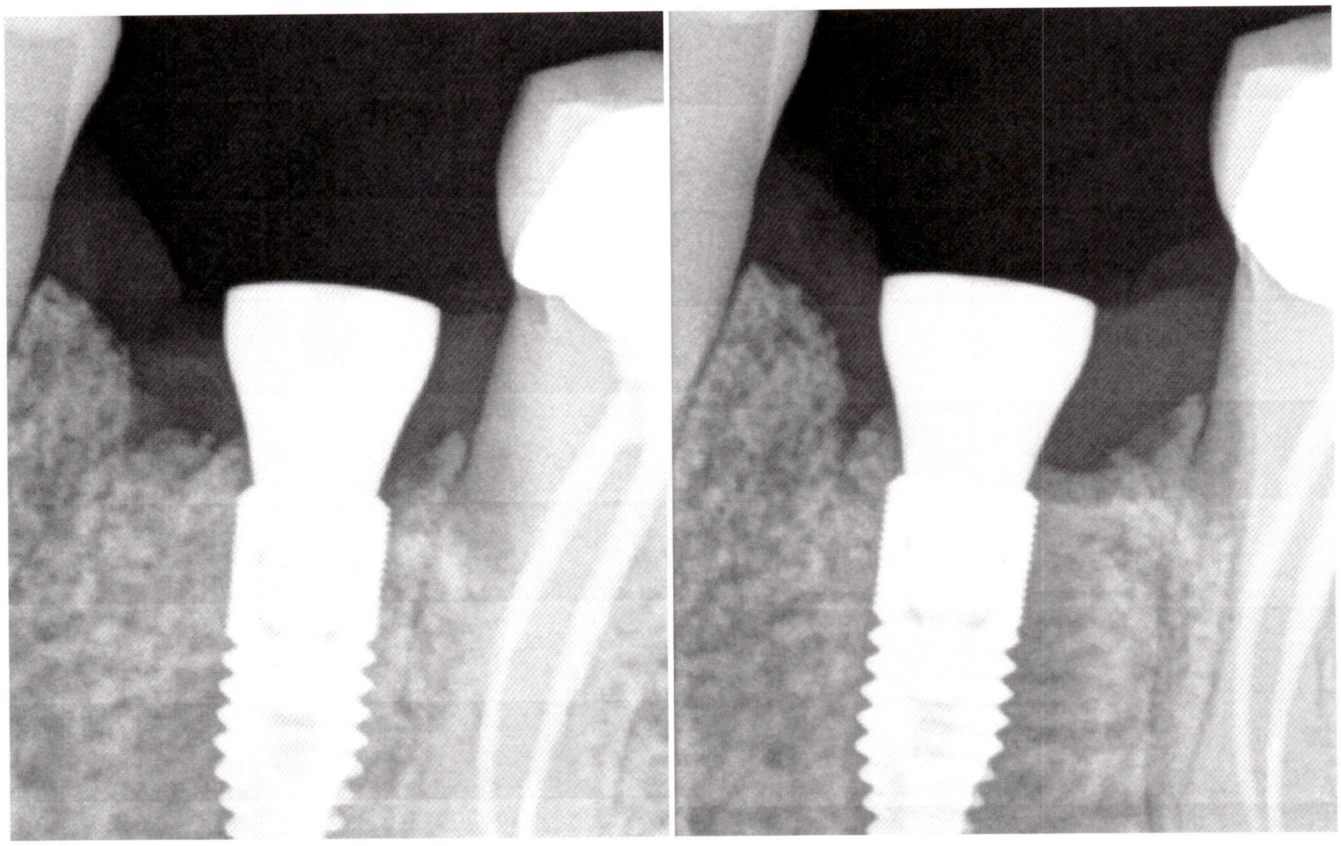

Figure 8-20 After taking a final PA (*left*), I wasn't happy with the implant position. I repositioned the implant (*right*) with a much better outcome. The final image can be another intraoperative image. If you don't like the implant's position, just change it.

Intraoperative PA images confirm angulation and positioning of the osteotomy usually with a drill or guide pin in place. They are most beneficial right after the initial osteotomy, giving you the opportunity to tweak the position with the remaining shaping drills. As with any radiograph, the orientation of the tube and the sensor can be misleading. The value of this image is in understanding the three-dimensional orientation of the osteotomy and the adjacent anatomy. It is easy to get fooled into thinking the osteotomy is off to one side or another if the radiograph is not perpendicular to the site (which at times is impossible, especially in the anterior). The goal is not a perfect looking radiograph, but an ideal implant.

Immediate post-operative periapical image

The immediate post-op PA radiograph is routine for most implant surgeons. It serves a few purposes. It verifies implant angulation, confirms complete seating of the healing abutment, and establishes a baseline image of the surrounding bone.

The angulation and position of an implant can look much different radiographically than it does intraorally. If it looks a bit off radiographically, cross reference with the clinical picture. Afterall, the patient doesn't smile or chew with the radiograph. The combination of radiographic and clinical confirmation is quite helpful. If you don't like the position, consider adjusting it. It is that simple at this point in the game. It becomes much more difficult as the site heals.

Confirming the complete seating of the abutment on the immediate post-op radiograph is important. If the abutment is not fully seated, it will fall out. Achieving adequate abutment torque is not sufficient. The abutment must engage the solid platform of the implant for the torque on the threads to securely retain it. It is possible for bone or soft tissue to get between the abutment and the platform, giving the sense that it is seated with adequate torque. But you can usually tell if a healing abutment is completely seated by how it feels with the last turn of the driver. This tactile sense is far more obvious with a typical hand screwdriver than a torque wrench or drill. As the abutment reaches the platform, it should feel like a very abrupt and definitive stop when the metal of the abutment contacts the metal platform of the implant. It is a crisp halt. In contrast, when there is soft tissue or bone impeding the abutment, it may still feel like it gets tight, it just does this in a more gradual and "sticky" feeling sort of way. It can be like the abutment is squeaking its way down, rubbing against the bone or tissue.

One key component of implant success is the stability of the surrounding bone. The immediate post-op PA serves as a baseline for this evaluation. If there is crestal bone loss or peri-implant lucency during or after initial healing, it is very helpful to have a baseline for comparison. Some remodeling is expected, especially if the implant is placed subcrestal. But without an initial image, it may be impossible to know if the bone is stable.

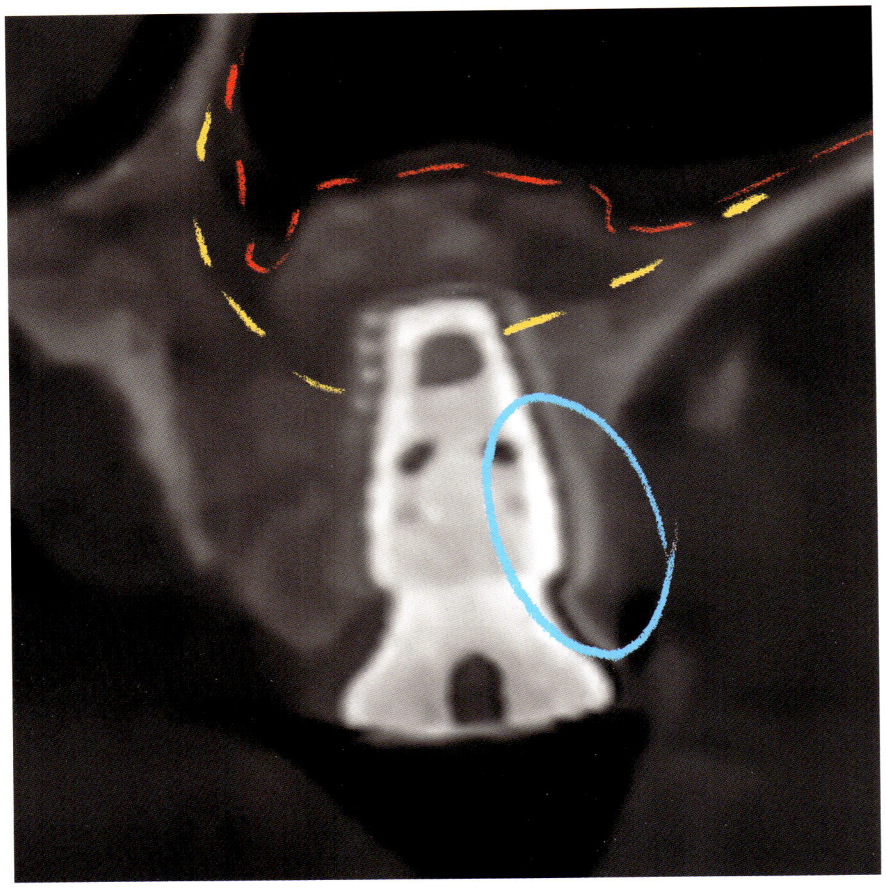

Figure 8-21 Post-operative imaging is particularly beneficial when performing sinus augmentation. It provides feedback on whether the lining remained intact and initial bone density. But it set off a false alarm. These images often underestimate the bone immediately adjacent to the implant. This image shows questionable bone (*blue*), but five minutes earlier I was looking at about 2 to 3 mm of nice bone.

Cone Beam Computed Tomography (CBCT)

Implantology has dramatically improved with the increased availability of CBCT imaging. There used to be a debate about whether every implant should have a pre-operative planning CBCT. Now the question is whether the risks outweigh the benefits of obtaining an immediate post-op three-dimensional image for every implant patient. We are becoming increasingly aware of the potential long-term complications of bone loss associated with implants. Buccal bone stability is of particular interest. This cannot be evaluated with two-dimensional imaging. Routine immediate post-op CBCT imaging is certainly a variation on the theme of operative imaging and is one worth considering.

Theme 7: Grafting and Timing

Patients want to know how long treatment will take, and they don't usually want to wait. Neither do we. We live in a world of instant gratification and immediate results that doesn't seem to be slowing down anytime soon. We all want the process to go as quickly as possible. But in implant surgery, we must obey biology. It has the final say.

As our understanding of biology continues to deepen, we are becoming more predictable in pushing traditional timelines. We now have a better understanding of what bone needs to succeed. We are able to promote faster healing through techniques and materials. And we are also gaining a better understanding of when we need to slow down to allow a bit more time for healing. Not everyone is an ideal candidate for an immediate implant. Before deciding when to place an implant, spend some time learning about the patient and the site. The final decision should be made when all the critical information is gathered. Make the best decision for the patient with all the information available. The bone and implant don't care what the patient wants. They just do what they do. We should set them up for success. It is our job to balance the resources and the needs of the 37 trillion celled human organism and the patient as a person.

It is helpful to have a general understanding of the timeline of bone and tissue healing to guide the process. This provides a framework that can then be tweaked for each case, depending on patient and site-specific factors. Implants have been placed successfully in all stages of healing: immediate, early and late. A basic understanding of the biology of bone healing can be leveraged in deciding when to place and restore an implant for any given situation. The available data in the literature is riddled with holes and contradictions. Some findings are very reproducible, and others are not. This decision-making process is guided by the biology of bone healing. It is tailored to the final prosthetic and esthetic needs of the patient. And it is influenced by patient and site-specific factors. When I think about all these things, sometimes I feel it is like mixing paint. If it all just gets combined and mixed together, it becomes a brown blah. But with training and practice, the right combinations produce a masterpiece.

Bone healing

On average, fairly stable bone is formed about three months after surgery. In the first week, the bone in the site is in the inflammatory phase. This transitions to the reparative phase around weeks 2 to 6, at which time the bone is generally remodeling and maturing. By weeks 12 to16, the bone has typically established a relative state of stability and maturity. Bone continues to remodel well beyond three months.

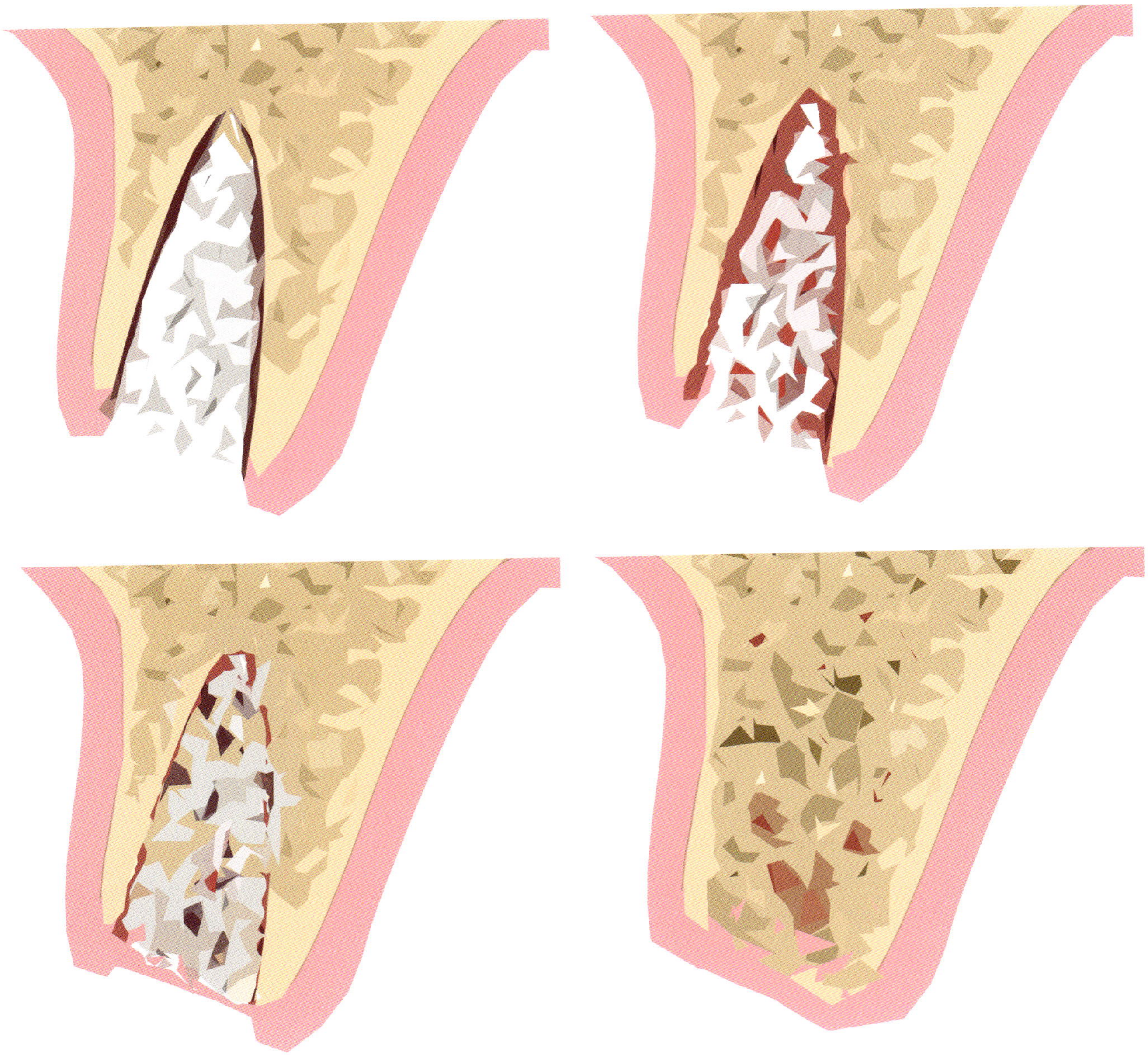

Figure 8-22 This is how I envision the healing of a ridge preservation site. Surgery (week 0). Inflammatory phase (week 1). Reparative phase (weeks 2 to 6). Remodeling phase (week 8+). This rough estimation of the timeline and site helps guide timing of subsequent steps. Depending on patient factors and anatomy, I may place an implant immediately or wait a couple months longer into the remodeling phase.

Patient specific factors

Some patients have great protoplasm. They are just built to heal and be well. A young, healthy patient with a non-restorable coronal fracture may have a shorter healing timeline with more generous response to grafting. On the other hand, an older patient with comorbidities may take much longer to heal. I could not find any published articles that provide a good, comprehensive timeline for the many patient factors. In my experience and study, I have found the following adjustments to be helpful rules of thumb for figuring out how long to allow a patient to heal before attempting the next stage of treatment.

Age/mileage

This is not just measured in years, but more like mileage on their body. How old do they seem? Act? Look? Feel? There are 75-year-olds who seem like they have the mileage of a 50-year-old. They are more likely to heal faster and better than the 50-year-old who seems 75. In general, after about 50 to 60 years, it seems like the bone and tissue start to take longer to reach the same level of maturity and remodeling. This may merit 1 to 2 months longer in each of the bone healing phases.

Comorbidities

It seems natural to split up medical comorbidities into a few categories when it comes to timing: Endocrine, Connective Tissue, Medication/Radiation and Self-Inflicted. With mild or well controlled conditions, it is reasonable to consider adding 1 to 2 months of bone healing time. When these patients have severe or uncontrolled disease, they may not be a good candidate for implant therapy, even with additional healing time. For these patients, proper expectations and informed consent regarding the potential impact of their overall condition on implant success are crucial. It may be even more important to discuss the potential impact of the implant surgery on their overall condition.

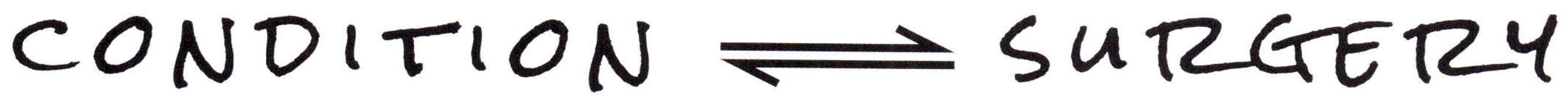

Figure 8-23 The patient's overall condition impacts the surgical plan. And the surgery has the potential to impact the patient's overall medical condition. A frail, elderly, diabetic patient's health could be significantly compromised by performing invasive grafting and implant surgery.

In patients with more severe comorbidities, staging the extraction and implant placement allows time to evaluate healing before committing to the implant. See how the patient responds to and heals from the extraction. If after three months the site looks inflamed and friable, consider re-evaluating after another three months or possibly pursuing non-implant options. If the tissue looks great after three months and the bone appears to be calcifying on the CBCT, they may be ready for the implant. For radiation patients in particular, it seems like there is a significant variation in healing potential. Some seem to heal well, and others have persistent soft and hard tissue defects years after an extraction. Let their own tissue and healing help inform your decisions. It is also very important to know their radiation mapping and understand the risk factors at varying doses. Similarly, with antiresorptive or bisphosphonate medications, you need to know the relative risk factors with the patient's history. But their own healing can help guide their treatment options with proper informed consent.

SOME IMPORTANT COMORBIDITIES TO UNDERSTAND

- Endocrine: Diabetes mellitus, thyroid issues
- Connective Tissue: Ehlers Danlos, lupus, autoimmune spectrum of diseases
- Medication/Radiation: SSRI, antiresorptive/bisphosphonates, radiation treatment
- Self-inflicted: Smoking (packs per day), alcohol, eating disorders (over and under)

History

When a patient has a history of complications with previous surgeries, especially oral surgery, get curious about what happened and why. Figure out as much as you can. Consider allowing an additional 1 to 2 months for bone healing. It can be tremendously helpful to ask a few questions when patients indicate previous healing issues. If a patient has had previously failed implants, consider burying the implant, staging the extraction, and allowing 1 to 2 months of additional bone healing time. Remove as many variables as possible from the equation. If the implant is placed into good bone and buried with ample time to heal prior to uncovering, the chances of success improve. This is the perfect time to set expectations with the patient. We want to learn each patient's own specific biology and tailor their care to achieve their own best possible outcome.

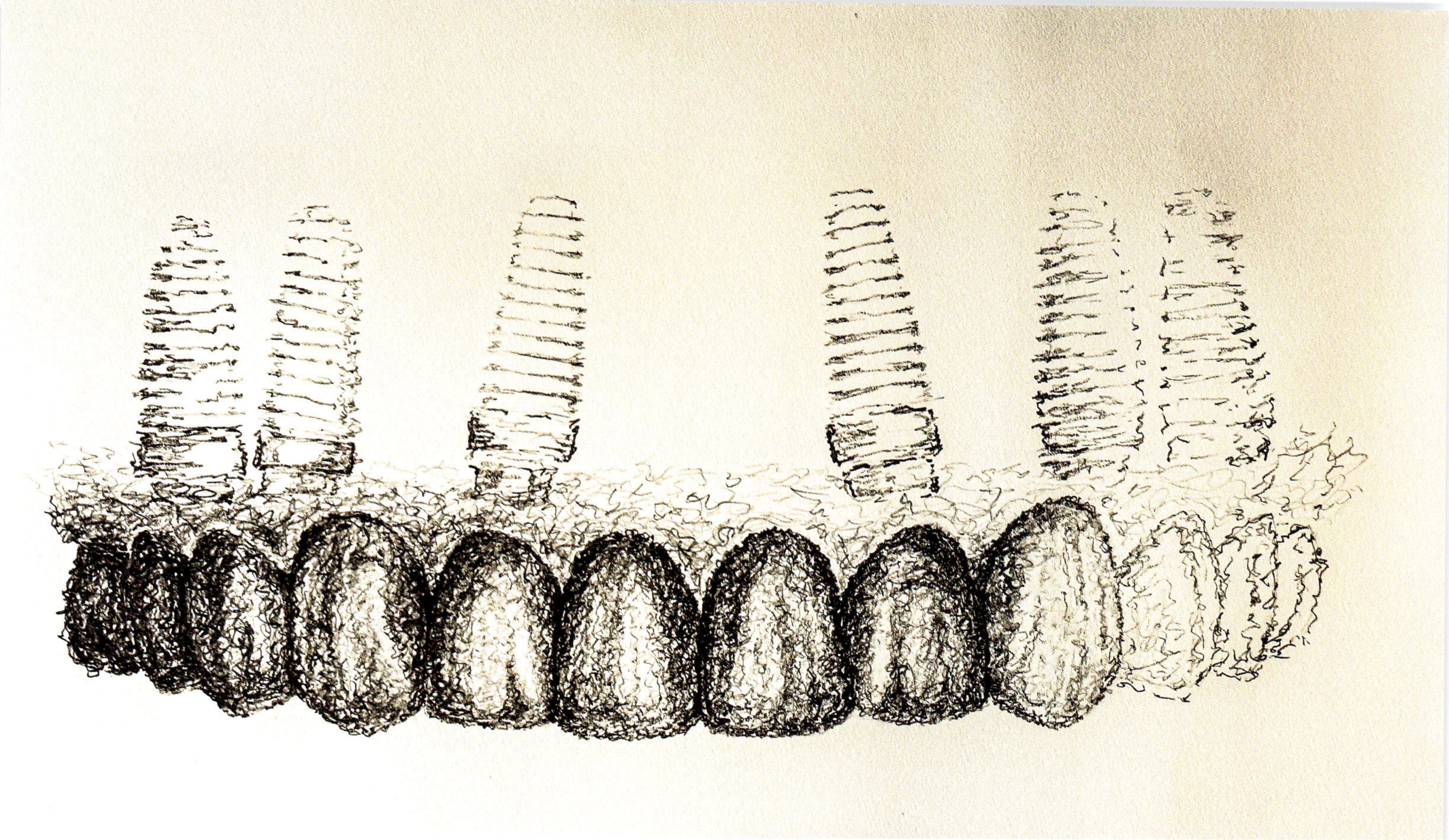

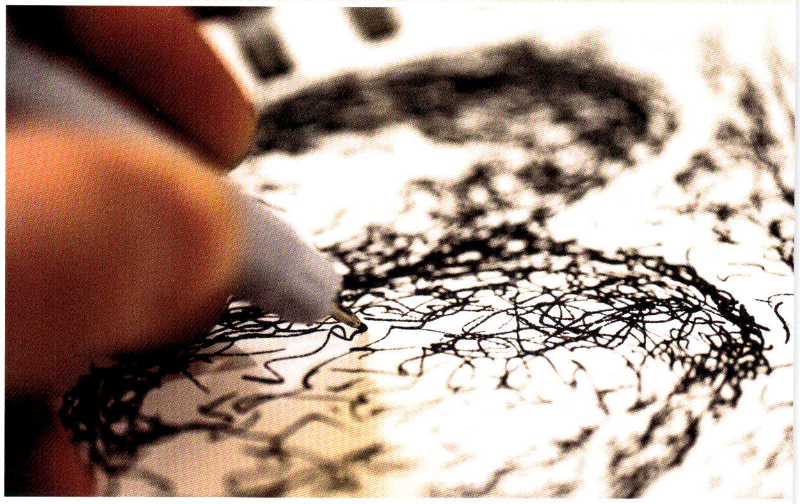

Figure 8-24 We all want to have our cake and eat it too. And how much more so if we were faced with the threat of losing all our teeth. In considering all of the various approaches to full arch implant restorations, it pays dividends to take your time at the drawing board, sketching out the options before deciding when to place and restore the implants. (Artwork inspired by Myron Sahlberg.)

Site specific factors

How much cellular regeneration is needed? How much is the site going to contribute to healing? The answers to these two questions help guide the healing timeline.

If you look at a site three dimensionally, you can get a general idea of how much healing and regeneration will be needed. The more grafted bone there is in a site, the longer it will take to remodel and be ready for implant placement. The greater the distance between the native tissue and grafted bone, the longer it takes to adequately regenerate. We need to give the tissue enough time to do what we ask of it, especially when we are asking a lot.

The tissue in a surgical site has a significant impact on how long it takes to heal. An extraction site with intact walls will provide significantly better resources for healing than a site with buccal and lingual defects. When the site requires significant healing with limited tissue support, consider adding 1 to 3 months for bone healing. Extra attention should also be given to evaluating bone density on a CBCT prior to scheduling implant placement.

A great example of this is guided bone regeneration. We are asking significantly more of the tissue and there are relatively limited resources for healing. In these cases, 4 to 6 months of bone healing time is a minimum. If the site appears questionable radiographically, consider allowing more time for healing. It is particularly important to have adequate stable bone in these cases for both short- and long-term success. Challenging immature bone with an implant that has limited protection and stability from the surrounding native bone can have disastrous consequences.

Sinus augmentation may also benefit from increased healing time. This is dependent on the overall sense of stability and healing resources of each particular site. A little crestal sinus bump for an implant with excellent stability may not need any additional healing time. In contrast, in the case of a direct sinus augmentation with limited native vertical bone height, the site may need an additional 1 to 3 months or more of healing before proceeding to the next phase.

Frequently, soft tissue grafting can be done in conjunction with the extraction or implant placement. This doesn't routinely require additional healing time, but it may require additional time if it is performed at uncovering or on its own. At uncovering, allow 1 to 2 months healing prior to restoration. If the implant is provisionalized, consider allowing more time for the tissue to mature. If soft tissue grafting alone is performed, 1 to 3 months healing is necessary prior to proceeding to the next phase of surgery.

Implant stability can also impact the amount of healing time needed to adequately osseointegrate. When limited torque is achieved, consider allowing 1 to 2 months of additional healing prior to definitive restoration.

This is an outline of what implant surgery timing may look like. We all develop our own opinions based on these principles. But this framework can help establish predictability for the patient, surgeon and team. When everyone is calibrated to the same general principles, the whole experience is enhanced. The restoring dentist, surgical assistant, implant treatment coordinator and scheduler can all have a relatively good idea of what to expect. That is a powerful team dynamic.

Immediate, early and late implant placement

Ultimately, we need to decide when to place the implant. Do we place an immediate implant? Place an early implant after allowing the soft tissue to heal and infectious risk to decrease? Or do we allow the soft tissue and bone to heal and mature, placing an implant into a healed site with the highest proven likelihood of success? What does the patient want? What does the patient need? What does the patient have to work with? It is ultimately up to you.

For more information on implant timing and risks, check out the consensus report published in the 2019 *Journal of Clinical Periodontology*. This group of experts did a nice job of summarizing the literature available at the time and making consensus statements to help guide decision-making[7].

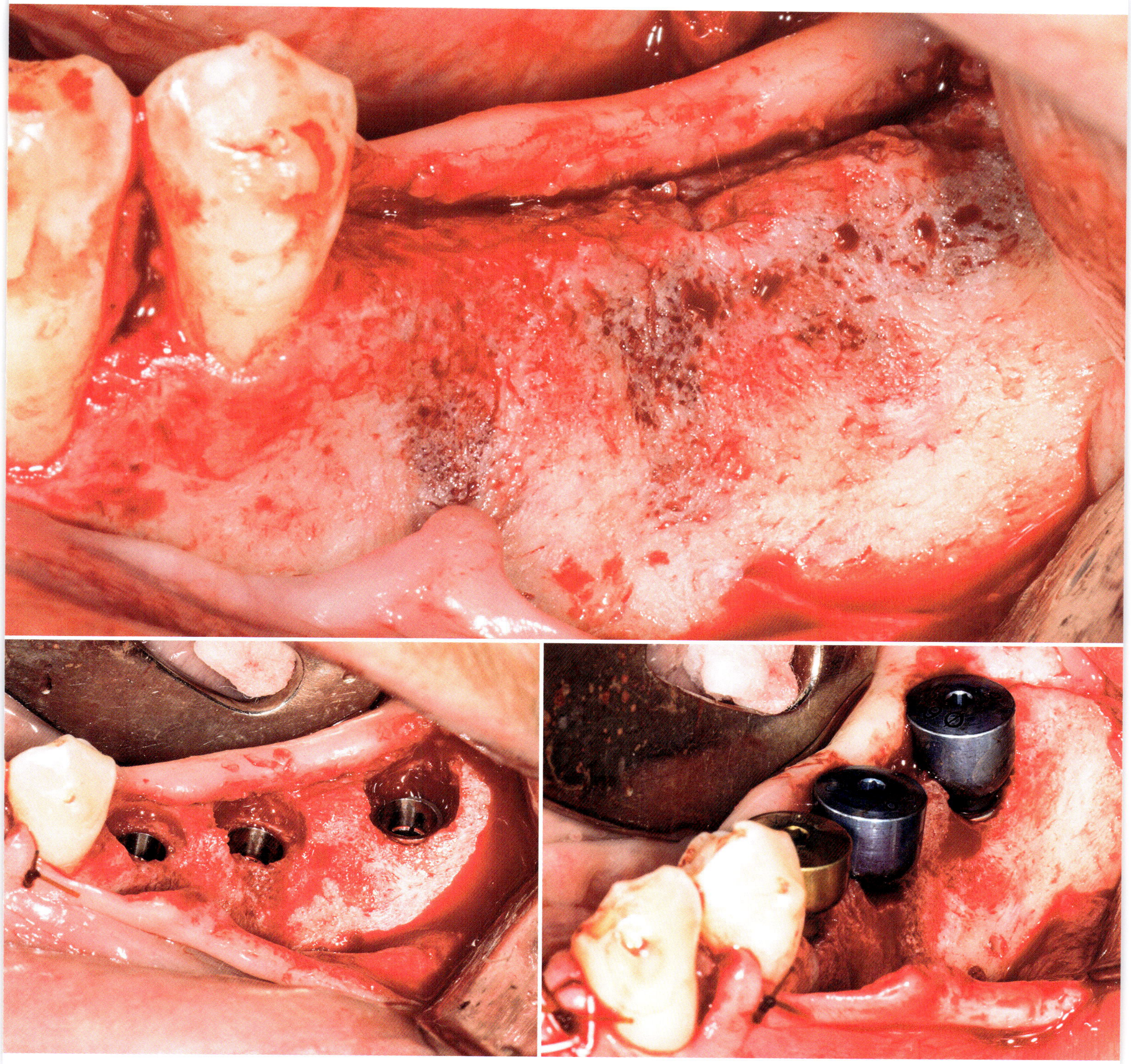

Figure 8-25 Healing is a process. Though this bone has healed enough for implant placement, you can still see the previous extraction sites. It is so cool to see the healing process taking place right in front of my eyes. It reminds me again that the body does all the healing. Notice the ridge anatomy and how the bone has been profiled around the platform to optimize the emergence and biologic width.

Theme 8: Immediate Implant

Planning

Immediate implant placement has been promoted heavily from the podium and in the literature. Many authors and speakers are showing equal or better results compared to staged implant placement in the right circumstances. It seems the body appreciates a shorter transition from tooth to implant. Some studies show improved hard and soft tissue results, but others share a different perspective, with a potential increased risk of failure and more compromised tissue outcomes[7].

The immediate implant is a complex dance, progressing from the extraction to the osteotomy and culminating with implant placement. There is a higher expectation from the outset and the pressure is on. The patient is hoping for fewer procedures, less treatment time, and a quicker definitive restoration. And the surgeon knows placing the immediate implant improves efficiency and profitability. It is a win-win.

Each step is directly preparing for the next step. Every step counts. At the outset, the site should look adequate radiographically and clinically for a possible immediate implant. The patient should be a good candidate. All the principles of exodontia and implants throughout this book apply. They may be even more critical in these cases. There are different and additional criteria that have been proposed for immediate implants. Here is a general outline of the main criteria that allows me to successfully offer this service to my patients.

▶

Figure 8-26 The immediate implant must engage the socket walls. It must be wider or longer than the tooth.

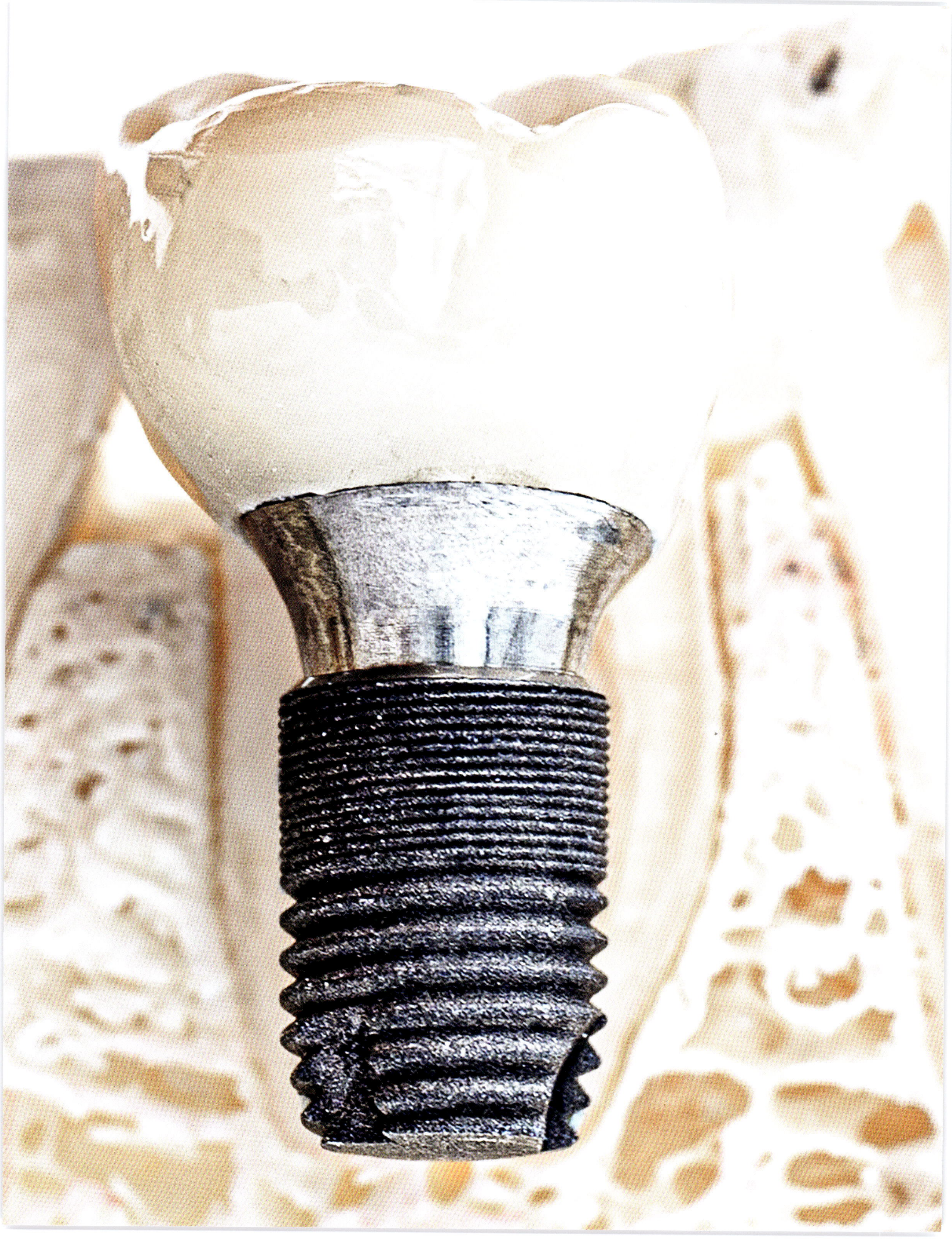

Radiographic

Adequate bone is necessary for the implant to achieve stability. It doesn't require complete circumferential bone contact, but enough of the implant must be engaging enough bone to immobilize the implant during initial healing. This can be assessed visually with a CBCT and some basic implant planning software. Place a digital implant in the site and envision how much of the implant is engaging bone. How well would an implant in that site resist displacing forces? In other words, how well will the bone hug the implant? There must be reasonable surrounding bone, both in quality and quantity.

The immediate implant inherently will not engage as much bone circumferentially as the staged implant because it is placed into an extraction site. There will be a "gap" somewhere between the implant and the socket walls. Because the implant is not engaging as much bone, it is critical there at least be enough bone and that the bone is of reasonable quality to stabilize the implant and promote osseointegration. Look at where the implant will engage the bone in all dimensions. This is more than just a calculation of percent of bone to implant contact. For optimal stability, the bone needs to engage the implant in multiple dimensions.

Understanding the design of the implant is key. The shape and thread design is engineered to engage bone at different levels and capacities. Implants with fully parallel walls primarily engage apical bone upon seating, whereas tapered implants may increasingly engage coronal and apical bone as the implant is

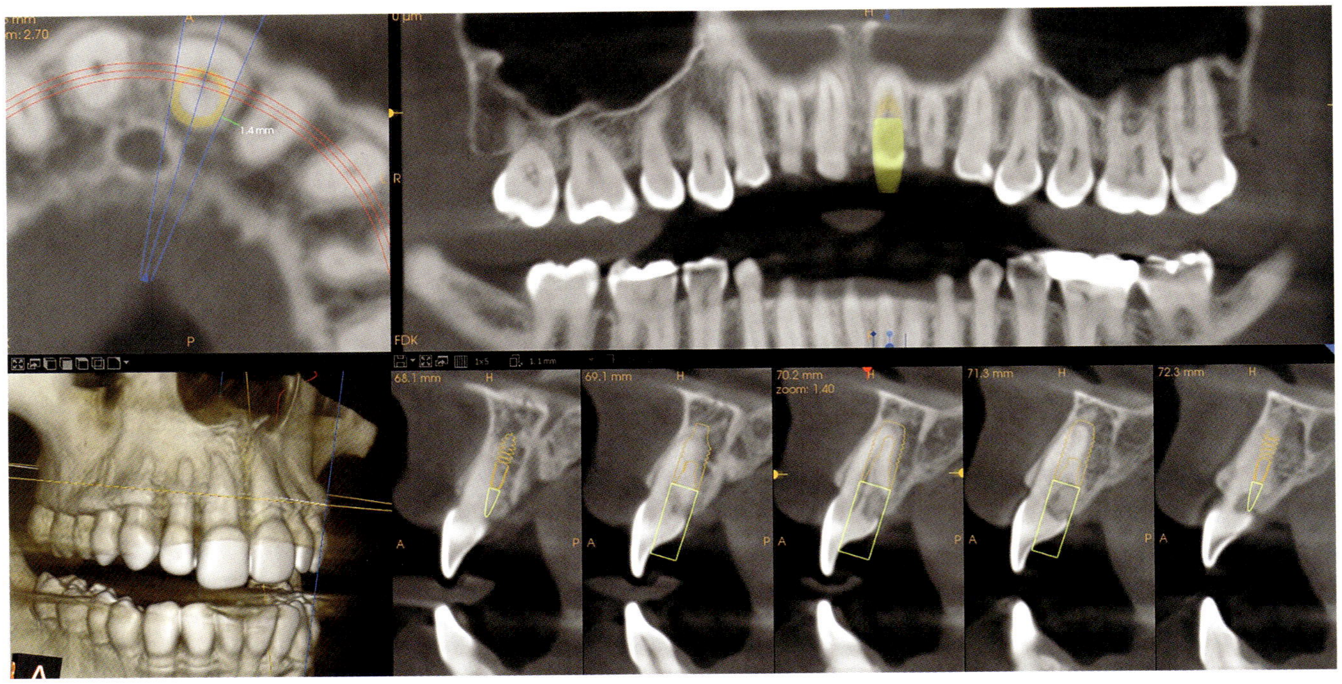

Figure 8-27 Planning software allows multiple views simultaneously to help evaluate whether there is adequate bone to engage the immediate implant. In this case, the bone was engaged as the socket narrows apically and beyond the apex. Multiple views on one screen help determine the condition of the bone and likelihood of stability.

inserted. Some implants have a reverse taper that narrows slightly at the platform. This will actively disengage the coronal bone as the implant is fully seated. Visualizing the specific implant engaging the bone is simple with current CBCT planning software. Implant libraries can be imported with the exact dimensions of the implant. This can be quickly and easily positioned and adjusted to visualize how any specific implant will fit.

With such a wide variety of comfort in immediate implant surgery, some surgeons are more aggressive with immediate placement while others may be more confident with staging an implant. Either way, the end result must maintain sufficient buccal bone. It seems to be well accepted that 1.5 to 2 mm of facial bone thickness is the minimum for consistent long-term stability. The immediate implant must be positioned at least that far from the facial cortex. Thicker facial bone is universally accepted as better than a thin facial plate. There is discrepancy in the literature and in practice on what qualifies as an adequate buccal plate for immediate implant placement. I want at least 1 mm, preferably 1.5 to 2 mm, of facial plate thickness and 2 to 2.5 mm total distance including the gap. Placing a narrower implant will increase the potential buccal dimension of bone. However, it also decreases potential socket wall engagement.

It is more critical for there to be adequate facial bone near the crest than the apex. Maintaining or regaining bone if it is deficient toward the apex is easier and more predictable than at the crest, as long as the implant doesn't extend outside the envelope of bone. When an immediate implant is placed in a site with an apical defect, attention must be given to ensure the area regenerates with bone and not soft tissue. Various membranes have been used to hold the tissue out of the socket. Simply placing particulate graft material may be sufficient. This depends somewhat on the anatomy and the condition of the apical tissue. It is worth the extra time and attention to ensure any and all soft tissue is removed or repositioned completely outside the socket walls and kept there with a membrane and/or particulate bone graft. In my practice, I routinely place some type of membrane if the tissue seems to keep trying to invade back into the socket. Otherwise, I typically just condense a particulate mineralized/demineralized allograft into the space to displace the tissue.

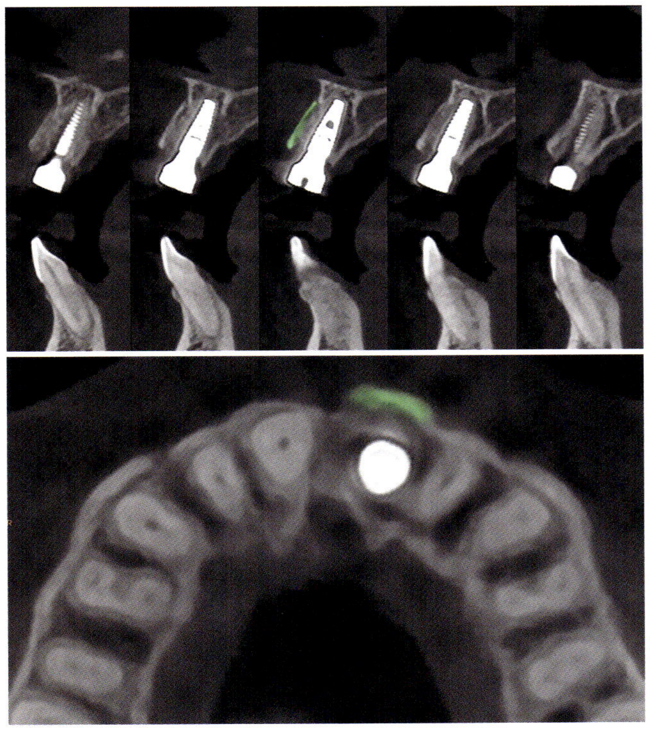

Figure 8-28 The facial plate was expanded during this extraction due to the osseous formation within the external resorption (note planning figure previously). The plate was displaced (as highlighted in *green*) but remained stable and served to augment the site nicely.

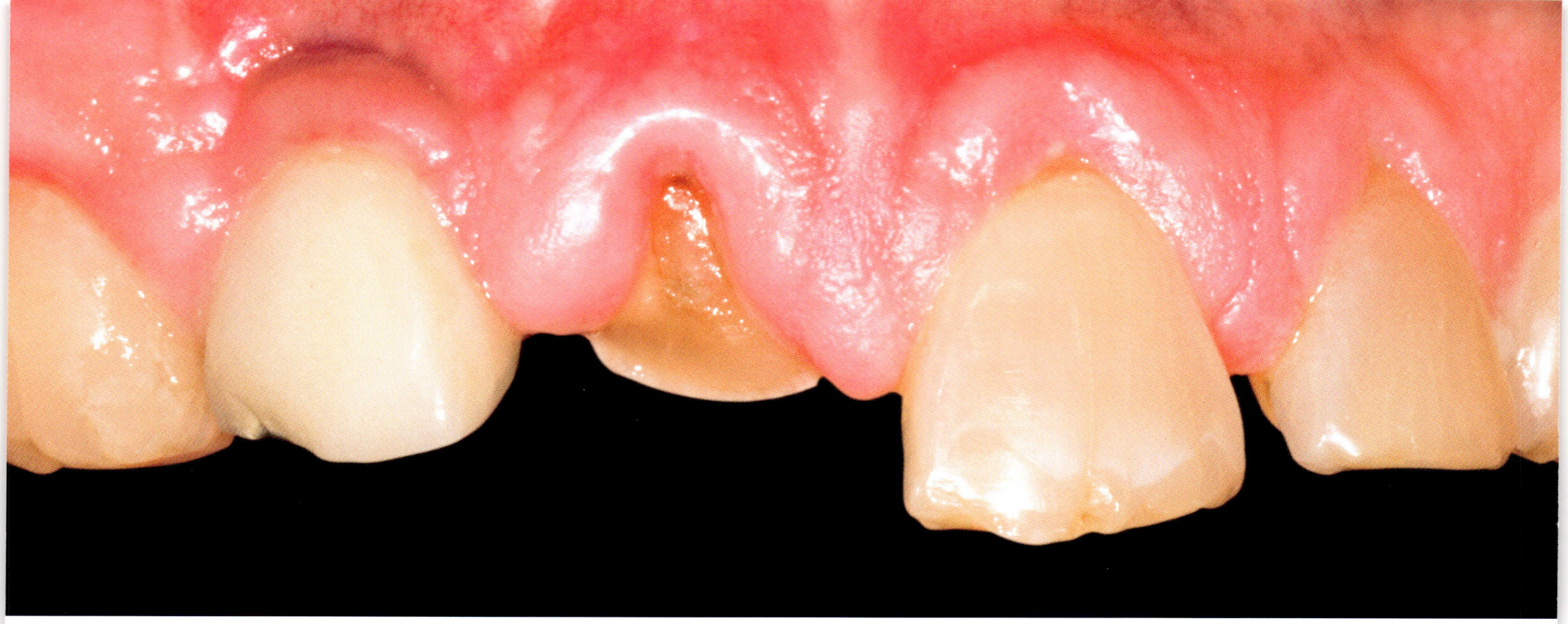

Figure 8-29 This thick gingival biotype is ideal for an immediate implant. The tooth fractured and the underlying bone is relatively intact.

It can be difficult to decide whether a site is amenable to an immediate implant. If you are not confident the bone would fill in well without an implant, it will not likely fill in better with an immediate implant. Try to visualize whether the defect is favorable or unfavorable and don't push the envelope too far. Simply put, immediate implant placement doesn't inherently improve regeneration of an osseous defect. Be careful to not ask too much from the site.

Clinical

Visual inspection is quite important in determining the treatment plan. The goal is not merely to achieve adequate initial stability in the bone, which is evaluated and determined based on the CBCT. The goal is to have long term stability, function and an esthetically pleasing result. Pay attention to the available keratinized gingiva. Limited keratinized or attached gingiva increases the chance the peri-implant soft tissue will be compromised over time. It can also negatively impact the esthetics. If soft tissue augmentation is anticipated, this may be an indication for staging the implant. It is more complicated to perform soft tissue grafting for an immediate implant than a staged implant. Some surgeons do it and do it well. They have built their confidence through a large volume of successful immediate implants and soft tissue grafting procedures. And they make it look so easy. So pretty. At least for them. For the rest of us, we may be better off taking our time and staging the treatment to optimize our outcomes and to better enjoy what we do.

Check out the surrounding soft tissue health. If there is significant inflammation that involves surrounding teeth, it is not likely a healthy environment for an immediate implant. It is more favorable to place an implant, immediate or staged, into a healthy periodontal environment. Consider performing ridge preservation and working with patients to optimize their hygiene before placing the implant. Patience is more than a virtue in this. It is a requisite.

An active acute infection may be a contraindication to immediate implant placement. If a site cannot be definitively cleaned and free from the infection and granulation tissue, it is better to stage the implant. If a site is contaminated, the risk and implications of an implant becoming infected and failing is much greater than that of a ridge preservation graft failing in the same circumstances. A contaminated biofilm forming on an implant surface can be the kiss of death.

Site preparation

Under preparing the initial osteotomy site for an immediate implant is key to achieving adequate initial stability. There is less bone to engage, and the remaining bone has likely been compromised at some capacity during the extraction process. It is common for there to be some expansion of the socket, compromising the socket walls, even with the various minimally traumatic extraction techniques. If the walls have been outfractured and destabilized, a significantly under prepared socket wall may blow out when the implant is placed. It is helpful to be aware of bone quality and how it responded during the extraction. It may be brittle, potentially fracturing upon placement if the outward or engaging force of the implant is too high. In this case, consider more fully preparing the osteotomy site or at least going very slow while placing the implant. If the bone appears to be fracturing, it may be salvaged if it is still stable and the osteotomy is enlarged to minimize the outward pressure. If the bone is not very dense, consider drilling a couple millimeters beyond the planned implant position and stopping much narrower than the implant. The implant system you use likely has its own "soft bone" protocols.

The bone left in the site may make it challenging to keep everything on course. When an implant is planned to hug the palatal aspect of the socket, it will likely get pushed facially upon insertion as it is engaging the palatal bone with no opposing facial bone to keep it straight. This can be compensated for by leaning the drills a bit more toward the palatal than the intended implant position. If the site is prepared too far palatally, it is very easy to reorient the implant toward the facial as there is no opposing bone. In contrast, it is far less likely that the implant could be adjusted toward the palatal at the time of insertion. The implant may also walk right out of the osteotomy site if too much lateral force is applied either by the surgeon or the adjacent bone. As the implant is inserted, the rotational forces tend to cause the implant to take a walk and roll right out of the site, especially if some course correction is needed or there is a very dense area of bone. Pay close attention to the palatal or lingual bone on anterior teeth and interradicular bone on multi-rooted teeth. Use caution and be patient in these instances to optimize predictability and the final position.

Drilling for an immediate implant can be quite tricky at times. The socket walls can be unruly, tending to deflect the spinning drill and throw it off course. It is nice to inform the patient, prior to drilling, that it may feel like the drill wants to jump around a bit. A quick heads-up may dispel some of the patient's questioning or concerns about your skills when the drill chatters on the interradicular bone. One patient told me it felt like hitting rumble strips on the highway, but inside his head. Employing a solid finger rest to support the drilling hand is helpful. It can also be helpful to use the other hand to stabilize the drill if it is getting deflected away from the planned position. Keep in mind this can make it more difficult for the assistant to evacuate the irrigation.

The smallest increments in drill size make it easier to stay on course from one drill to the next. With smaller steps, there is less chatter and more control of the drill tip. This allows you to better accommodate for the available bone or to course-correct if needed. It can be tempting to use a standard drilling protocol, but if the system has more stepwise drills, this is a good time to use them.

Higher speed provides more control. The drill is more likely to get deflected at a lower rpm. A higher rpm optimizes precise control over the drill. This seems most beneficial during immediate implants. For staged implants, I typically employ a very low speed for drilling and placement. My techniques on this have changed over the years and will likely continue to change in the future.

It is valuable to re-evaluate the bone in the site after drilling is complete, prior to implant insertion. Gently apply a bit of force, possibly with a curette, to the surrounding bone to check its stability. If the surrounding bone is grossly mobile, the plate may have blown out, significantly decreasing initial stability. At any point, if the site seems like it would have a better outcome by staging the implant, don't hesitate to graft the site and re-evaluate in a couple months.

A tapered drill shape makes it easier to increase the osteotomy size while controlling or manipulating the angle and position. The shape allows the drill to engage and follow the previous osteotomy. Tapered drills are also side cutting, improving control of the drilling compared to end cutting drills. Most immediate implant sites benefit from side-cutting drills. They are less likely to get deflected off course and more capable of being directed back on course.

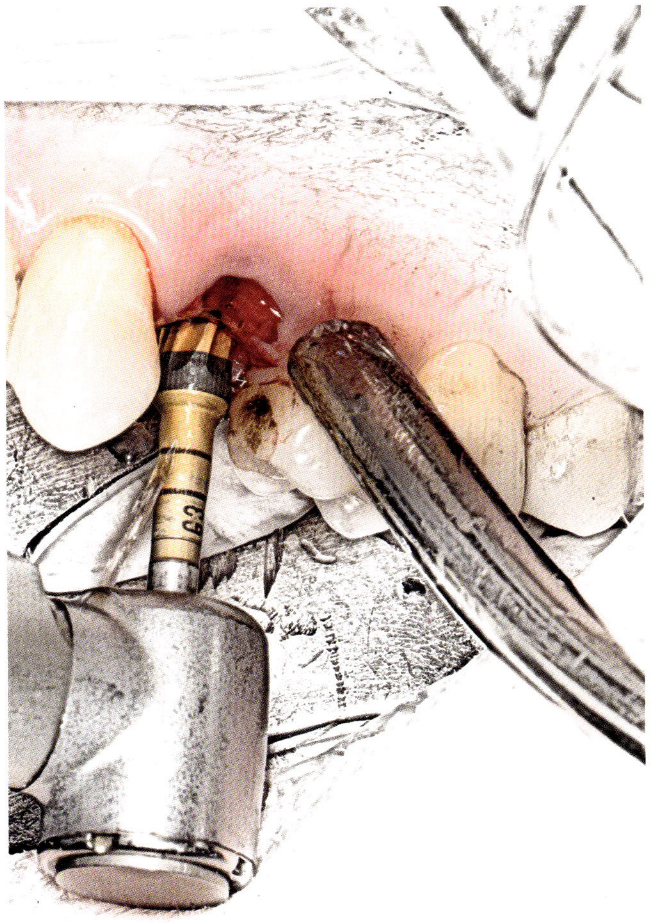

Figure 8-30 Tapered, side-cutting drills, like the Densah drills from Versah, help control the osteotomy in an immediate site.

▶

Figure 8-31 Pre-operative photos show the healthy appearing gingival architecture and the crown length discrepancy between tooth Nos. 8 and 9.

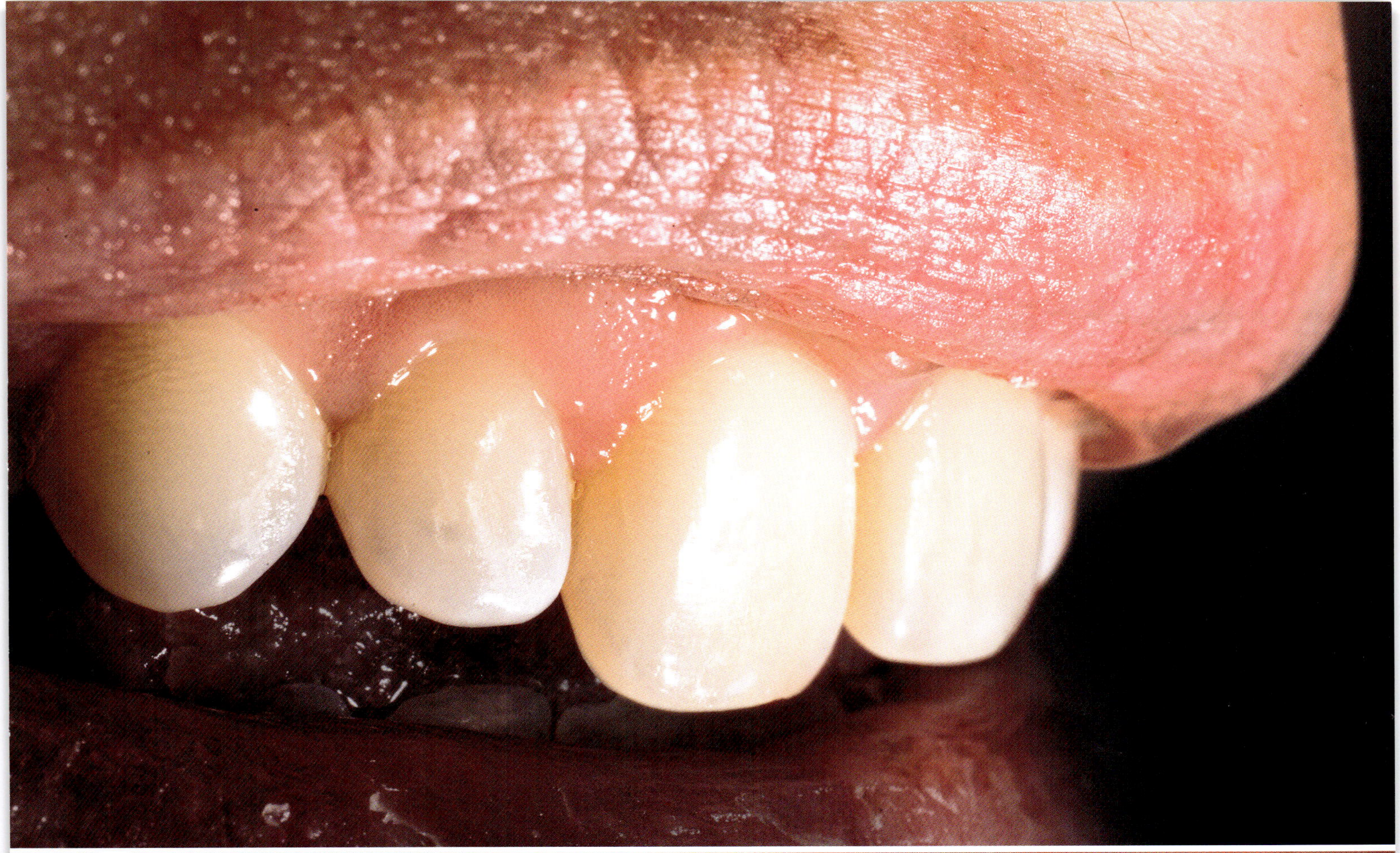

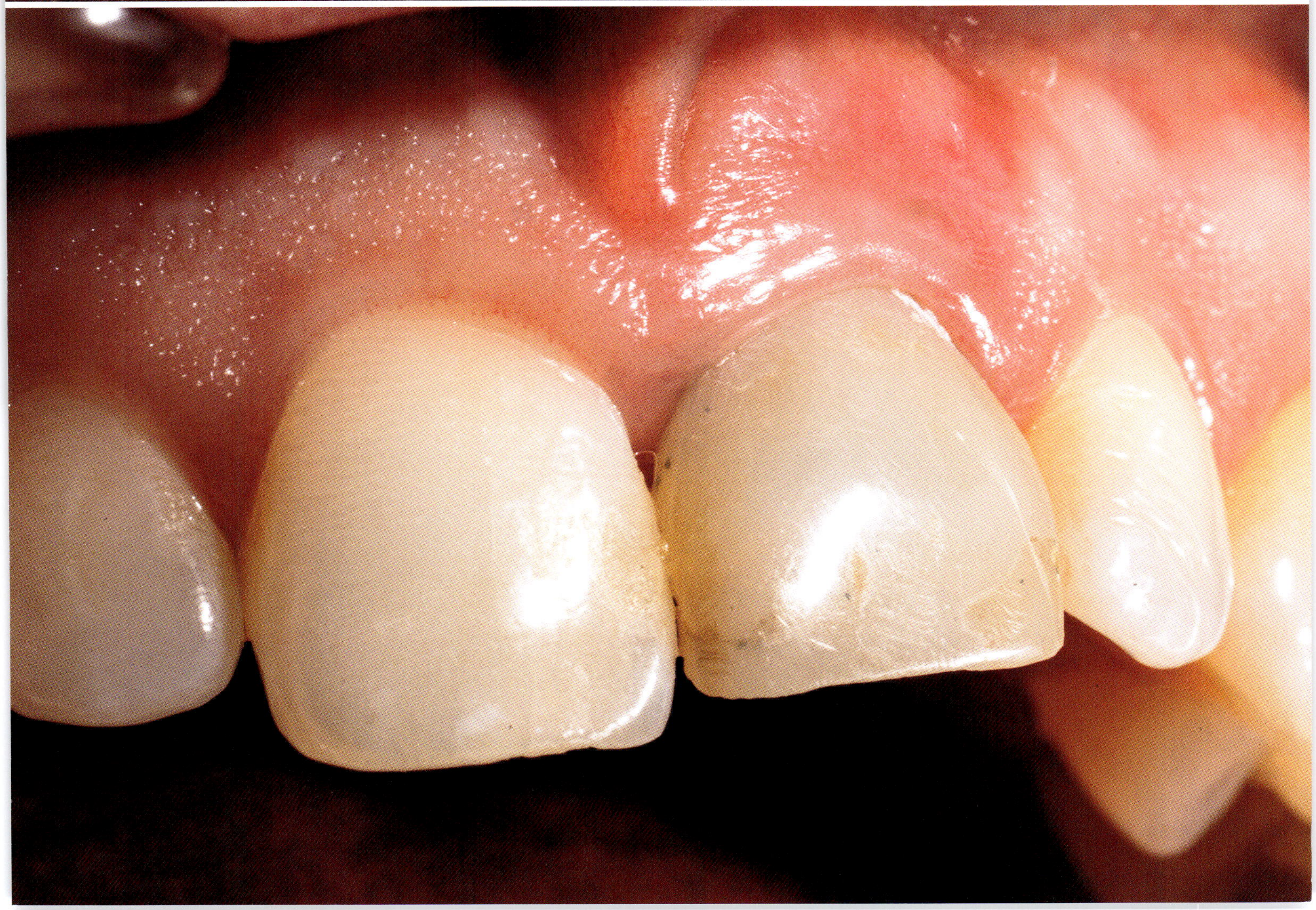

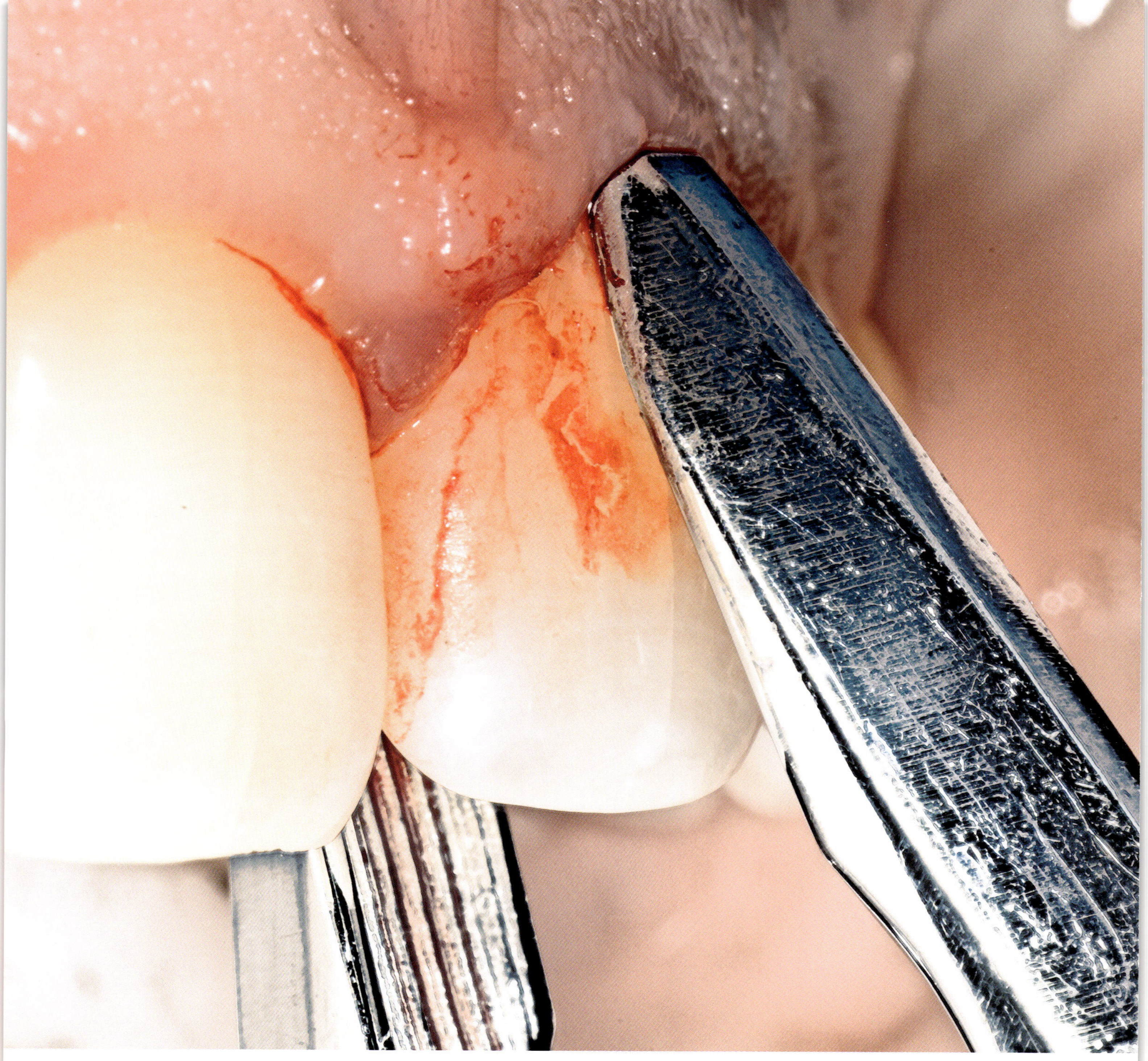

Figure 8-32 After separating the periodontal ligament with a periotome, the tips of the straight forceps can safely go under the gingival tissue to optimize engagement of the tooth.

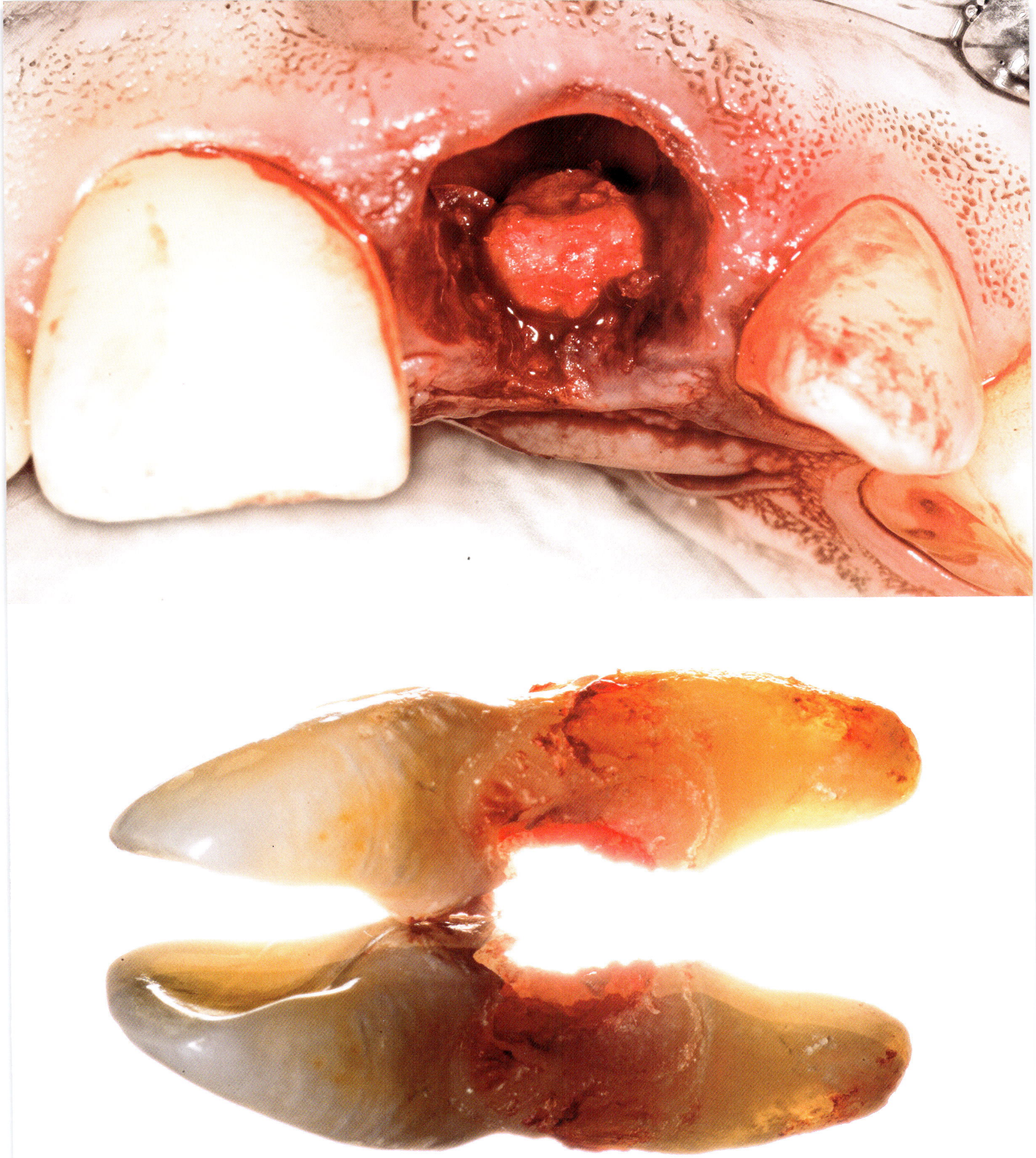

Figure 8-33 External resorption caused a significant area of bone growth within the socket that had to be removed when preparing the osteotomy. This beautiful photo shows the incredible destruction of the macrophages[8].

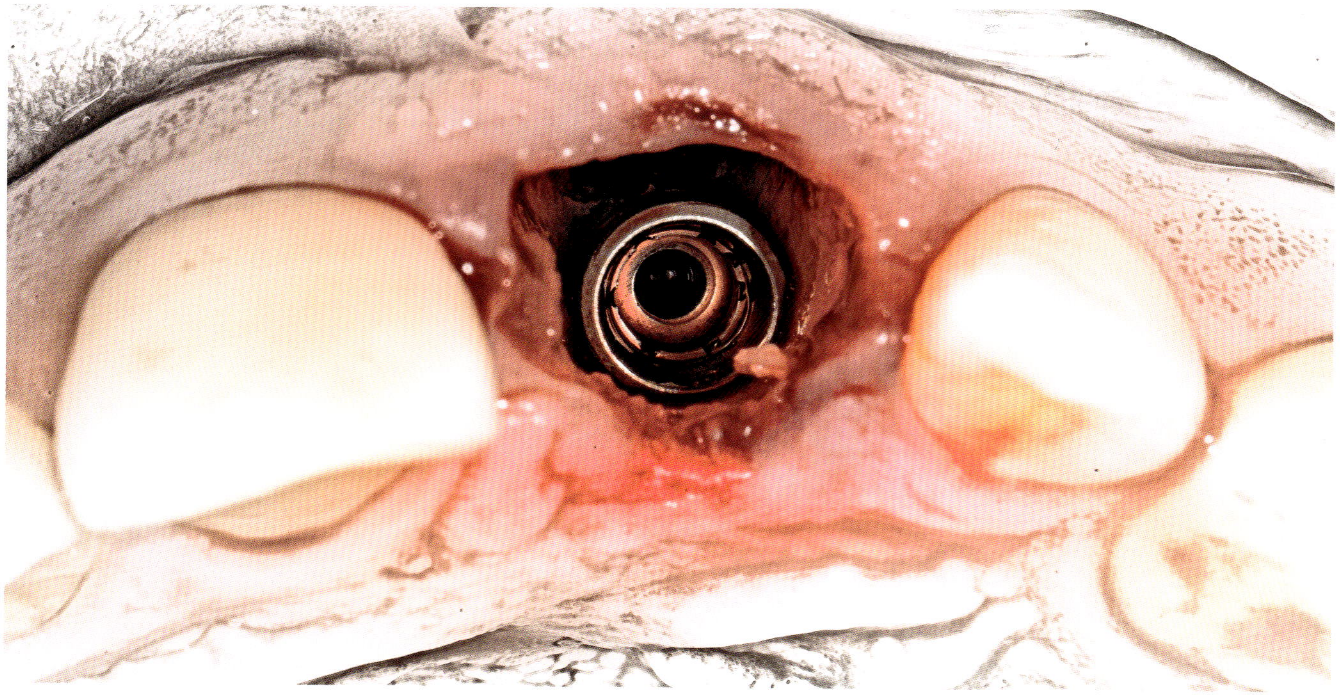

Figure 8-34 Osteotomy is prepped favoring the palatal wall. The final position of the immediate implant respects the facial contours and minimum dimensions.

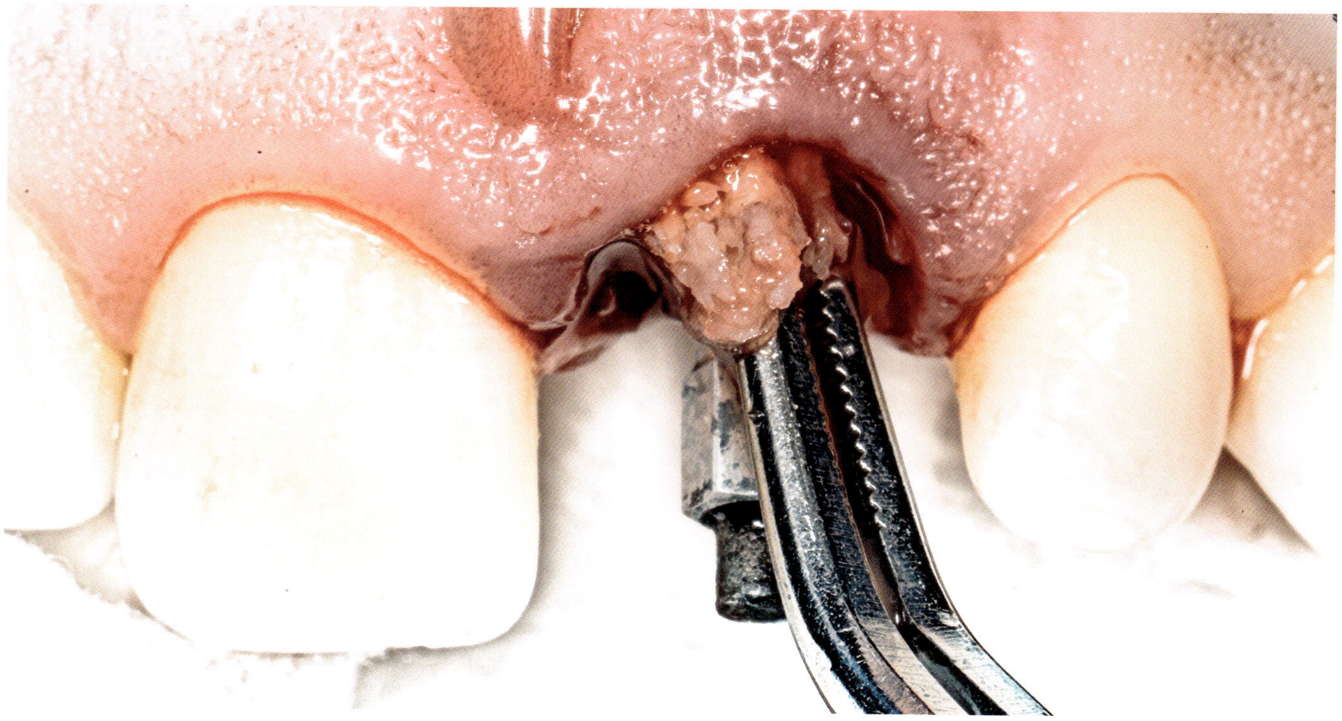

Figure 8-35 The facial gap is packed with allograft and PRF combination. Grafting with the Ostell peg in place protects the implant and allows more space to work than the abutment.

Figure 8-36 Crestal bone is contoured with a profiler to relieve the emergence profile, making room for a nicely contoured provisional restoration.

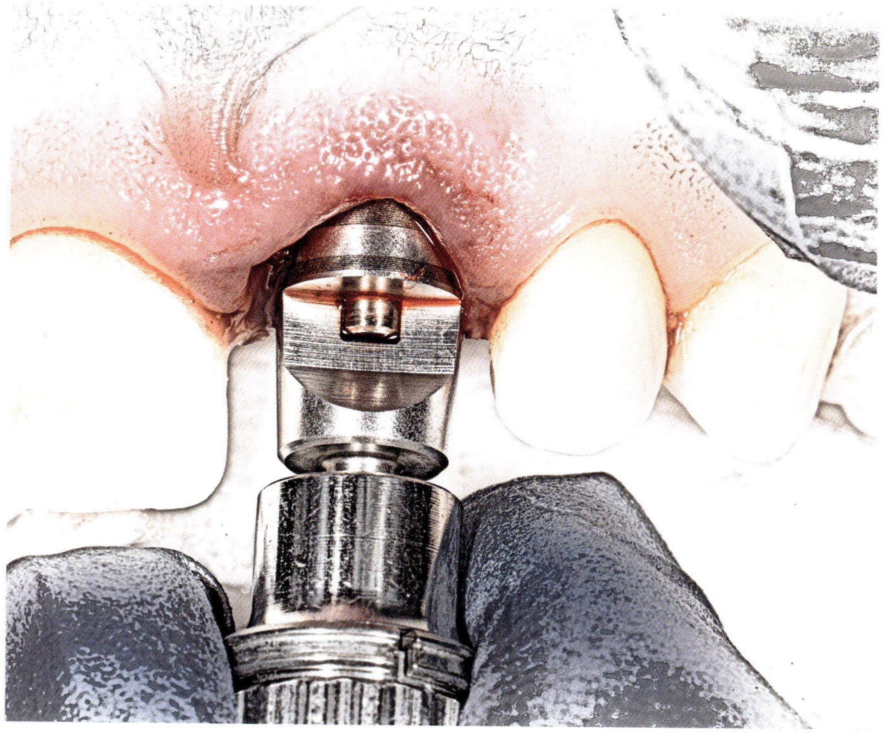

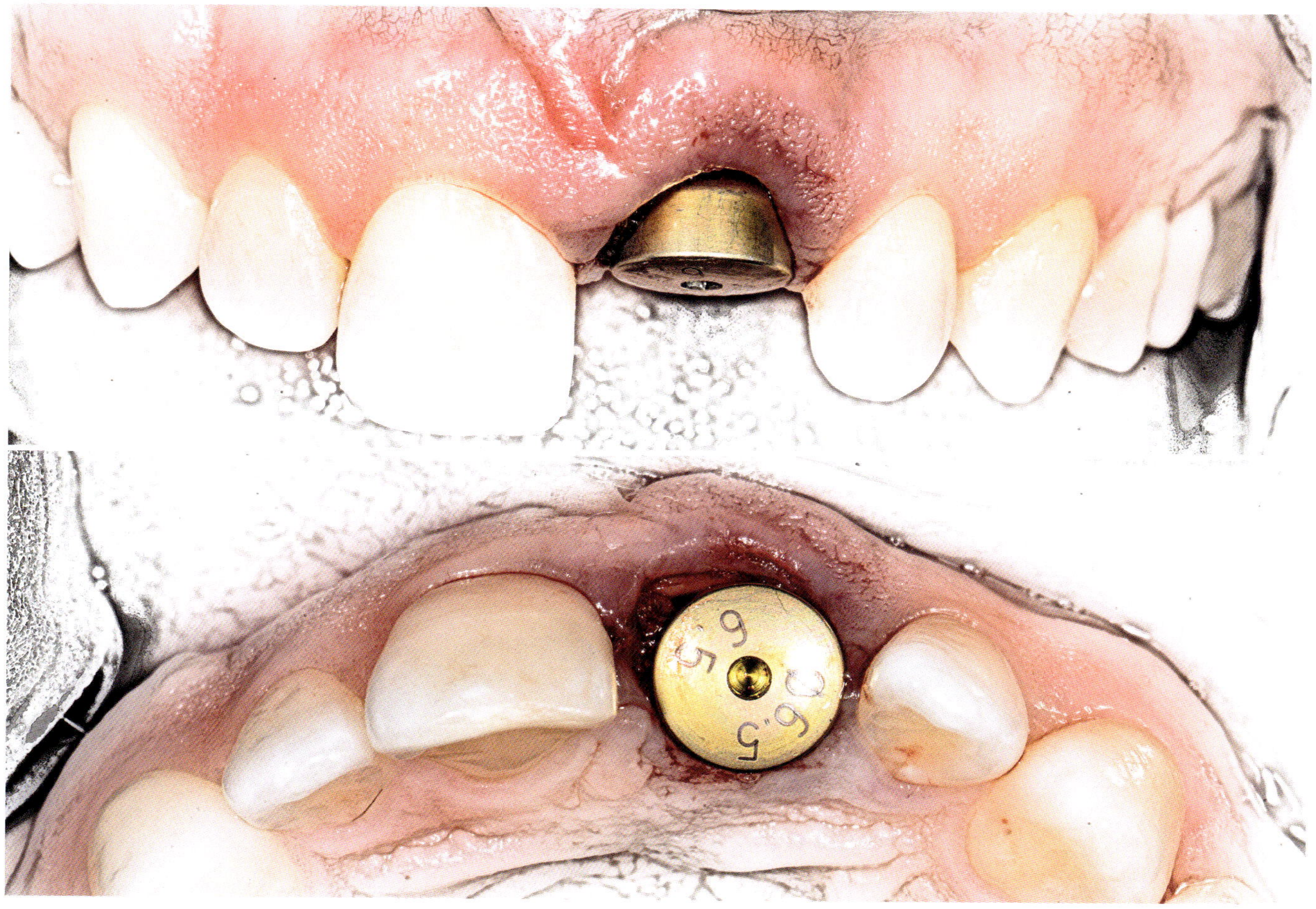

Figure 8-37 Healing abutment was placed for a few hours until the restorative dentists (Dr. Steve Zent and Dr. Sheena Zent) fabricated the immediate provisional restoration chairside.

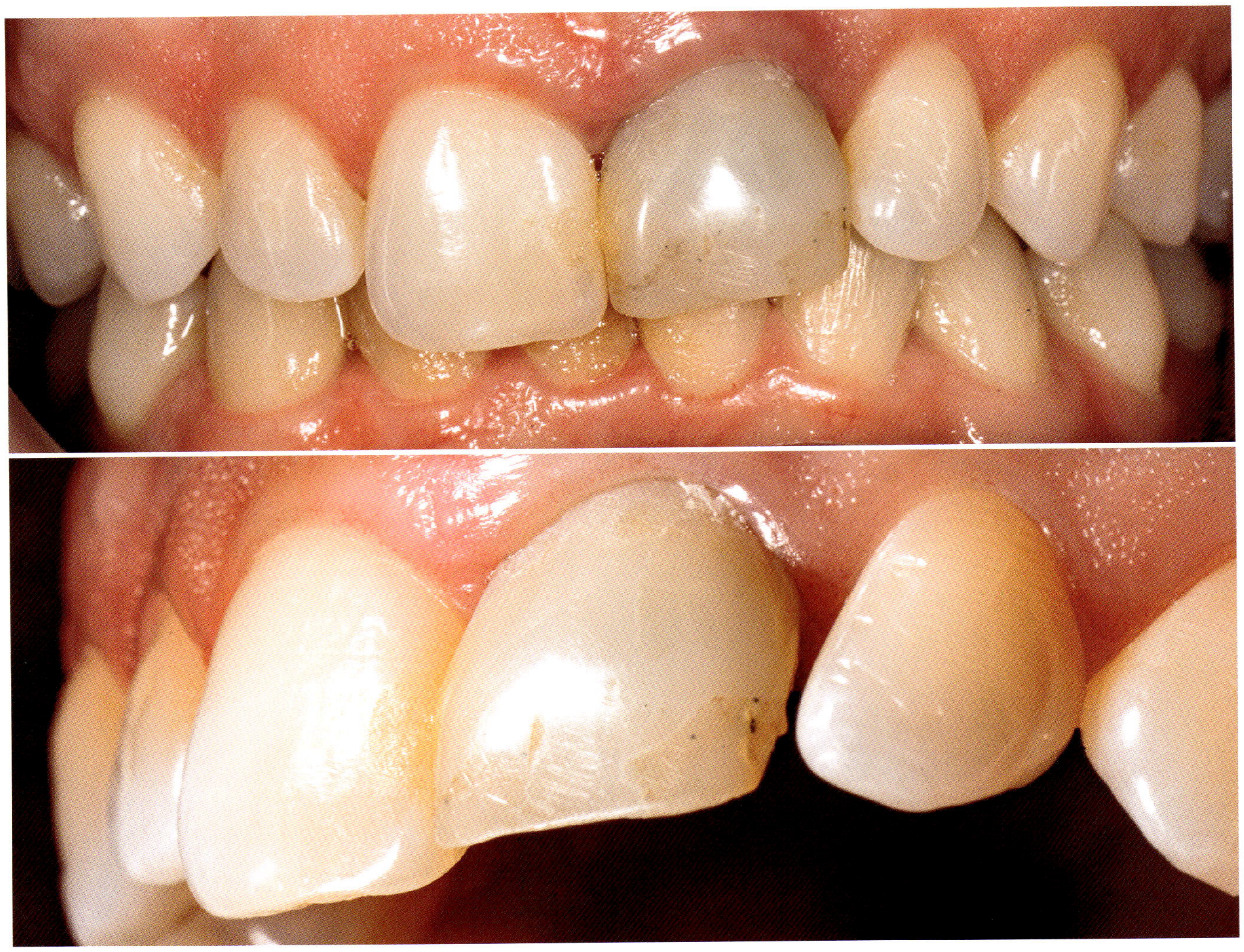

Figure 8-38 Immediate provisional No. 9 is out of occlusion. Notice how tooth No. 9 was also shorter than tooth No. 8 in the pre-operative pictures. The patient was delighted with this provisional.

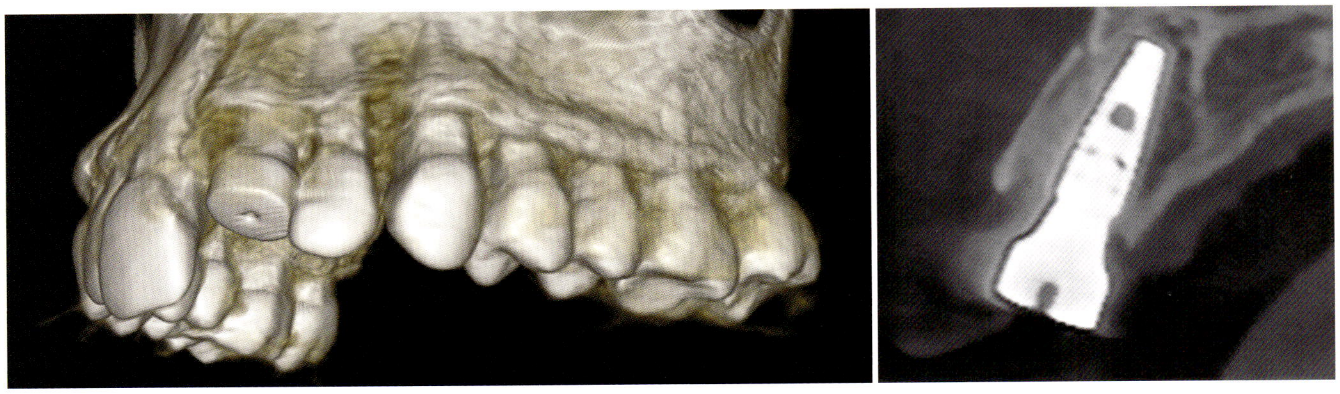

Figure 8-39 These radiographs show results of this immediate implant with ideal bone contours.

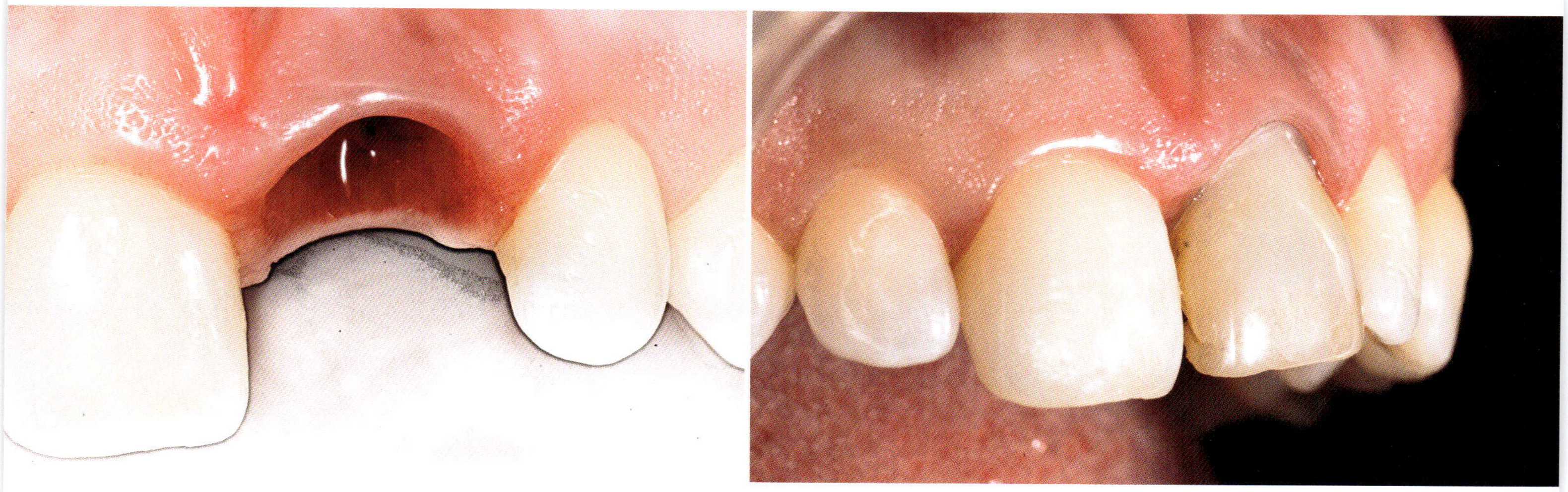

Figure 8-40 The soft tissue contours were maintained well. There is some inflammation in the sulcus likely due to the surface of the temporary restoration.

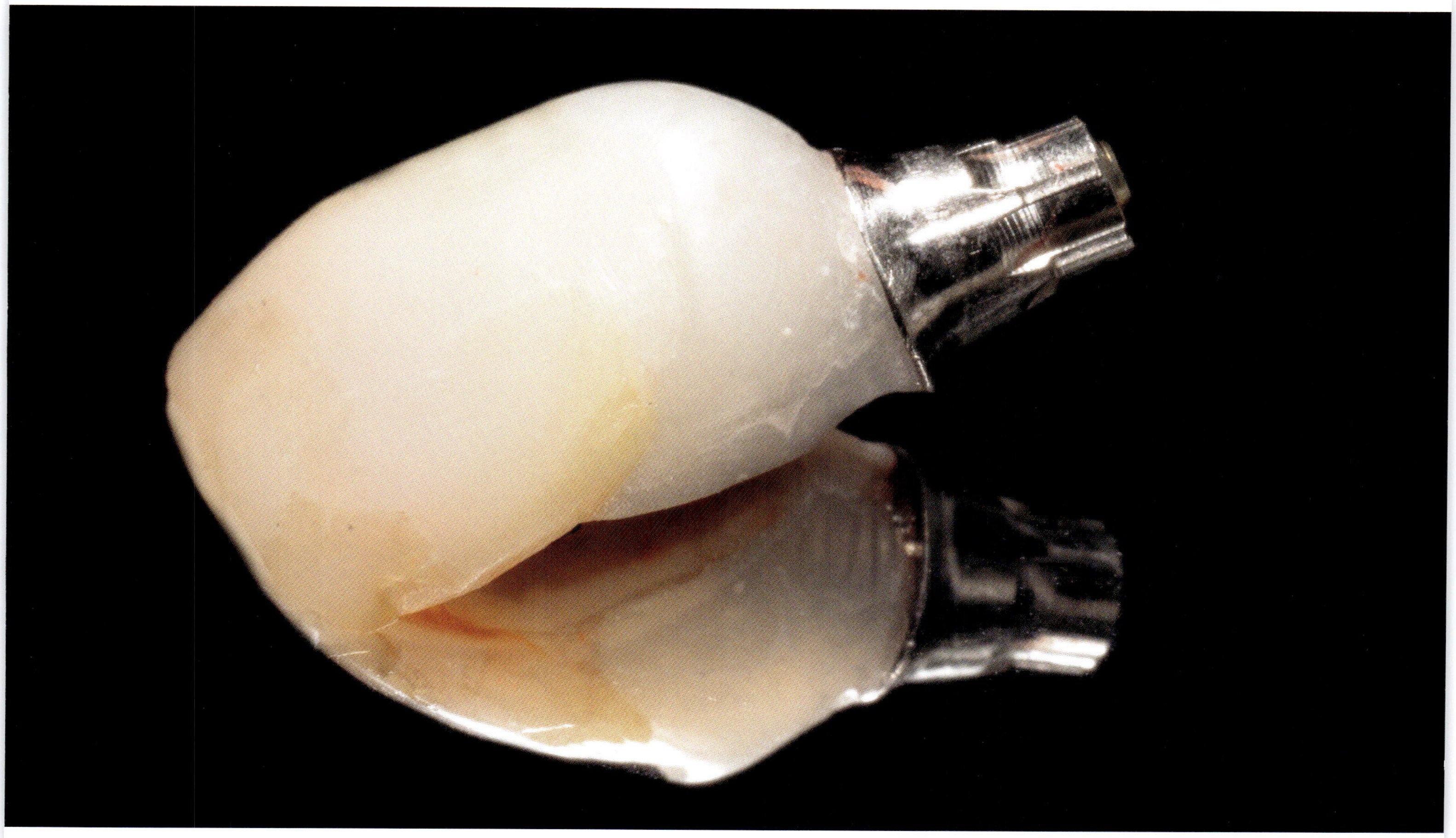

Figure 8-41 Smooth contours and refined margins are critical in guiding soft tissue healing around an immediate implant.

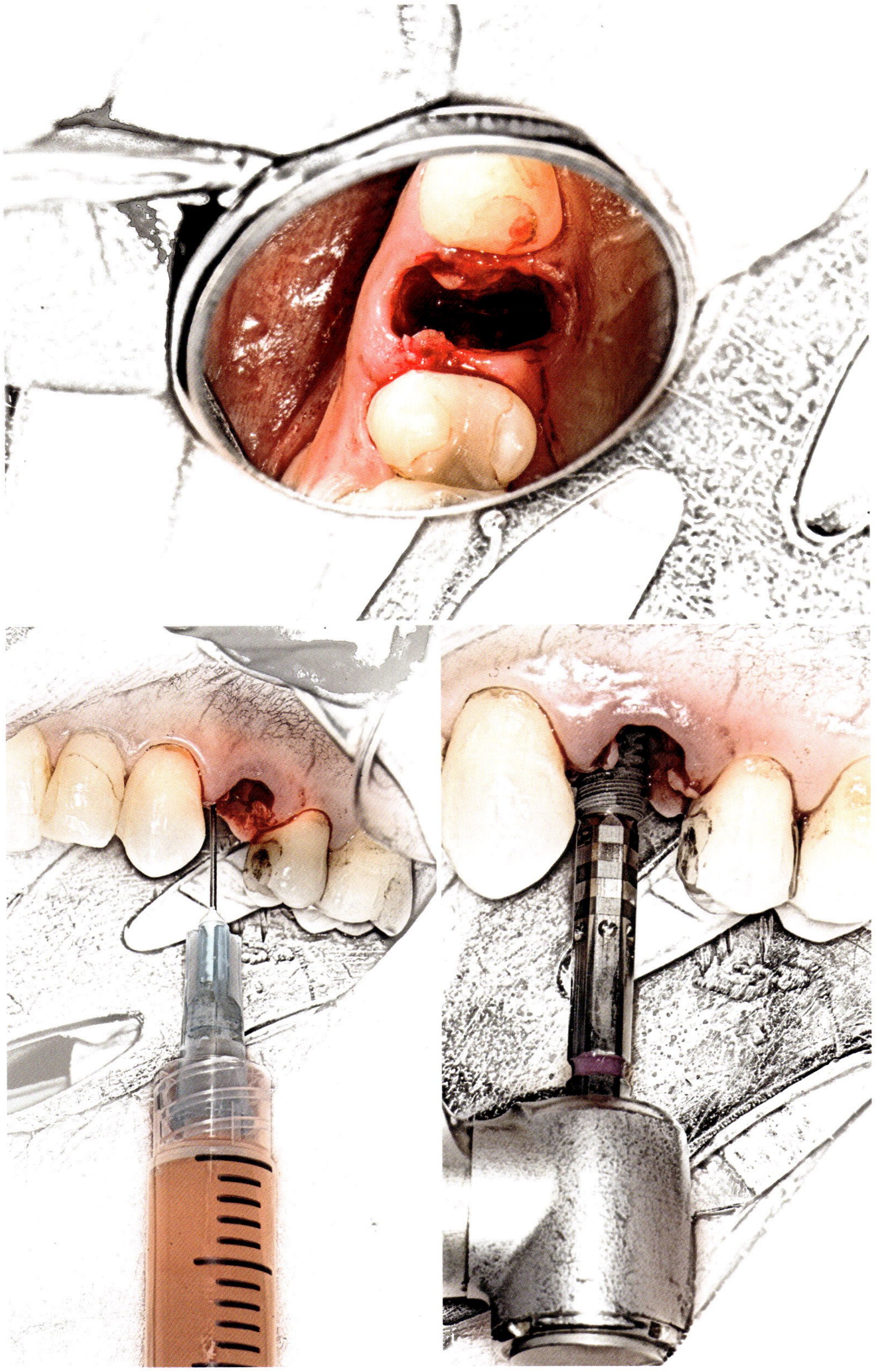

Figure 8-42 Using a mirror is helpful when examining and evaluating the site after the tooth is out. Administering i-PRF into the site immediately prior to implant placement wets the implant surface with bioactive material and helps optimize healing conditions for the implant.

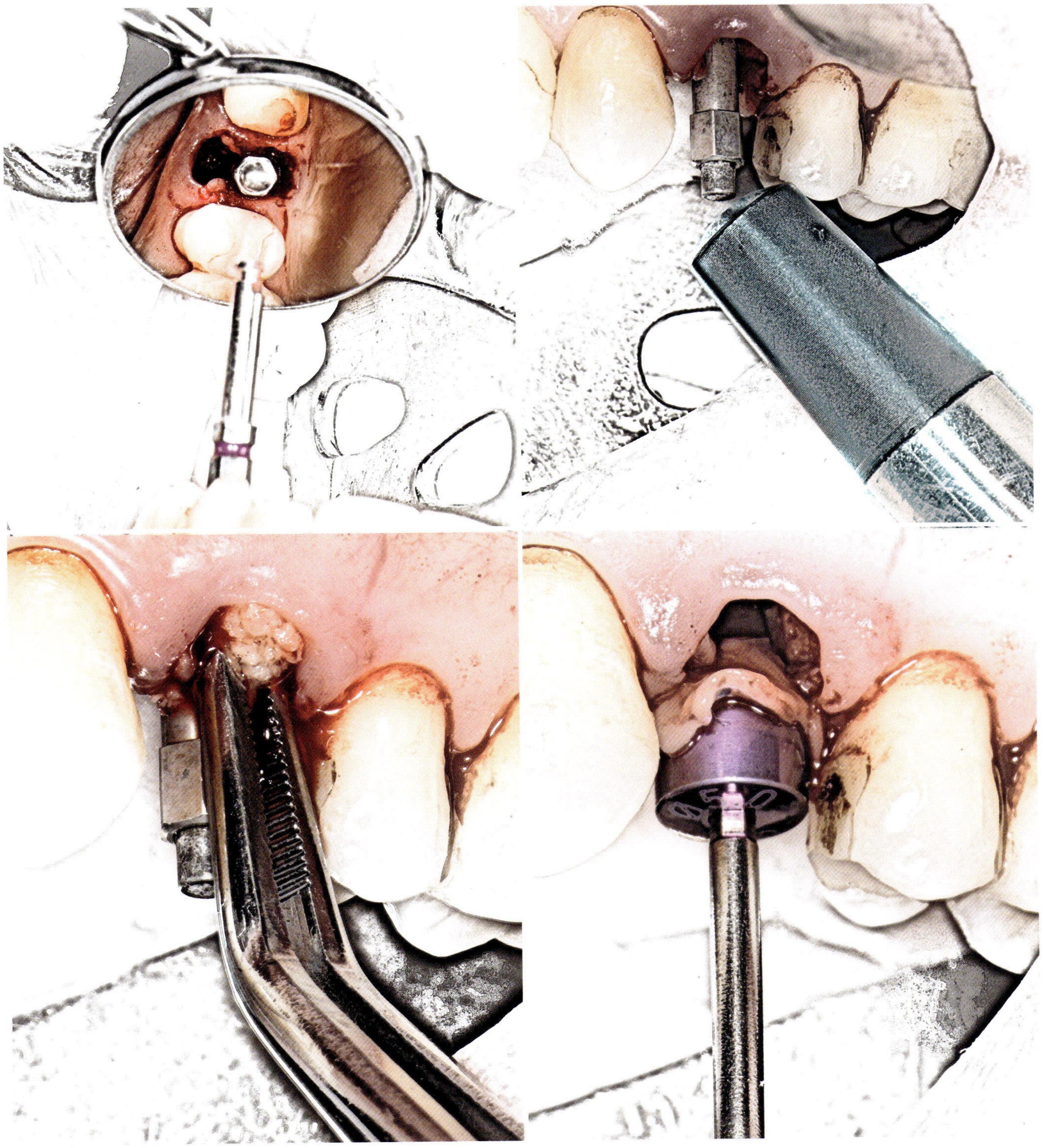

Figure 8-43 The gap between the implant and the buccal wall is grafted with a combination of cancellous freeze-dried bone allograft and minced PRF. This gap often leads to slightly lower implant stability due to lower bone to implant contact. I find the ISQ particularly valuable for immediate implants. The abutment is placed through a small hole in the PRF membrane and seated, containing the graft and socket beneath the membrane.

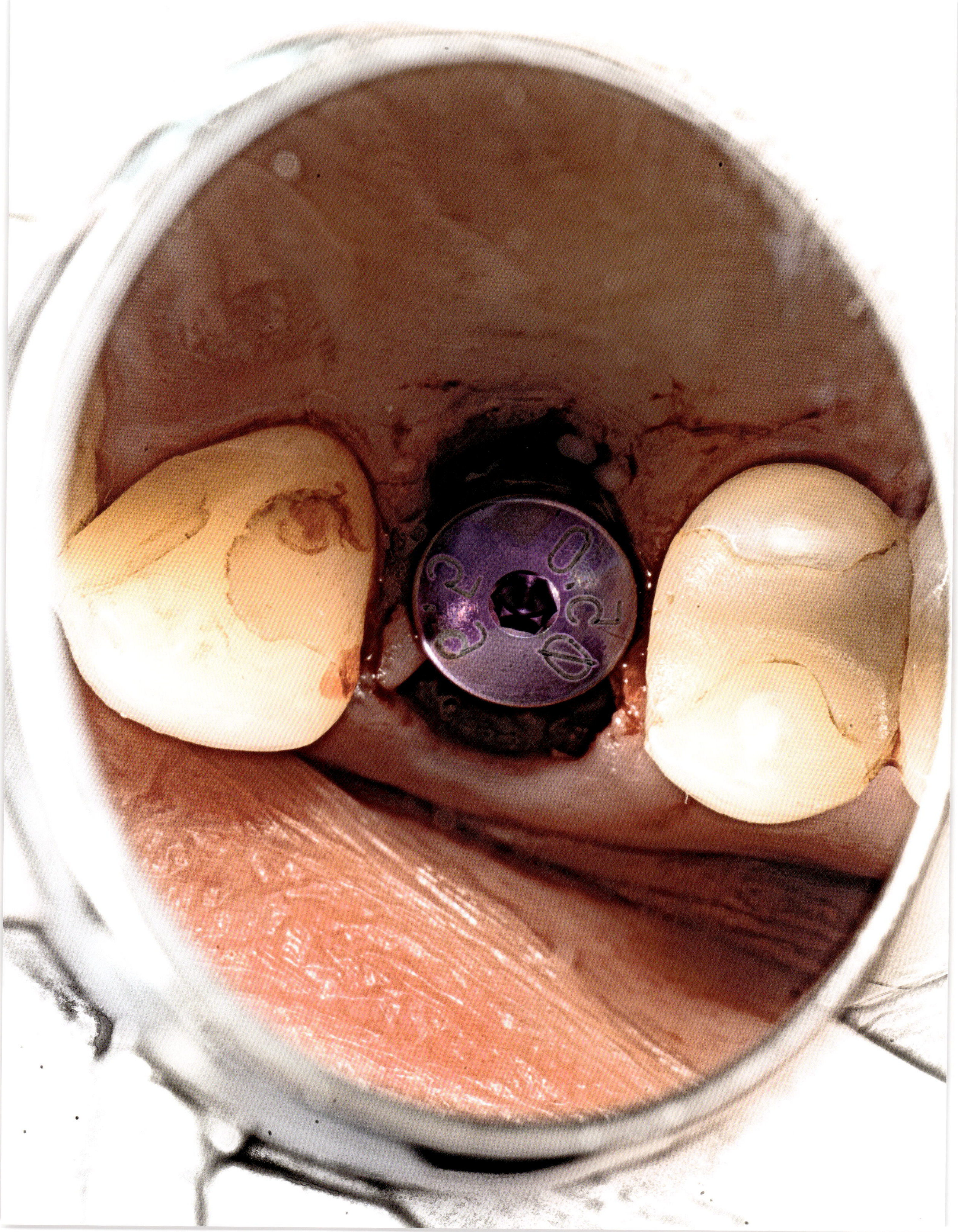

Immediate implants are a wonderful thing, but they are not for everyone. Not necessarily every patient. Not necessarily every site. And not necessarily every surgeon. Check the bone and soft tissue in the site. Do they look ready and willing to heal to the surface of rough titanium? Do they seem to have enough reserve in their tissue to absorb the insult and progress immediately to osseointegration? Does the hygiene and smoking habits of this particular lovely lady at age 76 push her over the edge to stage the implant treatment? These questions should be asked. I often tell patients "You could probably talk me into doing an immediate here, but given the circumstances, I just don't have as much confidence in my ability to get a stable implant or your ability to heal to an immediate implant. Let's consider playing it safe and going with my gut on this and extract, graft and come back after a few months healing to place the implant under a more controlled environment."

References

1. Block MS. How to Avoid Errors When Using Navigation to Place Implants – A Narrative Review. J Oral and Maxillofac Surg. 2023 Mar 1;81(3):299-307.
2. Mishra SK, Chowdhary R. Heat Generated by Dental Implant Drills During Osteotomy – A Review. J Indian Prosthodont Soc. 2014 Jun 1;14(2):131-143.
3. Abouzgia MB, Symington JM. Effect of drill speed on bone temperature. Int J Oral Maxillofac Surg. 1996 Oct;25(5):394-399.
4. Kraut RA. Clean operating conditions for the placement of intraoral implants. J Oral Maxillofac Surg. 1996 Nov;54(11):1337-1338.
5. Al Rezk F, Trimpou G, Lauer HC, et al. Response of soft tissue to different abutment materials with different surface topographies: a review of the literature. Gen Dent. 2018;66(1):18-25.
6. Furuhashi A, Ayukawa Y, Atsuta I, et al. Soft Tissue Interface with Various Kinds of Implant Abutment Materials. J Clin Med. 2021 May 28;10(11):2386.
7. Tonetti MS, Jung RE, Avila-Ortiz G, et al. Management of the extraction socket and timing of implant placement: Consensus report and clinical recommendations of group 3 of the XV European Workshop in Periodontology. J Clin Periodontol. 2019 Jun;46 Suppl 21:183-194.
8. Kamat M, Puranik R, Vanaki S, et al. An insight into the regulatory mechanisms of cells involved in resorption of dental hard tissues. J Oral Maxillofac Pathol. 2013;17(2):22833.

◂
Figure 8-44 Final examination reveals the graft contained beneath the PRF membrane collar and some slight soft tissue irregularities from the extraction. The final position is nicely within the occlusal table and centered between the teeth to optimize the emergence profile.

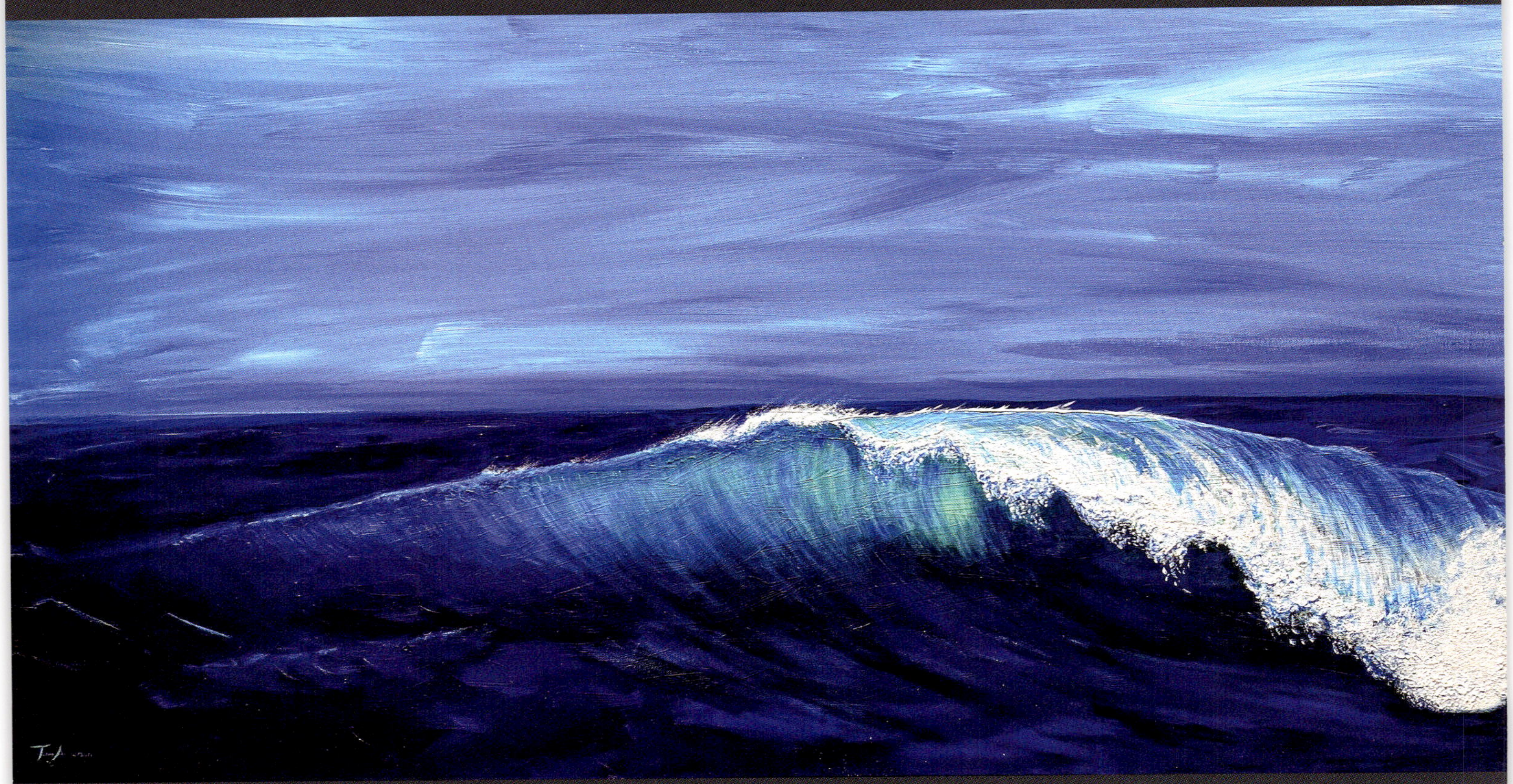

Through the Wave. (20x40 inch acrylic on canvas)
This painting hangs in my home as a reminder of two life lessons I learned sailing on big waters: sail *through* the waves and focus on the horizon.

CHAPTER 9

IMPLANT SITE DEVELOPMENT

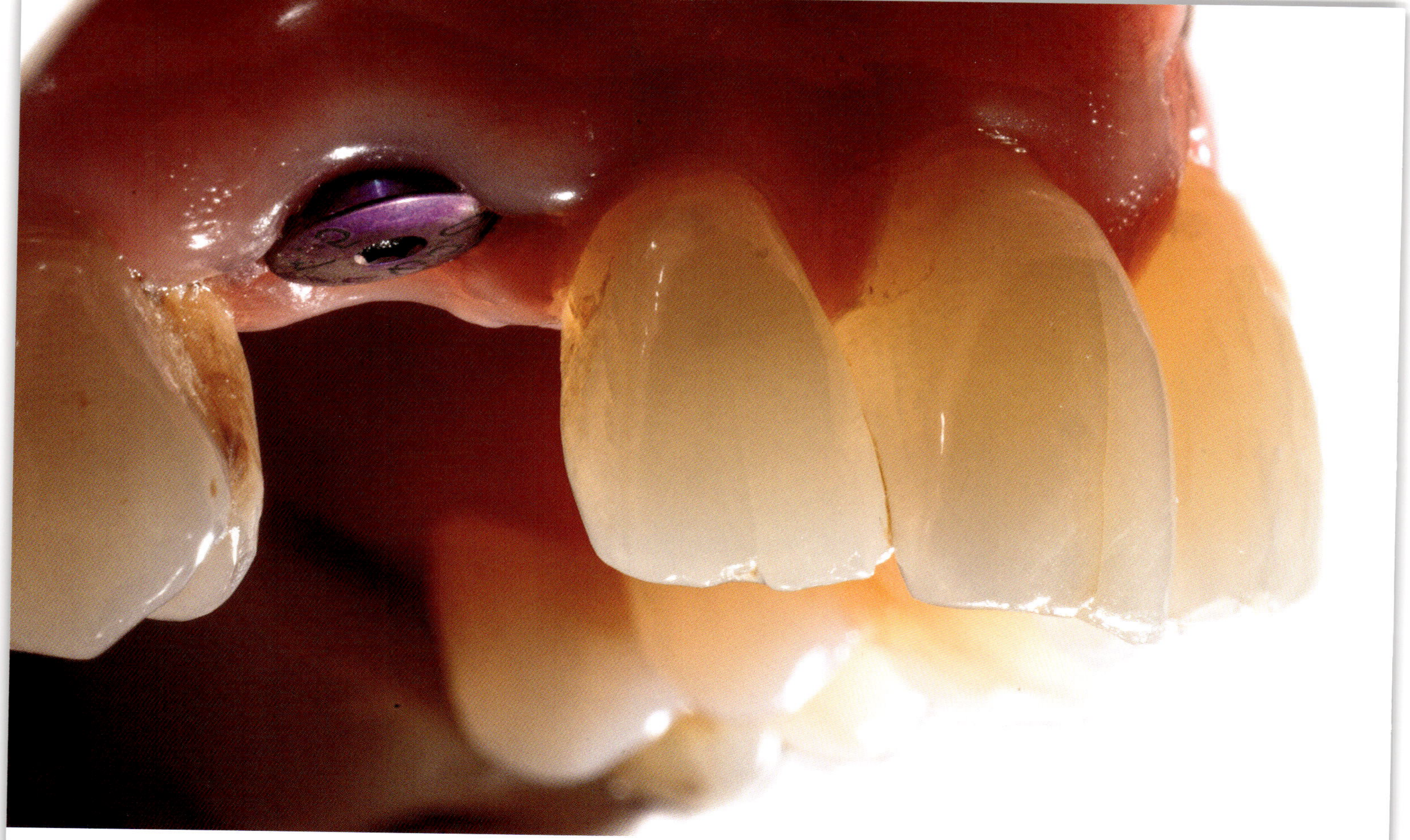

Figure 9-1

We are constantly pushing the envelope to achieve better results with ever increasing standards for success. Even if what we are doing seems fantastic to us by today's standards, we want to get better. Without a stable implant site, we won't have a stable implant. Bone and soft tissue work together in developing an implant site. They complement each other. Bone provides the structural framework for the overlying soft tissue. It can support and improve the soft tissue. Similarly, the soft tissue can sometimes compensate for limited bone. Ideally, we want to efficiently develop a site with great hard and soft tissue.

Hard Tissue Development

The moment a tooth is removed, the body begins the process of resorbing the bone to conserve resources. This happens to varying degrees in extraction socket healing as the ridge gets narrower and shorter. For some patients, almost no appreciable ridge resorption ever occurs. They just seem to keep a nice, broad ridge contour. But sometimes the body acts like a vacuum packer, sucking in all the tissue around the teeth and in edentulous areas.

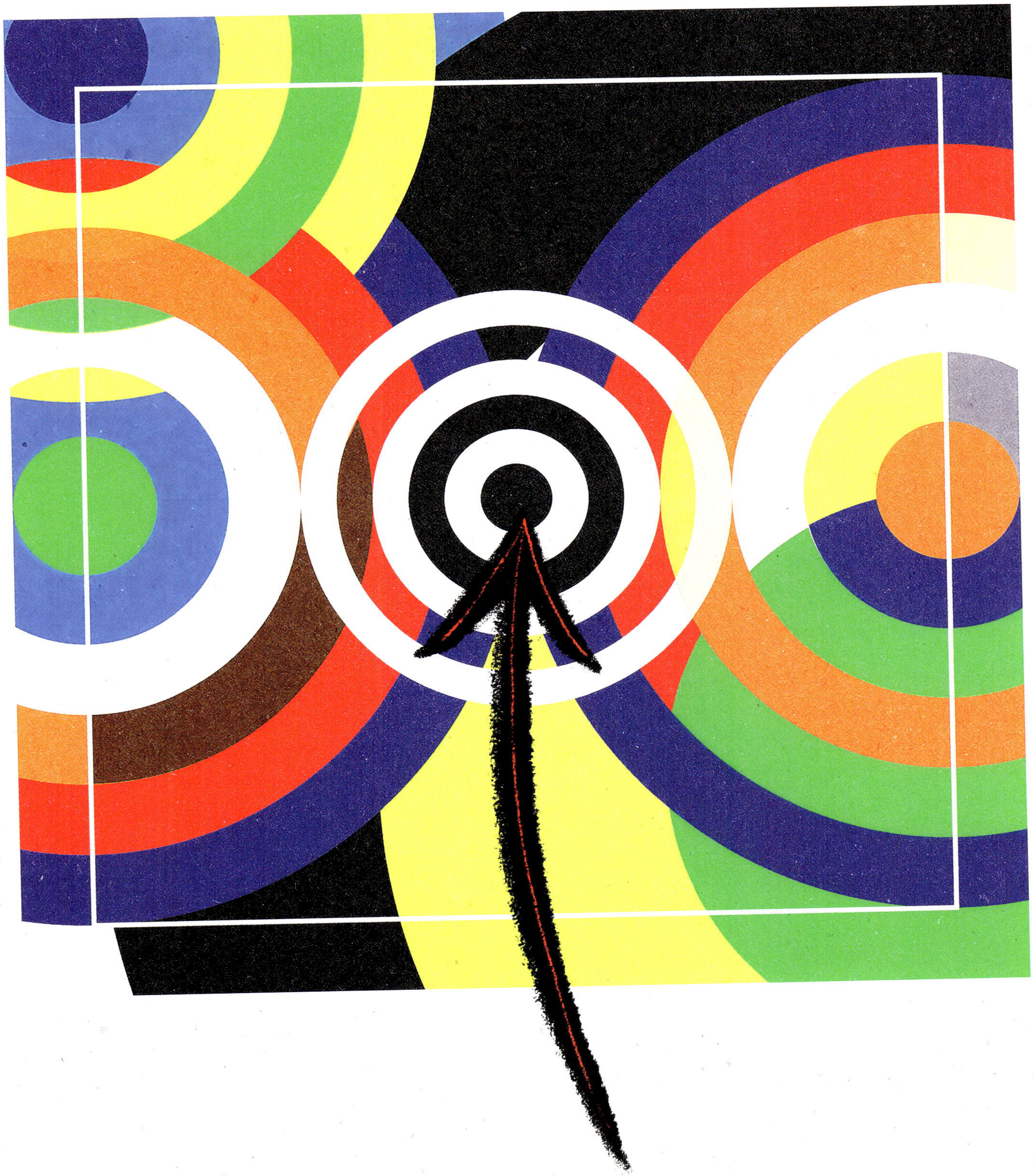

Figure 9-2 Optimizing hard and soft tissue is the goal for implant rehabilitation. Planning and careful tissue management are foundational to every surgery. We need to see how the factors influence each other. And we need to consider factors outside the box. (Artwork inspired by Frank Stella.)

These patients quickly lose width and height. For a clue on how the ridge may respond, pay attention to the general bone contours. If the bone is thin and scalloped around the roots or severely deficient in edentulous sites, there will likely be a lot of resorptive pressure on that site. Let that be an indication of how the body may try to heal. If ridge augmentation is needed, make sure to compensate for the increased pressure on the graft. The body has already declared it didn't want bone there. We have our work cut out to get it to keep any graft we place. It is our job to convince the body to do what we want it to do, not necessarily what it wants to do.

Hard tissue implant site development starts by minimizing trauma during extraction and optimizing bone in the healing socket. If needed, it includes horizontal or vertical ridge augmentation, sometimes including sinus augmentation. We'll look at some aspects of each.

When it comes to hard tissue management principles, we want to create and maintain space for the body to fill in with stable bone. It needs to be an environment that promotes bone healing, limits soft tissue infiltration, resists bacterial colonization, and maintains long-term stability around the implant.

Minimally traumatic extraction

Every surgeon's duty in every surgery is to minimize trauma. There is a lot of talk about atraumatic extraction right now. The idea of a truly atraumatic extraction is a bit of a misnomer. There is always some amount of trauma from an extraction. Our goal is to minimize trauma as much as reasonably possible. As I see it, there are three guiding principles for a minimally traumatic extraction: protecting the buccal plate, minimizing trauma to the surrounding bone and tissue, and preserving the periodontal ligament remnants as much as reasonably possible. This may require more patience and attention to detail than routine exodontia. It takes more time, but the persistent memory of the remaining tissue makes it worthwhile.

Protecting soft tissue protects underlying bone. For long-term success, this is especially important on the buccal aspect. The thin buccal plate inherently loses a big portion of its support and blood supply from the periodontal ligament when the tooth is removed. Atraumatic extraction is flapless, which preserves the periosteal blood supply. And it is kind to the buccal plate. Even microfractures can compromise the delicate intrinsic blood supply. Minimize lateral forces on the socket, especially in the buccal dimension.

The primary objective is to disrupt the periodontal ligament and float the tooth right out of the socket. The circumdental crestal fibers of the periodontal ligament can be severed with a scalpel or a controlled force on a thin elevator or periotome. These crestal fibers are oriented to be more resistant to extraction forces. The midroot or oblique fibers are more responsible for bearing the chewing load.

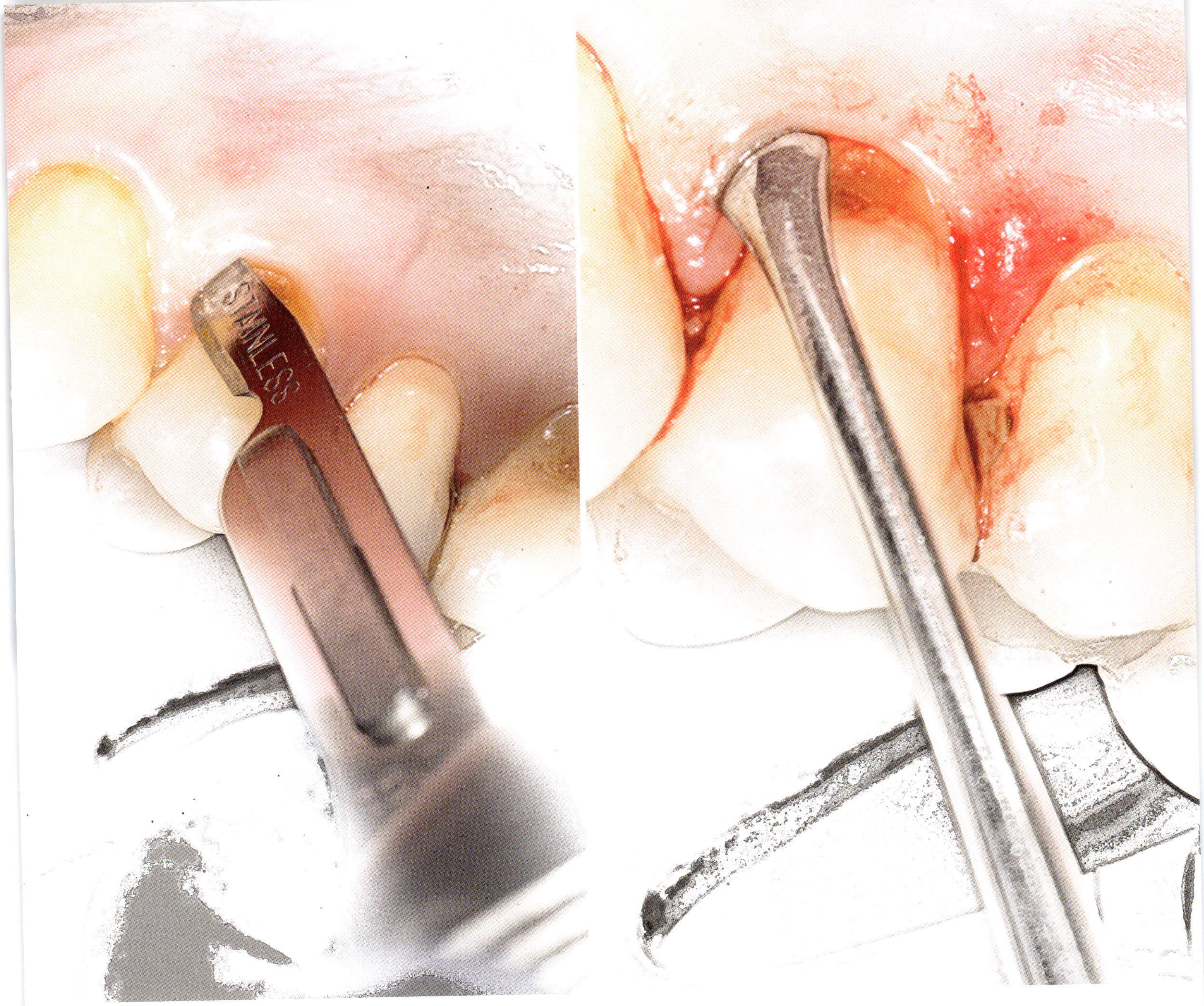

Figure 9-3 Incising the crestal periodontal ligament with a 15c blade and a Micro Buser helps minimize trauma and optimize healing.

Surgically severing the ligament as much as possible is the initial step in atraumatic extraction.

The periodontal ligament is designed primarily to sustain a loading force during chewing. It can experience catastrophic failure when the tooth is overloaded laterally and extrusively. After incising the crestal fibers, push the periotome into the ligament space with controlled pressure all around the tooth. This further severs the ligament and applies lateral and avulsive forces on the tooth. The ligament and bone are said to "creep" or change shape over time under the constant load of the instrument. This gradual change loosens the tooth by disrupting the ligament and gently expanding the socket. There is also a physiologic change leading to enzymatic breakdown of the ligament.

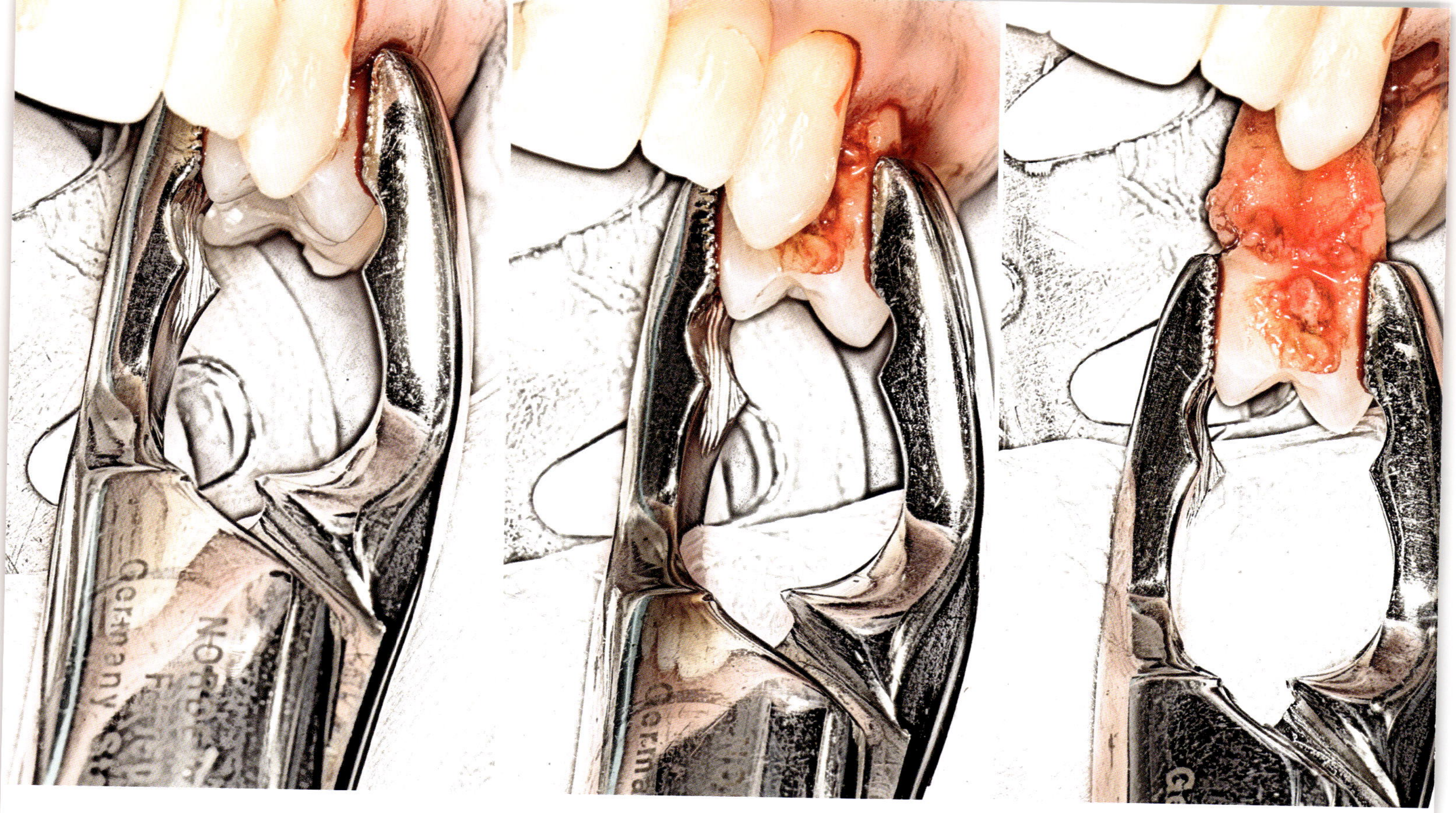

Figure 9-4 When the tooth has been adequately luxated and the periodontal ligament stretched, you can easily deliver the tooth with forceps using little force.

One particularly clever system designed to protect the buccal bone while applying these forces is the Physics Forceps™. The design applies a lever action on the tooth with the fulcrum widely spread on the buccal tissue, thus preserving and protecting underlying bone. There is an art to this technique that requires some experience to master. The general concept of severing the ligament and applying sustained, controlled forces to expand the socket and disrupt the ligament can be employed with many different instruments. Sometimes just giving the ligament time to respond to the stimulation will simplify the extraction. If a tooth seems to be particularly stubborn, consider subjecting it to constant luxating forces for 20 to 30 seconds in each of a few dimensions. Then, leave the tooth alone for a few minutes. If there are other teeth to remove, proceed with them and come back. Or maybe even step out of the room for a minute. Sometimes, after a few minutes alone, the tooth will be ready to come out with relative ease. Other times, it is still as stubborn, but at least you have a fresh perspective on it.

Respect the soft tissue. It can easily be crushed during extraction. An elevator can pulverize the papilla. The beaks of forceps can wreck the buccal tissue. This can be especially harmful when it destroys a thin band of keratinized gingiva. The quality of the tissue surrounding the extraction socket determines how it will heal. Good buccal keratinized gingiva stimulates the site to populate with good healthy keratinized gingiva. When you seat forceps, look to make sure the tips aren't going to harm the tissue.

There is collateral damage from the microscopic battle around many of the teeth we remove. The chronic inflammatory process has beat up the cellular structure of the tissue. Neutrophils have migrated through the leaky vessels into the area. In the fight, they have inadvertently begun destroying the collagen by releasing collagenase and other destructive enzymes[1]. The connective tissue holding everything together has been stretched by the increased fluid from edema. The tissue is ragged and weary, barely holding on. We often remove teeth in this environment. We step in to help the body heal through surgery. Be kind to this tissue. It needs all the help it can get.

Ridge preservation

Preserving the ridge from the inevitable resorption is a mitigation tactic. Some resorption will occur, we just want as little as possible. There are numerous techniques that reduce resorption. Many different types of graft material have been employed, from allograft and autograft, to xenograft and alloplastic material. Even native tooth structure can shield the buccal plate. This employs the retained periodontal ligament to provide stimulation, effectively fooling the alveolar bone into thinking there is still a tooth it needs to maintain. It tricks the body into doing what we want it to do, rather than what it is programmed to do.

While the specifics continue to change with the state of the art, the general concept is to place material into the site to support the bone and slow its resorption. The most common commercial products are allograft and xenograft bone. These mostly get turned over into vital bone with time. Some materials, such as xenograft, undergo a slower turnover process and have more graft remnants long term. Allograft undergoes more rapid maturation and, potentially, more rapid resorption. Depending on the situation, the properties of the different options can be leveraged to optimize short- and long-term outcomes. Where we want faster regeneration, allograft may be preferred. When there is more pressure for resorption, incorporating xenograft may help maintain the volume for longer.

In addition to graft material selection, there are multiple options for a membrane to cover the graft. Some research even questions the long-term benefits from any membrane at all, though this is debatable. Overall, membranes can be divided into resorbable and non-resorbable, synthetic, alloplastic, xenoplastic or autologous. Each of these options have shown unique benefits. While some have more benefits than others, clinicians owe it to their patients to understand the evolution of these materials and techniques to provide the best possible outcomes.

When an implant is planned, ridge preservation is almost always beneficial. Most of the time, the steps are quite simple. Remove the tooth. Remove any pathologic tissue from the socket. Place particulate graft material. Cover it with a membrane. Retain the membrane with a suture. This is simple and effective most of the time.

In situations where there is a large osseous defect, especially on the buccal, more advanced techniques are beneficial. Simply condensing an allograft into a site with a blown-out wall may improve the situation some but the soft tissue can quickly infiltrate the graft, leaving a residual defect. Restoring the alveolar volume works better by placing a non-resorbable or slow resorbing membrane over the buccal defect to prevent soft tissue infiltration into the graft. This is a situation where elevating the buccal tissue may be indicated, which contradicts atraumatic extraction principles. By carefully elevating the tissue at the margin of the defect, you can create space for the membrane to span the defect. This keeps the periosteum and soft tissue out of the socket.

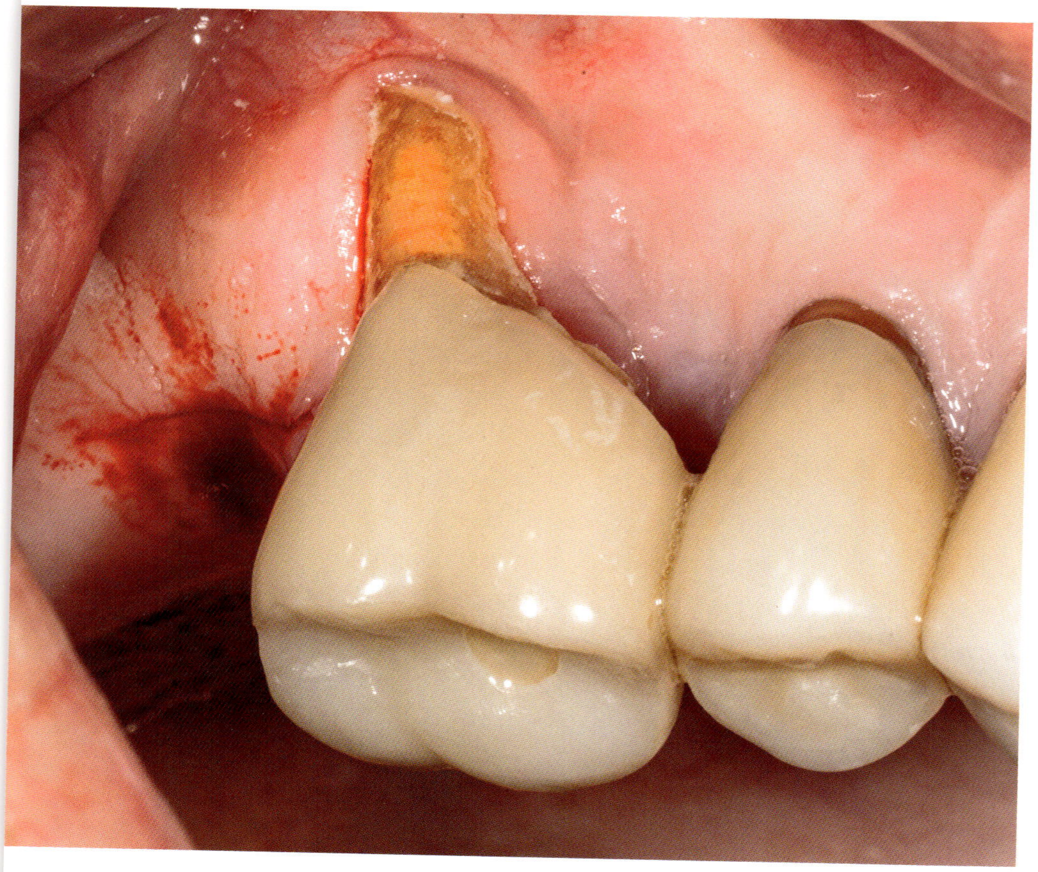

Figure 9-5 This recession defect has compromised the hard and soft tissue. The goal with this implant site preparation is to regain alveolar volume and keratinized gingiva. One predictable way of accomplishing this is ridge preservation performed with a non-resorbable membrane.

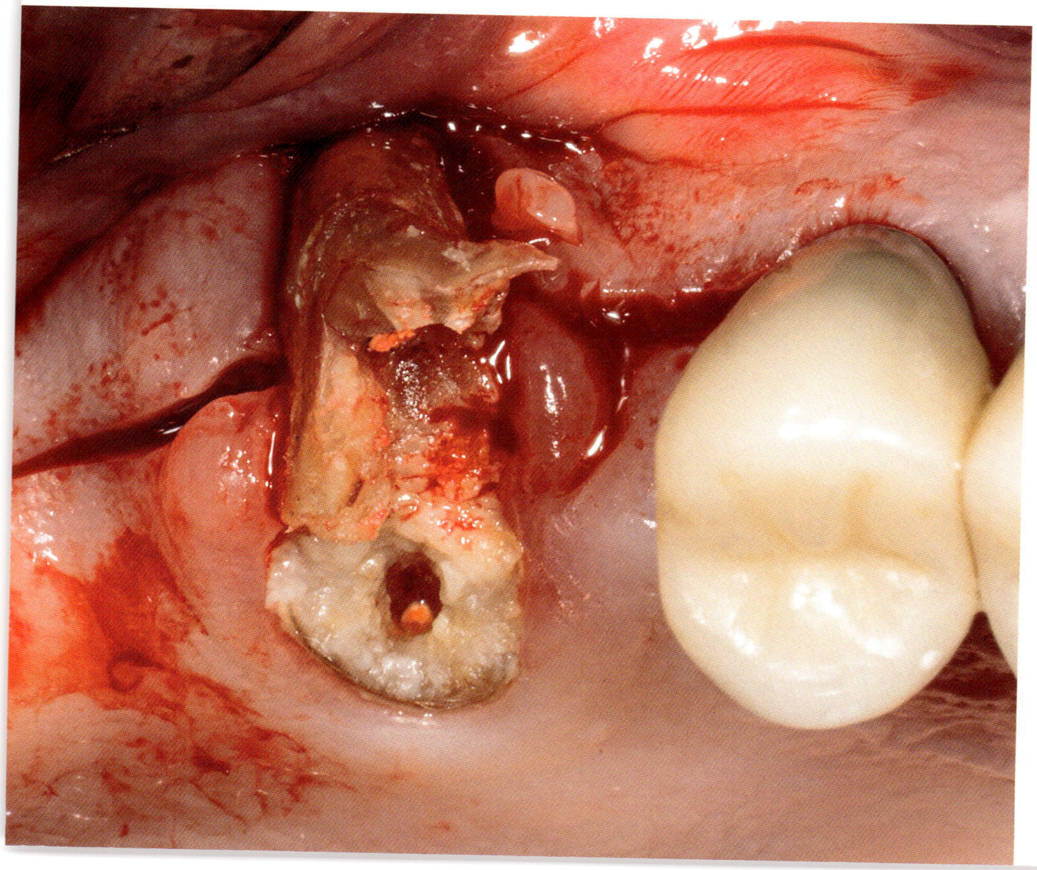

Figure 9-6 Access to the entire buccal osseous defect allows membrane placement across the defect. This is accomplished with a mesial and distal releasing incision.

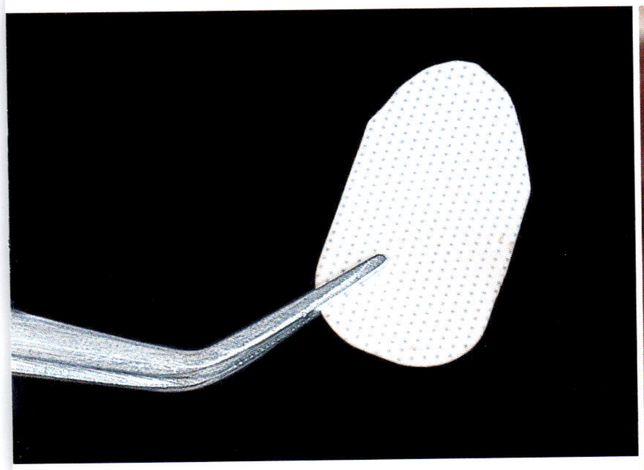

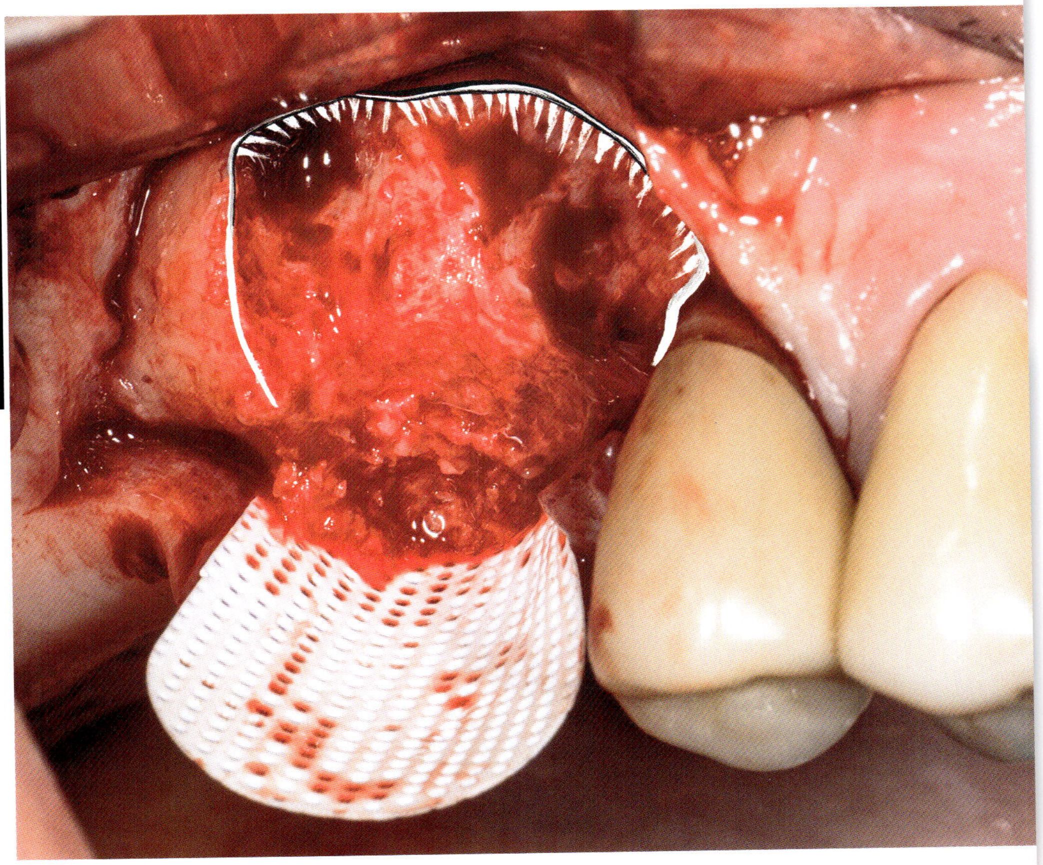

Figure 9-7 With the flap reflected, tooth removed, and site debrided, a PTFE membrane is contoured and tucked under the palatal periosteum. Trimming the membrane a bit can make it easier to tuck under the tissue. This flap must be subperiosteal to develop space for the membrane. The flap reflection and membrane should span the osseous defect. The site is then filled with graft material from the palatal toward the buccal. Notice the significant osseous defect we are trying to restore.

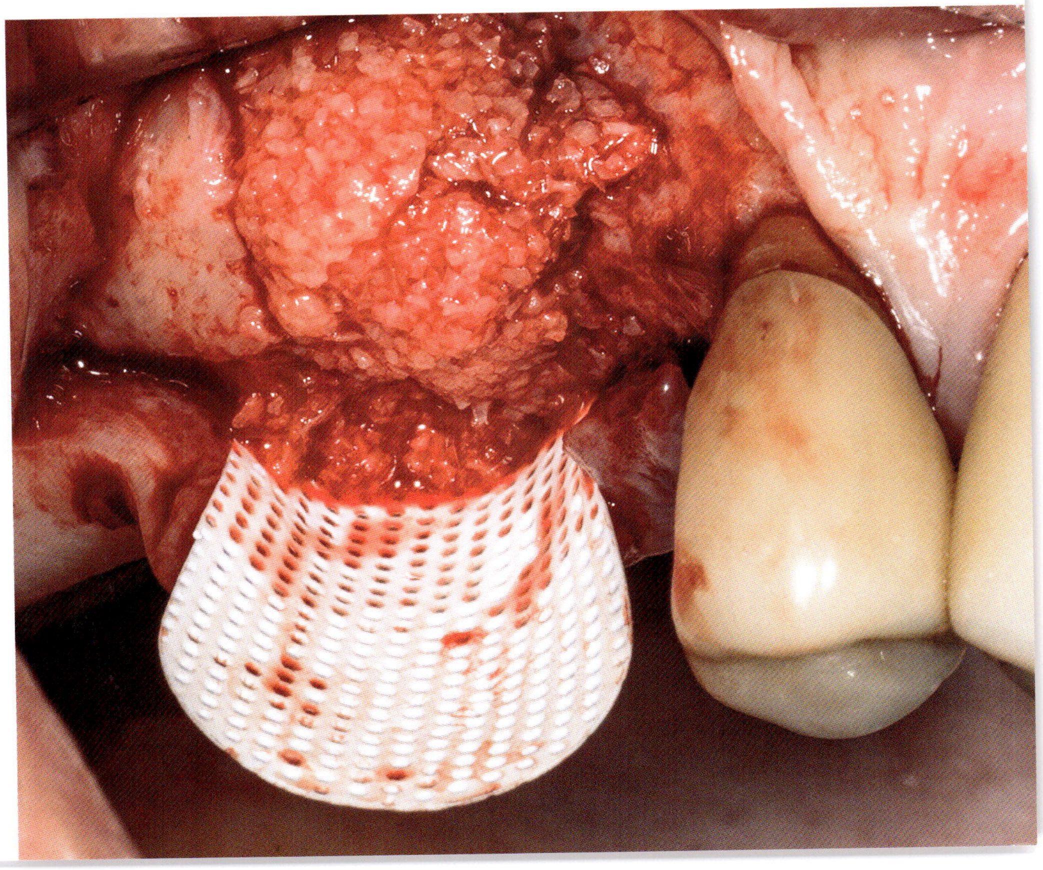

Figure 9-8 The graft can overfill the site slightly, especially on the buccal.

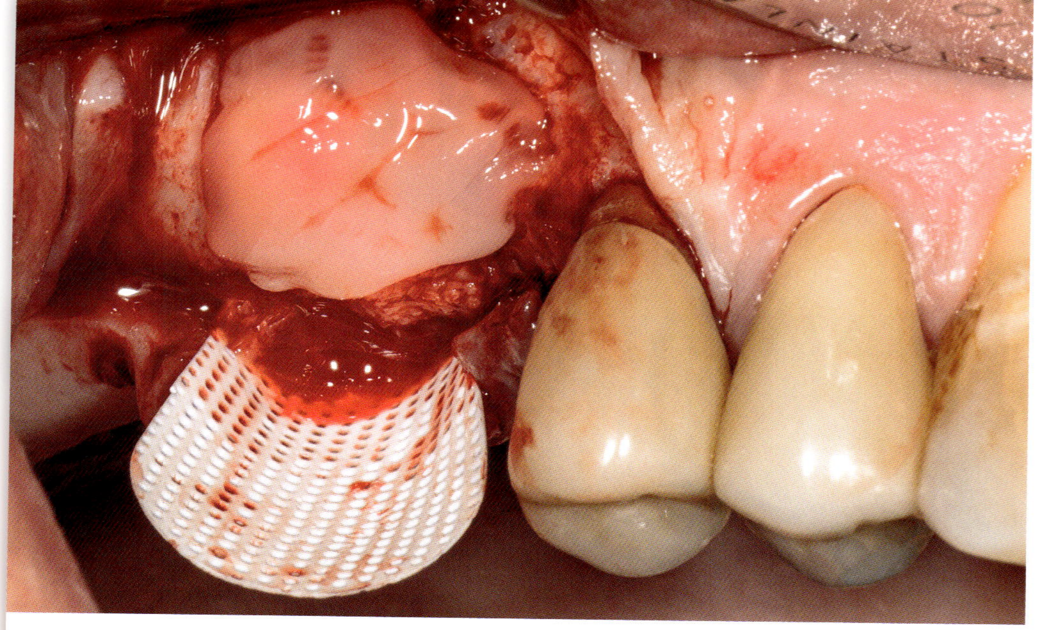

Figure 9-9 PRF membrane is placed over the graft material and under the PTFE membrane.

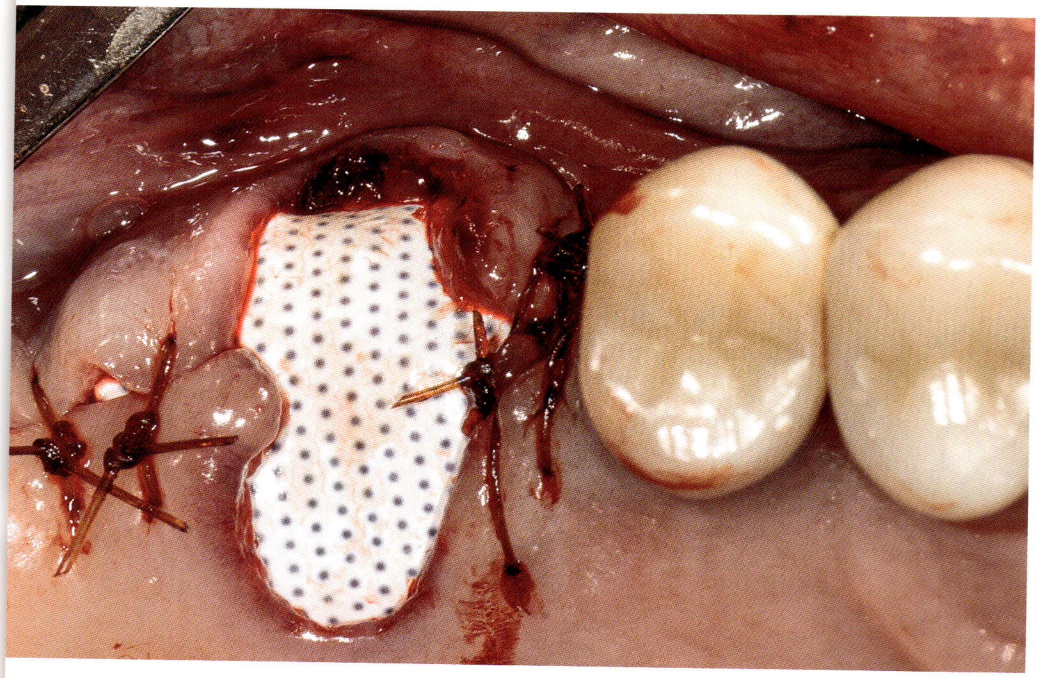

Figure 9-10 The PTFE membrane is tucked under the buccal tissue and sutures are used to reapproximate the flap. Note the exposed membrane. Keratinized gingiva will populate beneath this membrane in the weeks to come. The membrane must be passive under the tissue and should be flat with no folds. Primary closure should be avoided in these cases.

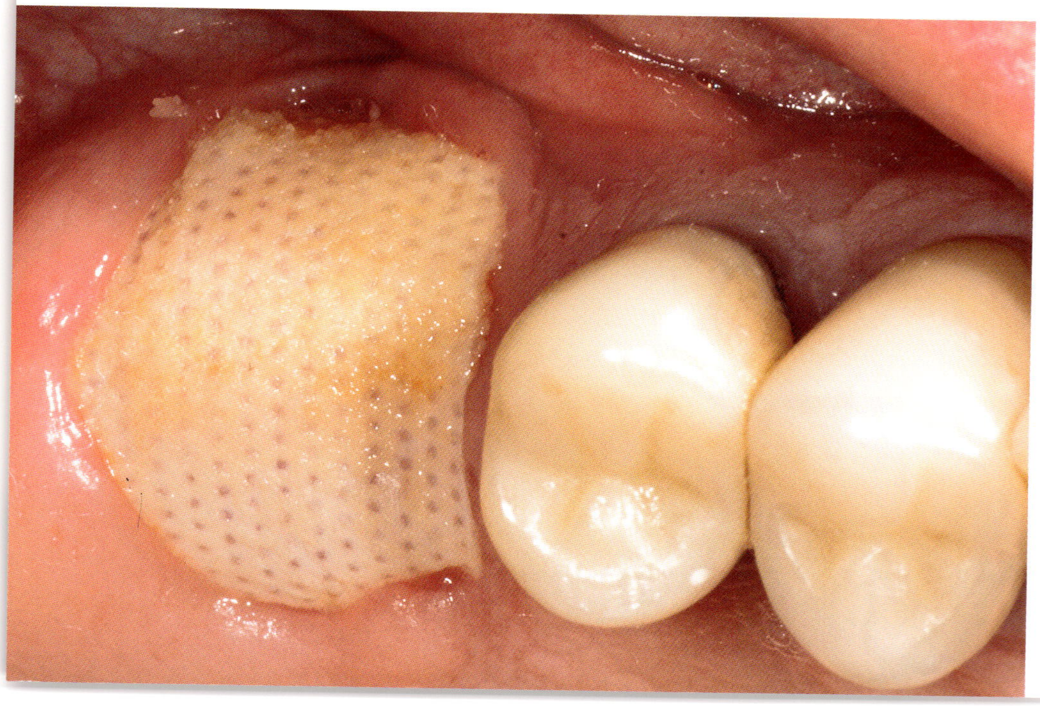

Figure 9-11 After one month of healing, the membrane remains exposed and is normally covered with plaque.

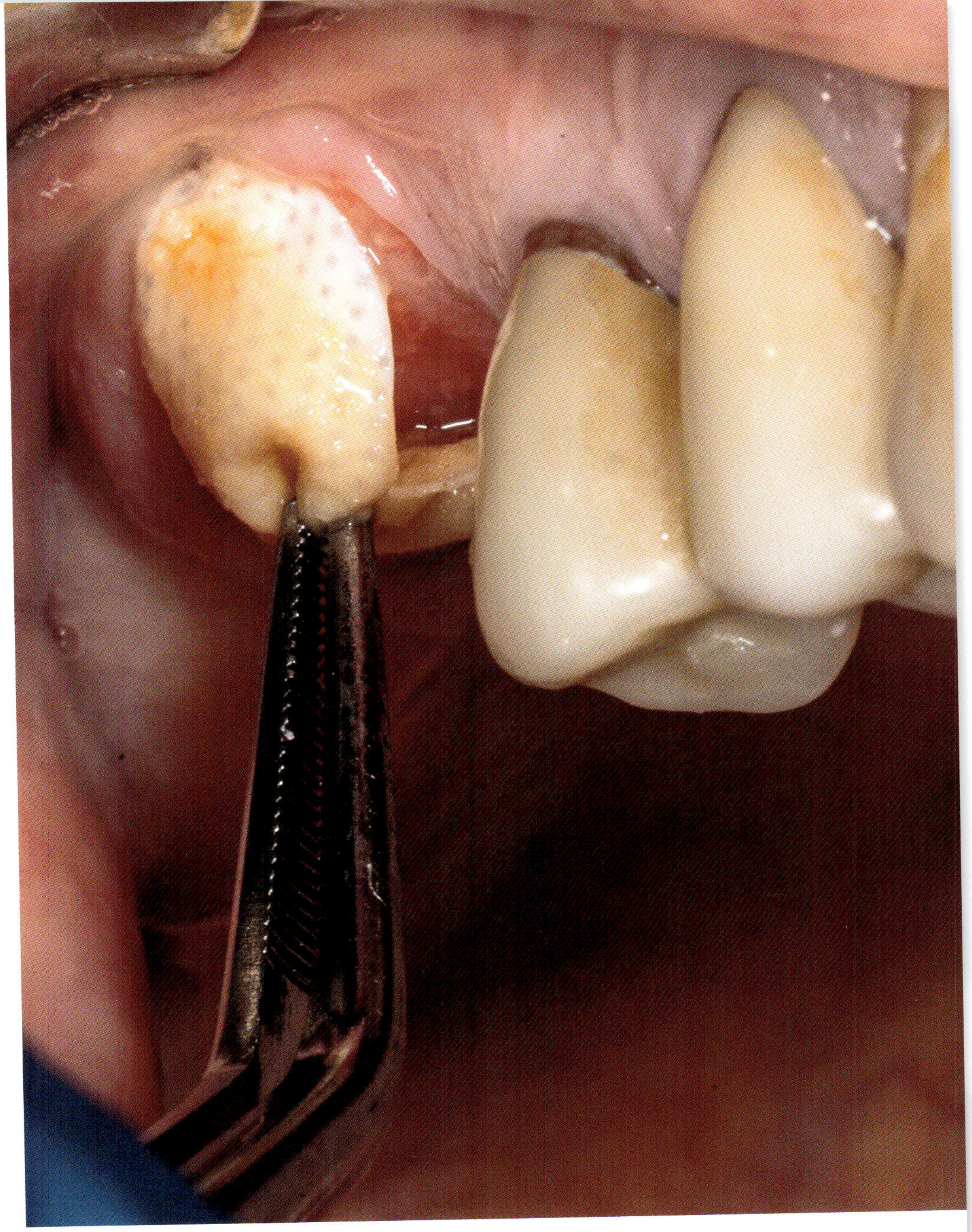

Figure 9-12 After about three months of healing, the membrane is easily removed without anesthetic. It feels like an odd tug to the patient, but seldom causes pain.

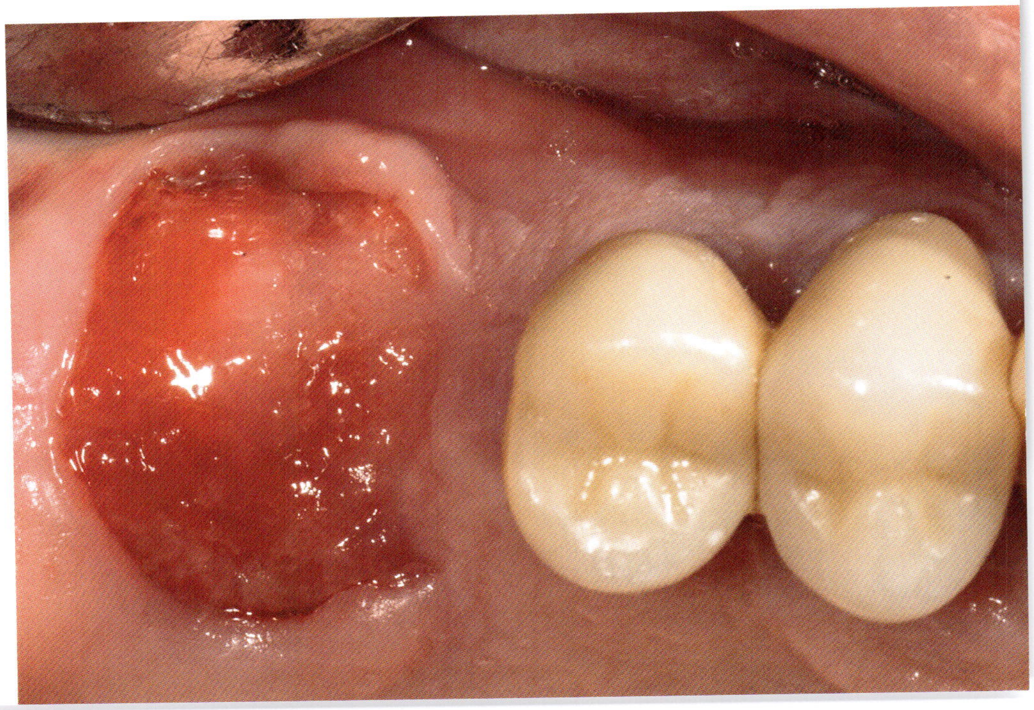

Figure 9-13 Upon membrane removal, the underlying tissue appears to be healing well. This entire site should fill in with keratinized gingiva. Sometimes, small bone graft fragments exfoliate from the site before it is entirely revascularized. When patients know this can happen, they are less likely to become overly concerned. This is healing very well.

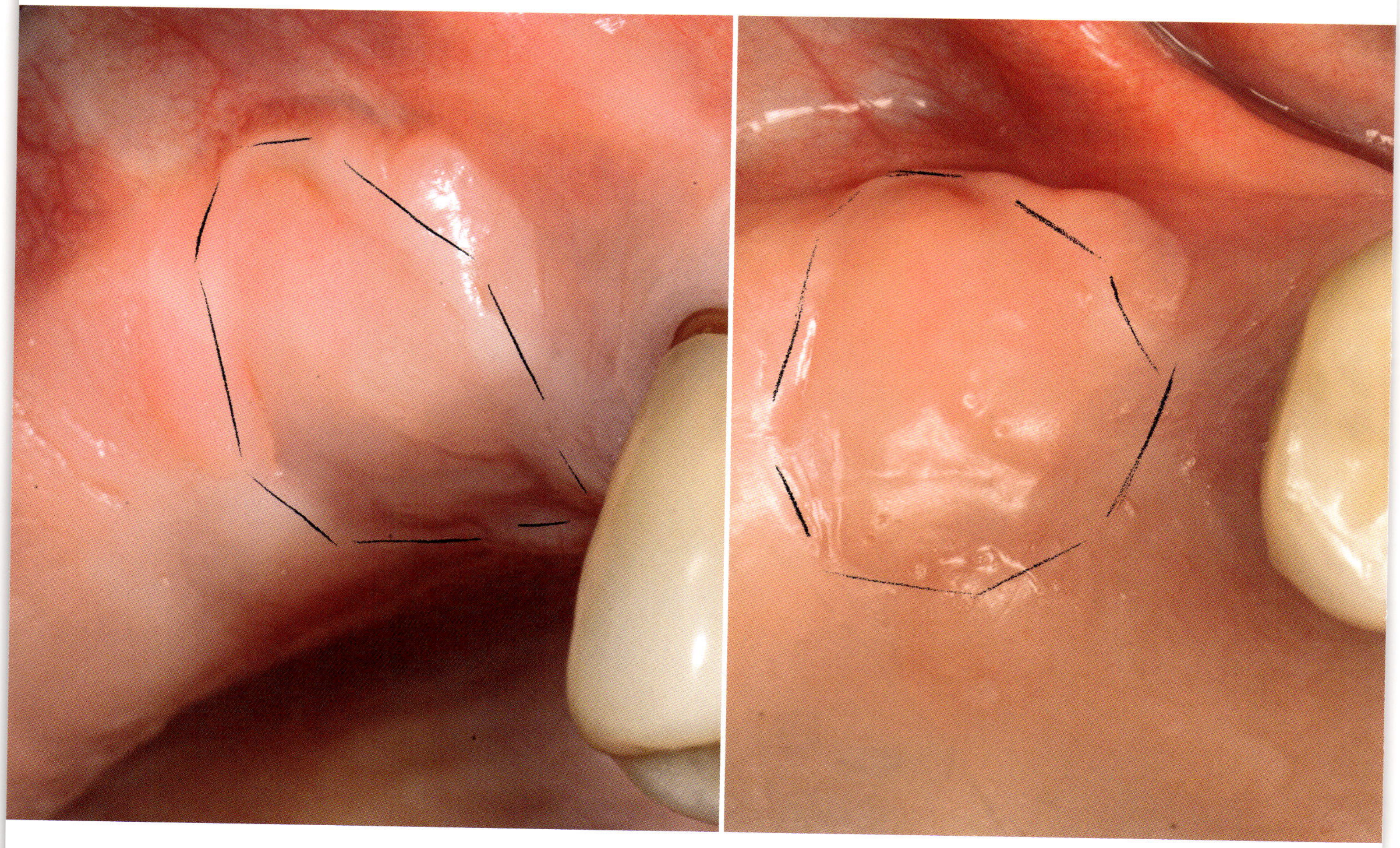

Figure 9-14 The entire area under the membrane fills in with keratinized gingiva. Look at how much the tissue improved!

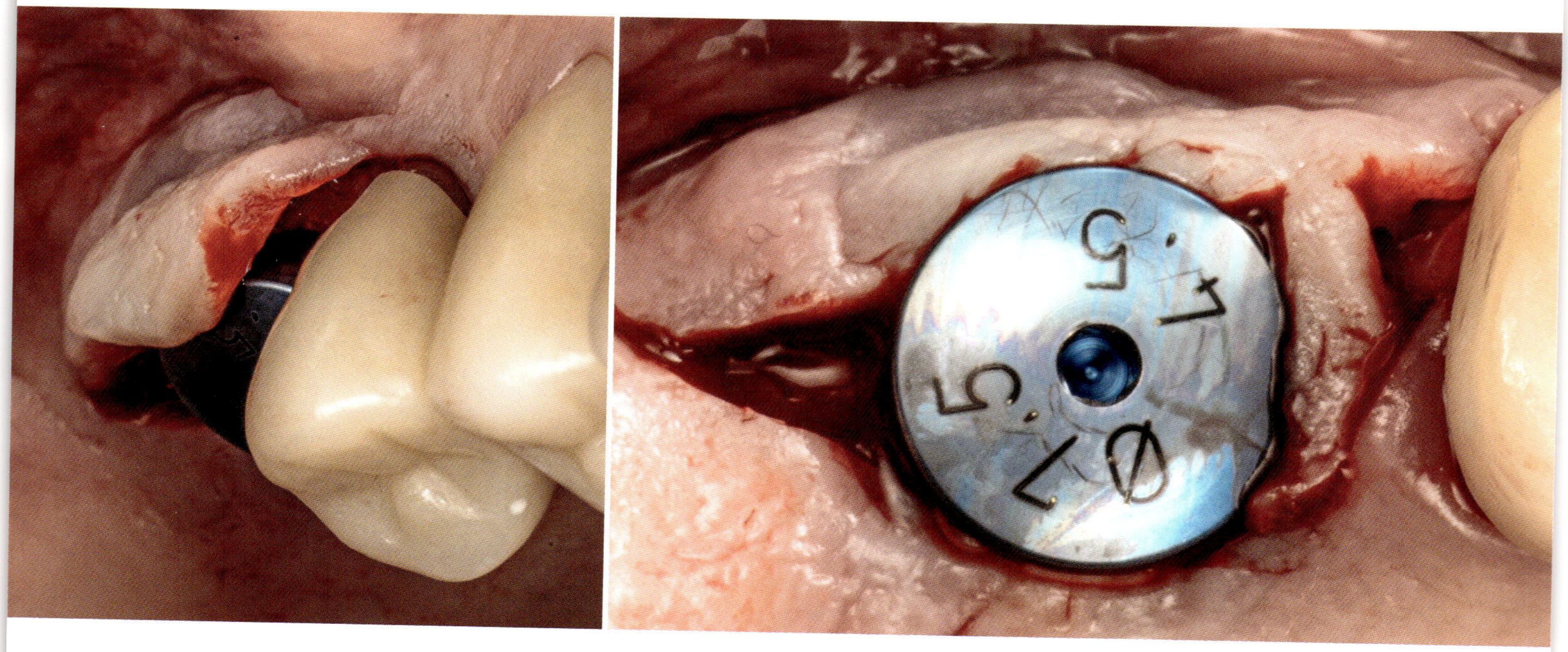

Figure 9-15 Notice the abundant soft tissue available at placement. This was optimized with a Palacci style rotational flap (*see Figure 9-59*).

Careful soft tissue management is critical regardless of which ridge preservation technique is used. Tissue strangulation from tight sutures negatively impacts healing. Excessive tissue elevation compromises blood supply to the underlying bone. Subgingival or subperiosteal membrane placement must be passive and non-irritating to the tissue.

Soft tissue manipulation is much more conservative in ridge preservation than in guided bone regeneration or other ridge augmentation procedures. The overall goal in ridge preservation is to limit site disruption. Preserve the surrounding tissue as well as possible and create a socket that facilitates bone formation. Less manipulation is better. Get in and get out with as little harm as possible. The socket can be covered or sealed with a number of different membranes. These typically granulate over, increasing the amount of keratinized gingiva. Primary closure is not part of ridge preservation. In contrast, guided bone regeneration relies on passive primary closure for success, with the tissue mobilized to completely cover grafted bone. Don't do that in ridge preservation. It will sacrifice valuable tissue and cause unnecessary pain for the patient.

Graft material can be gently condensed in the socket during placement. A bone graft syringe or carrier makes it easy to place the graft right into the site. When making sticky bone with platelet rich fibrin, the bone can be easily handled with cotton forceps and carried to the site. A large condenser seats the graft in the site. A smaller tip condenser can be used to push the bone to the depth of the socket and gently condense the graft material. We want the bone to be condensed enough so it is stable and non-mobile, but not so much it inhibits bone healing and angiogenesis.

Sticky bone. Platelet rich fibrin.

It seems more accurate for "sticky" bone to be called "stuck" bone. After it coagulates and sticks together, it doesn't stick to other things. It is only stuck to itself. If it gets separated or loaded in a syringe, it won't coagulate again in the socket when it is placed. The fibrinogen has already been converted to fibrin and formed the crosslinked mesh network. It is already stuck. (Platelet rich fibrin is briefly discussed in *Chapter 1: The Art of Healing*.)

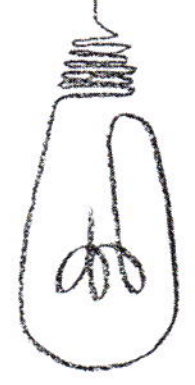

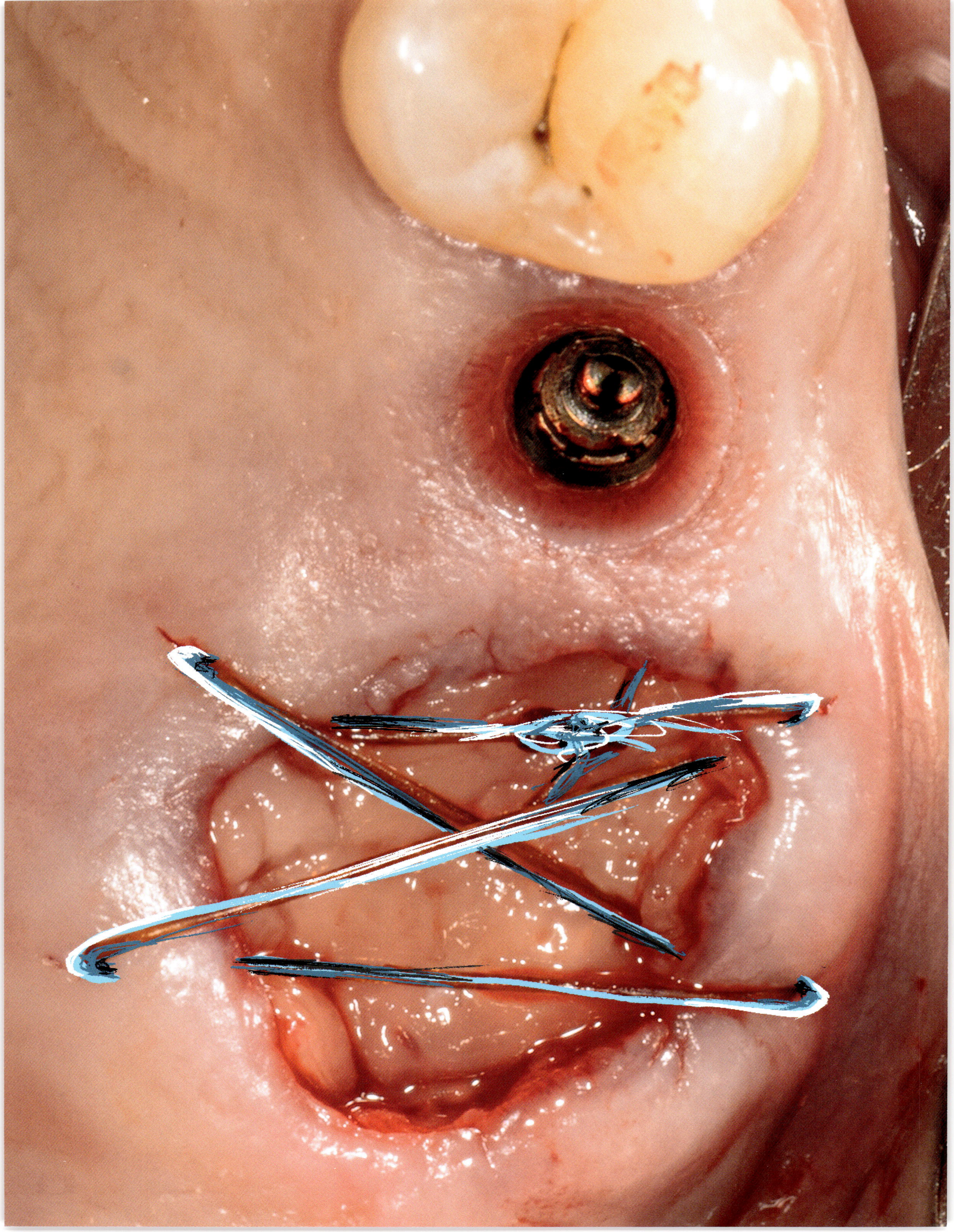

Ridge augmentation

The periosteum is the ticket for successful ridge augmentation. The body is programmed to generate and maintain bone beneath the periosteum and nowhere else. The periosteum has tremendous osteogenic capacity. When a subperiosteal space is created and maintained, it will fill with bone as long as soft tissue infiltration is prevented. The cells will differentiate along the osteoblast line and form bone. The main challenges with any of the techniques include: isolating the space from infiltration, maintaining the volume of the space, and promoting osteoid formation. To isolate the space, pay attention to the periphery of the graft. Soft tissue will try to infiltrate at the margins. Maintain the space by choosing a stable graft material and stable membrane. Consider other adjuncts, such as tenting screws or titanium reinforcement in the membrane. Promote osteoid formation by delicately handling the tissue, using osteogenic graft material and performing cortical perforations. Overcoming these three main challenges sets the tissue up for successful healing.

◂
Figure 9-16 Figure-eight suture for ridge preservation over the platelet rich fibrin membrane.

Block bone graft

Using a block of bone to maintain the subperiosteal space is one of the early ridge augmentation techniques. When the block is harvested from the patient, it transplants viable cells into the site, speeding the initial healing steps. This type of graft may be criticized for the morbidity of a harvest site as well as an increased rate of resorption. It is still a common technique and maintains its place in many skilled surgeons' repertoire for ridge augmentation. In an attempt to minimize morbidity, an allograft block of bone may be used. This forfeits some of the benefits of cellular transplantation and signaling, but it is still a viable option and common technique.

Guided bone regeneration (GBR)

Another technique that has stood the test of time is guided bone regeneration. This evolving technique seems to have surpassed block grafting as the most common and predictable ridge augmentation technique.

In principle, guided bone regeneration creates a subperiosteal space, protected by a barrier membrane, under which the grafting material promotes osseous formation and excludes proliferation of unfavorable soft tissue cells.

Vertical and horizontal augmentation can be achieved with this technique. Horizontal augmentation is easier and seems more predictable, both in the literature and in my experience.

SURGICAL PROTOCOL: GBR

Steps for success:

1. **Adequate flap mobility**.
   a. Incision design with vertical releases.
   b. Buccal and lingual tissue reflection.
   c. Periosteal release through periosteal incisions and dissection or soft tissue brushing.
2. **Thorough full-thickness tissue dissection.**
   a. Any remaining tissue remnants on the surface of the bone promote soft tissue infiltration of the graft, compromising the outcome.
3. **Cortical perforation.**
   a. Access for healing cells and blood supply to populate the graft.
   b. Consider harvesting the bone from the osteotomies with a bone collection filter.
4. **Space maintenance options.**
   a. Cross-linked collagen membrane.
   b. Titanium reinforced membrane.
   c. Stable graft material.
   d. Tentpole screw.
5. **Immobilizing the graft.**
   a. Immobilizing the membrane with tacks.
   b. Sticky bone graft (PRF).
6. **Passive primary closure.**
   a. Tension free with sling mattress sutures.
   b. Meticulous approximation of incisions.
      i. Over edentulous site.
      ii. Papilla and releasing incisions.

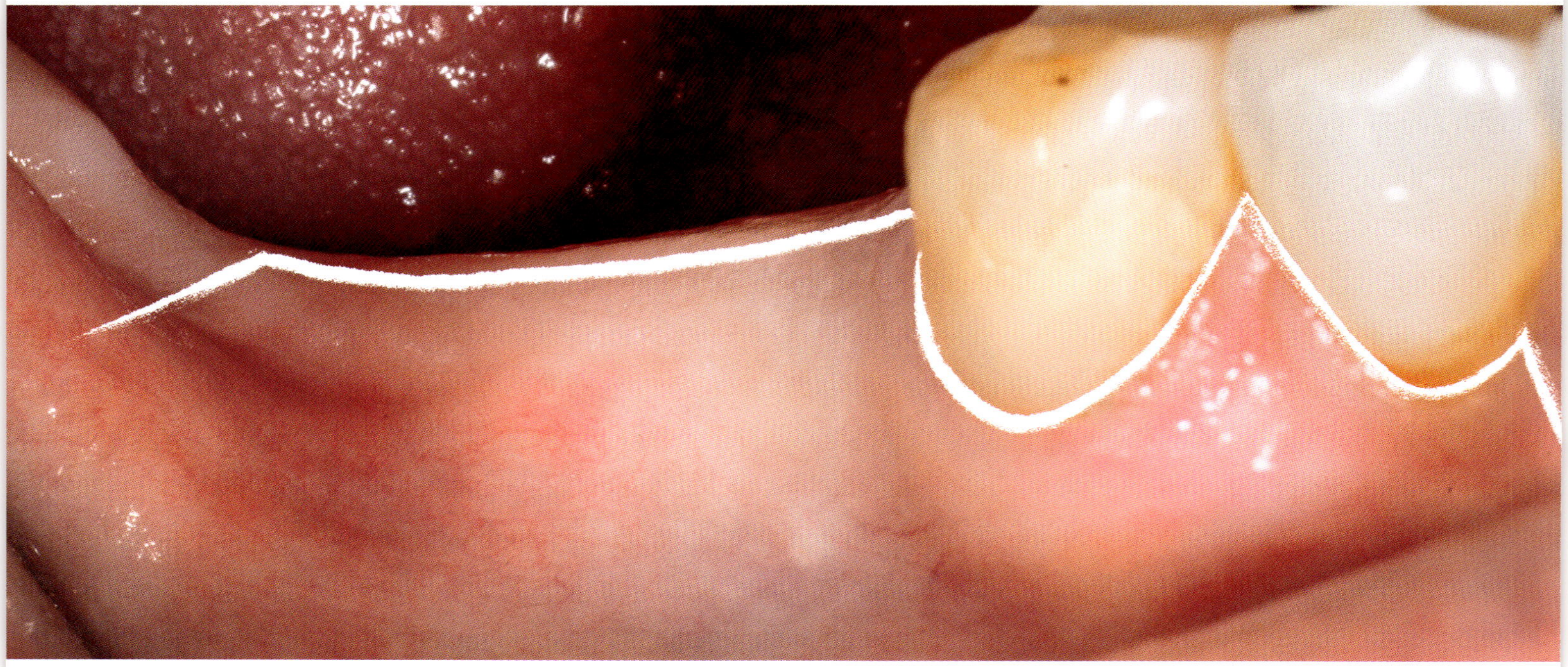

Figure 9-17 Incision design must allow for adequate vertical and horizontal mobilization of the flap. It is a three-dimensional graft that must accommodate a three-dimensional volume increase. The vertical releases are quite helpful and should be placed in good tissue, protecting the blood supply of the flap.

Figure 9-18 The flap must be developed mobilizing both the lingual and buccal tissue. Periosteal releasing incisions significantly increase mobility. They must span the entire length of the flap. The flap can be manipulated and advanced with tissue pick-ups to determine where further dissection is needed.

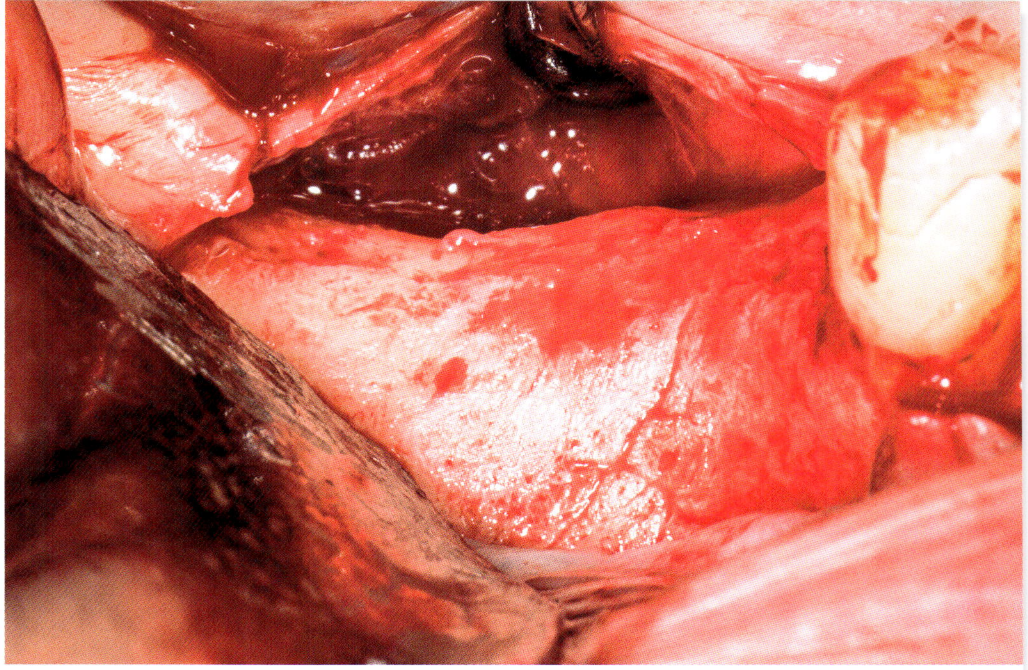

Figure 9-19 Full thickness dissection removes all remnants of tissue from the surface of the bone. This helps decrease the potential for soft tissue infiltration. Multiple cortical perforations improve cellular and vascular access to the grafted bone. The bone removed from these sites can be harvested with a bone filtration system on the suction. Note the different sizes of the perforations. The larger holes help harvest more bone and improve vascular and cellular access, but they do not retain the tacks. Consider anticipated placement of the tacks when performing the corticotomies with smaller holes around the periphery. The size and position also should be factored in when using tenting screws to accommodate the ideal position and stability.

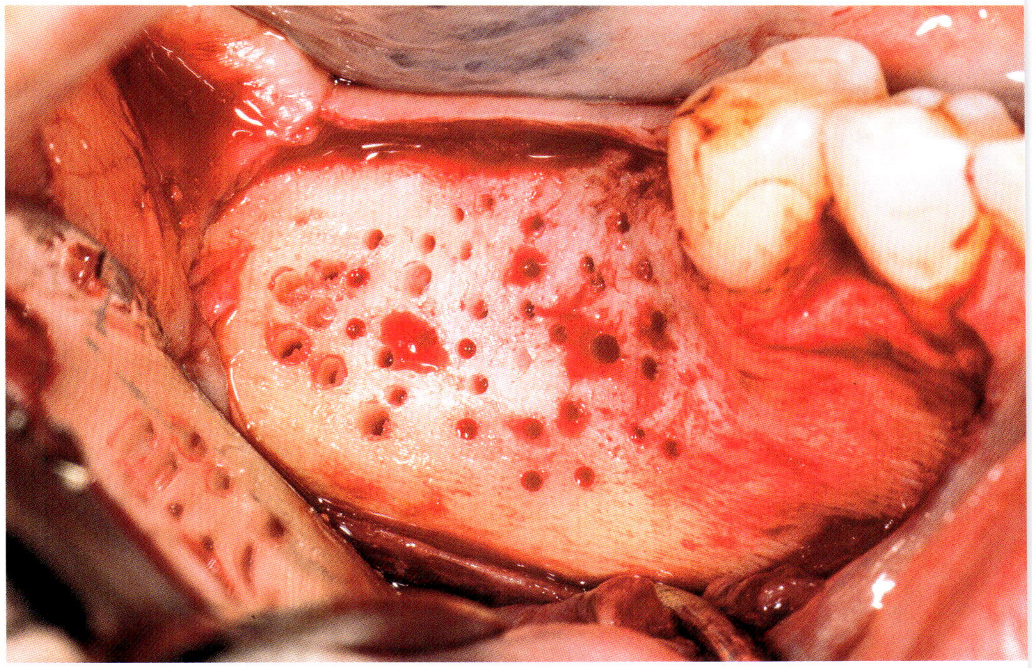

Figure 9-20 Multiple options are available for membrane material. They all need to keep out infiltrating soft tissue and remain long enough to allow bone graft maturation. These can be non-resorbable or resorbable, as in this case. The membrane and underlying graft material must be stabilized. Sticky bone, tacks and a screw stabilized this graft. It was covered with PRF membranes prior to closure.

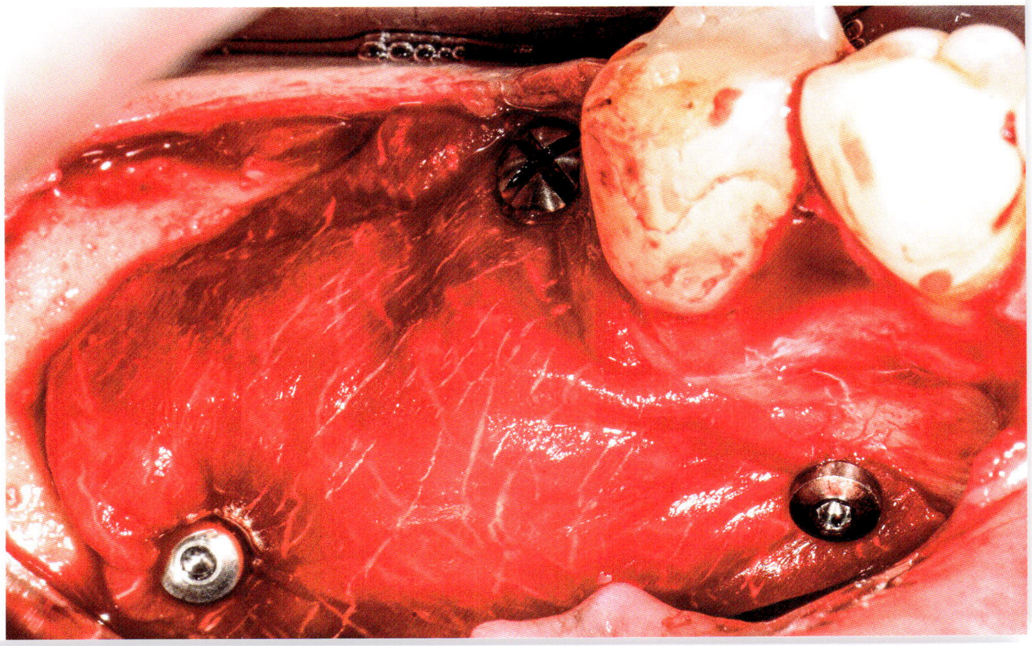

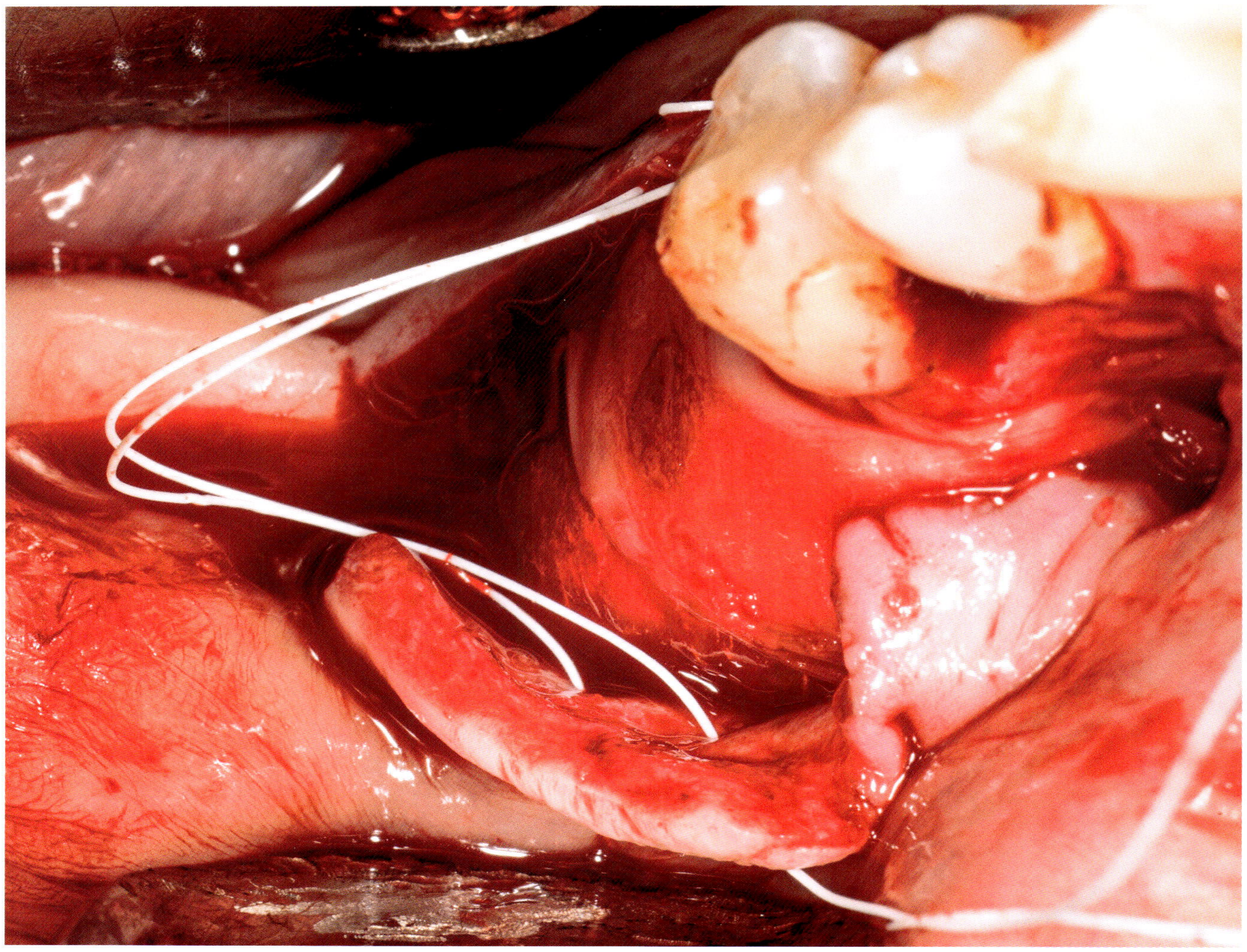

Figure 9-21 Passive primary closure is critical to success. The non-resorbable sling suture is a horizontal mattress design that brings the wound edges together prior to final closure. This supports the tissue and re-approximation during the critical first few weeks of healing.

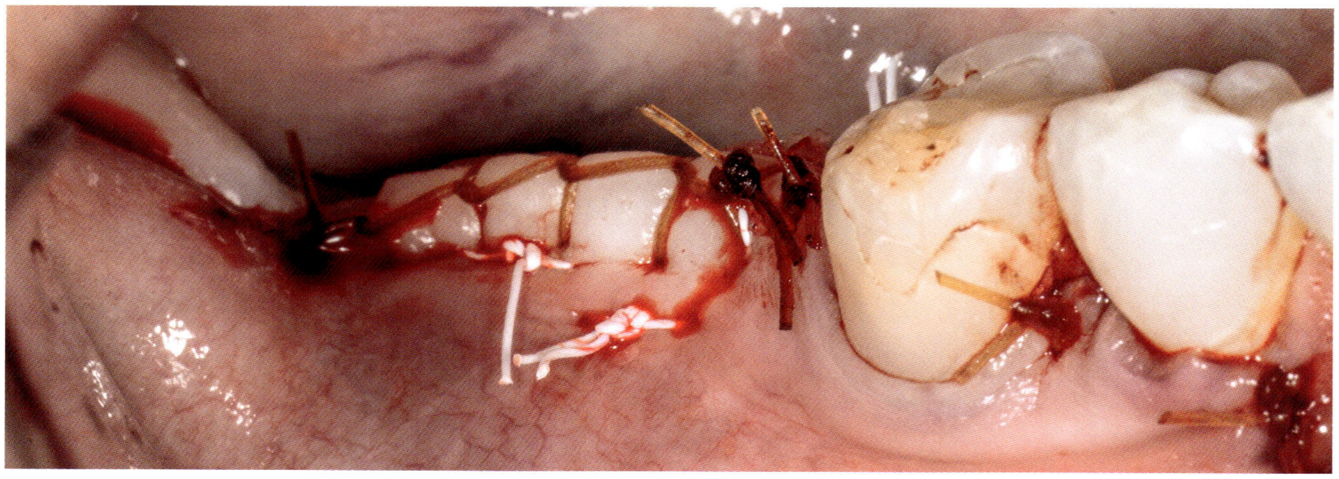

Figure 9-22 The edges of the incision are everted on themselves with no tension. This passive primary closure is critical for healing. We are asking the body to increase the volume of bone and overlying tissue. We don't want to leave any memory of how it was. Tension on the incision threatens to expose the underlying graft during healing. It also retains some memory of the previous dimensions, increasing resorption during healing.

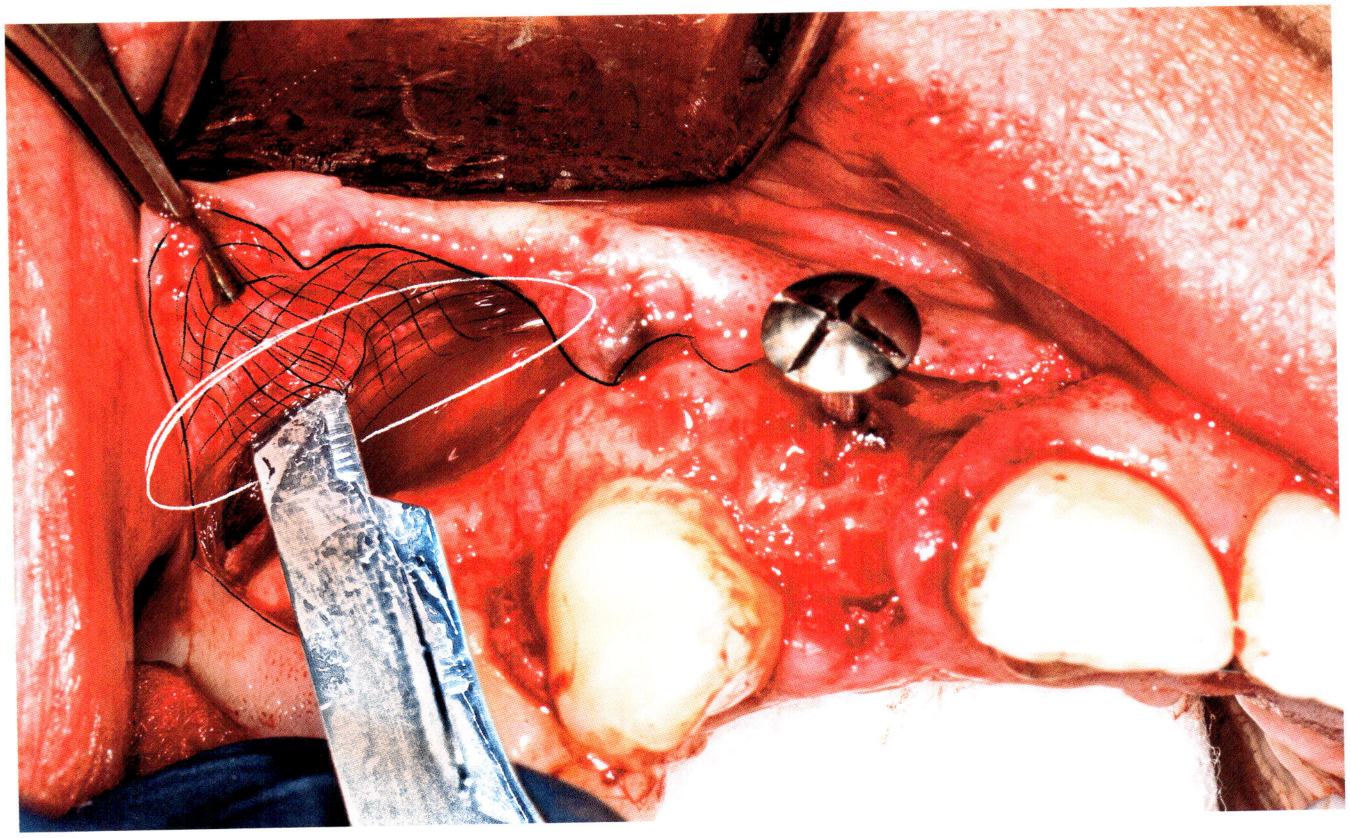

Figure 9-23 A periosteal releasing incision optimizes flap advancement. With the tissue taut, a scalpel can cut through the periosteum along the flap. Care must be taken to avoid perforating through the mucosa in the vestibule. Mobility can also be achieved through the soft tissue brushing technique.

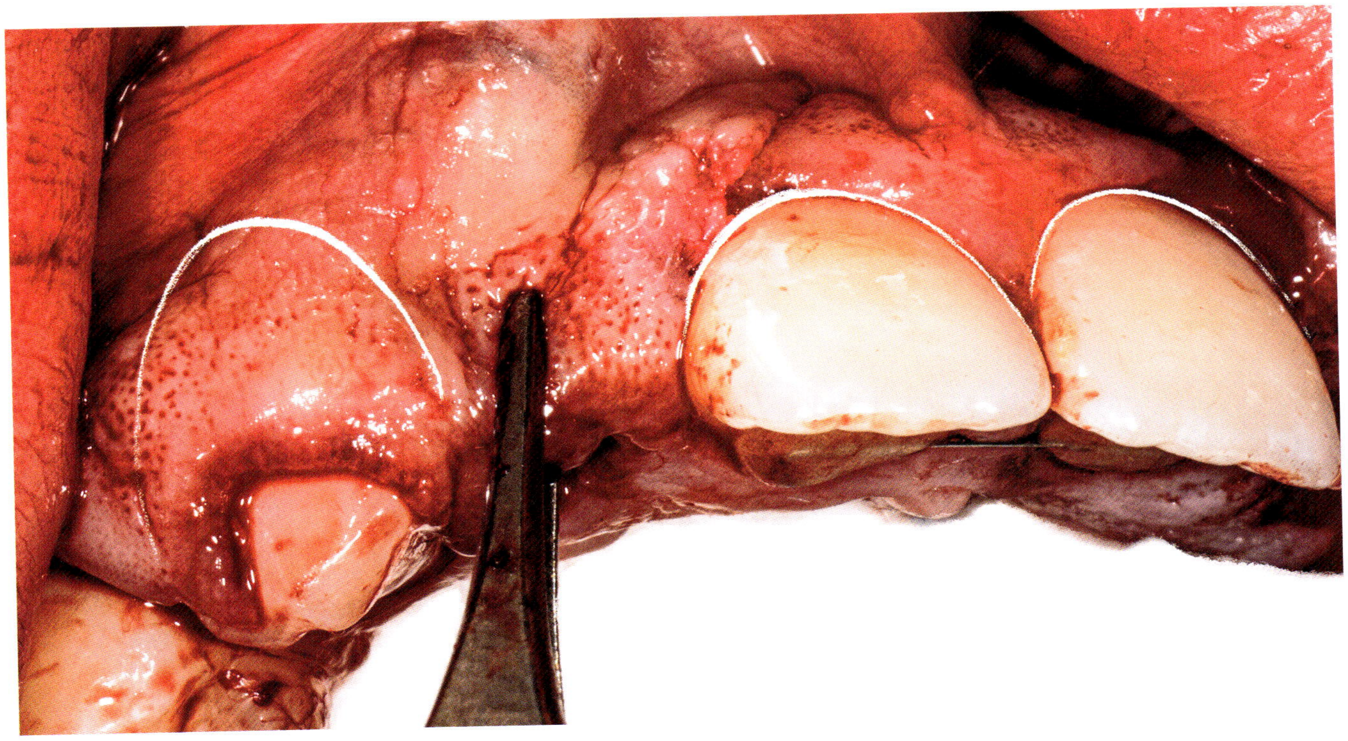

Figure 9-24 Mobilizing the flap to extend far beyond the margins allows for passive closure with graft material. Note how far the flap advances over the approximate position of the adjacent teeth.

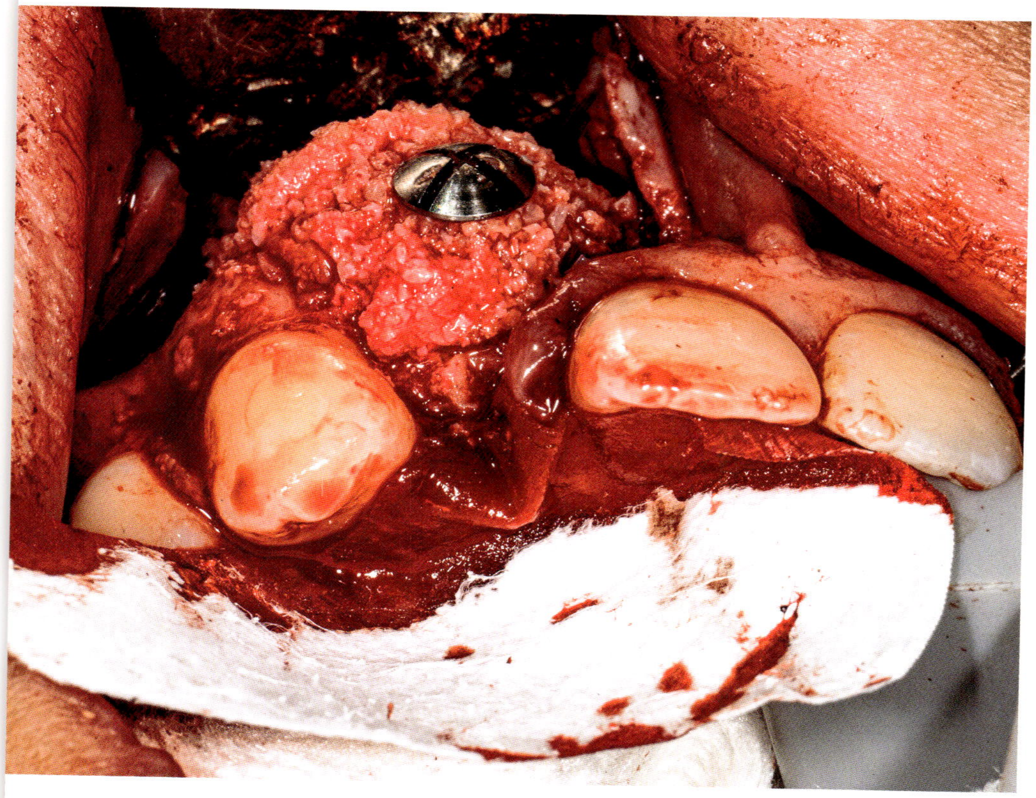

Figure 9-25 The cross-linked collagen membrane is tucked under the palatal tissue and graft material is placed around the tenting screw, filling the site slightly beyond the needed amount. The excess will help compensate for the resorption that will occur.

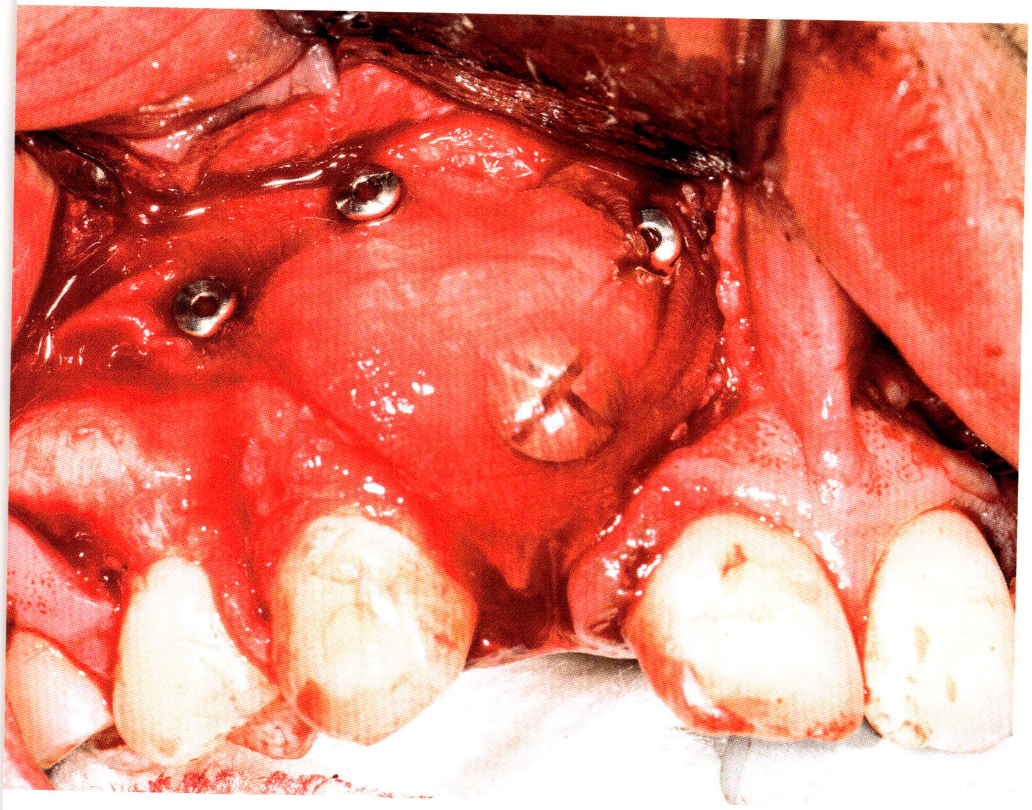

Figure 9-26 The collagen membrane is pulled over the graft and secured with monocortical tacks. Some manipulation of the shape can be accomplished by pressing and molding it with finger pressure.

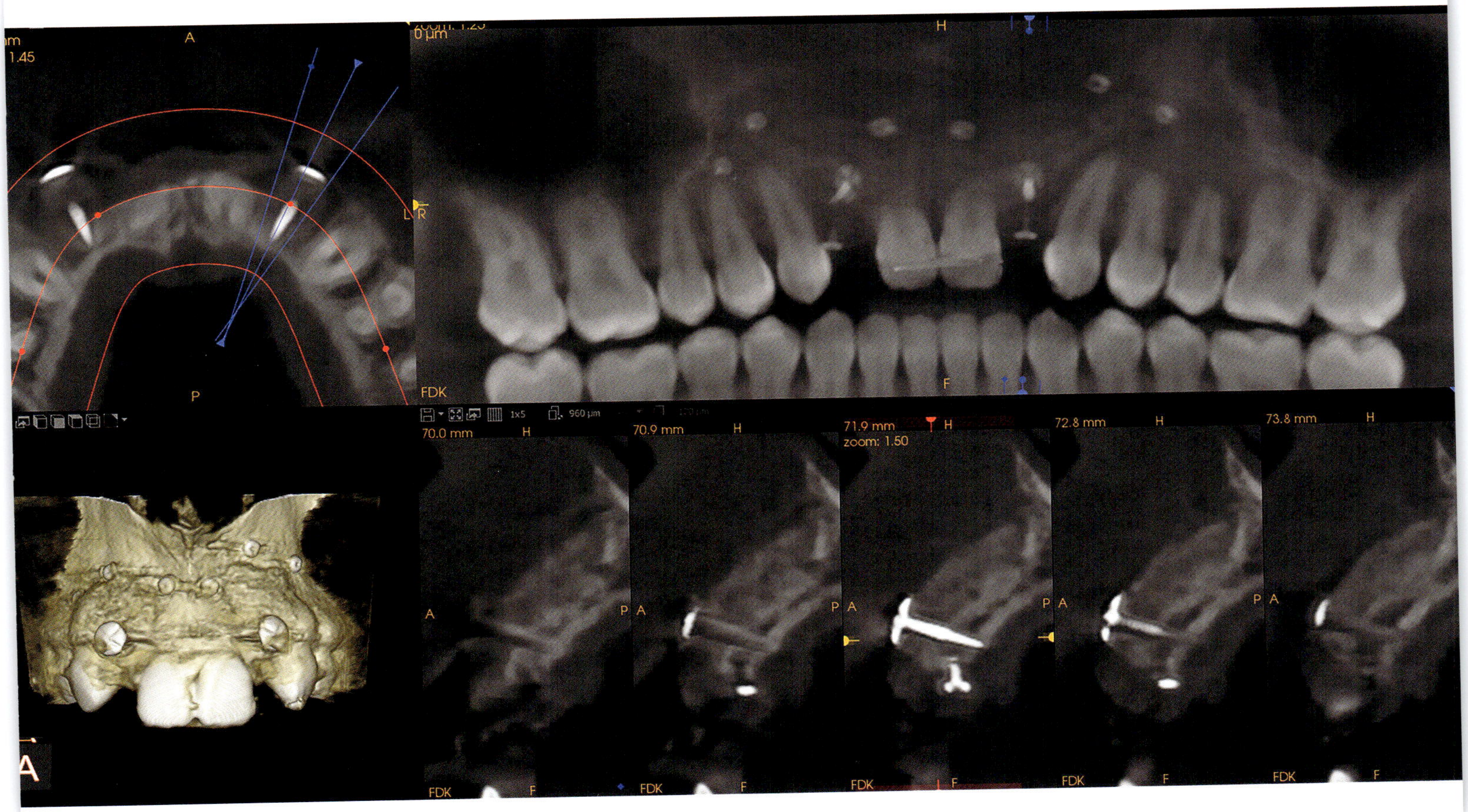

Figure 9-27 Tacks stabilize the membrane and the tenting screw defines and maintains the space.

Ridge preservation and guided bone regeneration employ very different techniques for managing soft tissue. With ridge preservation, the soft tissue socket should have about the same dimensions as the tooth. There should be a void the size of the tooth that will fill-in with keratinized gingiva. The less soft tissue disruption the better. With guided bone regeneration, on the other hand, a wide envelope of subperiosteal dissection needs to be performed to mobilize the flap and achieve passive primary closure. If guided bone regeneration principles are applied to a ridge preservation procedure, you sacrifice the potential development of several millimeters of keratinized gingiva.

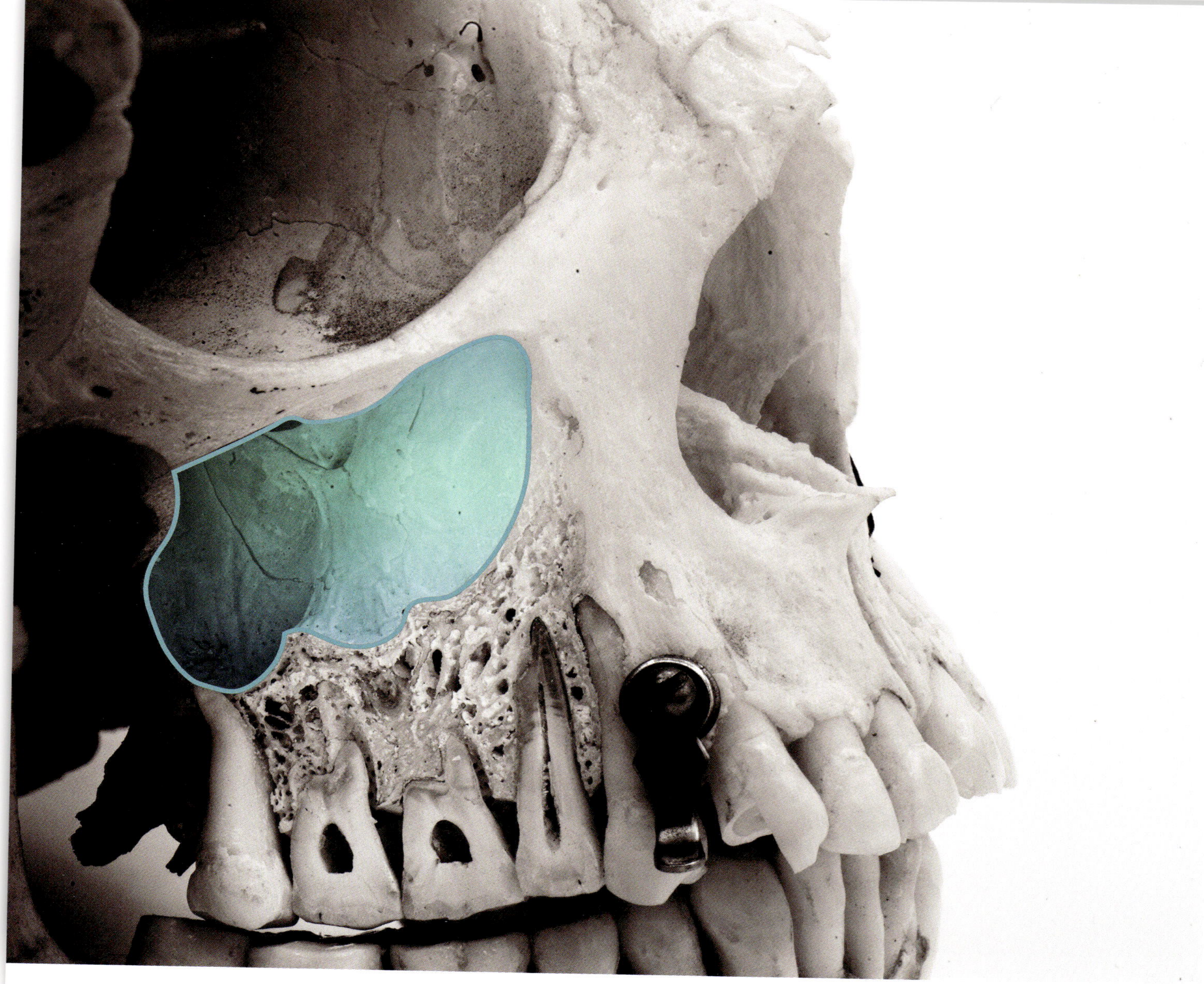

Figure 9-28 The anatomy of the maxillary sinus has very little impact on the teeth, but can have tremendous impact on implants.

Sinus graft

The evolution of the maxillary sinuses in homo sapiens seems to have served a few purposes. As part of the upper airway, sinuses help condition inhaled air on its journey to the lungs. They serve as an airbag for the brain, protecting it by sacrificially fracturing in traumatic situations that we see on call as oral surgeons. (They help extend the modern dentist's career by decreasing the load of the large cranium on the cervical spine.) But the maxillary sinus didn't seem to consider dental implantology in its evolution.

The low position of the maxillary sinus often impacts implant placement in the posterior maxilla. Sinus floor augmentation is routinely performed to increase the vertical height for an implant. This can be done directly through the lateral wall of the sinus in a Caldwell-Luc approach. It can also be done indirectly through vertical elevation of the floor through the crest of the implant osteotomy. The main indication for these approaches depends on the amount of additional bone needed. Less than 3 mm additional height can be accomplished predictably with an indirect sinus lift. More than 3 mm usually requires a direct sinus lift. This all depends greatly on the surgeon's comfort level and experience with the different approaches, as well as case specific factors.

It is possible to perform direct or indirect sinus augmentation at the time of implant placement, as long as the implant is stable. Implant stability is dependent on implant design, bone quality and preparation technique (see *Chapter 7: Implant Architecture*). Generally, a minimum of 5 mm of vertical height is necessary to achieve adequate stability for simultaneous sinus lift and implant placement.

Think of sinus augmentation as a form of guided bone regeneration. We are asking the body to form bone where there is none. A space between the bone and the overlying soft tissue (sinus membrane) is filled with osteogenic material, setting the site up so the programming of the body will generate bone in the site. At its core, sinus augmentation consists of three steps. The space for the graft needs to be defined, filled and maintained. Defining the space for the graft material is the most technically demanding step, whether through a direct or indirect approach. The lining is thin and fragile. It must be respected and handled gently. It needs to be lifted away from the floor, preferably without tearing it.

Pay attention to sinus dimensions as they impact where the blood supply and bone cells will come from. It takes longer for bone cells and vascularity to populate a graft with a wide sinus. Robust alveolar bone has more potential to supply the components for healing than thin bone does. The width and height of the sinus and alveolar bone are important factors to consider in determining timing and potential resorption post-operatively. As is common to all surgery, the more we ask of the body, the more time and attention we need to give to the plan, execution and follow up.

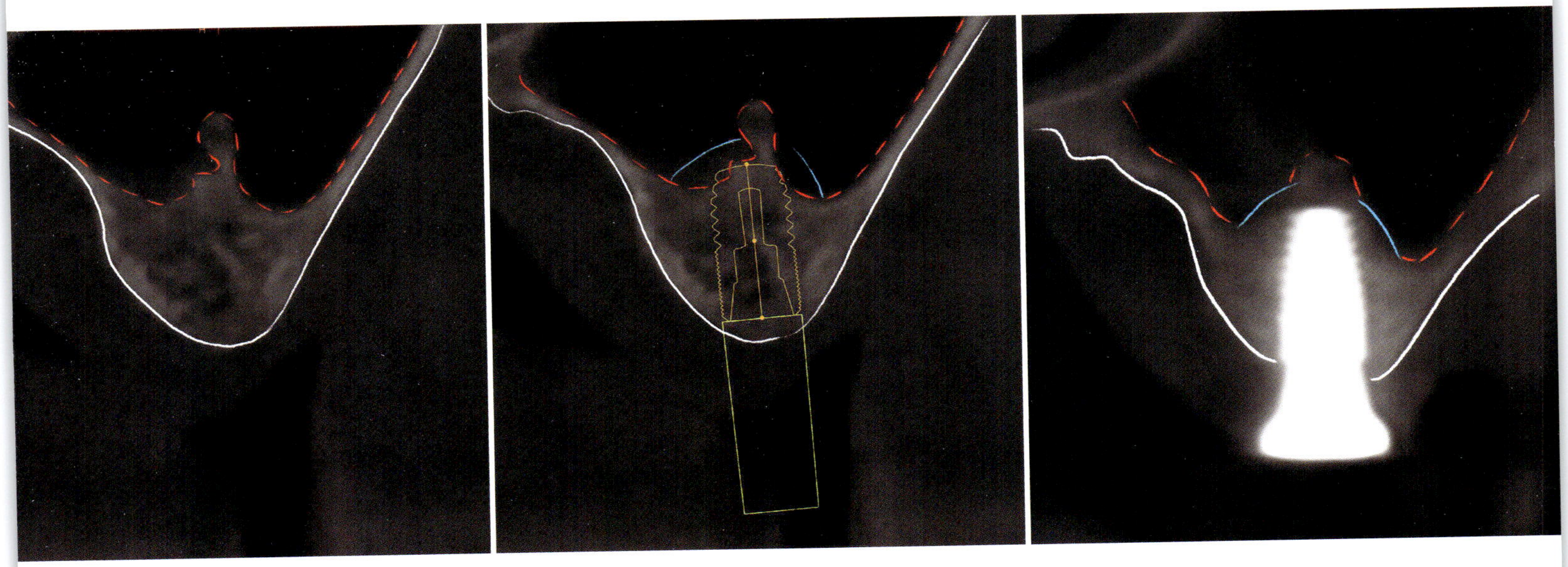

Figure 9-29 Indirect sinus augmentation can be much easier than direct sinus augmentation when there is significant irregularity in the sinus floor, like in this case. It seems to be nearly impossible to negotiate such tight corners around sinus septae with the direct approach. With the indirect approach, these septae can be advantageous by improving implant stability.

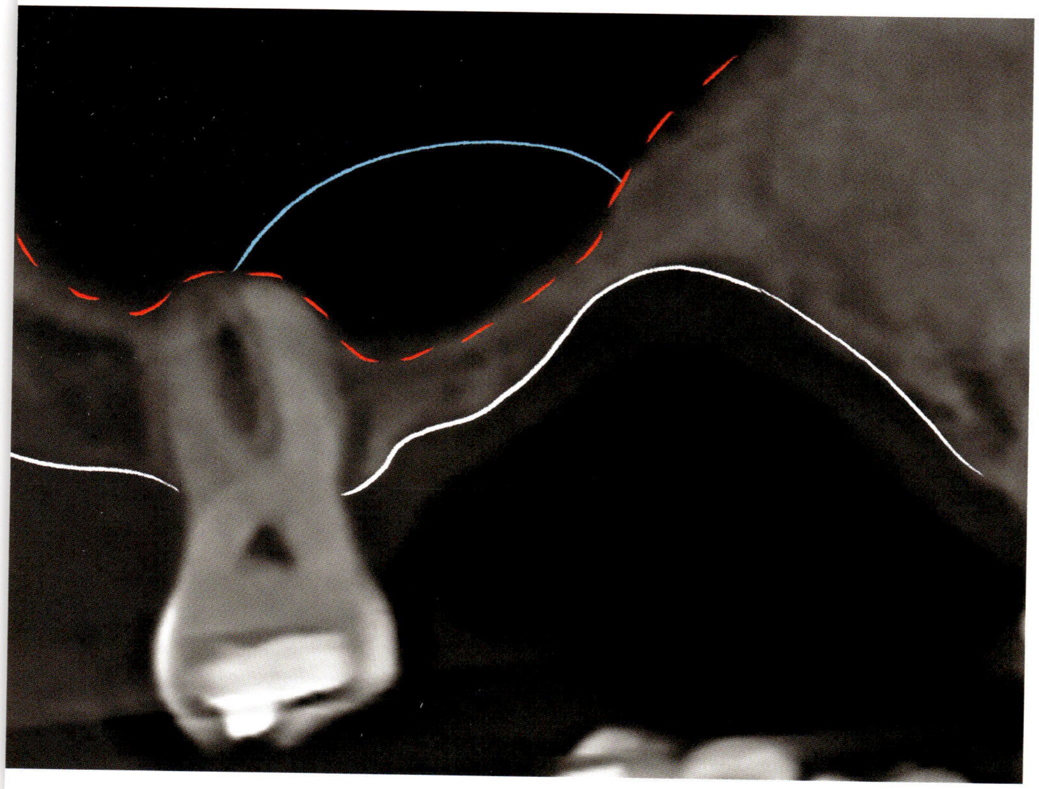

Figure 9-30 Direct sinus augmentation is required in this case, along with several months of healing before implant placement. The vertical ridge atrophy here caused a significant defect that can be addressed with ridge augmentation or prosthetic design, depending on the patient's goals and needs.

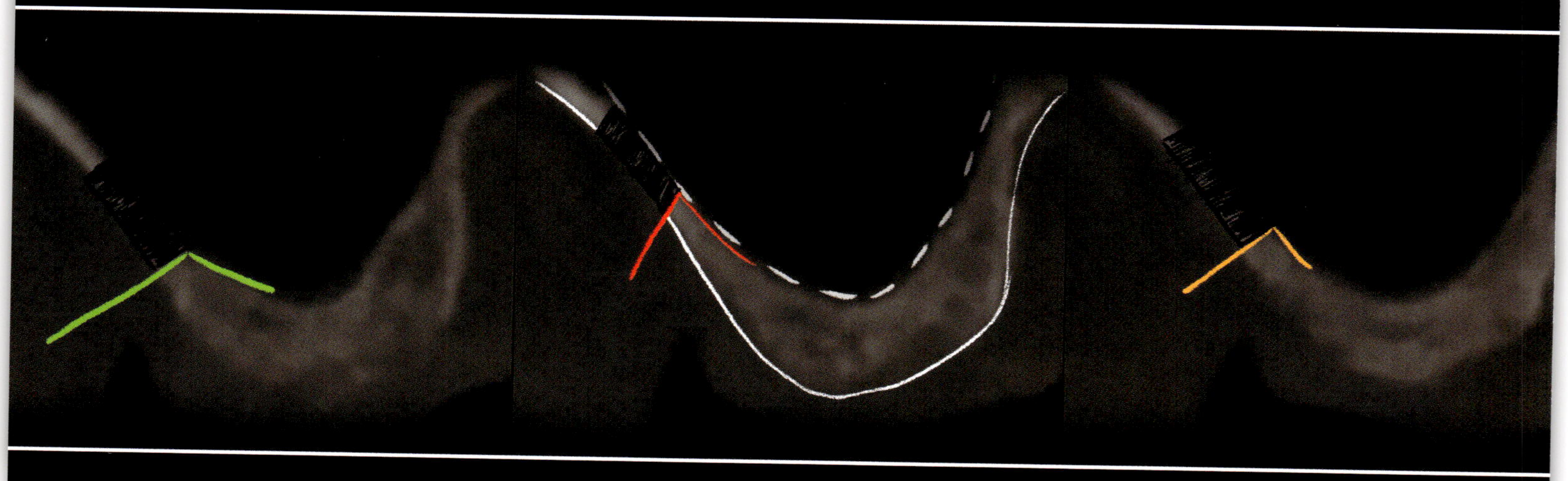

Figure 9-31 The angle of approach to the floor of the sinus impacts the difficulty of the procedure. The position of the antrostomy can impact the angle. The higher the window, the more acute the angle. Approach the sinus as low as possible to simplify the dissection and improve visualization. This can be limited by the anatomy and adjacent teeth.

Surgical protocol

Direct sinus lift

Three-dimensional sinus evaluation can help plan antrostomy location, optimize the angle of approach, and visualize any sinus floor irregularities to avoid during the procedure. (Dynamic navigation can be tremendously helpful in guiding this procedure.) This can be a technically demanding procedure. Don't make it harder on yourself by creating a small access. Give yourself room to see and work.

The incision can be crestal or vestibular. I usually make a crestal incision if I am placing implants at the time of the sinus lift. If the implants are going to be staged, a semilunar vestibular incision in the mucosa provides great access and keeps the surgical trauma away from planned implant sites. The semilunar incision should be made below the planned antrostomy site, and it should extend far enough anterior and posterior to reflect the flap above the site. Full thickness dissection must be extended through the periosteum to the margins of the incision to optimize exposure. Care should be taken to protect the soft tissue flap and avoid traumatizing it with the periosteal elevator or Minnesota retractor by keeping the tip firmly on bone.

The antrostomy can be performed with rotary and/or piezo instrumentation. Either or both can be used. I have found a round bur in a surgical handpiece makes quick work of the bulk of the osteotomy. As I approach the Schneiderian membrane, I switch to the piezo surgical handpiece with a round diamond tip to minimize any trauma to the membrane and to decrease the risk of perforation.

Figure 9-32 With the antrostomy completed, the sinus membrane is teased up off the sinus floor over the planned implant sites.

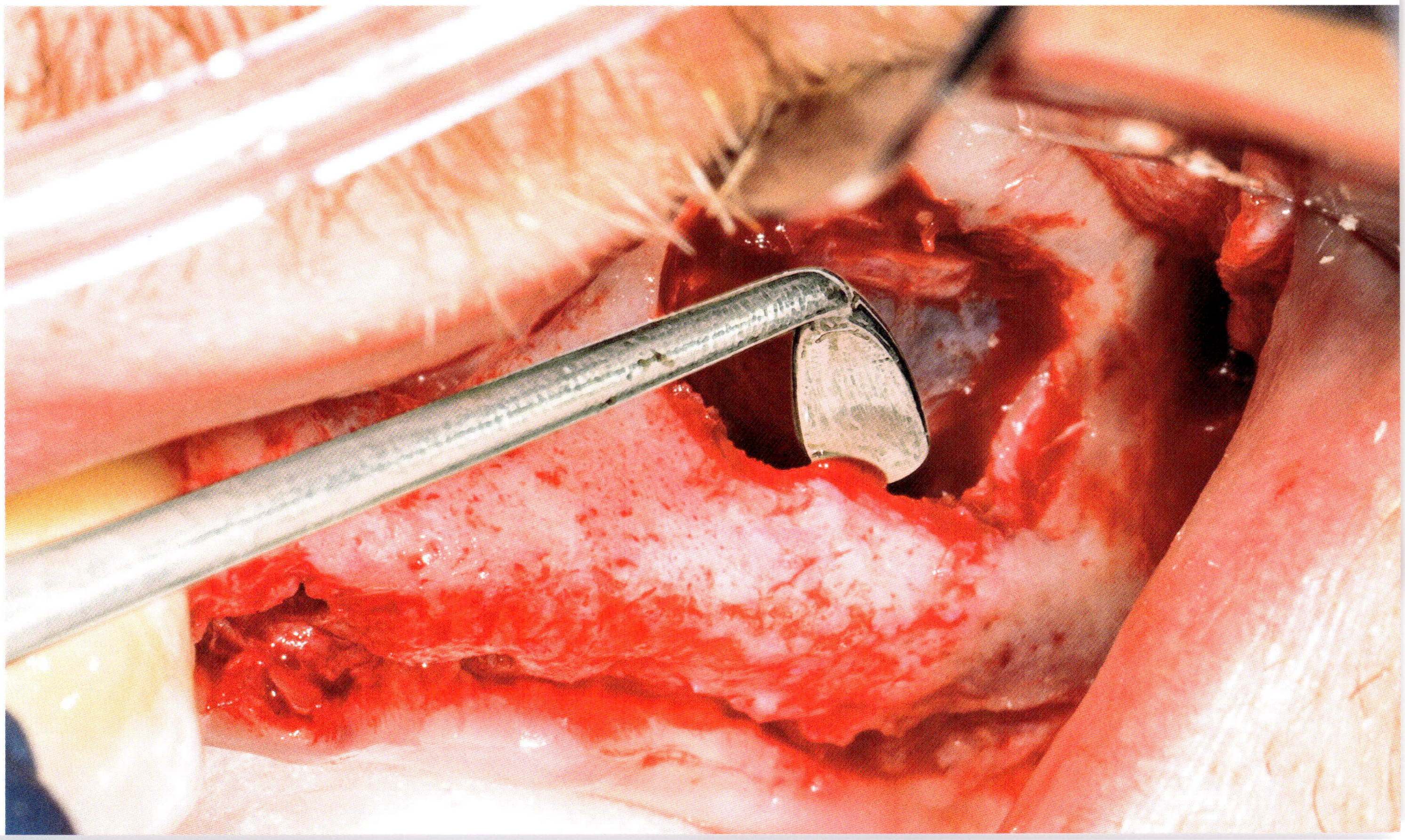

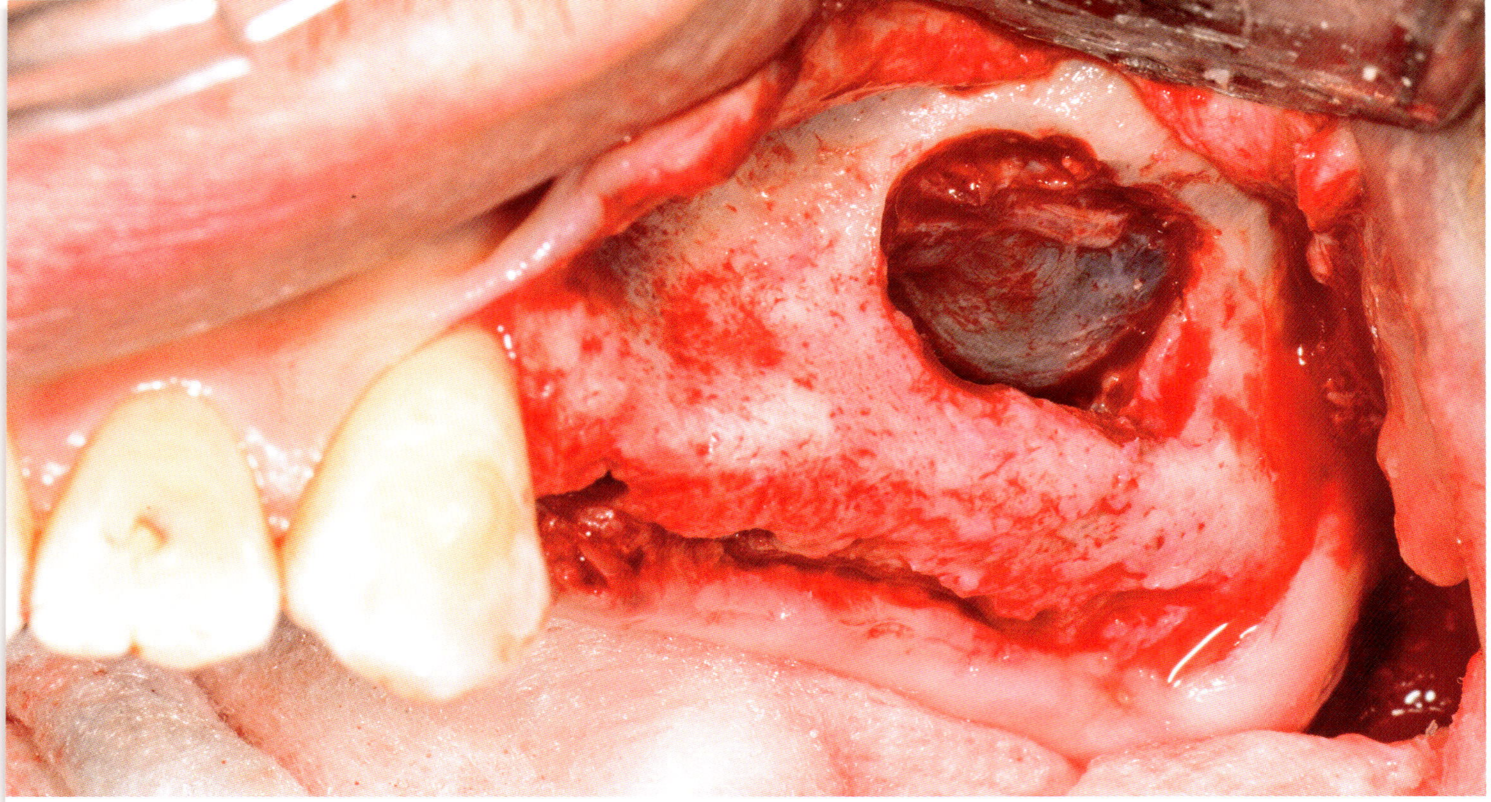

Figure 9-33 A mobilized sinus lining moves with each breath. This is a good sign that the lining remained intact.

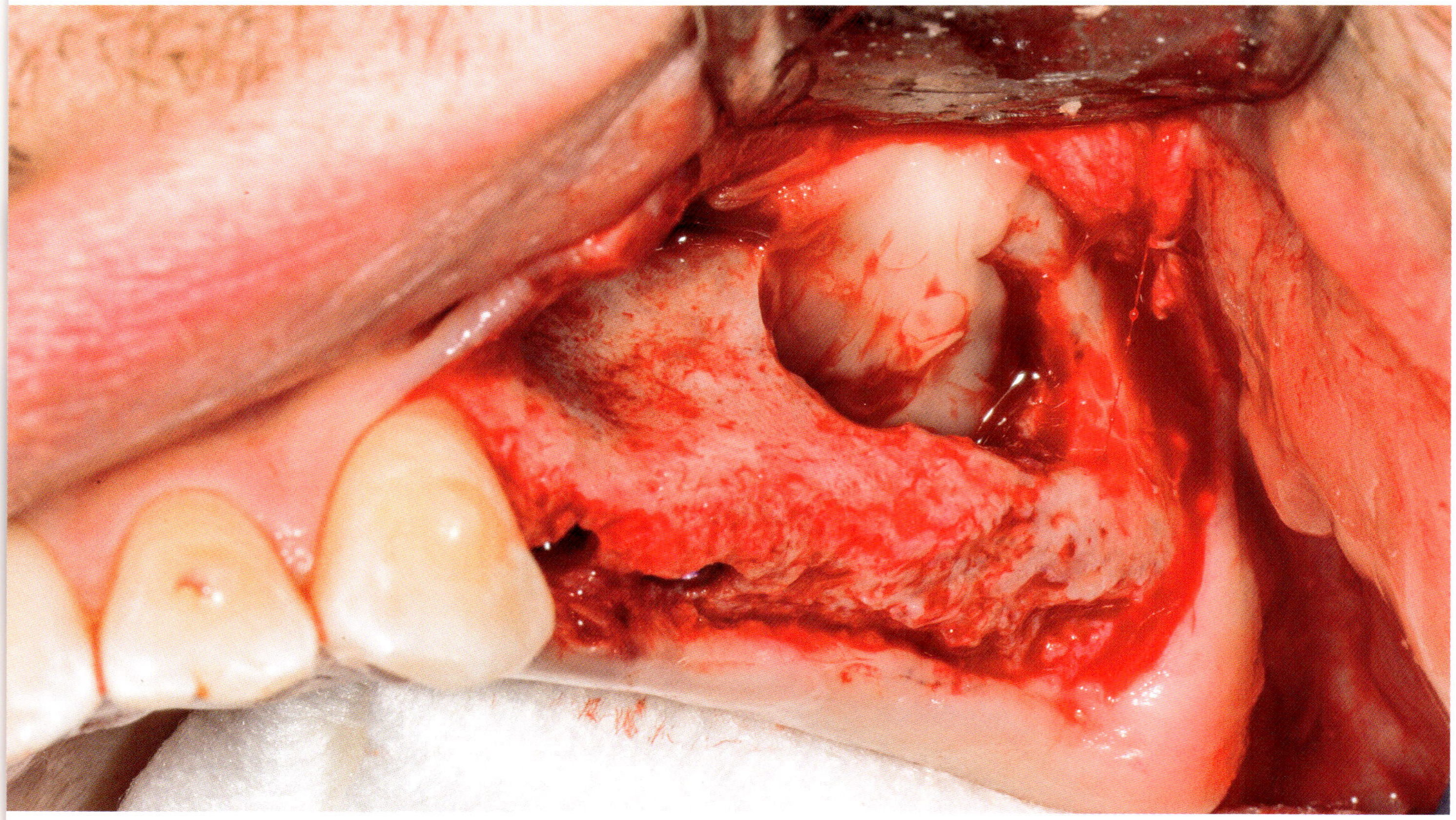

Figure 9-34 A PRF or collagen membrane can be placed under the sinus membrane to further protect the graft from any compromise in the sinus lining. If it is long enough, the tail can be pinned in place with the tip of the Minnesota retractor. This tail can be draped over the graft before closing to help keep the graft material in place.

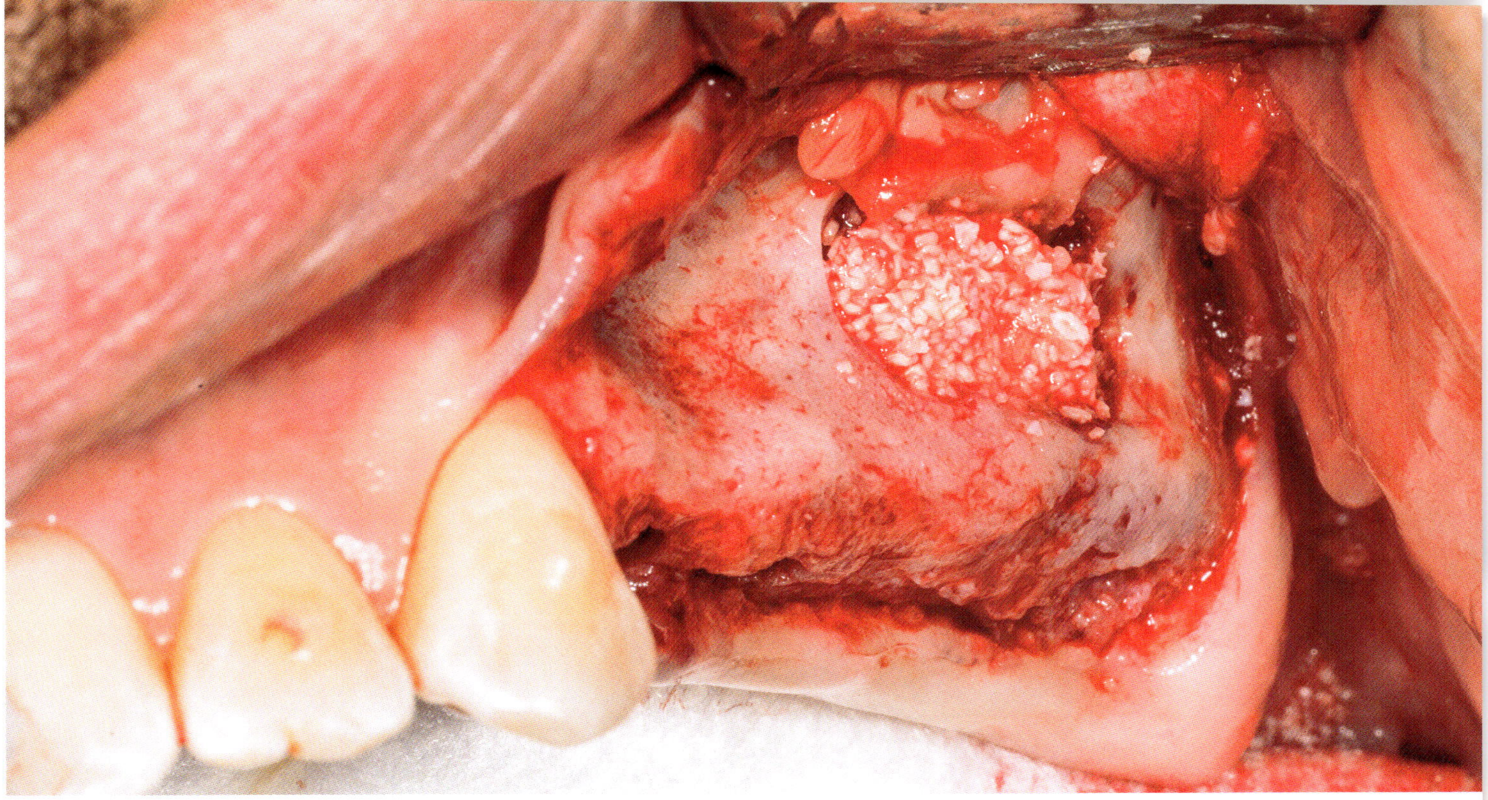

Figure 9-35 A combination of allograft, xenograft and PRF is placed. Gently condensing the graft material can help ensure adequate fill as well as confirm the sinus lining is intact. If the graft material seems to be disappearing into the site, it is possible the lining is torn, and the graft is going directly into the sinus cavity.

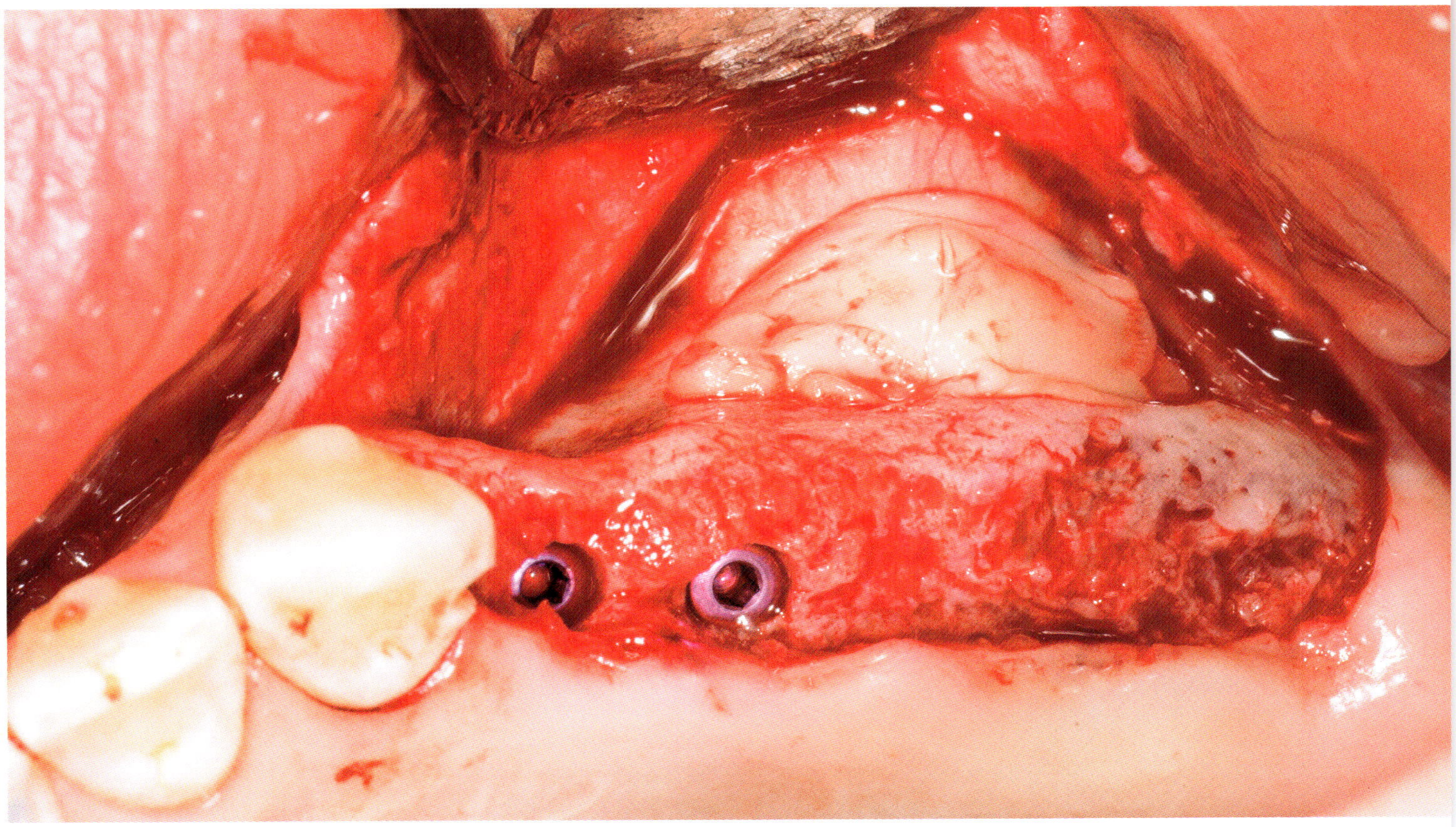

Figure 9-36 With adequate graft in place, the tail of the initial membrane is folded down over the buccal portion of the graft. Another PRF membrane is placed over the lateral antrostomy. The two implants in the premolar areas did not require sinus augmentation. The sinus lift was staged with planned implants at the molar sites after healing.

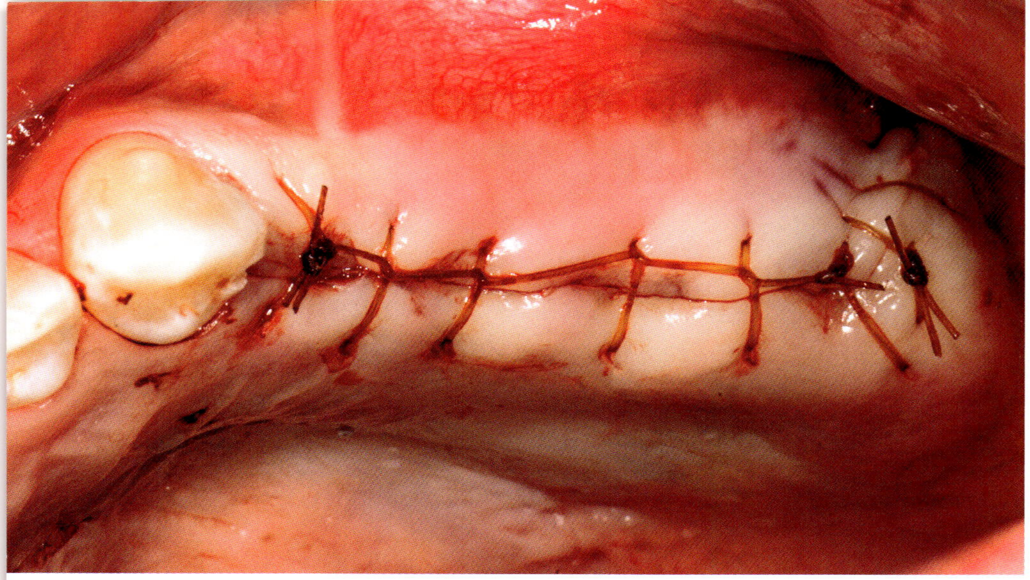

Figure 9-37 A few key sutures at the corners help line up the incision. A running suture can close the remainder of the incision.

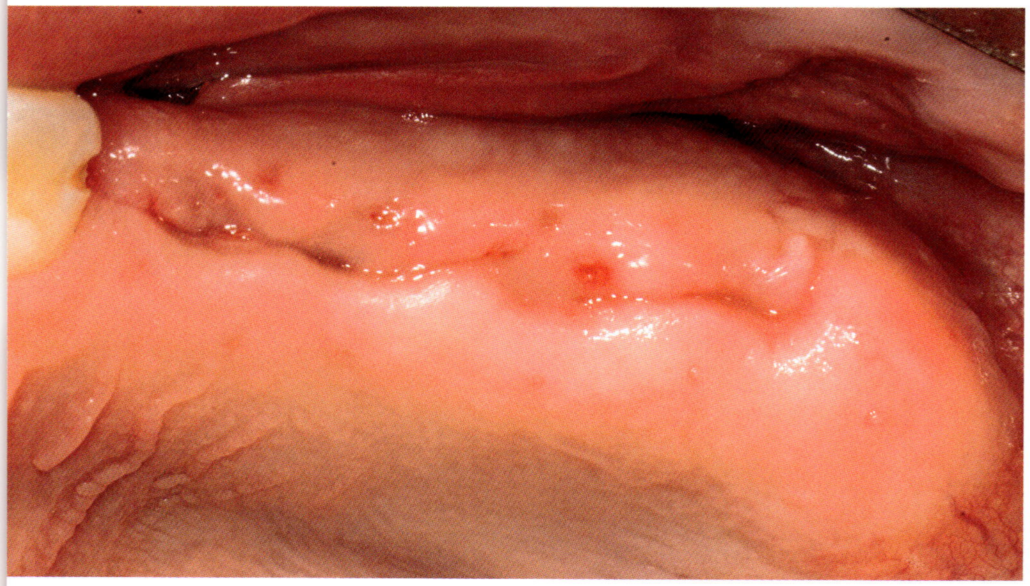

Figure 9-38 Two weeks after surgery, the incision is intact, and the site appears to be healing well.

▸ **Figure 9-39** The angle of engagement is key to successful membrane elevation. The tip of the instrument must maintain contact at an acute angle to elevate the membrane or the membrane will tear.

Delicate pressure is needed when making the lateral antrostomy. When the sinus wall's dense overlying bone finally gives way, the bur may suddenly drop into the sinus, disrupting or tearing the thin membrane. Pay attention to how the bone looks and feels. It will often start to feel slightly spongy as the central portion of the round cutting instrument approaches the membrane and the sides of it still engage bone. The membrane becomes visible as the bone thins. It darkens, has a different sheen, and may reveal a vascular network differentiating the membrane from the bone.

There is a tactile sense that helps guide membrane elevation. When the instrument tip engages bone, there is crisp feedback indicating the membrane is being elevated. If the instrument tip is not definitively engaging the bone, it begins to feel soft or dull. The membrane may be getting pinched or is likely to be torn or perforated. Keep the tip definitively on the bone.

Create only the space needed for the graft. It is not beneficial to elevate the membrane beyond the scope of the graft. When placing bone, it should fill the prepared site. This stabilizes the graft material and improves healing.

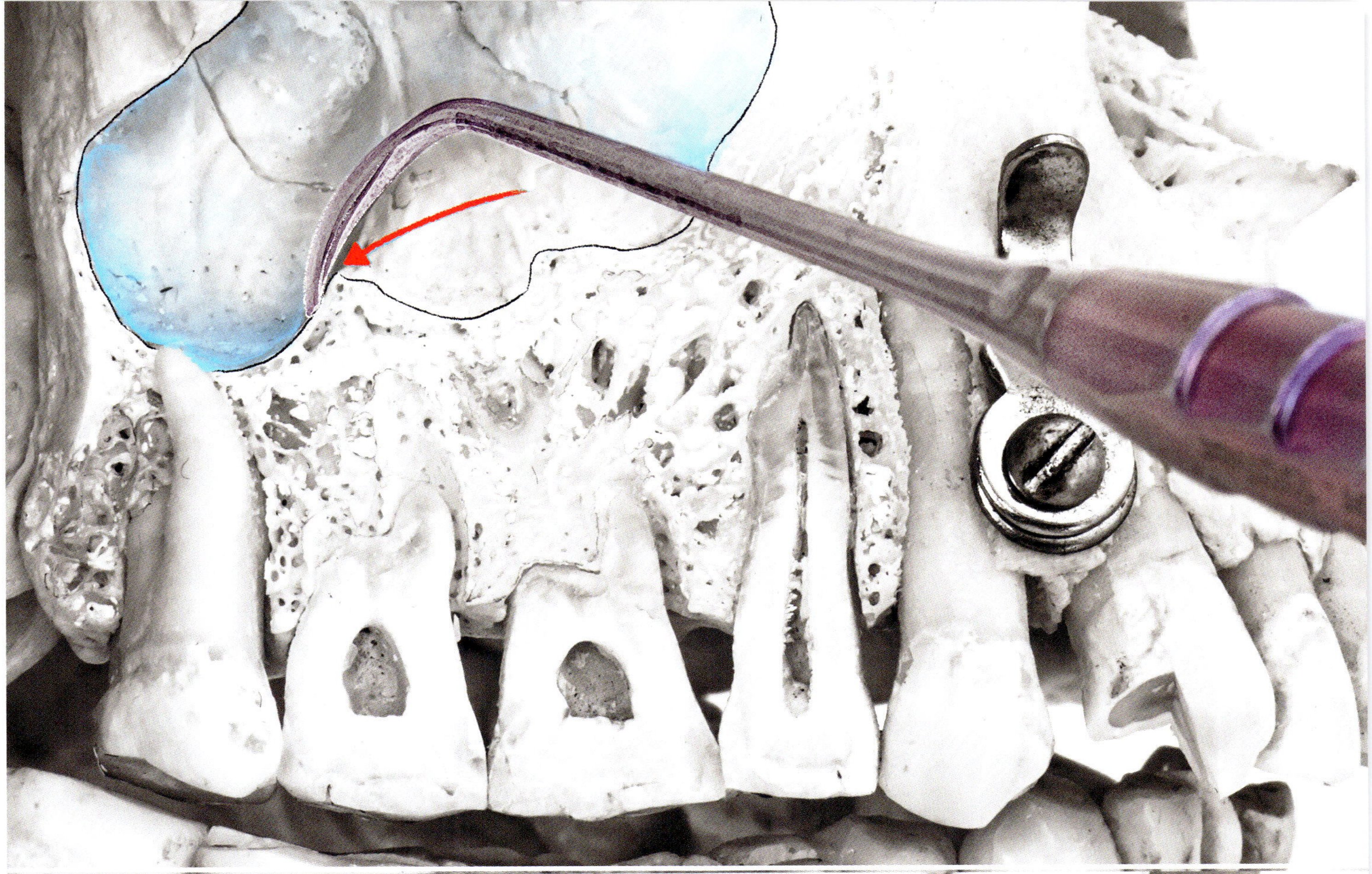

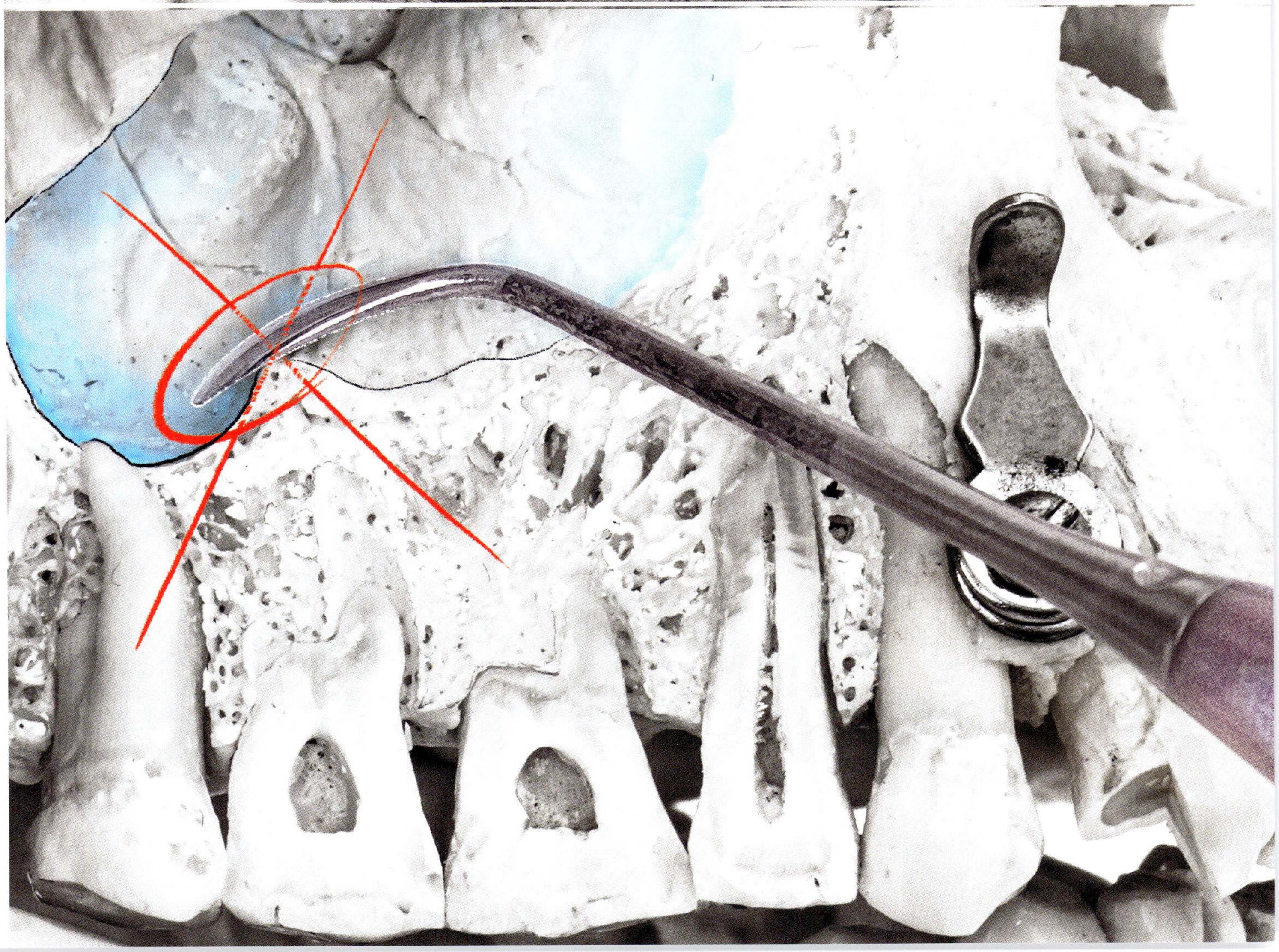

It is more challenging to reflect the membrane when the angle between the access and the sinus floor is acute. The instrument tip must be kept in tight contact with the bone to avoid a tear. The tighter this angle, the more challenging it is. Three-dimensional imaging provides information on bone thickness and the angle of approach to the sinus floor. Extending the osteotomy inferiorly usually opens that angle, simplifying membrane elevation. The piezo instrument is the safest way to widen the osteotomy, improving angles and increasing access. It also has attachments and settings to gently begin membrane dissection. The vibration of the flared blunt tip can begin teasing the membrane loose at the margin. This frees the marginal tissue, beginning the tedious work of elevating the membrane.

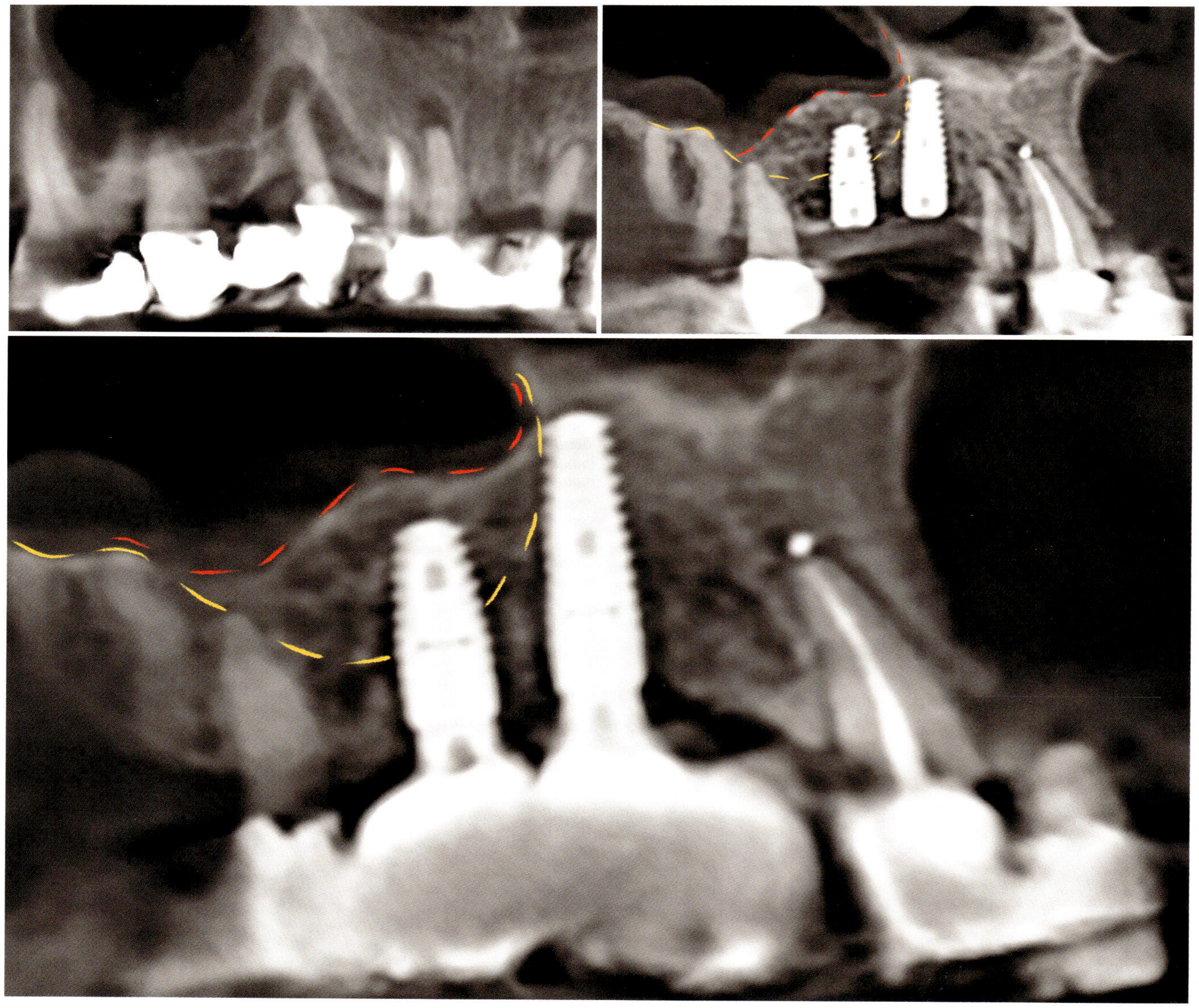

Figure 9-40 Tooth No. 5 had significant bone loss and needed to be removed. It was ultimately sinus grafted and implants at Nos. 5 and 6 retained a cantilever at No. 7. The sinus graft is still stable one-year post-operatively.

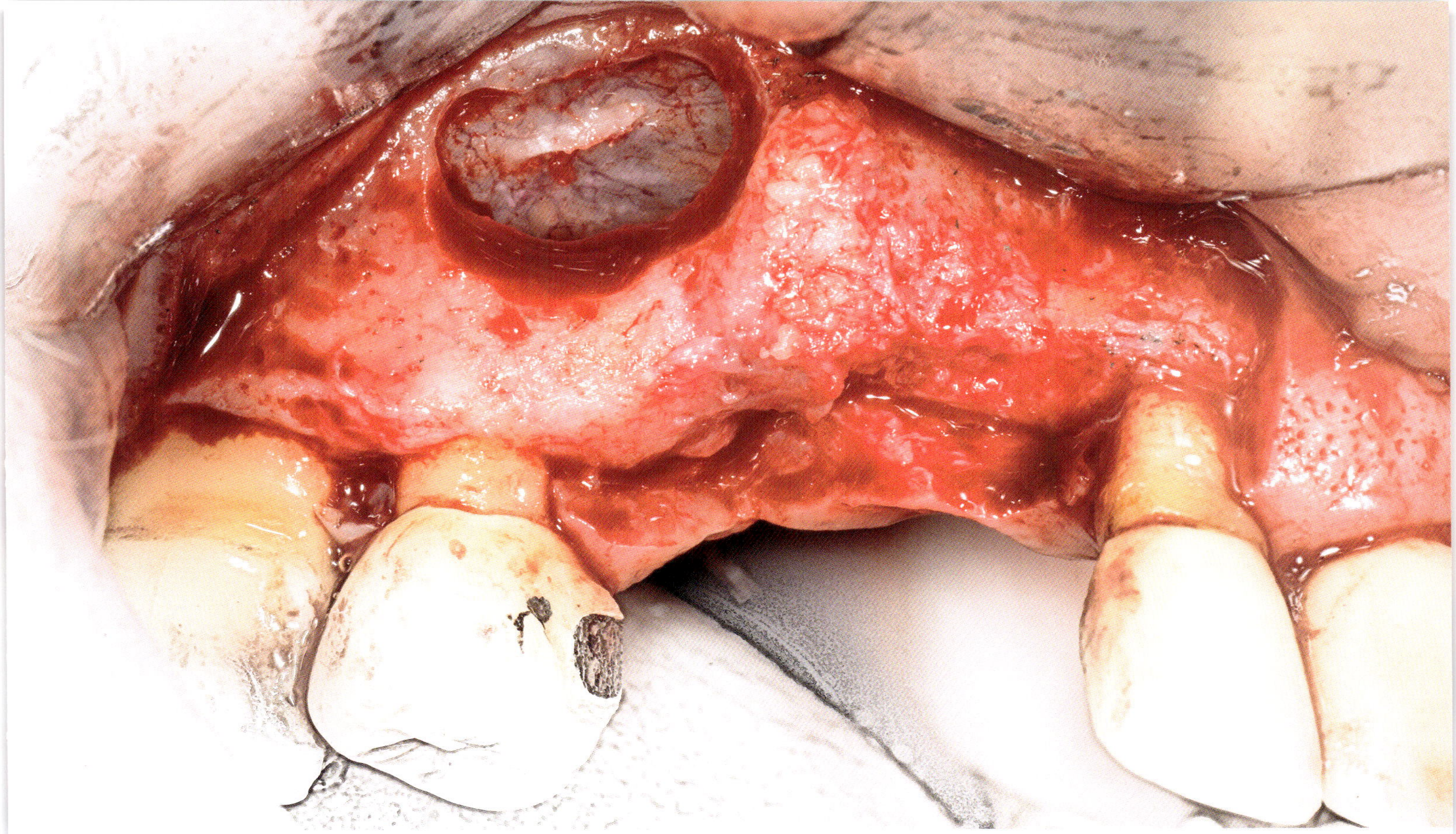

▲
Figure 9-41 You can usually see the membrane appear as the overlying bone is removed. Gently touch the tip of the piezo instrument on the central bone to determine whether it is free or still attached. If it is not mobile, retrace the osteotomy with the piezo to relieve any remaining intact bone. This central portion needs to be free to access the sinus and elevate the lining.

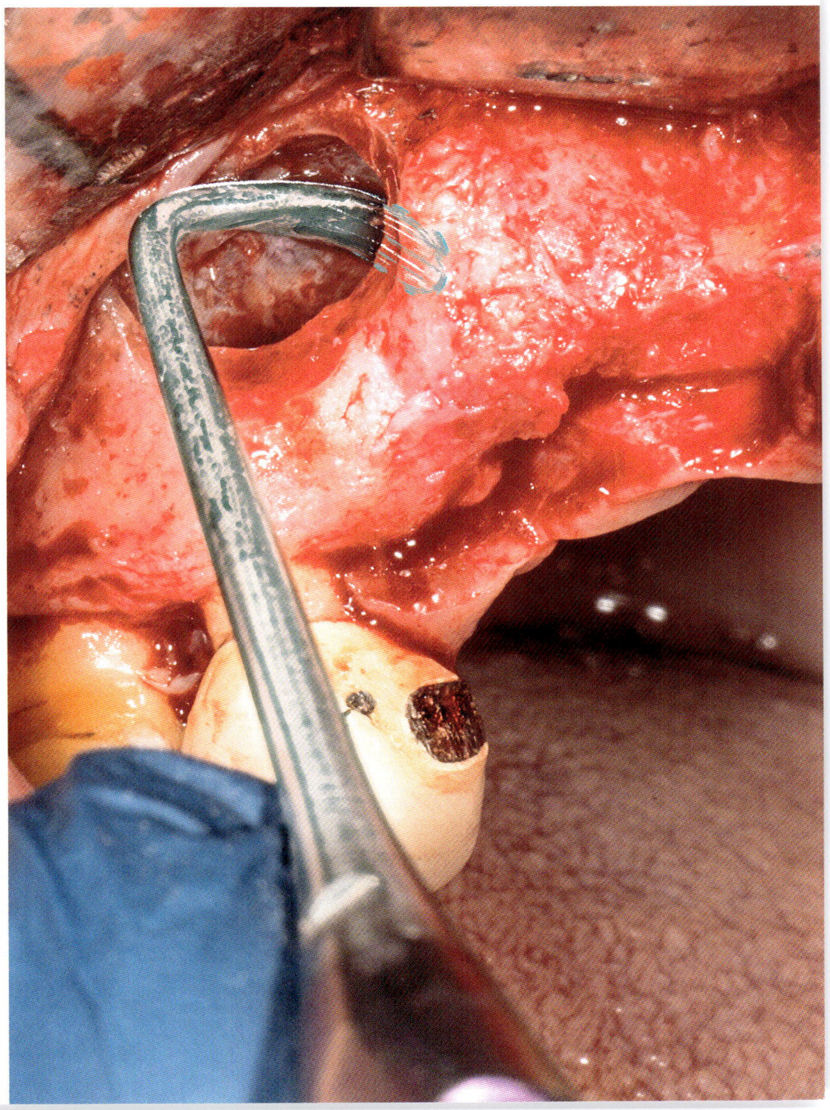

▸
Figure 9-42 The best place to start elevating with the sinus curette is usually along the inferior margin of the antrostomy. Other areas may be easier to begin elevation depending on the angle of approach and angle of the sinus curettes. Be flexible and explore the options for each case.

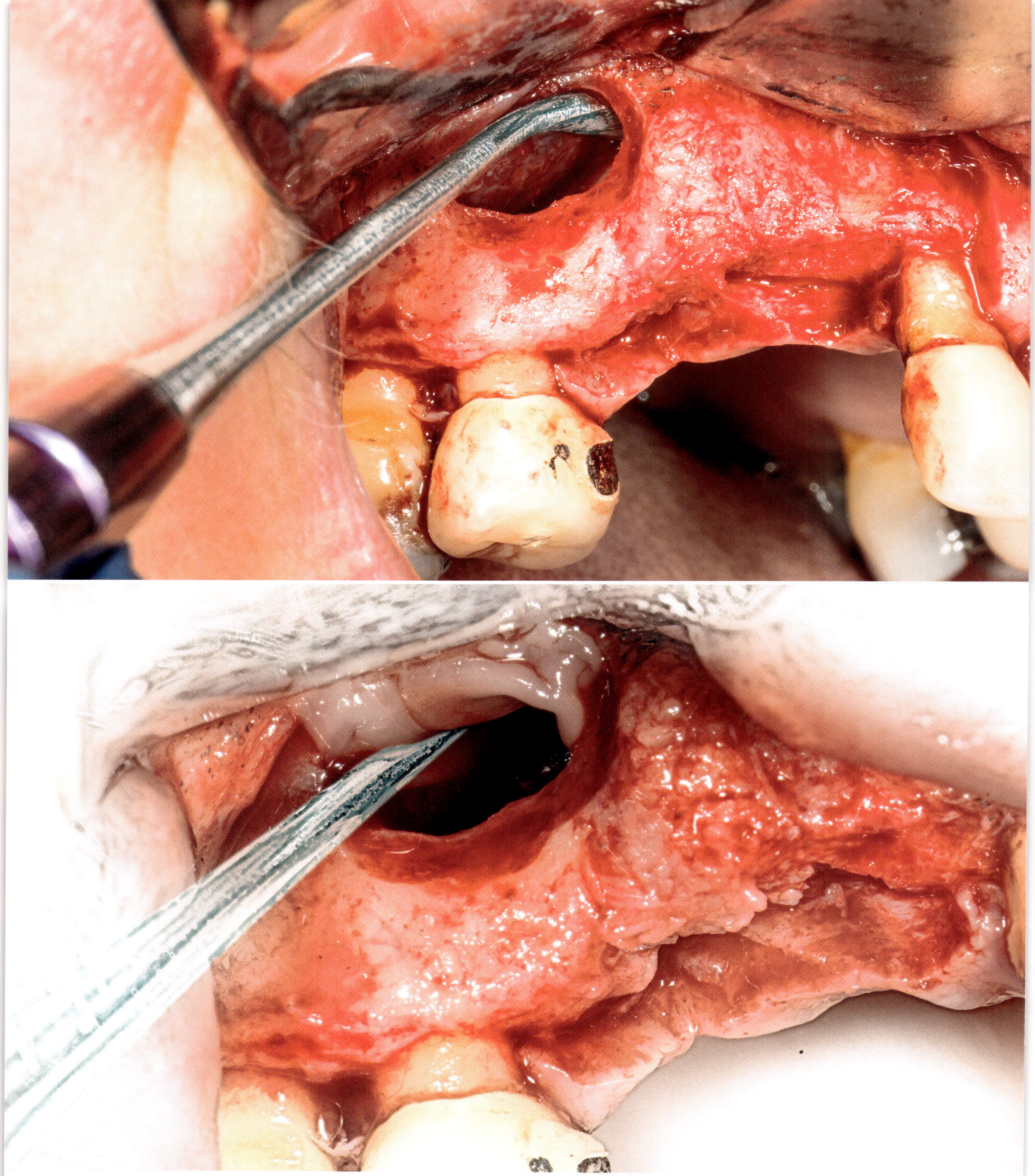

Figure 9-43 A platelet rich fibrin membrane extends out of the osteotomy as it is placed over the retracted sinus lining. The membrane is long enough to cover the graft internally and drape over the antrostomy. This isolates the graft material in the site.

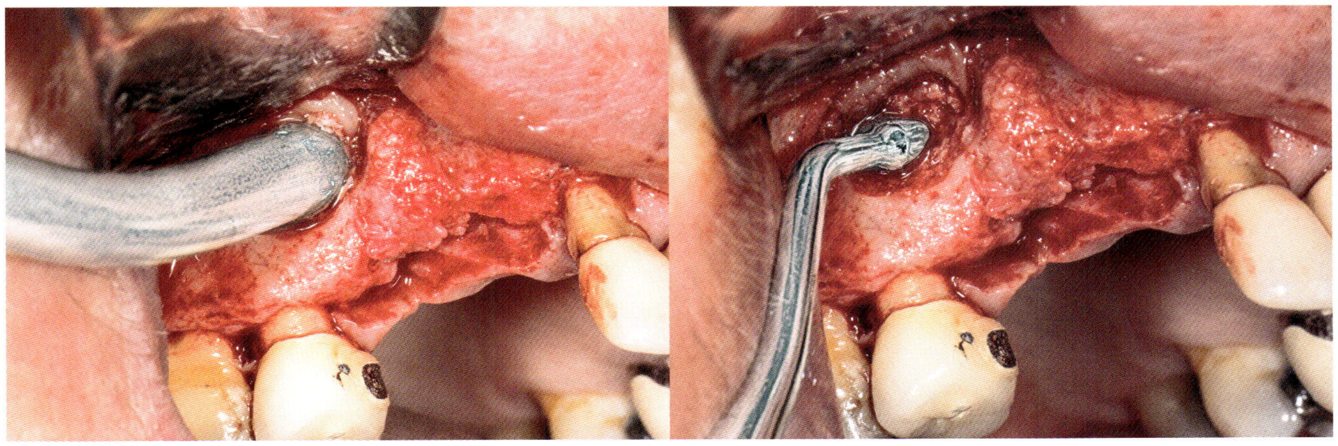

Figure 9-44 Blended allograft, autograft and xenograft is combined with liquid platelet rich fibrin and a minced membrane to make sticky bone. This is inserted with a bone syringe and positioned with a condenser. Make sure the graft extends to the blind spot in the anterior portion of the sinus. It is easy to miss this area when placing the graft.

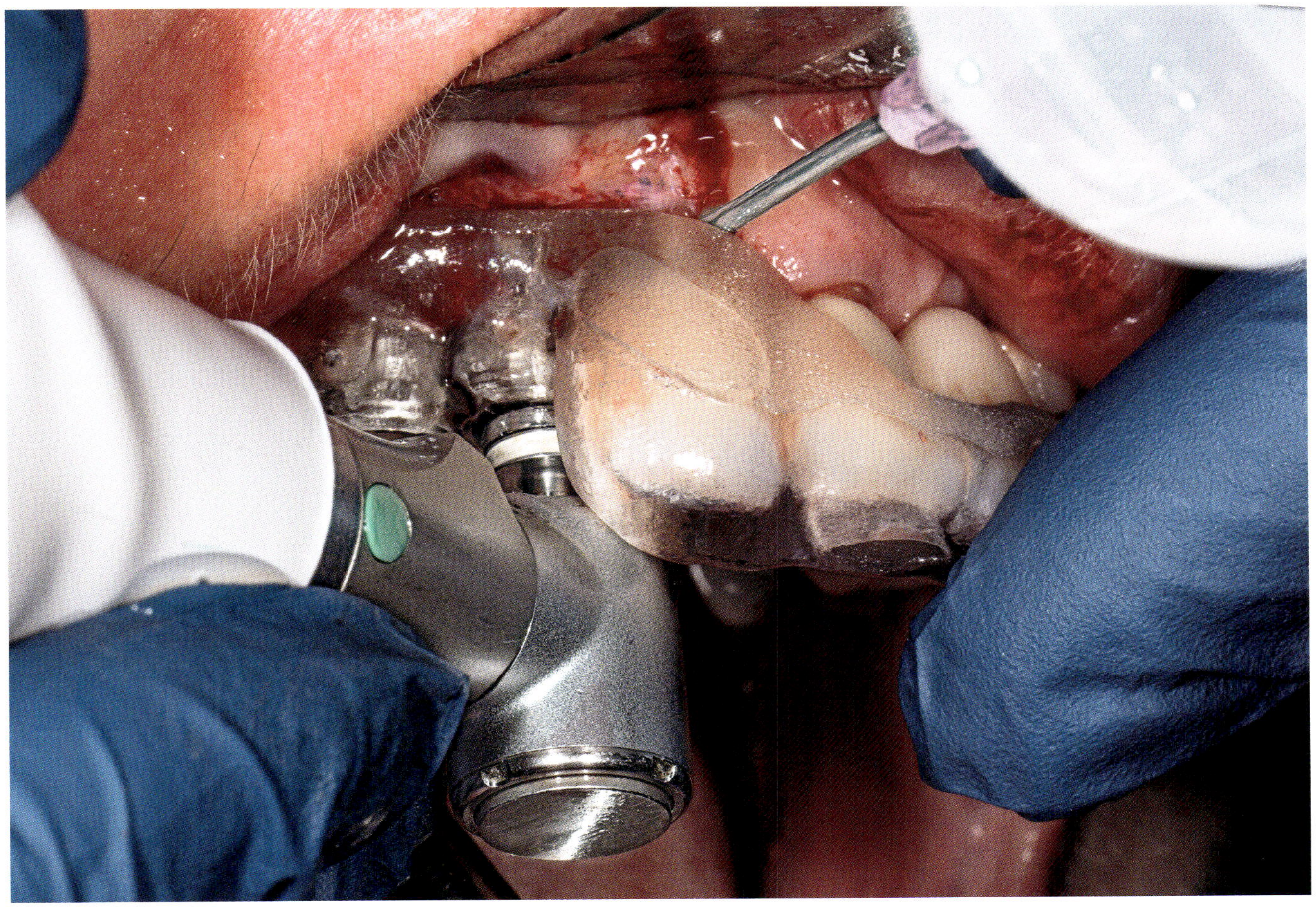

Figure 9-45 After the sinus site was developed, a static guide was used to begin the implant osteotomies. Irrigation was best applied beneath this guide with an irrigating syringe.

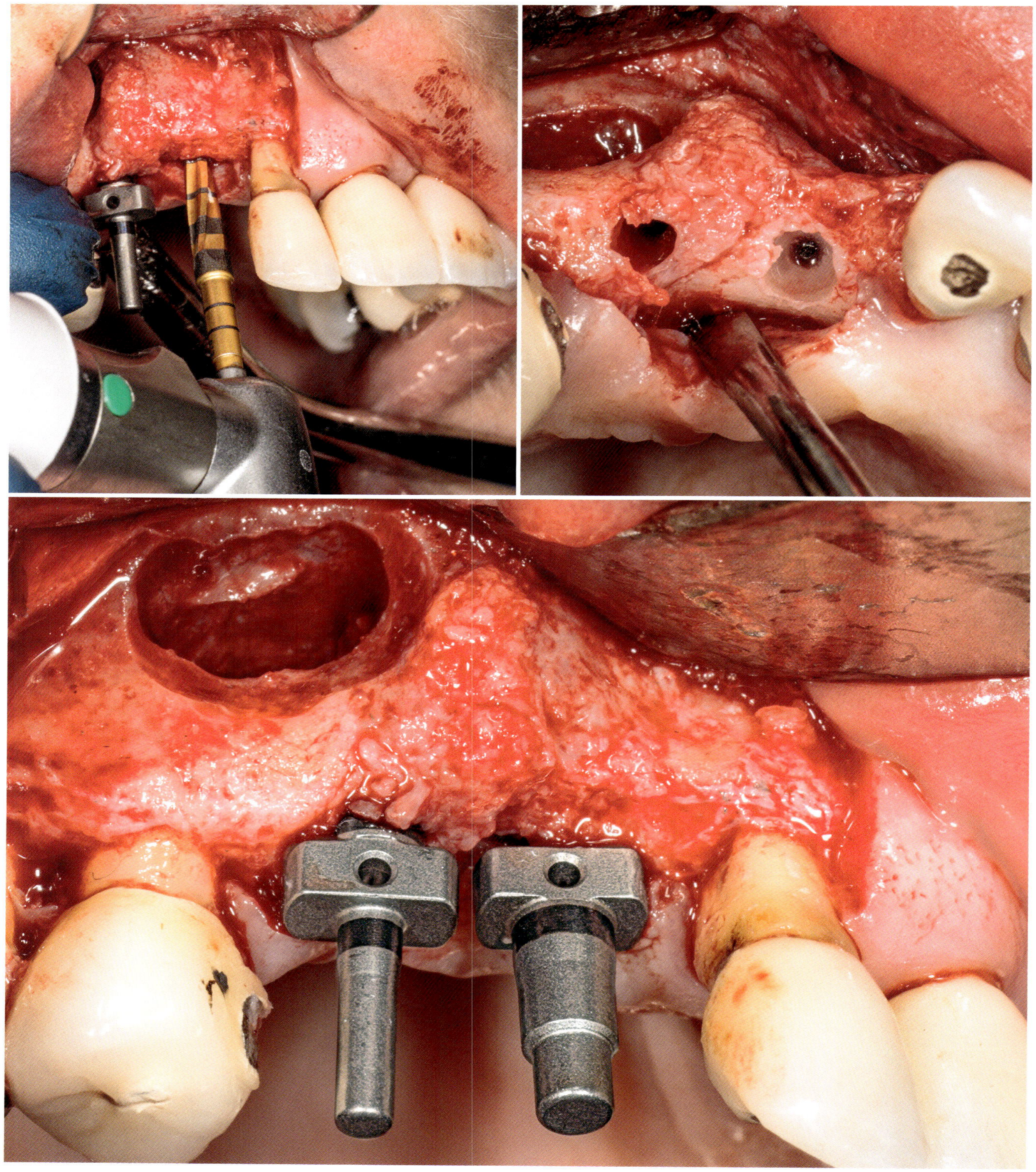

Figure 9-46 The lining was protected from perforation when drilling. Guide pins are helpful to ensure proper alignment, even when the initial pilot drill was guided. Note how this osseodensification drill appears to have increased the density in the osteotomy on the right.

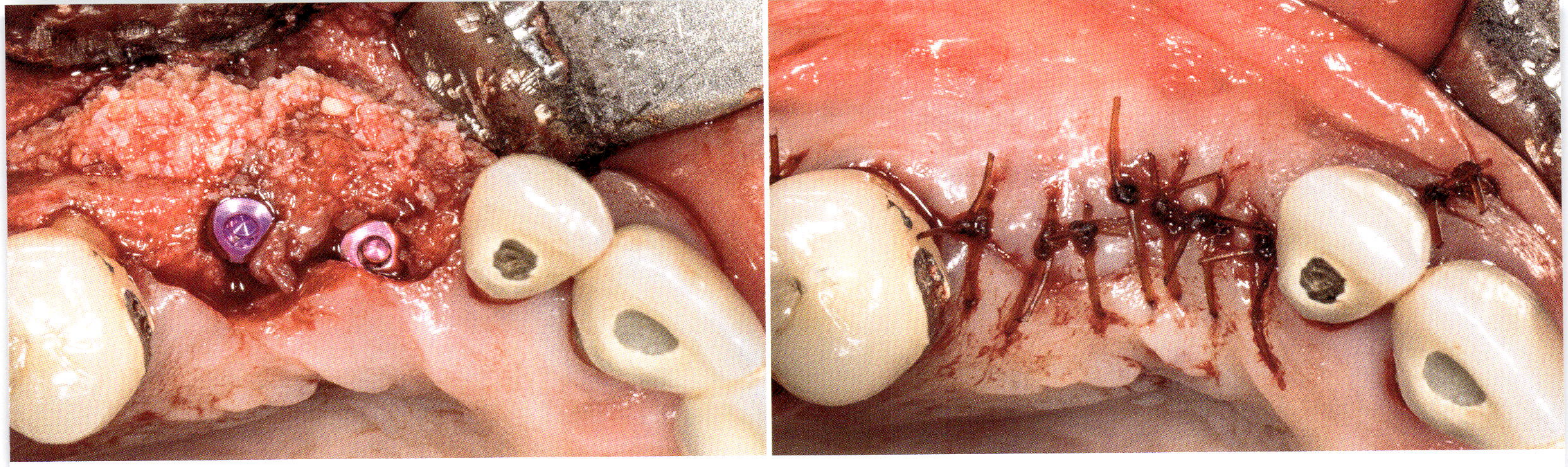

Figure 9-47 In this case, further augmentation was performed with the same allograft, xenograft and autograft mixed in a milieu with platelet rich fibrin. This was covered with a cross linked collagen membrane and passive primary closure was obtained.

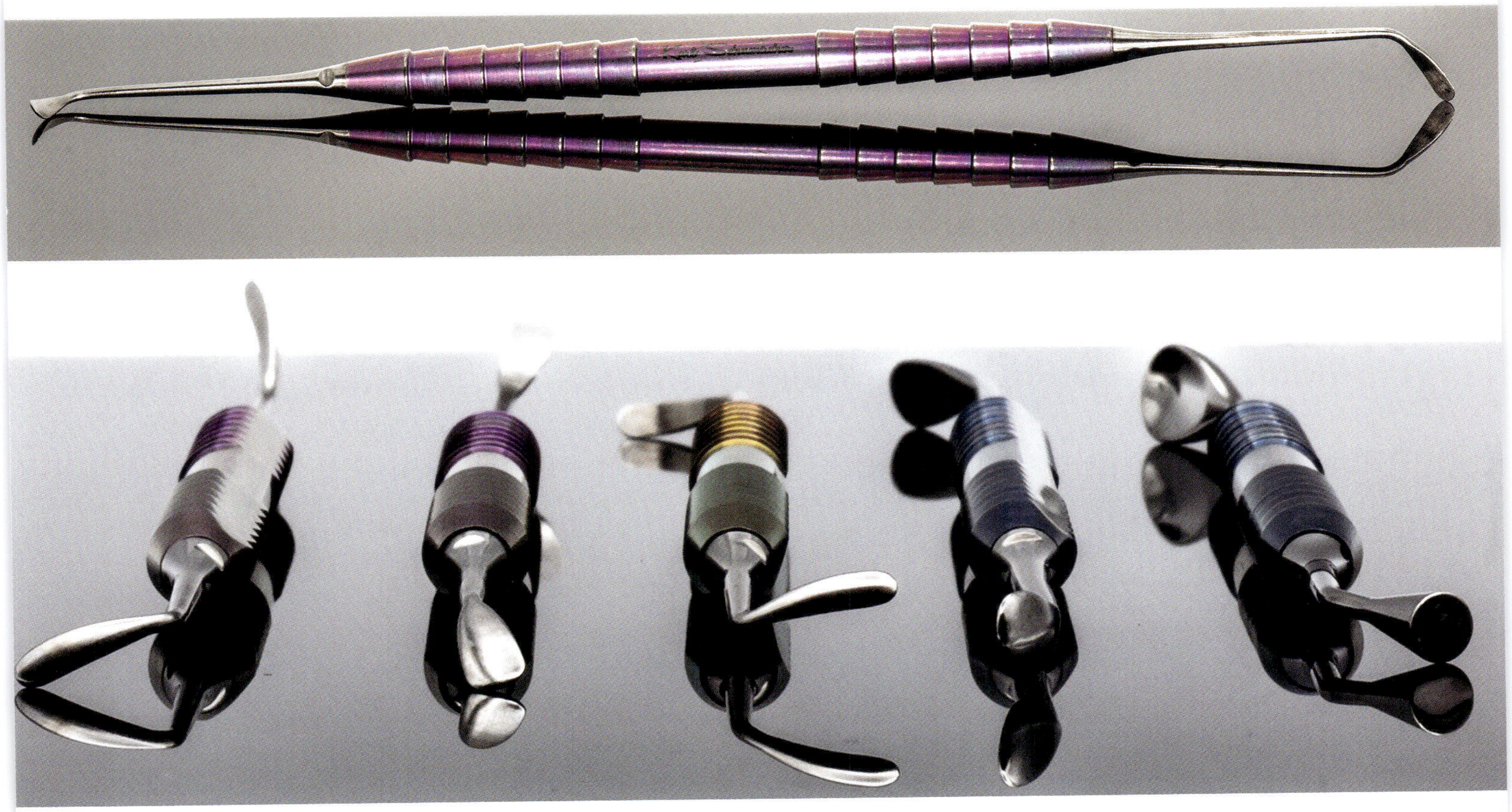

Figure 9-48 The sinus lift has unique needs, leading to the development of specific instruments to elevate the sinus membrane. The tight angles and restrictive access require off-axis dissection. Some instruments have a sharper tip (*purple*), beneficial for clean dissection of the sinus membrane. Others have a blunter tip (*yellow* and *blue*) for manipulating the membrane and graft material.

When simultaneous implant placement and sinus grafting are performed, implant osteotomy follows membrane elevation. Depending on the site, it may be beneficial to retract the membrane to protect it while drilling for the implant. It also can be beneficial to make the osteotomy narrower to increase initial stability in the limited bone. Graft material can be placed through the completed osteotomy, ensuring it is directly over the implant site. It can then be gently placed and condensed through the lateral window to fill the space. With the bulk of the graft in place, the implant is inserted to its final position.

As a principle, grafted bone must be contained. If it migrates out of the site into the surrounding tissue, it can cause inflammation and tissue may treat it like a foreign body. The ensuing neutrophil activation, giant cell formation, and ultimate fibrous encapsulation adversely affects the site. Meticulous care must be taken to ensure no granular graft material is left floating in the soft tissue prior to closing. Look around under the flap with a small tip suction to remove any remaining fragments.

Ideally, after the site has been inspected, the lateral aspect of the graft should be covered by a membrane. This further helps contain the graft material within the site and promote soft tissue healing. Many different resorbable membranes work well. A platelet rich fibrin membrane has become my preference. In addition to excellent handling properties, it optimizes coagulation, promotes stem cell activation, and stimulates osteoprogenitor cell migration to the site. The platelet rich fibrin membrane seems to help wound healing but is not a replacement for proper wound closure.

Primary watertight closure is critical to healing. A semilunar incision can be tricky to reapproximate accurately. The difference in the radius of the cut edges makes it easy to end up with an uneven closure, resulting in a dog ear at the end. While this can be revised by extending the incision and placing a few more sutures in a standard "dog ear revision" technique, proper tissue management will obviate the need for this added step. The easiest way to avoid tissue mismatch is to place a single resorbable suture in the middle of the incision, bisecting the wound. Then, either continue bisecting the remaining wound with multiple interrupted sutures, or consider running the suture, with or without locking. Any of these are reasonable options with a proper suture placement and knot tying technique.

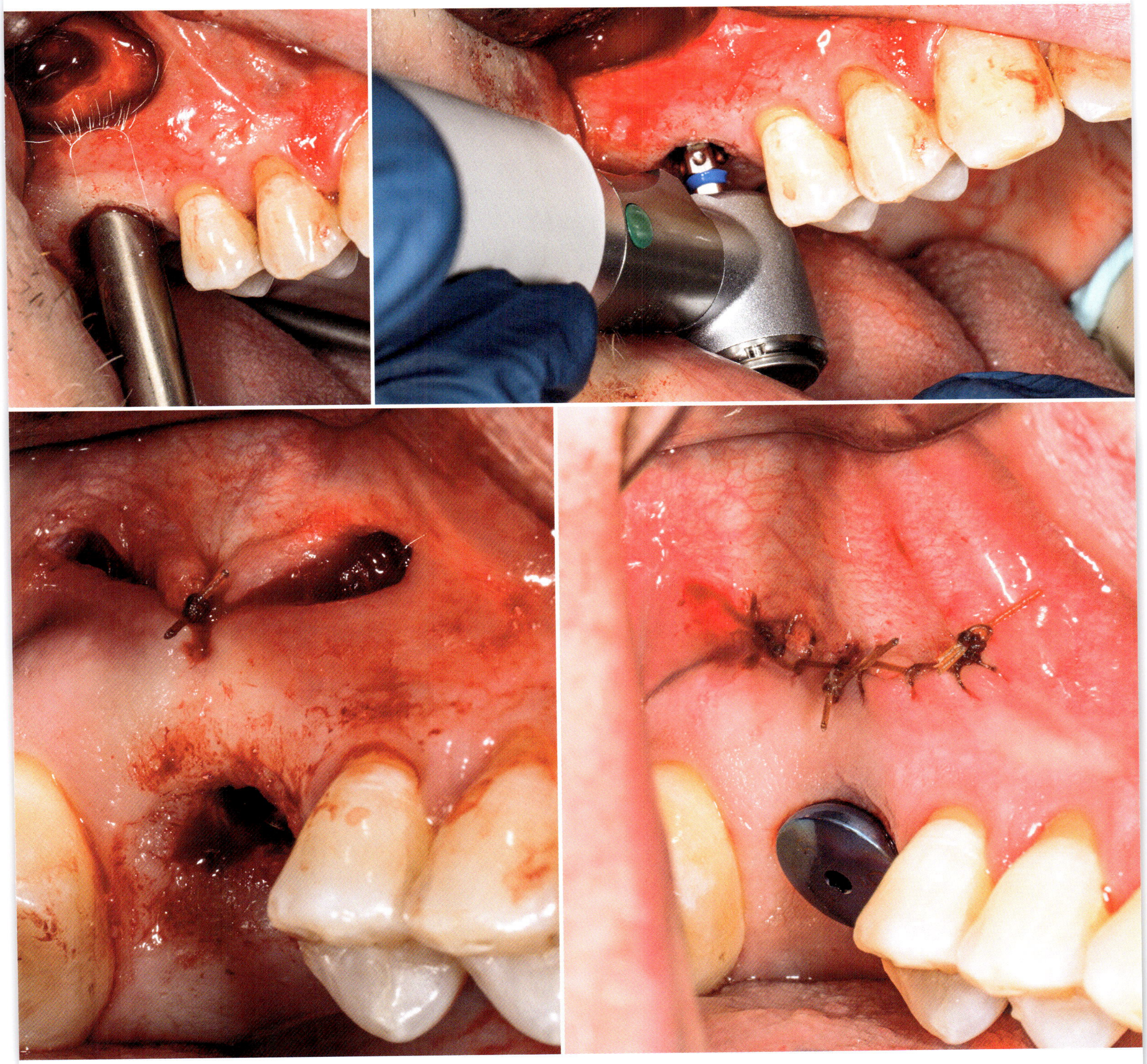

Figure 9-49 Placing bone graft through the implant site, in addition to the lateral window, helps ensure it will be adequate around the implant apex. I like to place a single suture in the middle of the incision to make sure it closes well. After the midline approximating suture, I usually run a locking stitch along the entire incision.

Indirect or crestal approach

The crestal approach blindly elevates the sinus floor during implant placement. Force is applied through the implant osteotomy to displace the sinus membrane, with or without the osseous floor intact. There are many variations to this approach. Sequential osteotomes can be whacked with a mallet, upfracturing the floor. Hydraulic dissection can gently elevate the membrane, creating space for graft material. The bone itself can be densified and displaced into the sinus to make room for the implant. These and other crestal techniques all serve to increase vertical bone for the implant.

Figure 9-50 The indirect sinus lift can be performed by tapping sequentially larger osteotomes into the implant osteotomy, fracturing and effectively lifting the sinus floor. This is quite technique sensitive with risk of tearing or perforating the sinus membrane due to the limited control and focused pressure. Alternative techniques, such as osseodensification, maintain better control.

▸ Figure 9-51 These offset osteotomes have a slightly concave tip to push bone from the walls into the sinus. They have depth markings to help avoid perforation. Tapping with a mallet provides a relatively controlled upfracturing force. These instruments seem less controlled than other methods, such as osseodensification.

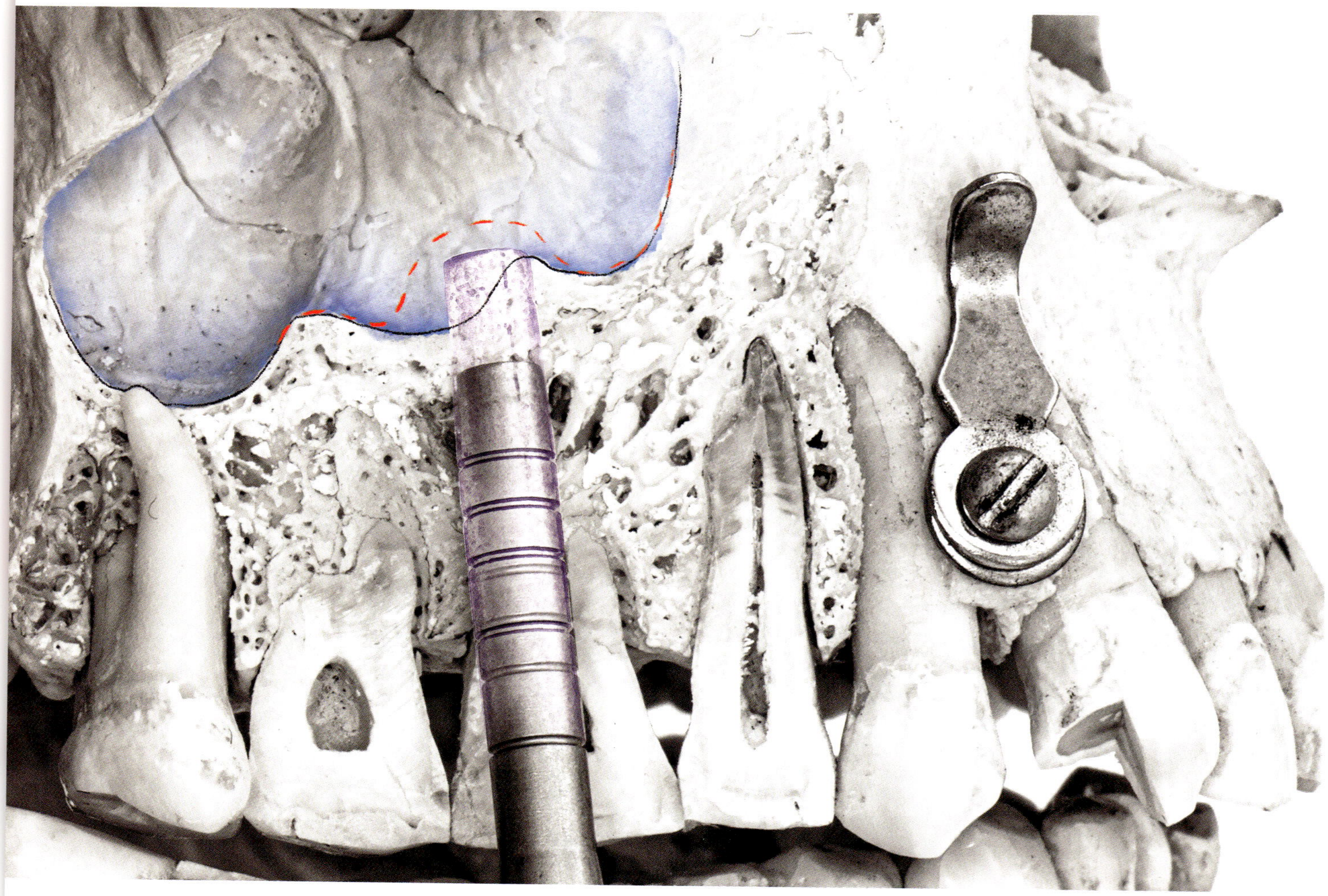

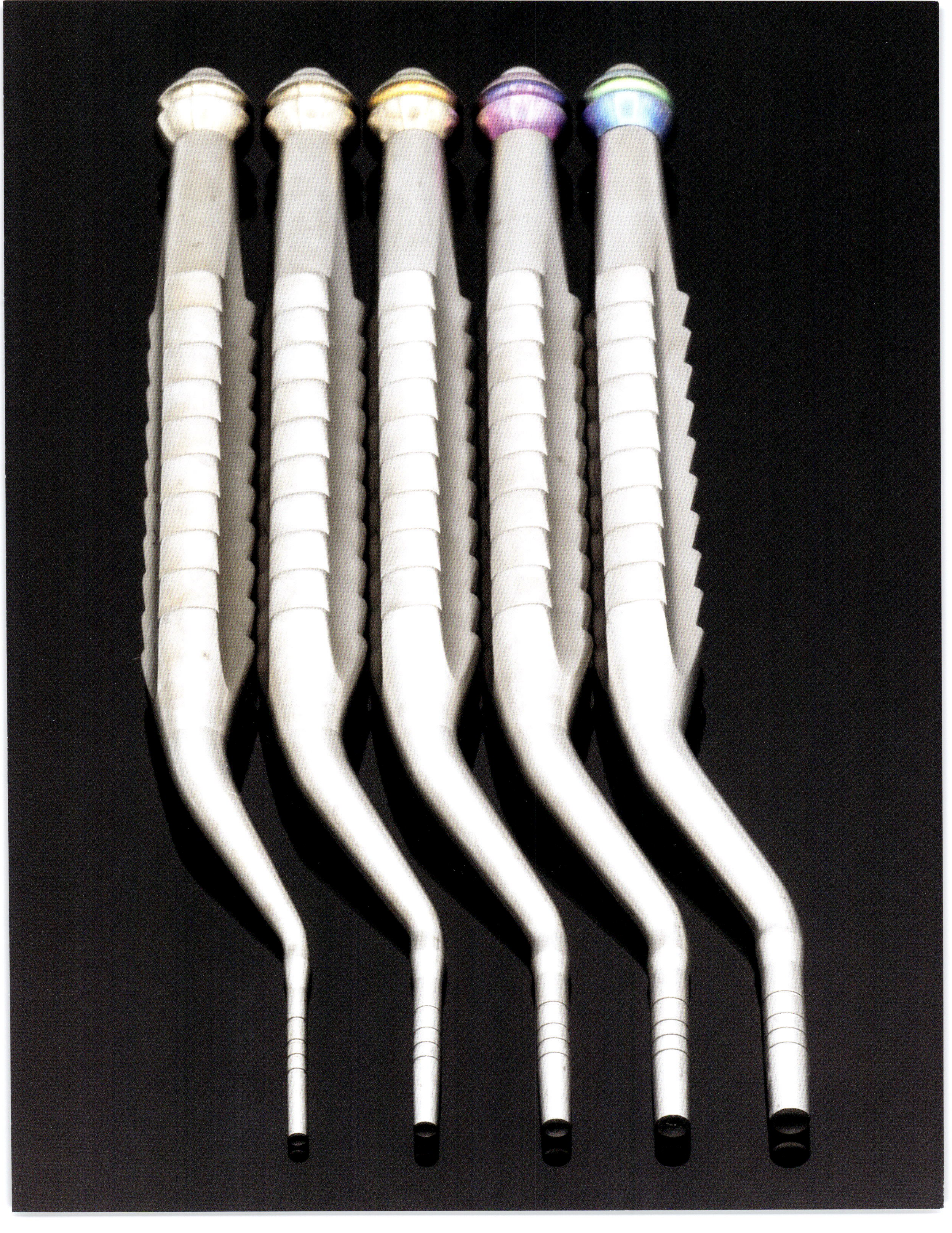

A word of caution regarding these techniques. While they are less invasive than a direct sinus lift, they are all blind approaches. The integrity of the membrane may be compromised without warning. When learning these advanced sinus grafting techniques, it would be prudent to gain competence in both direct and indirect approaches. Understanding each technique's nuances improves planning and the surgical outcome.

Sinus augmentation intraoperative complications

Membrane perforation

The most common intraoperative complication associated with sinus augmentation is perforation of the Schneiderian membrane. Small perforations pose a small risk while larger perforations carry higher risk of graft failure and potential sinus infection. In the big picture, prevention is key. Taking extreme care when elevating the membrane, directly or indirectly, helps to avoid perforation. If there is a small tear, try to get around it and prevent it from becoming bigger. If the margins around the perforation can be identified, it may be possible to cautiously elevate the membrane all around the defect and cover it up. Sometimes this works well and other times the tear seems to worsen. A small tear can often be managed by covering it with a membrane such as crosslinked collagen or platelet rich fibrin. This may also be possible with larger tears, but it is more challenging and less likely to be successful. Either way, the membrane absolutely must completely cover the graft and span the defect. Lifting the membrane around the perforation can be tricky. The challenge is to free up the margins without worsening the tear. It can be helpful to increase the osteotomy size to provide a fresh new area to approach the membrane. The pseudostratified epithelial lining of the sinus needs a guide for secondary healing. If the graft is not separated from the sinus properly, the chances of further complications, including infection and graft failure, increase dramatically.

▸
Figure 9-52 This patient had a 2 mm sinus perforation noted when elevating the membrane in a direct sinus lift (*upper middle*). The lining was elevated around the perforation. A PRF membrane was positioned covering the sinus floor well beyond the perforation (*upper right*). The membrane was large enough to drape outside the osteotomy to surround the entire graft prior to closing (*middle right*). This patient also had a significant apical granuloma involving the first premolar that was removed, debrided, grafted and covered with a crosslinked collagen membrane to reconstruct the defect. The final restoration reconstructed the premolar defect and achieved a great result with the molar implant.

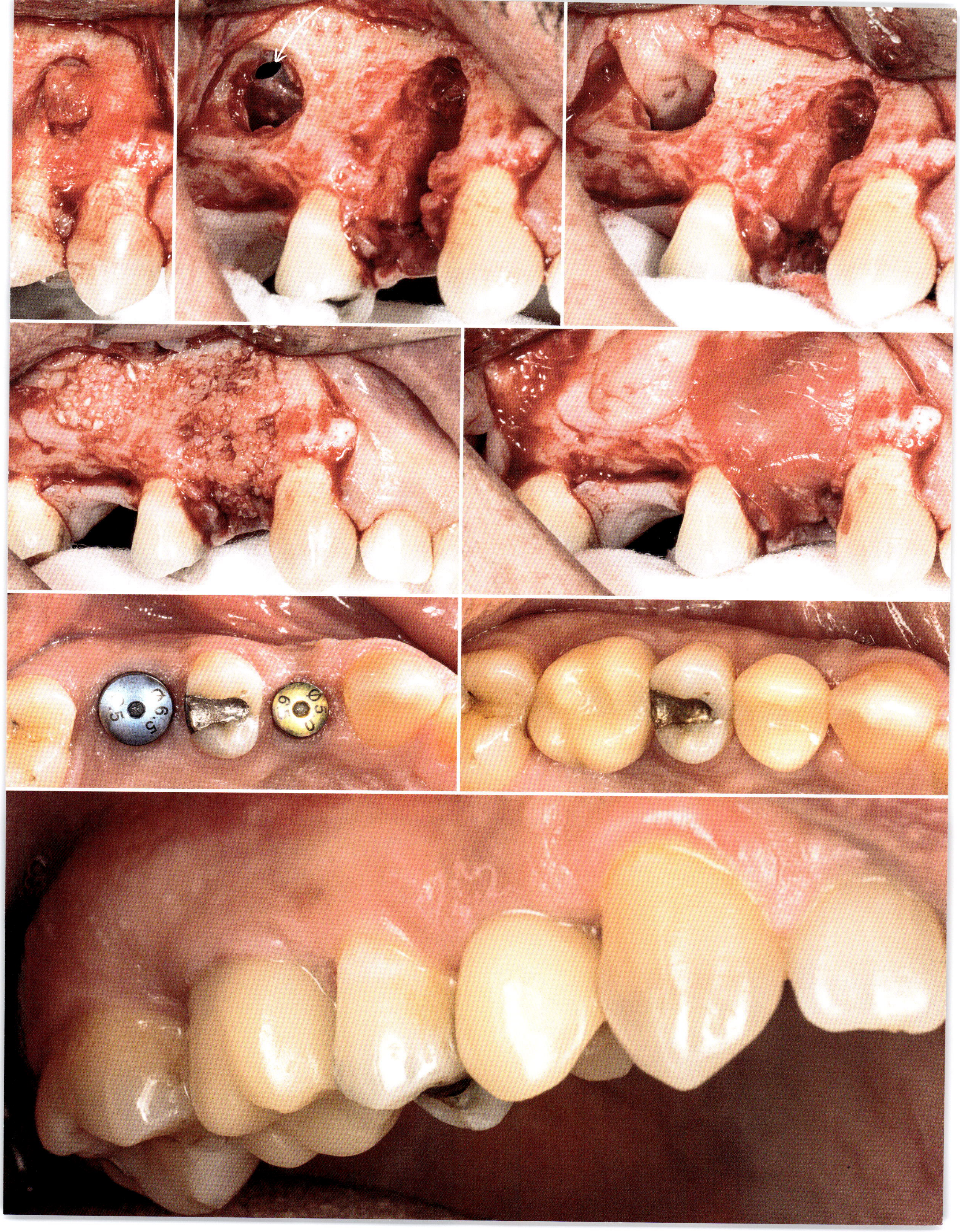

Bleeding

When performing sinus augmentation, hemostasis can be a challenge. It may be difficult or impossible to apply pressure to the bleeding site when it is occurring within the sinus. The posterior superior alveolar artery and alveolar antral artery are two of the most common vessels encountered during sinus augmentation. Carefully evaluating the CBCT will often reveal the position as a visible canal in the antral wall or floor. When encountered surgically, this small terminal artery can instantly flood the surgical site, impeding progress and potentially compromising the outcome. When the vessel is identified radiographically, the surgical plan could possibly be altered to avoid it. At times, significant vasculature is discovered during antrostomy. If possible, the osteotomy may be adjusted to avoid the vessel. Look for it and try to work around it.

If the vessel has already been compromised and bleeding must be managed, first identify the exact source and location of the bleeding as well as possible. With good suction and irrigation, the lumen of the vessel may be visible. Arterial bleeding may at times be managed with firm pressure for five or more minutes, but that is often inadequate. Other options include compressing the vessel by crushing the overlying bone, occluding it with bone wax, or cauterizing with a laser or electrocautery. If an arterial bleed seems to be manageable with pressure alone, beware. The post-operative arterial pressure may overpower the clot, resulting in significant bleeding.

When the site bleeds post-operatively, it is not just a nuisance for the patient. A hematoma can be temporarily disfiguring and alarming. If the bleeding distends the tissue containing the graft, it could compromise the graft. It can also compromise the soft tissue closure and potentially blood supply, making it more prone to infection. The amount of bruising can also be impressive. In patients more prone to bruising, especially elderly patients, the colorful array can paint the tissue for weeks, blossoming from a black eye through the cheek to a purple neck.

Figure 9-53 This vessel was notable radiographically but was obvious clinically. The antrostomy was shifted lower to avoid the vessel. This sinus lift was performed at the time of extraction.

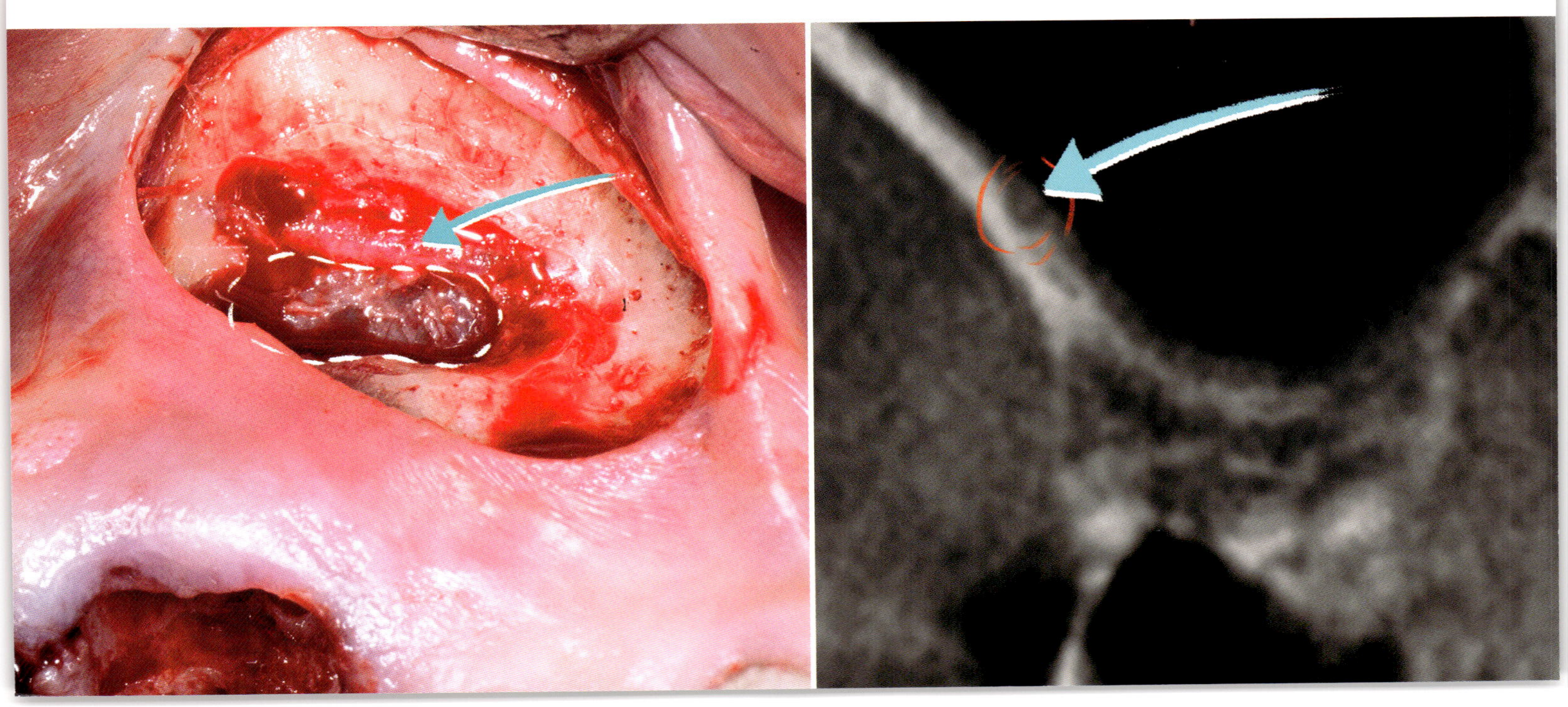

Inadequate implant stability

Implant stability is a critical component to success. In simultaneous sinus augmentation, it can mean the difference between a healthy implant and a potentially migrating foreign body trapped within the sinus cavity. While this seems to be rare, it can be quite the problem to retrieve. If the implant doesn't achieve reasonable stability, at least 10 Ncm or greater, consider completing the sinus augmentation and staging implant placement after the graft heals. This may be an inconvenience, but it is far more palatable than retrieving an implant traveling through the patient's sinuses.

Soft Tissue Development

There are many simple and elegant procedures and techniques to optimize soft tissue and develop an implant site. It feels good to see the soft tissue take form around an implant. When my patients need more extensive soft tissue grafting, such as free gingival grafts, I collaborate with my periodontists. Collaborating with them is rewarding and always beneficial. I have a tremendous level of respect for the artistic work my periodontist friends do every day. But I like to keep it simple and successful. Here are several ways I approach cases with high and low esthetic demand.

Tissue manipulation

Begin with the end in mind. We almost always want more buccal tissue in the end. That is where the tissue resorbs the quickest. In the body's attempt to conserve resources, it reduces ridge volume when a tooth comes out. When we measure the actual bone and tissue volume, we often have more in an edentulous space than when the tooth was present. But the overall ridge has a defect. We can push the tissue back outward, like it was before the tooth came out.

The ideal incision depends on ridge shape and tissue contours. We want thick, robust tissue all around the implant. Implants are prone to getting food impacted because of their narrower emergence and limited tissue. Optimizing the gingival contours has both esthetic and functional benefits.

There are many classifications available to evaluate and plan alveolar ridge soft and hard tissue management. You can find an incredibly elaborate and beautiful decision-making table on pages 648-649 in *Plastic-Esthetic Periodontal and Implant Surgery*[2].

In my daily practice, I try to keep it simple. If the underlying bone is adequate, I look at the soft tissue in a simplistic way. Is there enough? Almost enough? Not enough? Or is there a significant deficiency? If there is enough tissue, it looks green in my mind. Almost enough is yellow. Not enough looks orange. And if there is a significant deficiency, it looks red in my mind. No matter what formal or informal classification you use, figure out a plan to establish adequate tissue or the results won't be great.

Table 9-1 The type of incision and tissue manipulation depends on the ridge form. More precisely, how much tissue is present and how much we need.

	How much tissue is present?	How much tissue gain do we need?	Incision type
Green	More than enough	None	Punch
Yellow	Almost enough	Need a bit	Elliptical
Orange	Not enough	Need a bit more	Small fap
Red	Significant deficiency	Need a lot	Palatal roll or tissue grafting

Figure 9-54 Is the ridge wide enough? There may be more than enough tissue (*green*), almost enough (*yellow*), not enough (*orange*) or a significant tissue deficiency (*red*). Visualizing the final implant position helps determine how much tissue manipulation is needed to optimize the site.

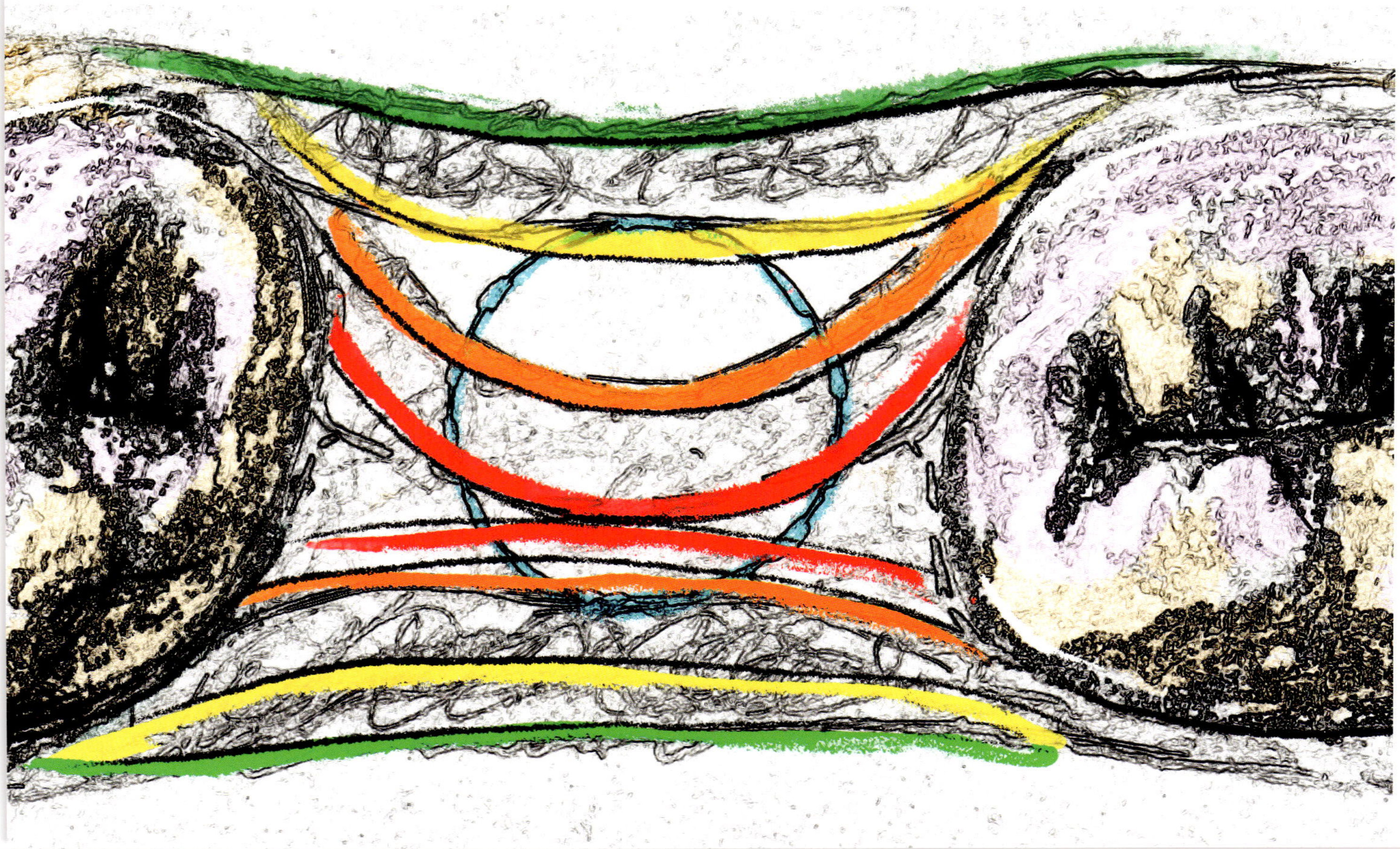

Green: Enough ridge

If the site has more than enough tissue already, a tissue punch can make a perfect circular incision for the implant. This is lovely when it works. It is the quickest and least traumatic way to expose the osteotomy site. But this technique does nothing to improve the tissue contours, so the case has to be just right. There is usually room for at least some improvement in the soft tissue contour.

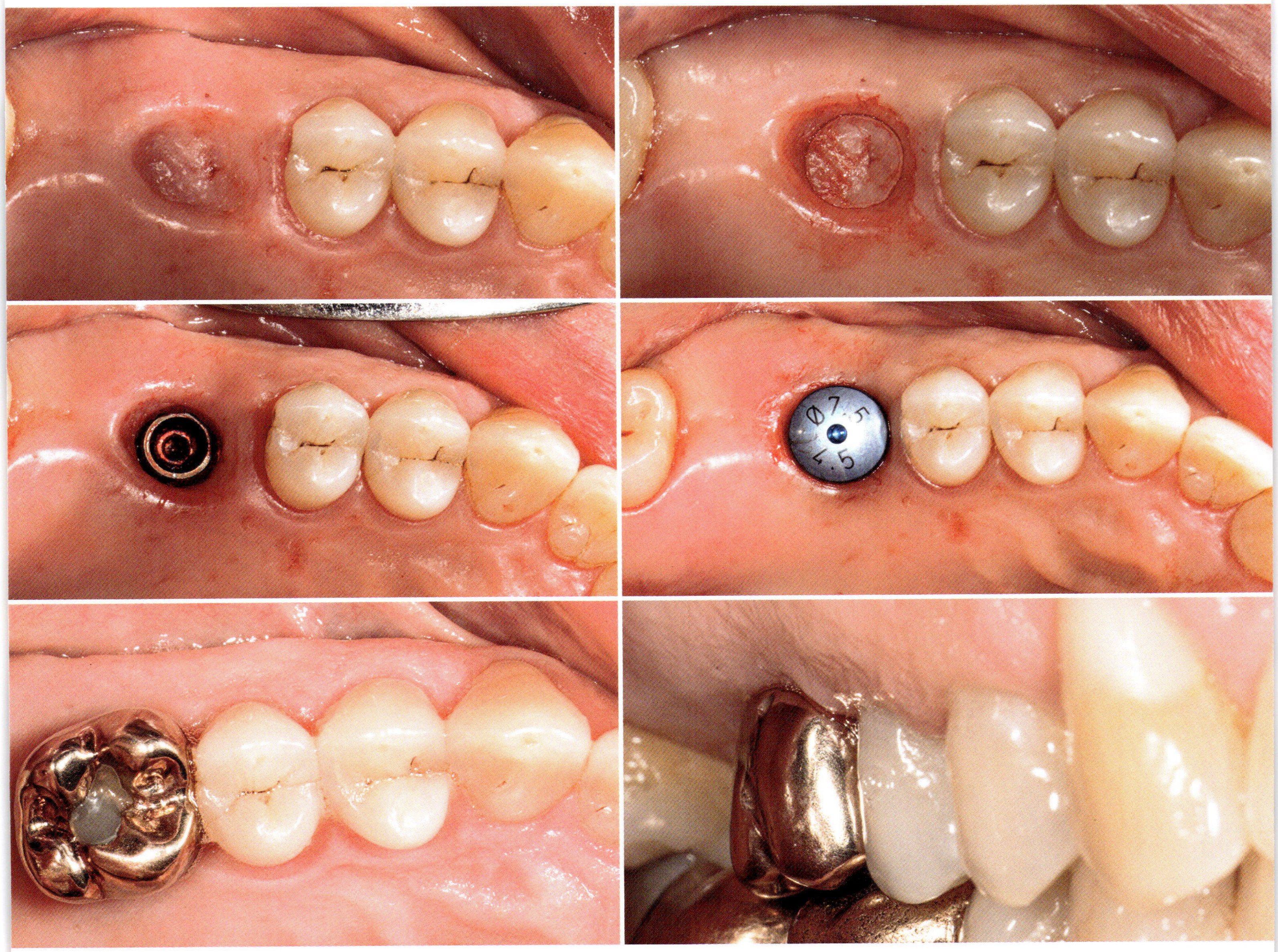

Figure 9-55 When there is ample bone and soft tissue, a circular tissue punch works well. In this case, the center of the implant was marked with the starter drill under dynamic navigation. A small 1 mm adjustment was made, moving the implant distal (this is the advantage of dynamic navigation). The circular incision was made, site prepared and implant placed. The final restoration has great ridge form and contours. The gold restoration works well with the opposing gold restorations.

Yellow: Almost enough ridge

If the site has almost enough tissue and ridge shape, an elliptical incision is a slick way to improve the tissue contours with minimal trauma. The tissue can be pushed buccally to the extent that the width of the incision is narrower than the abutment. A 3 mm wide ellipse with a 7.5 mm wide abutment will increase the tissue over 2 mm on both the facial and lingual. To move, the tissue must be freed from the underlying bone. Reflecting a small flap accomplishes this easily. This design can also be beneficial when the tissue at the center of the site is not yet fully mature. It will excise the soft tissue with the granular graft infiltration that remains, leaving mature tissue behind at the periphery.

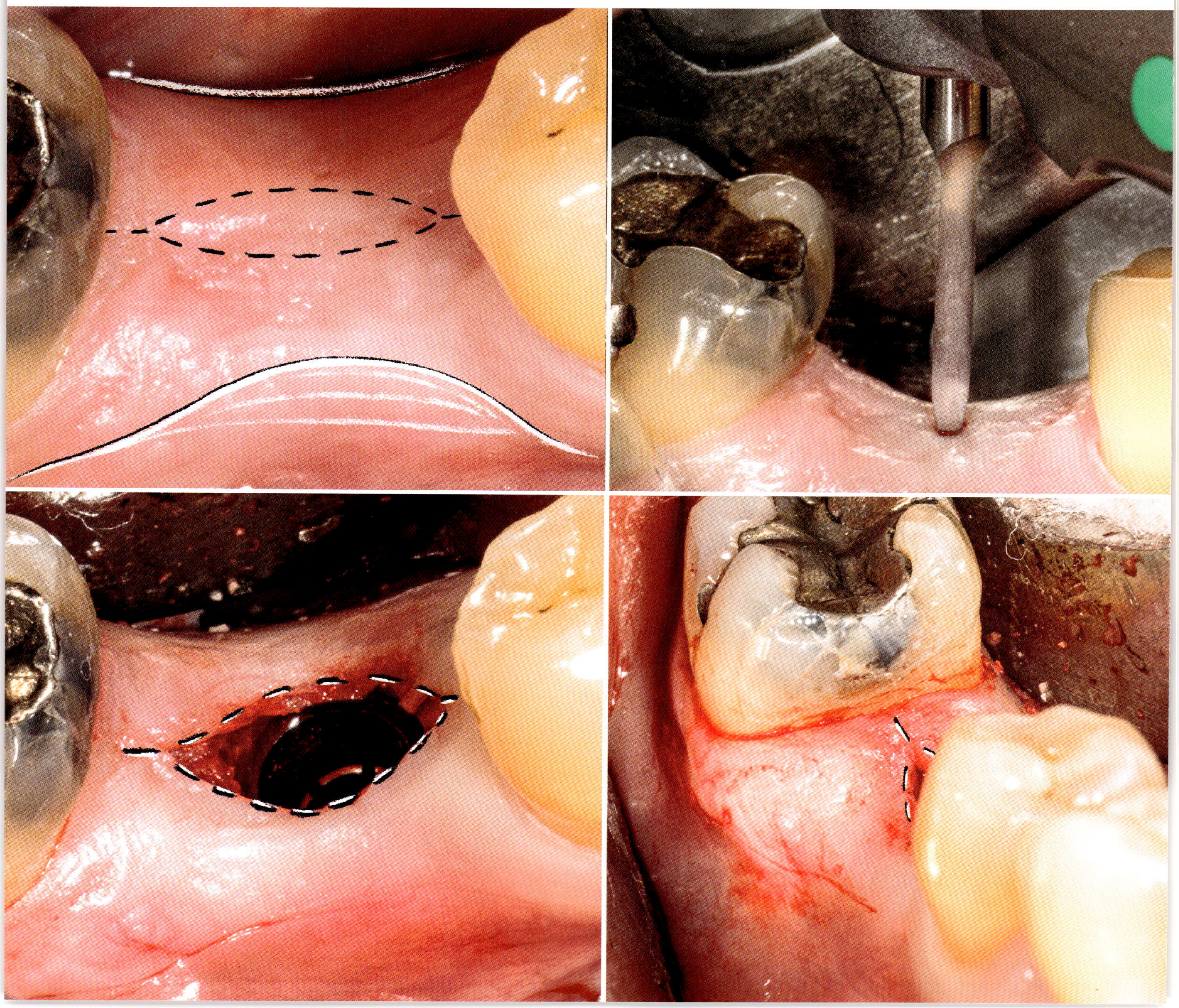

Orange: Not enough ridge

If there is not enough contour and tissue volume, a small flap can be made that repositions the tissue toward the buccal by placing the incision at the abutment's most palatal or lingual aspect. To do this, visualize the implant position and abutment flare. That line is where you cut. This preserves all the tissue the body has worked at growing since the tooth came out. We can't grow the tissue as surgeons. It is the body that does this. Let's respect its efforts and appreciate its incredible ability. Poke the starter drill into the tissue to mark the site. Figure out where the abutment margins will be. The incision should follow the palatal extent of where the abutment will sit. Reflecting a small flap is necessary to mobilize the tissue and reposition it.

The tissue can then be contoured around the abutment on the buccal to control the shape and optimize hygiene. If it is left high on the buccal, it usually will remodel and retract. But hygiene is easier when the abutment is exposed. Excising a small wedge of tissue can improve the final contours. This can be done with the edge of a tissue punch or a fresh blade. Either a V-shaped wedge or curvilinear incision can work well, depending on how the tissue will come together. Dr. Patrick Palacci described a clever technique in which this excess buccal tissue is not excised, but rather rotated to augment the papilla[3]. I find this technique effective and love how it looks when completed. It feels good to repurpose that tissue so nicely. See Figure 9-60.

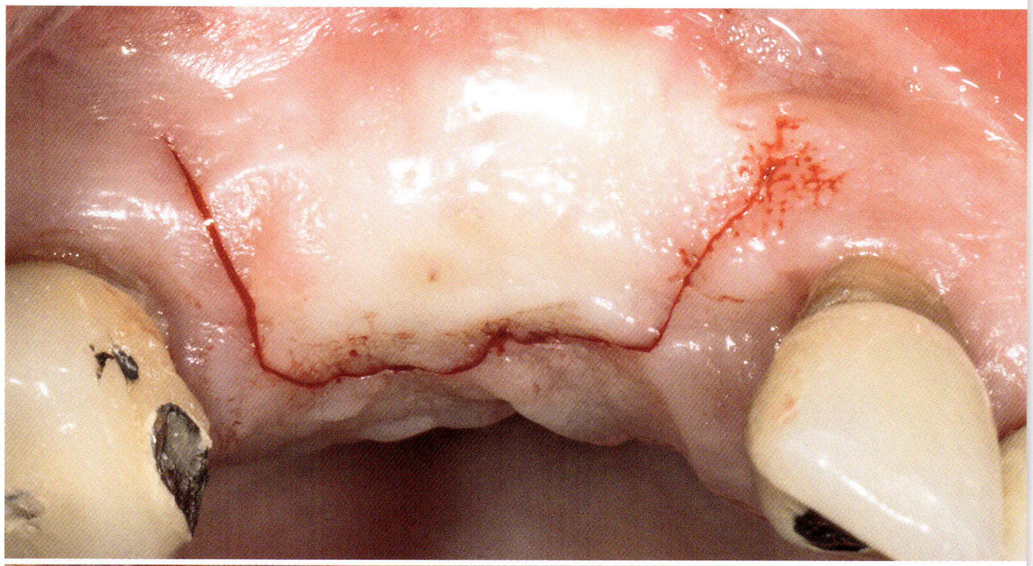

◄
Figure 9-56 A slight increase in ridge width would be ideal in this case, so an elliptical incision is planned. The starter drill is lined up in the planned position with dynamic navigation to mark the tissue. An elliptical incision is made, and the implant is placed.

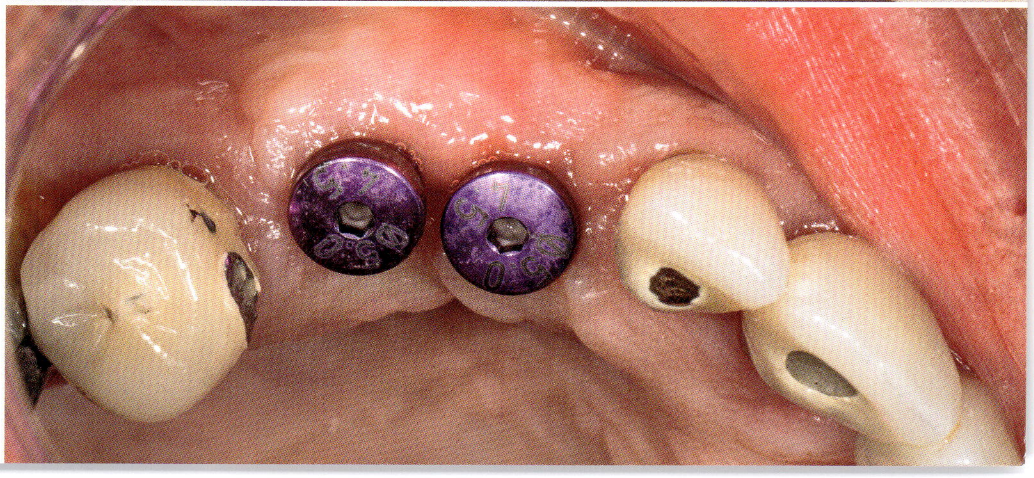

►
Figure 9-57 This incision design promotes an apically positioned flap, favorably moving the keratinized gingiva facially and helping to restore contours.

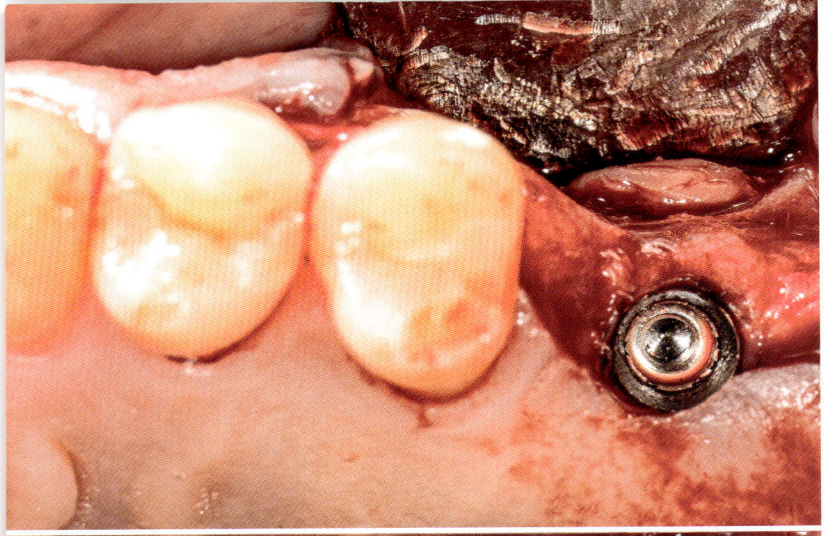

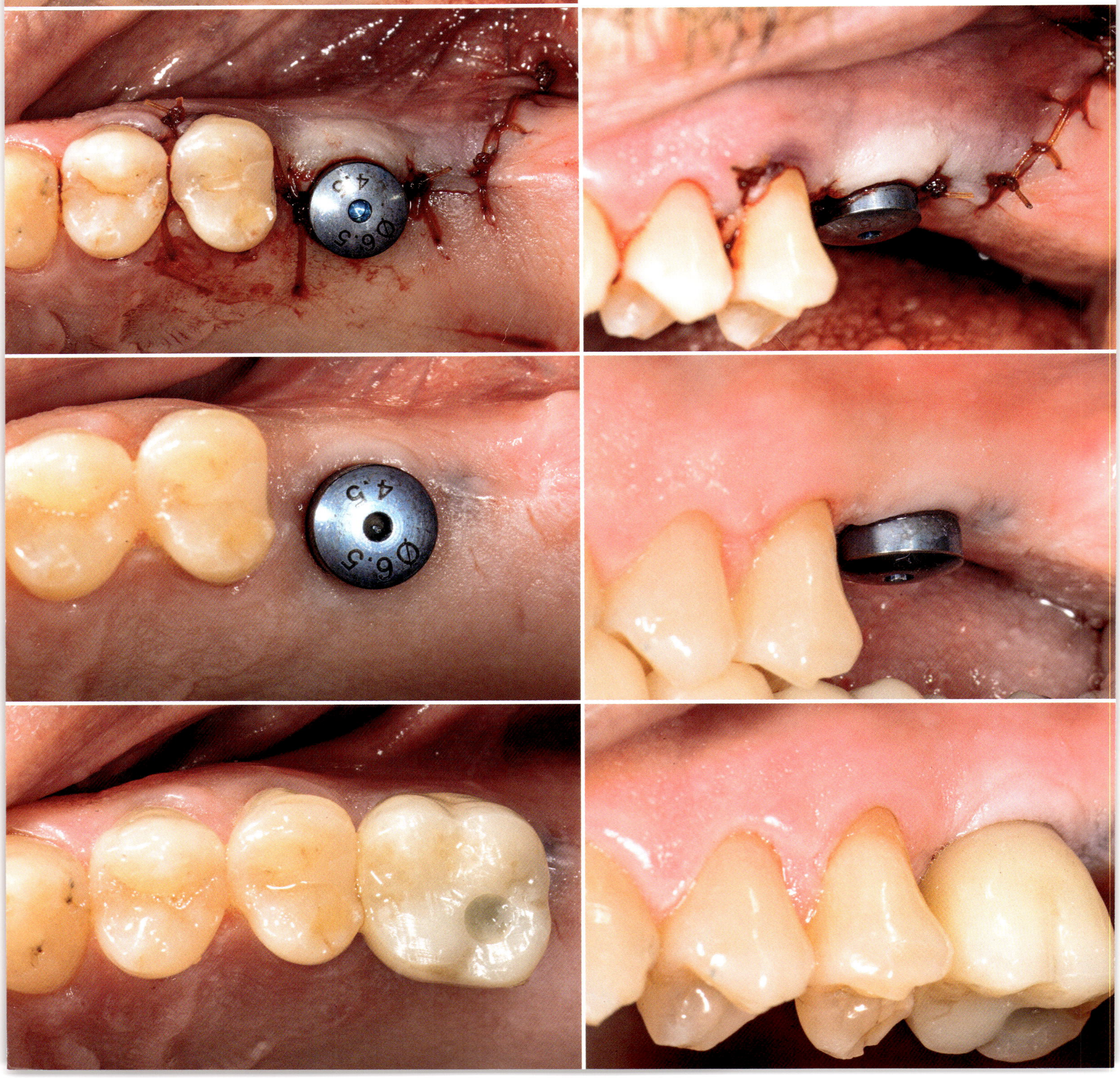

Figure 9-58 This incision design followed the palatal contour of the planned implant position. This preserves tissue that can then be used to bulk up the facial contours and optimize the site. The incision was extended back and up into the vestibule to access the direct sinus augmentation. At the three-month clearance appointment, the tissue contours appear stable.

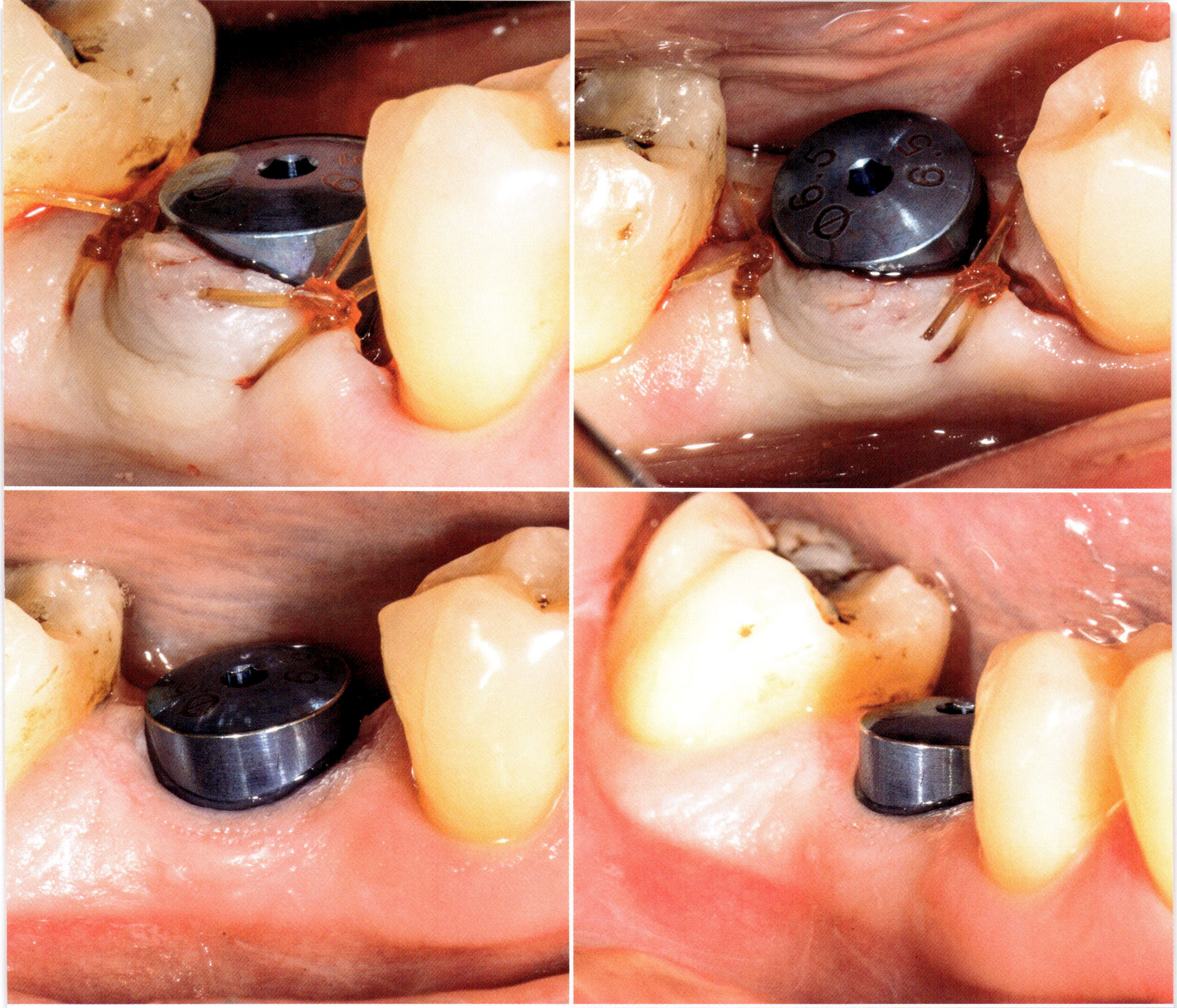

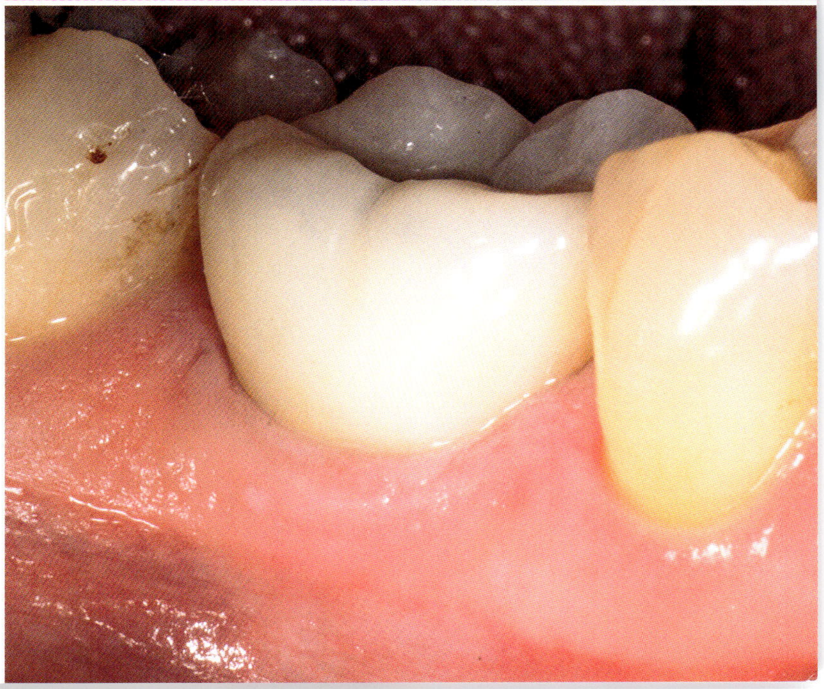

Figure 9-59 Facial gingiva may overlap the abutment at placement. It can be recontoured surgically, but it often remodels well on its own. Two weeks later, the tissue has adapted some. Ten weeks later, at the clearance appointment, the tissue has remodeled and looks great.

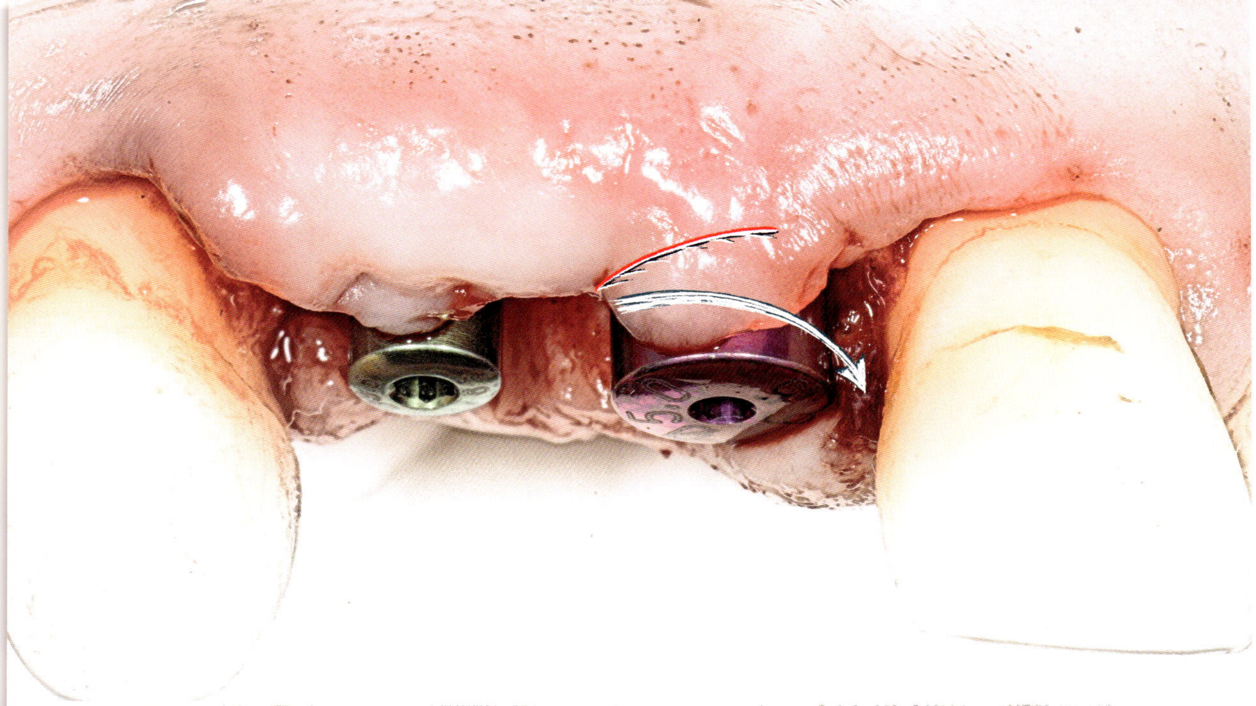

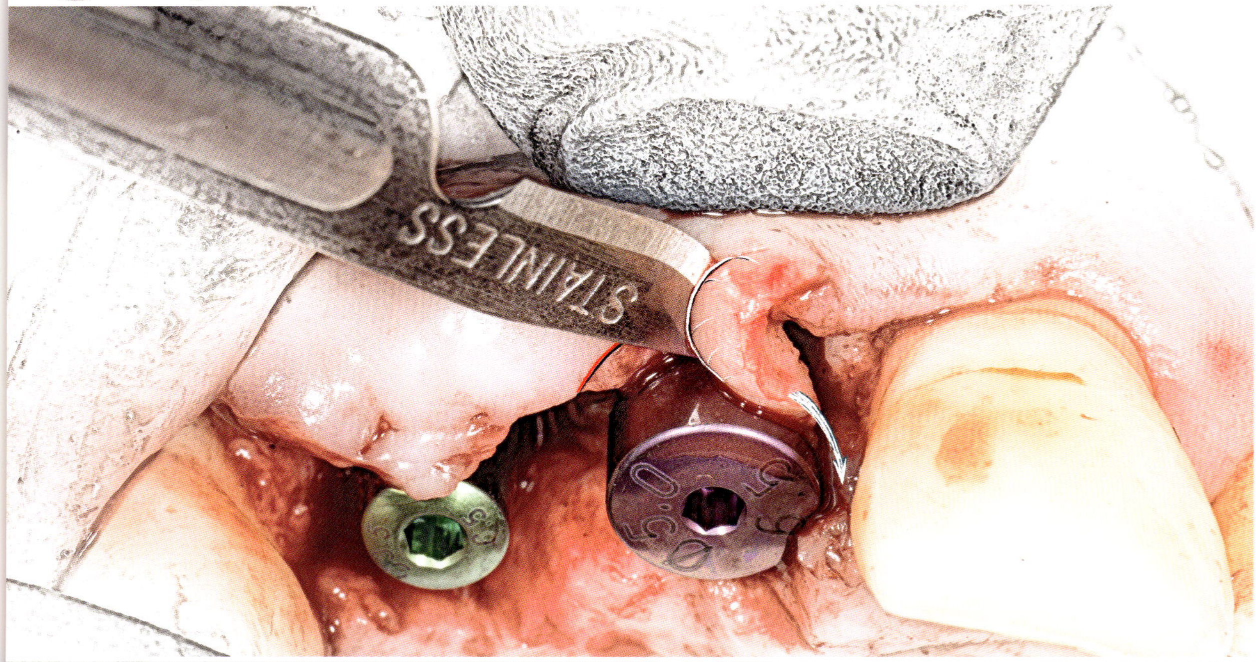
STAINLESS

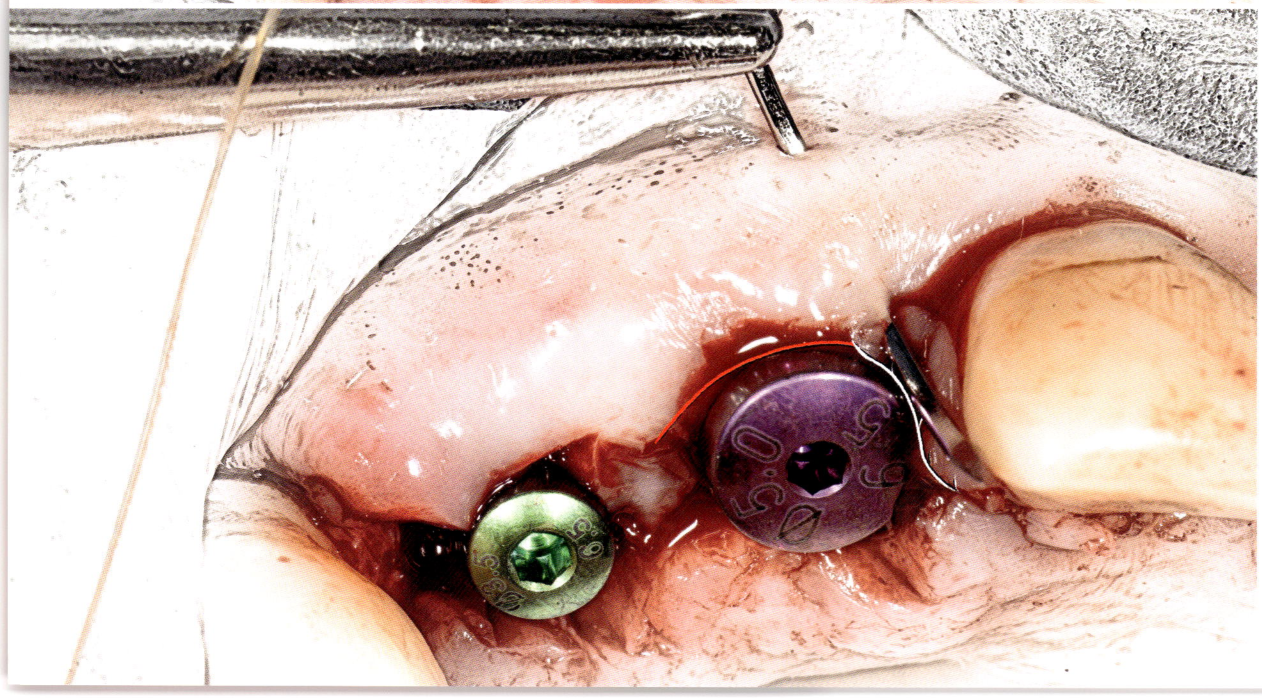

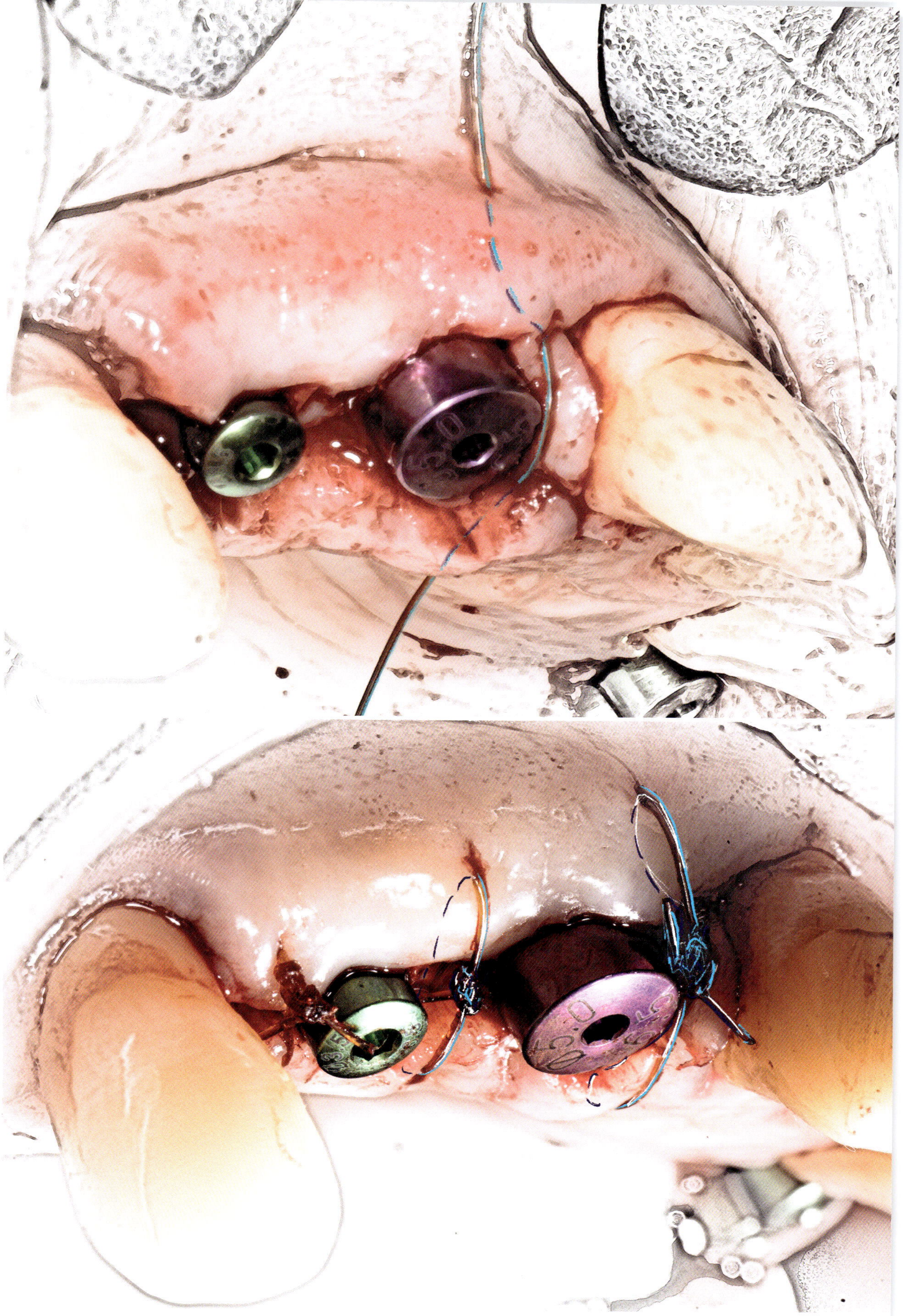

Figure 9-60 Palacci style gingival management rotates the midfacial gingival tissue mesial or distal to augment the soft tissue of the papilla[3].

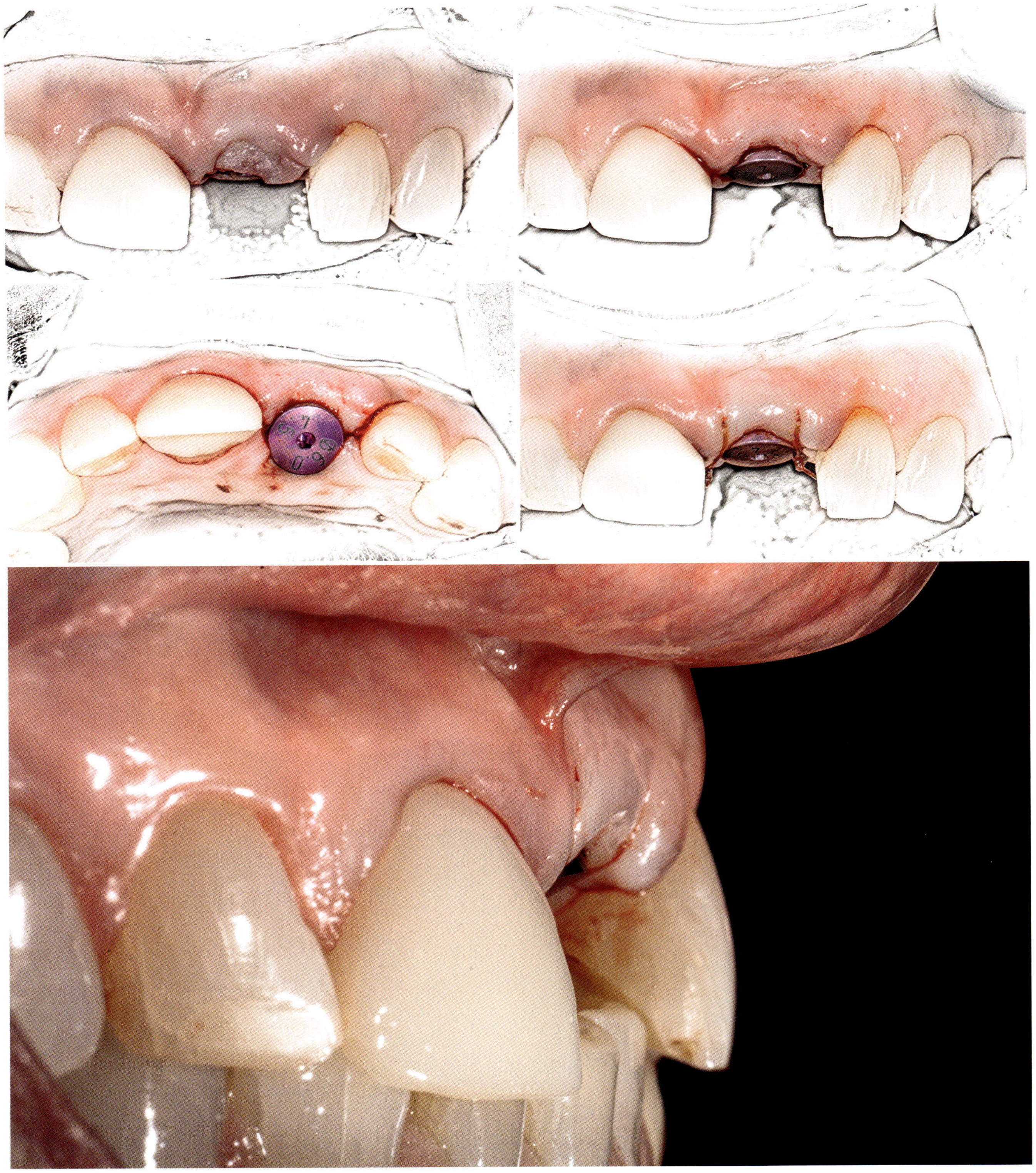

Figure 9-61 When a palatally favored flap is elevated, there is often some excess tissue on the facial. It can be recontoured and adapted to augment the site without excising the tissue or performing a full palatal roll.

Red: Significant deficiency

If we have a more significant defect, the palatal roll or palatal island flap is the second to last stage before gingival grafting. There have been numerous modifications to this technique that Dr. Abrams first described in 1980[4]. This fun procedure steals some of the adjacent underlying palatal connective tissue in the anterior maxilla and rotates it into a pouch under the facial tissue. It forms a lovely contour resembling a root eminence. It also helps cover the underlying titanium implant from shining through. And this is all done with minimal trauma and no untoward effect on the quality of the overlying gingival architecture. I collaborate on with my periodontist for gingival grafting when needed.

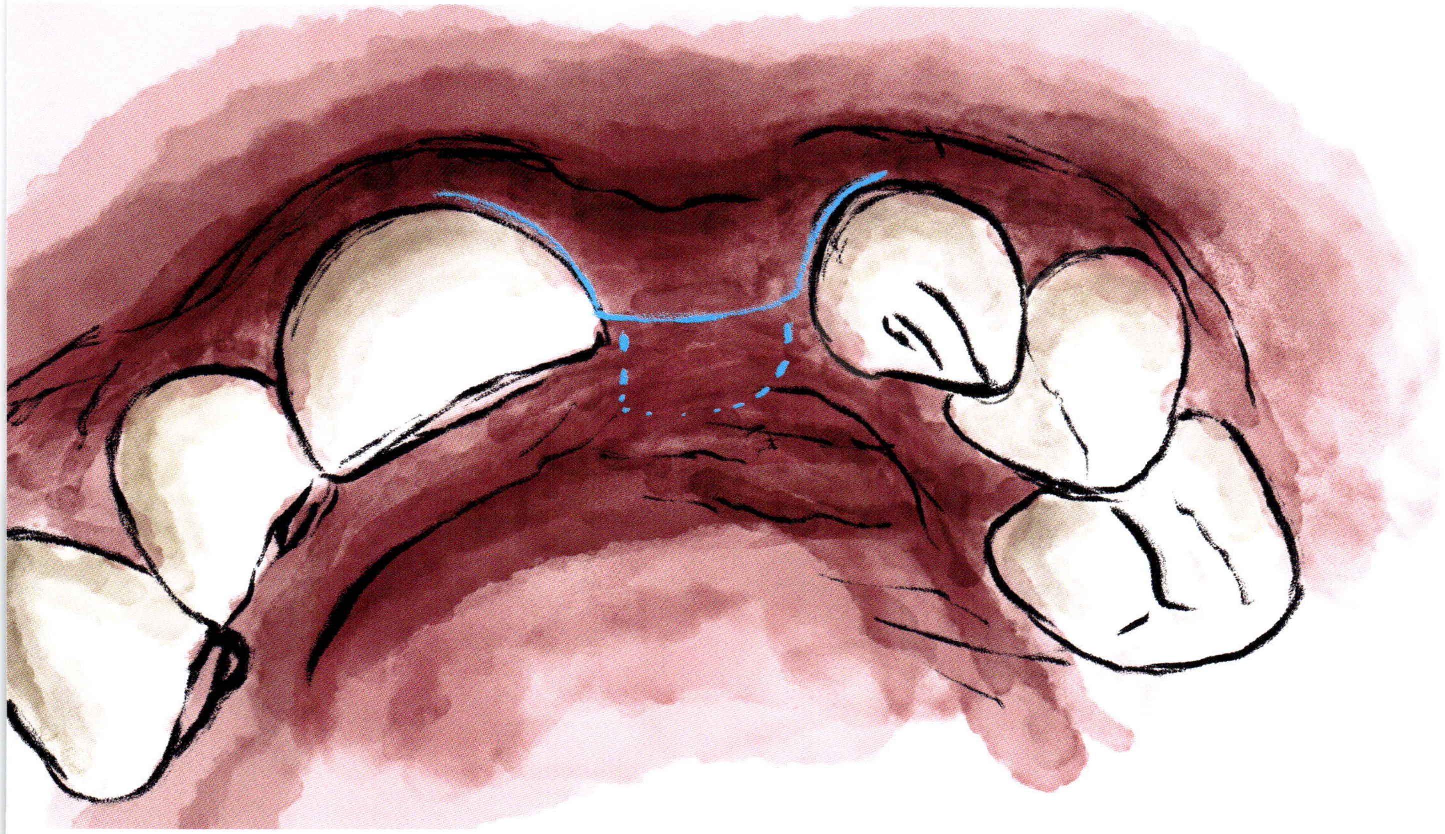

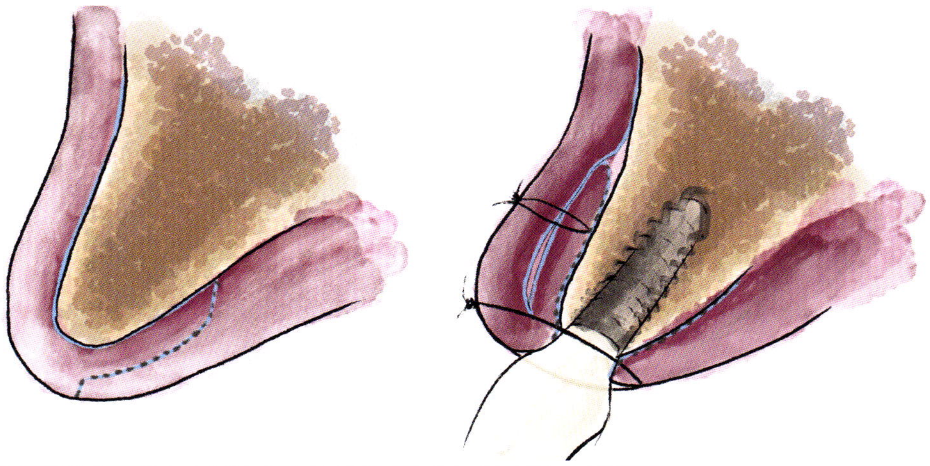

Figure 9-62 Palatal roll. The split thickness incision mobilizes the connective tissue on the palate, tucking it under the facial tissue. This can significantly increase facial tissue thickness with natural surface appearance. Because of the shape, it also gives a nice appearance of a root eminence.

Simple tips for soft tissue development

Use the tissue you have. Employ it. Get creative with it. It is your biggest asset. Don't cut away any tissue you could use. A generous and thoughtful incision improves the options for the final results.

Mind the gap

The flap margins around implants often have a gap that, if tended to properly, can be used to your advantage. When the tissue margins are stable, a type of guided tissue regeneration can occur. The epithelial cells on either side of the gap direct the ingrowing tissue type. Keratinizing stratified squamous epithelium will reproduce at the wound margin, filling in the gap with the best type of tissue. The gap can trip things up if it is left untended. If the tissue isn't stabilized, it doesn't fill in as well. Or if both margins don't have keratinized gingiva, the gap may fill with nonkeratinized tissue. Mind the gap and take advantage of its potential.

Keratinized epithelium has a layer of protein armor absent on normal mucosal epithelium. Keratin is the durable protein structure that makes fingernails and antlers so tough. The form it takes on epithelium is obviously different from that of a horn, but it is still quite protective in nature. Respect it and appreciate it. It is your friend. It improves masticatory gingiva durability and that improves peri-implant health. Healthy peri-implant soft tissue is vital. Keratinized and attached tissue improve hygiene and decrease the risk and complications inflammation brings.

Figure 9-63 Keratinization is like armor for the cells beneath. Considering the microscopic battle that ensues with constant mechanical and biological assault, the added layer of protection seems like a really good idea.

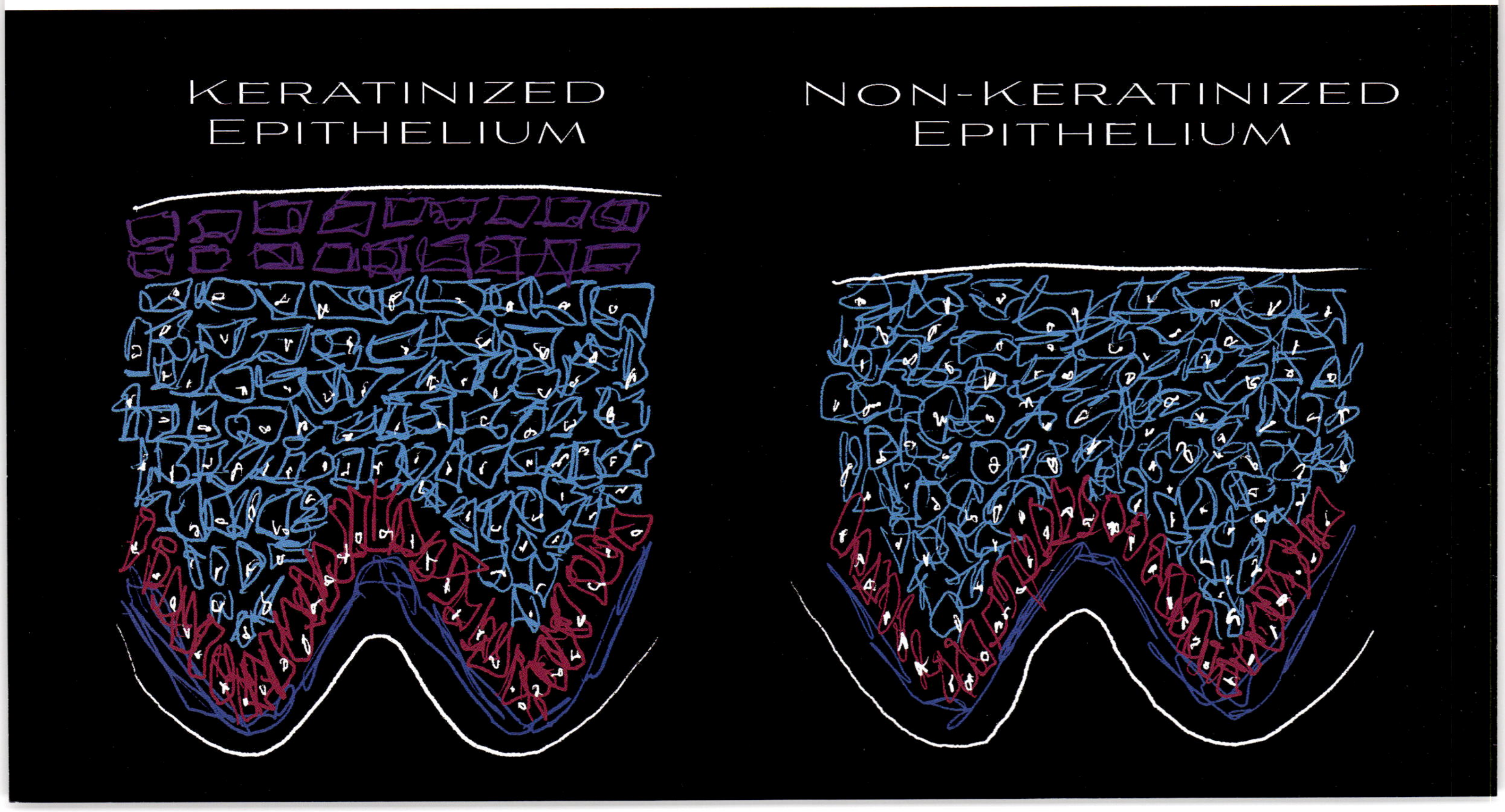

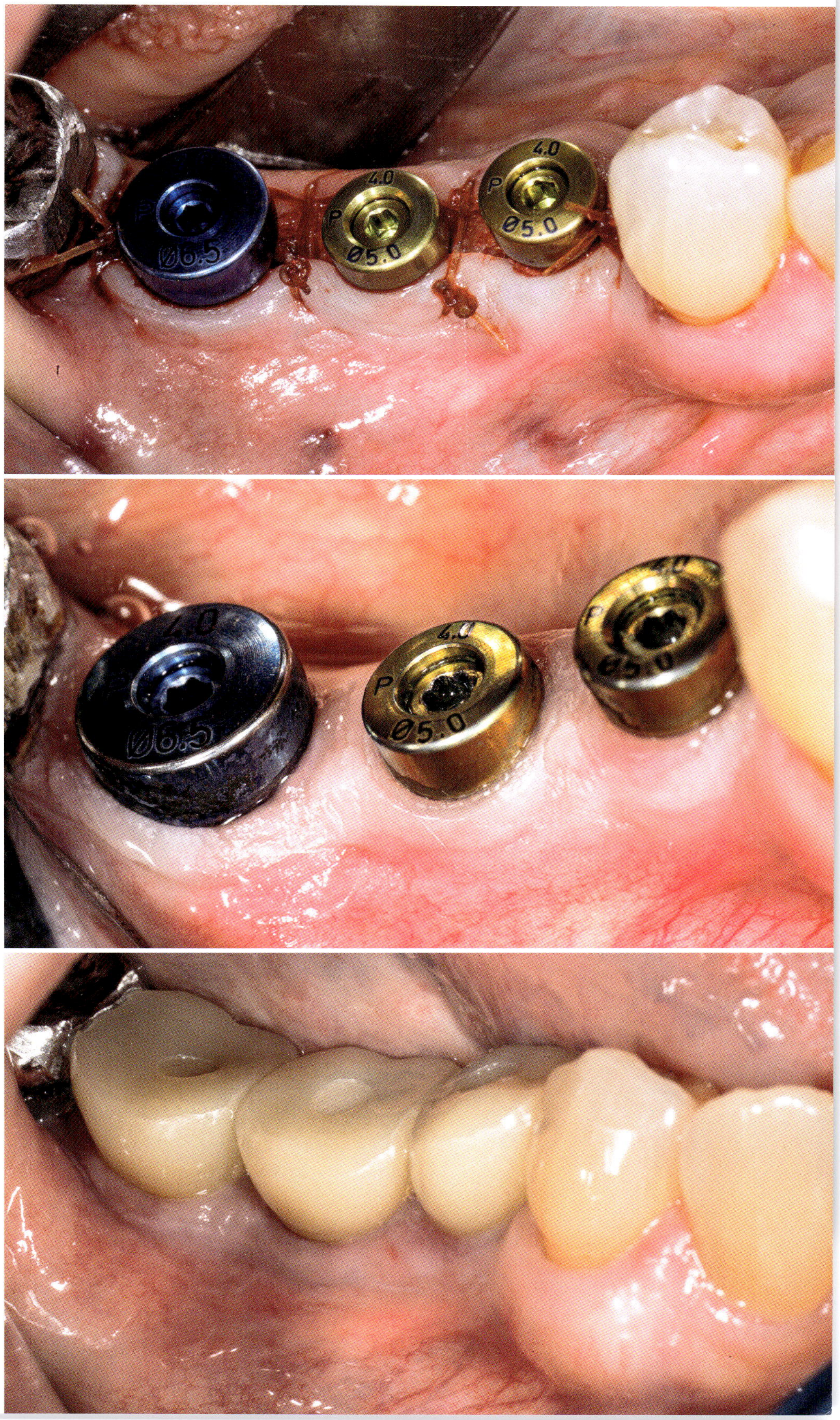

Figure 9-64 When there is keratinized gingiva on either side of a gap between implants (*top*), it fills in with keratinized gingiva after a few months of healing (*middle*). Primary closure between these implants would sacrifice much of the potential gingival architecture. This patient could have benefited from ridge augmentation. In lieu of further bone or soft tissue grafting, handling the soft tissue this way optimized the results with keratinized gingiva surrounding the implants (*bottom*).

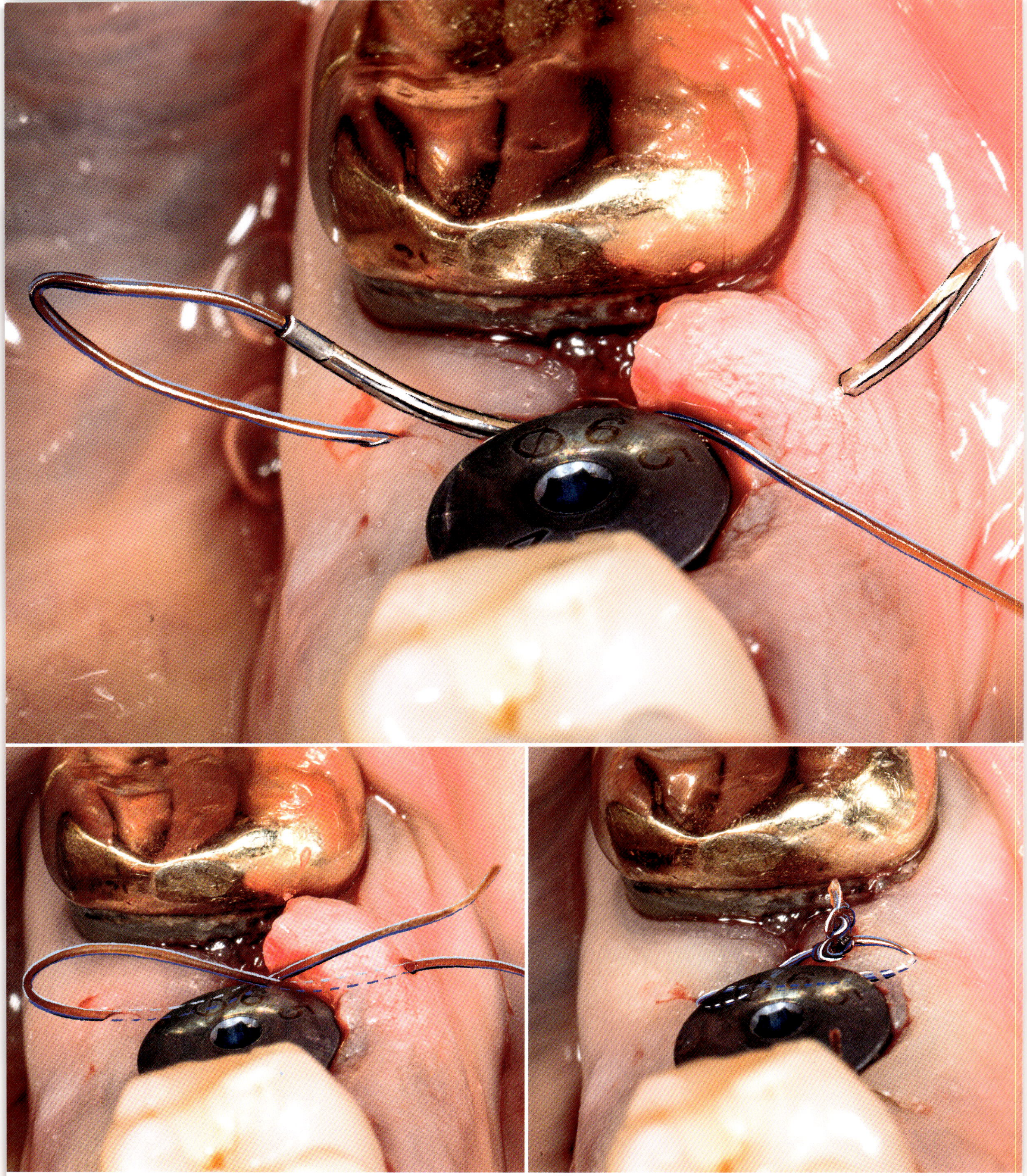

Figure 9-65 Passing the needle from the inside out creates a vertical figure-eight suture that pulls the margins downward, effectively tucking them in under an abutment or in an extraction site.

Stabilize, don't strangulate

The bone relies on the overlying periosteum and soft tissue blood supply. If it is sutured too tight, the capillaries and microvasculature get compressed. If the blood pressure within the vessels in the tissue is unable to force blood through a collapsed or compressed lumen, the tissue will suffer. Sutures are meant to stabilize the tissue, not strangulate it. Some tension is good. But the art is finding just the right amount.

Tuck in the tissue

When a small flap has been elevated or the papilla has been released, the soft tissue often wants to slide up over the abutment. A simple vertical figure-eight suture can lasso that tissue and drop it down into place very nicely.

Split the difference

Tissue width is often limited with multiple edentulous spaces, especially in the posterior mandible. There may only be a few millimeters of keratinized or attached tissue to work with. In these cases, split it down the middle. If the tissue is adequate, the gap will fill in nicely.

Make space for the tissue

Implants are surrounded by bone and project into the oral cavity through the soft tissue. It is comprised of the junctional epithelium and attached connective tissue. The junction between bone and soft tissue has been extensively studied. We refer to it as the "biologic width." If the abutment rests directly on the surrounding crestal bone, it must resorb to make space for the connective tissue and epithelium. That is the last thing we want the bone to do. It is so much easier for the surgeon to reduce the bone than the bone to resorb. It takes less than a minute for you, but I bet it takes weeks to months for the bone. The inflammation and irritation associated with this bit of "exposed bone" and resulting resorption is simply unnecessary. Just make the space. If the abutment doesn't passively seat with a solid feel on the implant platform, there is most certainly not enough clearance, and the bone should be reduced.

References

1. Rathee M, Jain P. Gingivitis. In: StatPearls [Internet]. Treasure Island (FL): StatPearls Publishing; 2023 [cited 2023 Apr 23]. Available from: http://www.ncbi.nlm.nih.gov/books/NBK557422/
2. Zuhr O, Hürzeler MB. Plastic-Esthetic Periodontal and Implant Surgery. A Microsurgical Approach. 1st edition. Chicago: Quintessence, 2012.
3. Palacci P. Aesthetic treatment of the anterior maxilla: soft and hard tissue considerations. Oral Maxillofac Surg Clin North Am. 2004 Feb;16(1):127-37, vii.
4. Abrams L. Augmentation of the deformed residual edentulous ridge for fixed prosthesis. Compend Contin Educ Gen Dent. 1980 May-Jun;1(3):205-213. PMID: 6950834.

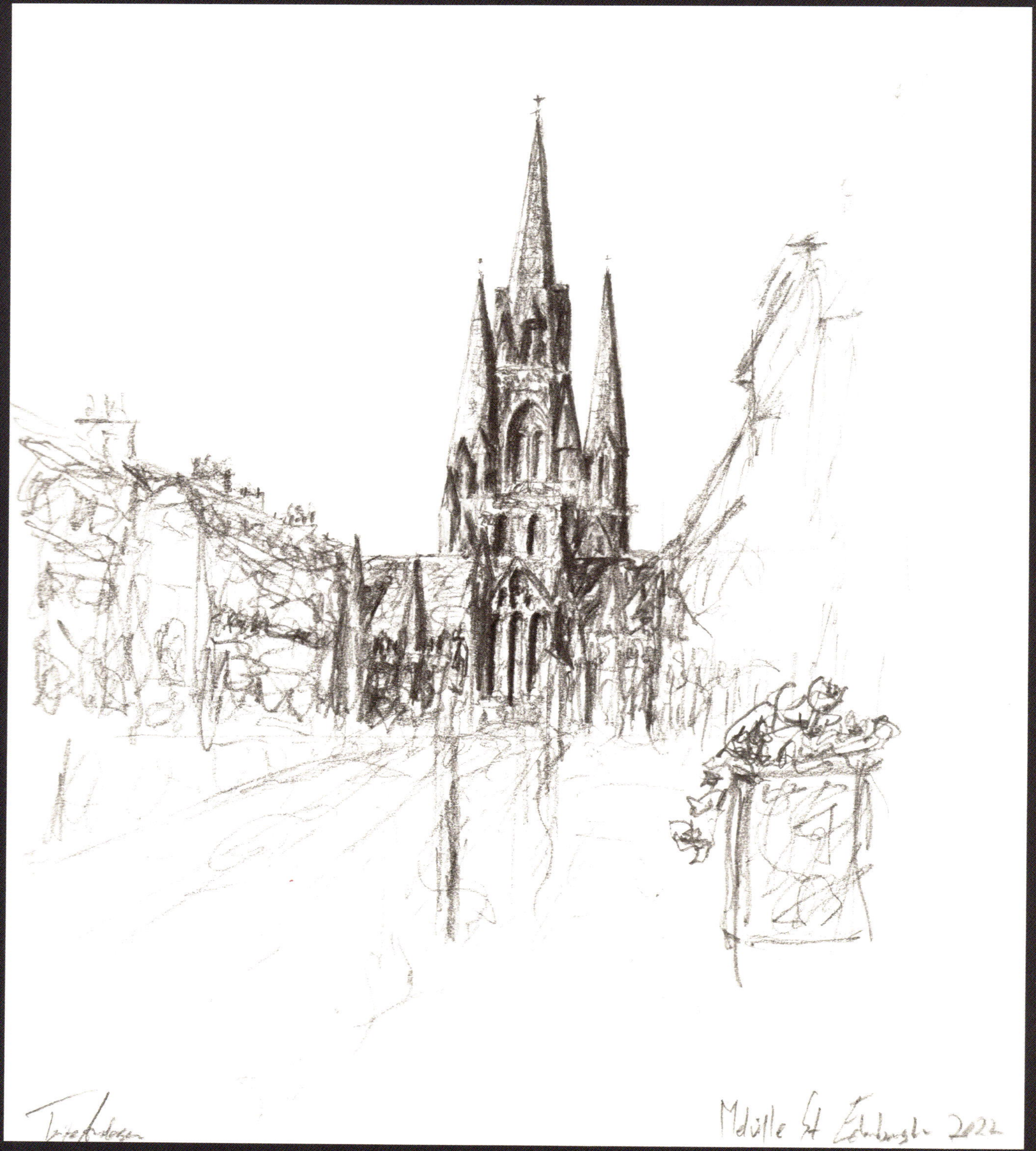

Perspective. Sketch what's there, not what you think you see.

On a trip to visit the Royal College of Surgeons in Edinburgh, I sketched what I saw while eating breakfast at a café on Melville Street.

I was surprised that afternoon when my perspective of St Mary's Cathedral changed. From atop Edinburgh Castle, I could see in the distance the main spire of the cathedral was in front of the two side spires, opposite of what I thought I saw that morning. It didn't make sense when I sketched it.

I couldn't help but laugh as I showed my friend Dr. Wael Garine my realization from our perch on the historic castle wall.

CHAPTER 10

THE ART OF INFECTION MANAGEMENT

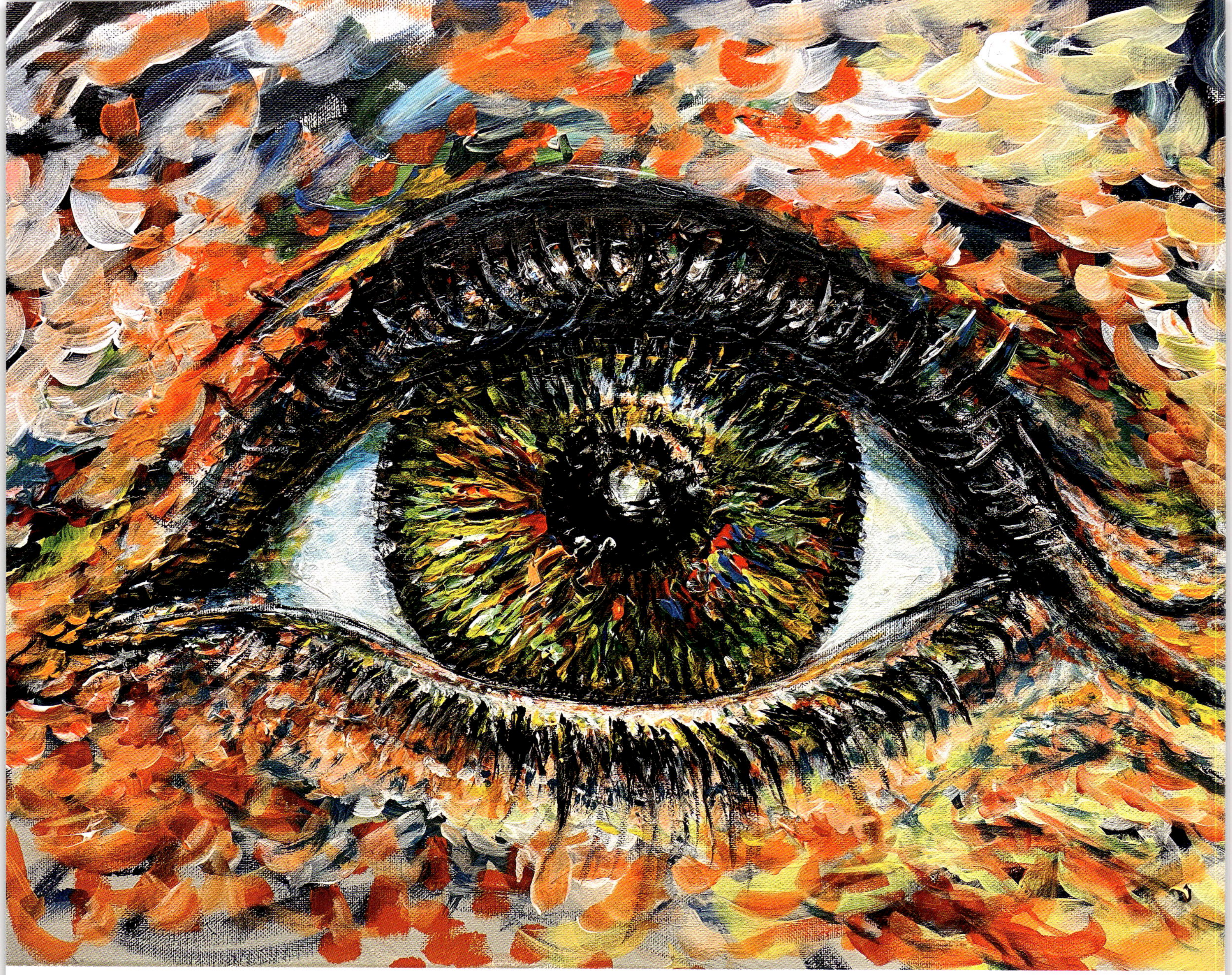

You only see what you know. You don't have to know everything, but you do need to know what to look for.
(Acrylic on canvas 16x20 inches. Artwork inspired by Jordan Anderson.)

There is a constant struggle for power in the synergistic relationship between humans and bacteria. They need us and we need them. Our responsibility as their host is to manage their environment to keep them at bay, while their entire existence revolves solely around reproduction. There have been more than 700 species of bacteria identified in the human mouth, with the average person hosting about 300 strains[1]. Many bacteria are so frail and dependent on their host that we haven't been able to culture them yet. But the common bacteria responsible for orofacial infections are normal oral flora, and they have been studied well[1-4]. An infection occurs when there is an unhealthy reproduction of a harmful microorganism within a host. This requires both a capable microorganism and a suitable host environment.

We study infections to understand their behavior. The art of oral surgery is not to memorize the different strains of bacteria that are most likely to cause an infection. Rather, we want to know how to prevent our patients from getting an infection and how to treat an infection quickly and effectively. The goal is to help return our patients to a healthy microbiological balance.

The human species has evolved with bacteria. In fact, we coexist quite well together. Even more than that, we have become dependent on them for our survival. But bacteria need constant supervision or they revolt. When they are isolated from the watchful eye of the host immune system, they can quickly produce an invasive army. A necrotic tooth is a common chamber for a bacterial uprising. It is like a bunker, a protected shelter from the guard. Within the fortified chamber of a necrotic tooth, bacteria reproduce and mount their invasion into the surrounding bone. As long as the bacteria control and occupy the chamber, they are protected from the immune system and they remain a threat. If the tooth is removed or the chamber obturated, the bacteria on the front lines no longer have support from their bunker and the war may be over. If, however, they have spread enough within the tissue, their reproduction may outpace their destruction. They may continue to advance, threatening the host's health and well-being. This is the story of a common apical abscess.

This overall storyline is similar in other types of infections. In pericoronitis, the protection and breeding ground for the bacteria (the bunker) is in the pericoronal tissue around an impacted tooth. An infected implant provides refuge for bacterial forces within a biofilm that forms on a contaminated surface. An infected bone graft harbors the bacteria in the "No Man's Land" within the graft where the blood supply has not yet reached. Any incision can potentially become a source of infection. When the superficial tissue layers are incised, bacteria are transported behind the host's first lines of defense. When an abscess forms, the central portion gets farther from the threat of the immune system and antibiotics. The abscess, in and of itself, can become a bunker for bacteria. Bacteria with a bunker are a real threat. When dealing with an infection, we must eliminate or overthrow the bunker to restore the healthy balance of power in the microbiome.

Management Principles

Eliminate the source of infection and **eradicate** the invaders. These are the two main objectives of both the immune system and the surgeon.

The casualties of an infection can range from minor pain, debilitation and localized tissue destruction to major airway compromise, sepsis and even death. To survive, our bodies have developed extraordinary systems to deal with the constant threat of their symbiotic companions. The intricacy and precision involved at the atomic level is simply beyond comprehension. Even a subtle shift in pH upends an entire bacterial defense mechanism. The transfer of a couple of electrons can disassemble the entire bacterial DNA structure, destroying the organism.

We ease pain and suffering when we partner with our patient's own immune system to fight an infection. We study and learn to improve our skills and the tools we have. This is our gift, our contribution to the world. As surgeons, we don't need to kill every single microorganism in the infection. We just need to help kill enough of them. We assist and augment the patient's immune system to alter the course from illness to health. There is an art to deciding when to engage in the battle and when to withdraw and allow the patient to finish the job.

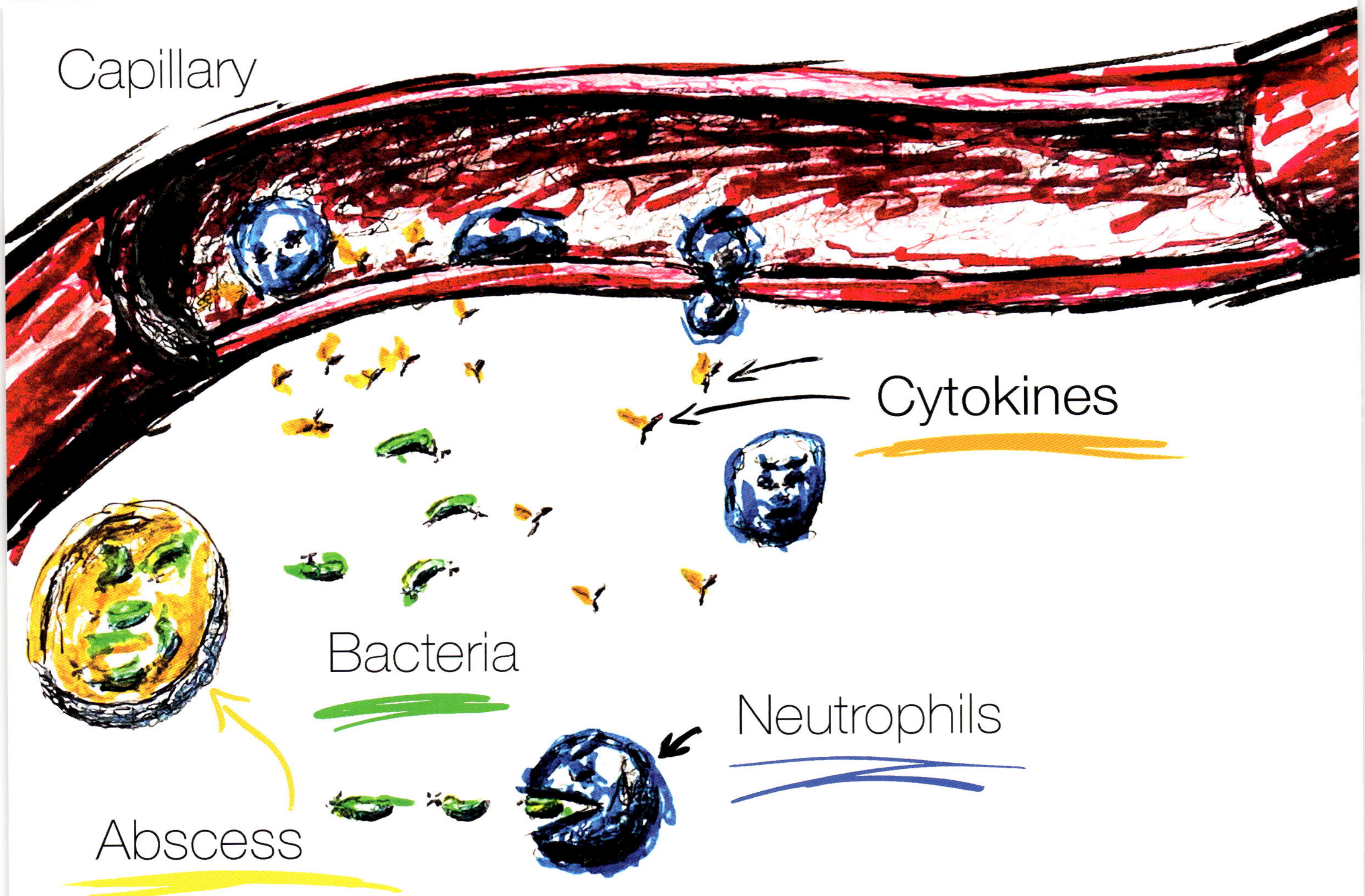

Figure 10-1 Neutrophils (*blue*) are attracted to an infection site by cytokines (*orange*). They squeeze out of the capillaries and go toward the signal. The tagged bacteria (*green*) are phagocytized and destroyed by the activated neutrophils. To contain an infection, the body can create a wall around the bacteria (*yellow left*). This can also protect the bacteria from the attack of the neutrophils and antibiotics. This is an incredibly oversimplified description of how the body responds, but it is helpful in discussing infection management and treatment.

The body's inherent defense

It is the immune system that destroys and eliminates the bacteria. Lymphocytes produce antibodies that identify and mark bacteria for destruction. Neutrophils are summoned through the release of inflammatory mediators. Upon arrival at the scene, neutrophils engulf and destroy the marked bacteria, gobbling them up like Pac-Man.

In an attempt to eliminate the source, the body can encapsulate an infected foreign object, such as an implant or bone graft. It can form a cystic wall or a fibrous barrier around it. While this is often an effective technique for self-preservation, it can be detrimental to the fight at times. The wall of protection can isolate bacteria from the immune system. With a cystic lining, it is as though the host and the bacteria set up a truce for a time; they may temporarily postpone the fight, but the war is not over. The bacteria have their protection and will continue their invasion attempt over time. That is just what they do. Such is the case in an infected apical periodontal cyst that can be asymptomatic for years.

Much of the devastation from an infection is collateral damage from the battle. Bacteria have an arsenal of destructive toxins and enzymes capable of dismantling the basic cellular building blocks of life. This contributes significantly to the debilitation and spread of an acute infection. But it is the immune response deploying resources to fight the infection that causes most of the injury from the infection. The capillaries dilate and become permeable. Extravascular tissue fills with fluid containing white blood cells and inflammatory mediators. This outflow of fluid stretches the tissue, causing edema. The pain typically associated with an infection is from inflammation and internal tissue expansion. Thus, the common symptoms of an acute infection are produced: pain (dolor), swelling (tumor), redness (rubor) and heat (calor). (Celsus first used these terms to describe inflammation in the early second century A.D.)

The surgeon's armamentarium

The surgeon's armamentarium mainly includes surgery and antibiotics. The most effective weapon is "cold steel and sunshine." Physically open it up or cut it out and expose the bacteria to the light of day. (Of course, it isn't the light of the sun that actually impacts the bacteria.) Surgery can remove an infected foreign object, drain an abscess, or physically flush away the bacteria. We can effectively wipe out the bunker. Surgery alters the delicate environment that has allowed the bacteria to thrive. Antibiotics are our other main tool. They chemically disrupt the stability or reproduction of bacteria, helping the immune system ultimately subdue the infection.

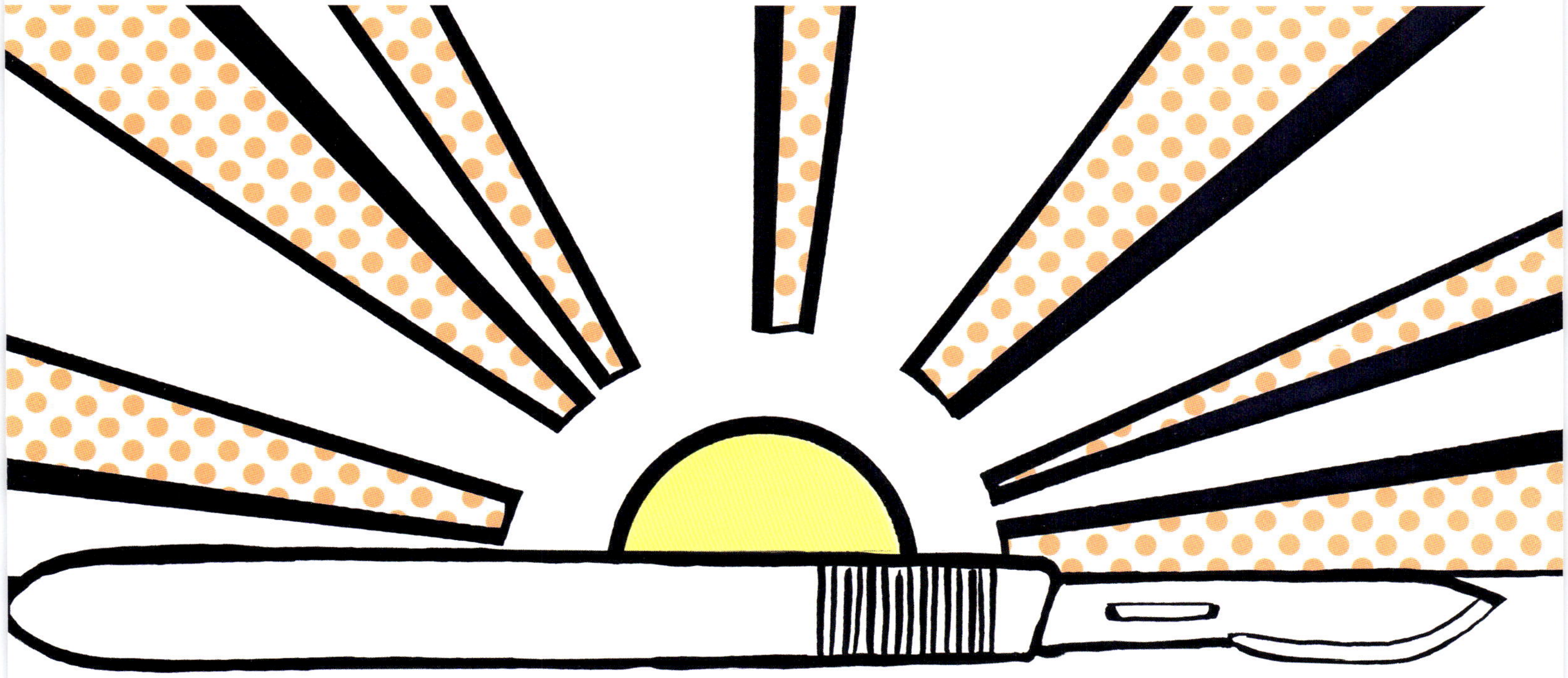

Figure 10-2 Cold steel and sunshine. (Artwork inspired by Roy Lichtenstein.)

Practical Classification

We can't physically see the bacteria that make up an infection. Patients can't tell us if they are growing more aerobic or anaerobic bacteria. We see the signs and listen to the patient describe the symptoms. It is precisely what we see and what we hear that guides us in clinical practice. Setting up a framework for classifying an infection allows us to apply sound principles in treating each individual patient and their own unique infection.

The art of infection management is to restore our patients safely and effectively to health. This requires an overall understanding of each individual situation: the patient, the bacteria and the circumstances. The force we use should match the resistance. The more powerful, swift or dangerous the infection, the greater the need for immediate surgery and robust antibiotic therapy.

In the clinical practice of oral surgery, it is helpful to classify an infection by the source, course, duration, onset and location. It is also important to know the level of functional impairment and systemic involvement. The most basic questions I ask are: Is there something causing the infection that needs to be removed? Is there pus? How long has it been going on? Is it progressing rapidly? Is it spreading? Is the patient immunocompetent? These questions help determine the source, course, onset and location of the infection. Let's look at each of these in more detail.

Table 10-1 Source: primary vs secondary

Primary	Secondary
Bacterial inoculation and colonization within the tissue itself without a foreign-body source.	Bacterial colonization of an object within the tissue. Presence of a foreign object or material supporting bacterial reproduction.
Example: Abscess formation after injection of local anesthetic, persistent infection after extraction, incision site infection.	**Example**: Apical abscess, infected implant or graft material, acute odontogenic abscess.
Treatment considerations: Primarily antibiotic therapy. May consider surgery depending on the course and progression of the infection.	**Treatment considerations**: Remove the source if possible. May consider non-surgical management in the case of an infected implant or graft when we want to retain the infected object.

Table 10-2 Course: chronic vs acute

Chronic	Acute
An infection with purulence without significant inflammatory symptoms.	An infection with inflammatory symptoms, often with purulence.
Clinical presentation: Asymptomatic draining abscess or radiographic lucency.	**Clinical presentation**: Pain and/or swelling.
Treatment considerations: Less aggressive. Surgically eliminate the source: endodontic, periodontal, or extraction therapy.	**Treatment considerations**: More aggressive and time sensitive. Potential to progress more rapidly. Must address pain.
Antibiotics will not resolve the infection. The source must be directly addressed.	**Antibiotics and/or surgery indicated**. Antibiotics may help resolve acute symptoms by reducing the bacterial load and thus reducing the body's inflammatory response. Surgery is typically the most definitive treatment.

Purulence/Pus

The body throws a lot of resources at fighting an infection. A collection of thick fluid called pus or purulence can accumulate in the middle of all the action. Pus consists of cellular debris from the fight, mostly dead white blood cells and the offending bacteria. This is an abscess. The fluid builds osmotic pressure and draws in more fluid. The body also sends resources bringing fluid to the fight. The collection of pus within tissue is known as an abscess. As it continues to grow, it increases outward pressure on surrounding tissue. When the pressure exceeds the strength of the tissue containing it, pus pushes into an adjacent space and the infection spreads. Sometimes the weakest area is superficial, allowing the pus to spill out through the skin or into the mouth. This becomes like a pressure relief valve that significantly decreases the risk of the infection spreading inward, which can be a real threat.

Acute infections can be further classified by duration, onset and location

Duration: cellulitis vs abscess

Infections typically progress from cellulitis to abscess formation over the course of several days. The bacteria change the environment, and the changing environment impacts the bacteria. Infections don't always follow this pattern, but it is an important concept in guiding our decision-making.

Table 10-3 Duration: cellulitis vs abscess

Cellulitis	Abscess
Infection spreading through the fascial planes without a distinct collection of pus.	Infection involving a localized collection of pus. As an infection organizes and progresses, it often develops a centralized area that becomes abscessed.
Clinical presentation: Typically early stage of infection, precedes abscess formation. Generalized swelling and tenderness to palpation.	**Clinical presentation**: Purulence often develops a day or two after symptoms begin. It can have a similar presentation to cellulitis. An abscess can also have associated cellulitis. Soft tissue CT imaging often identifies an area of fluid collection and associated surrounding cellulitic changes. The larger an abscess gets, the more obvious it becomes.
No fluctuance: When an infection progresses to form an abscess, the previous cellulitic changes don't necessarily resolve. There is often non-purulent spread through the fascial planes beyond the borders of the abscess. Often the first day or two of facial swelling is cellulitis. Beyond the third day, it typically will have formed an abscess.	**Fluctuance**: Sometimes fluctuance can be clinically appreciated as the fluid moves like a wave when you push on it. In clinical practice I have found fluctuance is often imperceptible as the fluid in the tissue is tense and exquisitely painful to palpation.
Treatment considerations: Antibiotics are often the primary treatment for an infection in the cellulitis stage. Antibiotics can more effectively penetrate and combat bacterial cellulitis than a bacterial abscess. The source of the infection also must be treated.	**Treatment considerations**: Drainage is much more helpful for a typical abscess than cellulitis. Although many acute abscesses respond to antibiotic treatment without drainage, surgically disrupting the abscess and removing pus is very helpful. Smaller abscesses often respond well to antibiotics. The larger they become, the more protected they are from the host immune system and from antibiotic treatment.

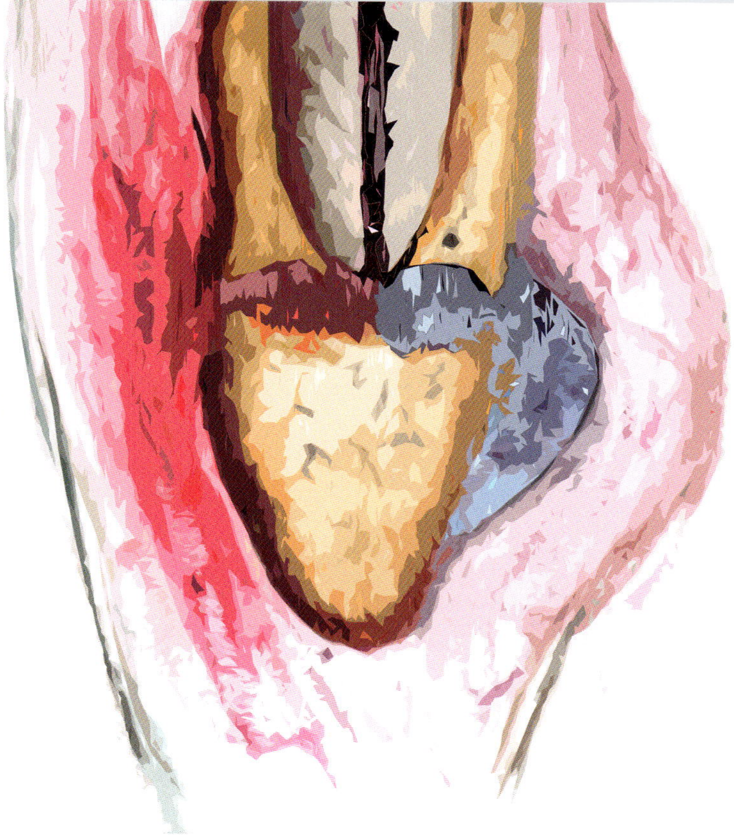

Figure 10-3 An odontogenic abscess forms when there is a collection of pus (*blue*). Cellulitis spreads through the tissue without a formal collection of pus. Sometimes, cellulitis precedes an abscess. Sometimes it never progresses to form an abscess.

Onset: slow vs fast vs severe

How fast is the infection progressing? This is different from the duration, which is how long it has been present. Onset describes the acceleration by relating the amount of time the infection has been brewing to the extent of the involvement. If it rapidly progresses to a large, multi-space infection overnight, the onset is severe. Like it is stomping on the gas pedal, accelerating the infection.

Table 10-4 Infection onset

Slow onset	Fast onset	Severe onset
Increasing swelling and symptoms over the course of several days or weeks.	Swelling and symptoms progressed significantly in the past day or two.	Significant increase in symptoms within hours or a day. When symptoms progress rapidly, this may indicate more virulent bacteria or a more compromised host.
Treatment: Less aggressive. May respond to initial antibiotic therapy, allowing postponed definitive intervention like endodontic treatment or extraction.	**Treatment**: More urgent surgery and higher-level antibiotic therapy.	**Treatment**: Swift and definitive surgical management and broad-spectrum, high-level antibiotic therapy. Consider IV antibiotics. Close follow-up is recommended in case further treatment is necessary.

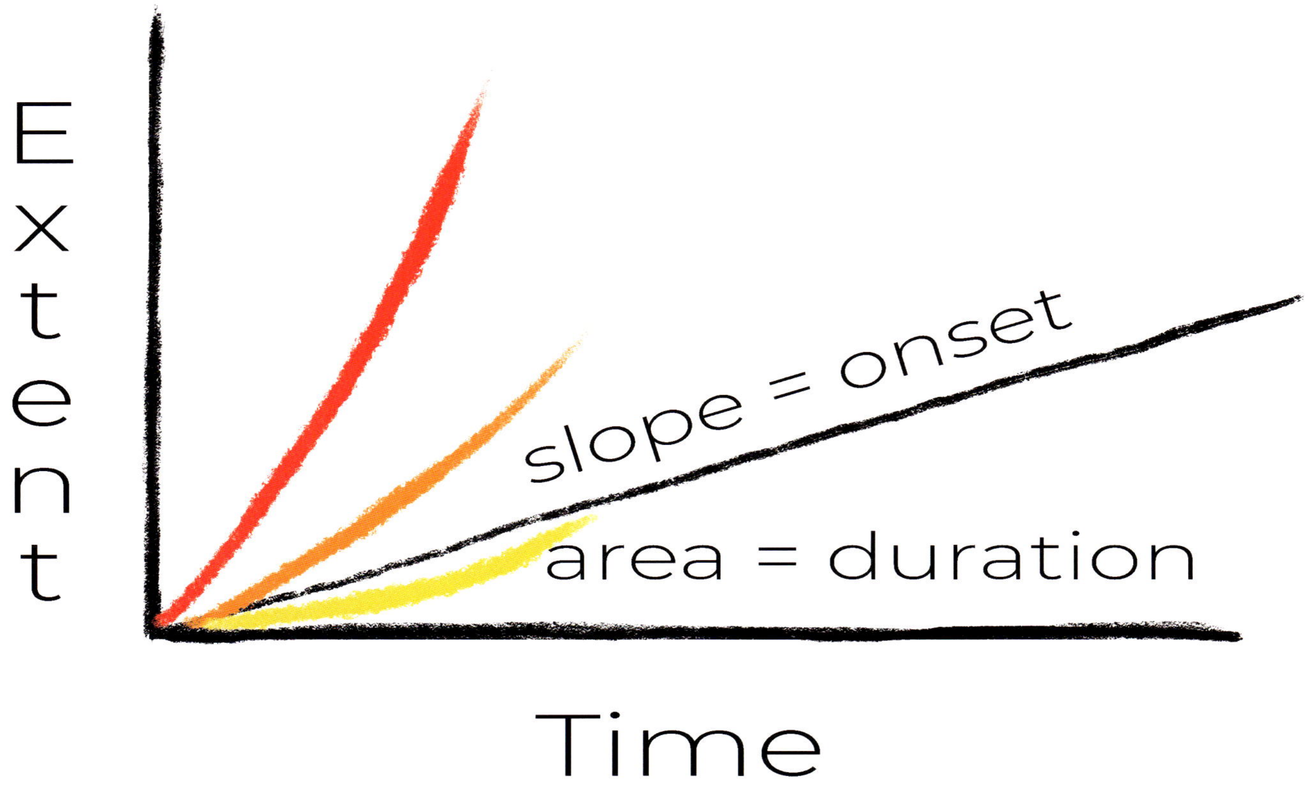

Figure 10-4 Duration vs onset. The duration is the area under the line. The slope of the line is the onset. The steeper the slope, the more severe the infection.

Table 10-5 Infection location

Localized	Spreading
Infection is isolated to the location of the source or inoculation.	Infection has moved beyond the immediate site and is involving adjacent spaces.
Clinical presentation: Swelling and pain are contained within the immediate surrounding area of the infection source.	**Clinical presentation**: Multiple spaces involved. This can be spreading cellulitis or abscess. Spreading mandibular infections more frequently compromise the airway and are often more critical. Spreading maxillary infections can look more severe with significant facial swelling, but less frequently result in critical compromise (though they too deserve respect).
Treatment considerations: Potentially less aggressive treatment is needed. All infections start out locally. You won't know how it will respond until it either progresses or resolves.	**Treatment considerations**: Aggressive and immediate intervention indicated. Risk of infection spreading and compromising the airway and adjacent structures can cause significant morbidity and potential mortality.

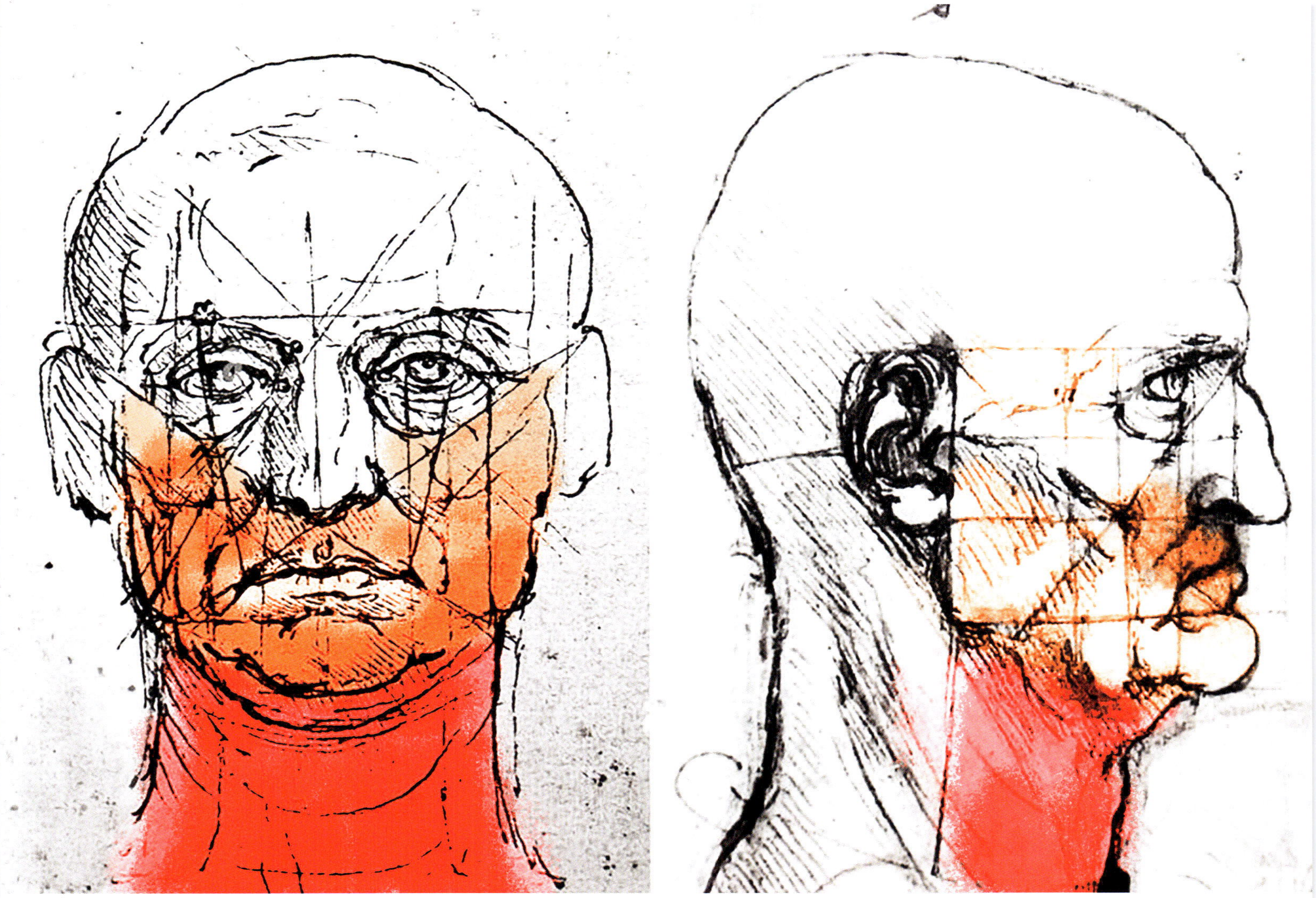

Figure 10-5 Infection severity increases as it spreads below the mandible, heading toward the clavicle and mediastinum. It also increases as it approaches or surrounds the airway posteriorly. (Artwork inspired by Leonardo da Vinci.)

Spreading: fascial planes

Let's look at how infections progress and spread. Ground zero is the source of the infection. The necrotic or partially impacted tooth is where it all begins. The rest of the story is dependent on the path of least resistance. An infection applies outward pressure as it grows. When it meets resistance, it squeezes through wherever it can. For example, when an apical abscess perforates through the bone into the surrounding tissue, it travels along fascial planes. Fascia is the connective tissue that encases or surrounds all the bones, nerves, vessels and organs in our bodies. It is the partition that provides internal structure and separation between organs. It begins forming when we are only three weeks old inside the womb. (It is fascinating to think about our development and growth, especially how it impacts what we do.)

The fascia surrounding muscles is mainly what limits and influences the spread of dental infections. Fascial planes wall off and contain the abscess, but the abscess applies pressure and can press through between fascial planes. Bacteria also have more sinister means of spreading. They can produce enzymes and toxins that can break down and penetrate connective tissue. For example, common gram-positive strains in dental infections produce hyaluronidase, which is an enzyme that helps destroy the tissue. While the effects of hyaluronidase are well known, its mechanisms are not well understood yet. But the production of this enzyme significantly impacts the virulence and spread of these infections. This and other enzymes seem to nearly dissolve the mortar holding the cellular framework together. In cases of necrotizing fasciitis, the infection seems to just melt the tissue away. It is truly awful.

Understanding fascial planes helps build an understanding of how and where an infection is likely to spread. For instance, an apical infection must perforate through the cortical bone to spread out into the soft tissue. Where it perforates the bone determines where it will spread first. The first location of spread outside the bone is called the primary space. Two main structures determine which primary space will be involved: the buccinator on the lateral aspect of the maxilla and mandible and the mylohyoid on the medial mandible. When an odontogenic abscess outgrows this initial space, it moves into one of the multiple secondary spaces: masticator, lateral pharyngeal, infratemporal, superficial temporal, deep temporal, and retropharyngeal. This book doesn't delve into the details of complicated infection management. There are other sources available for that.

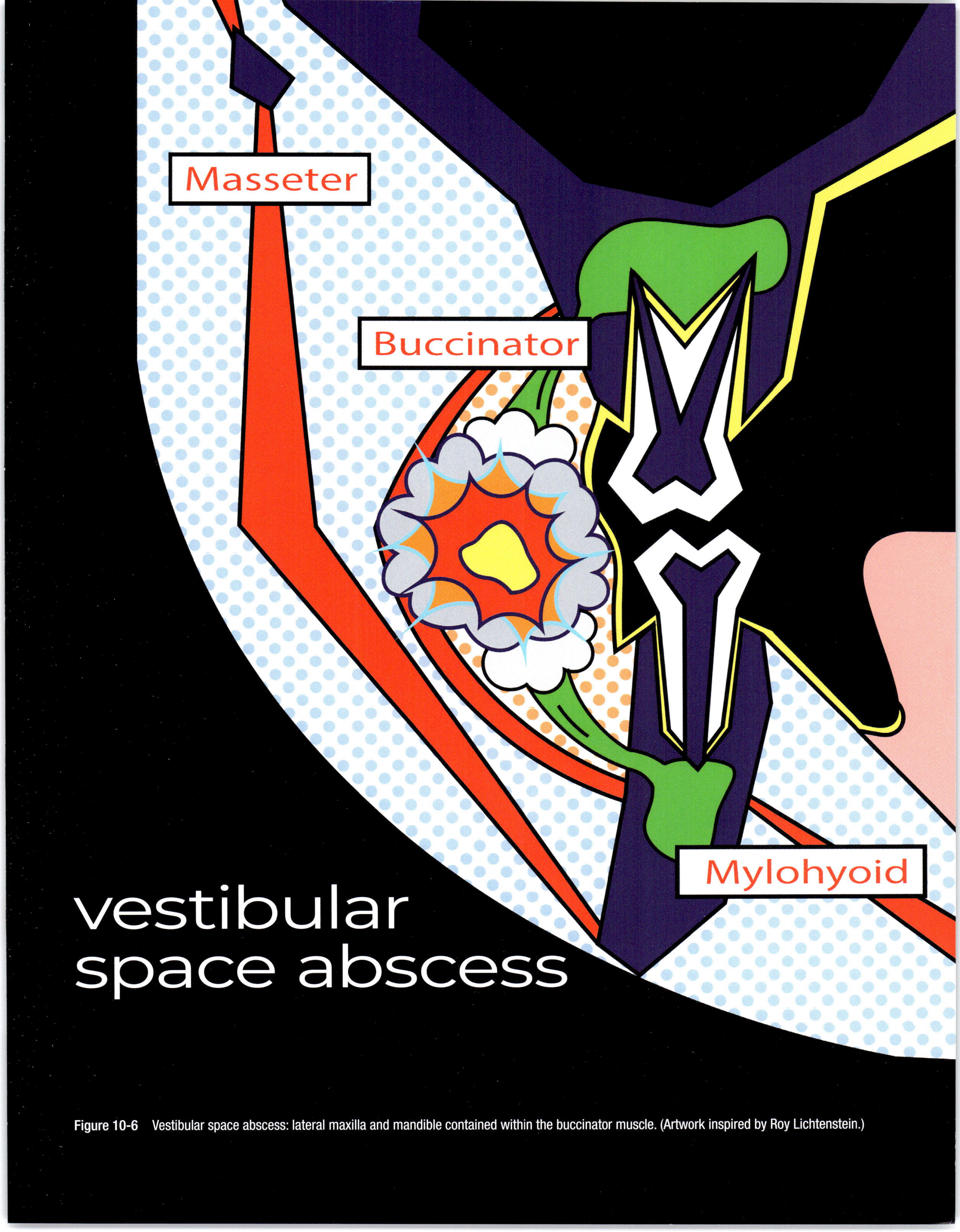

Figure 10-6 Vestibular space abscess: lateral maxilla and mandible contained within the buccinator muscle. (Artwork inspired by Roy Lichtenstein.)

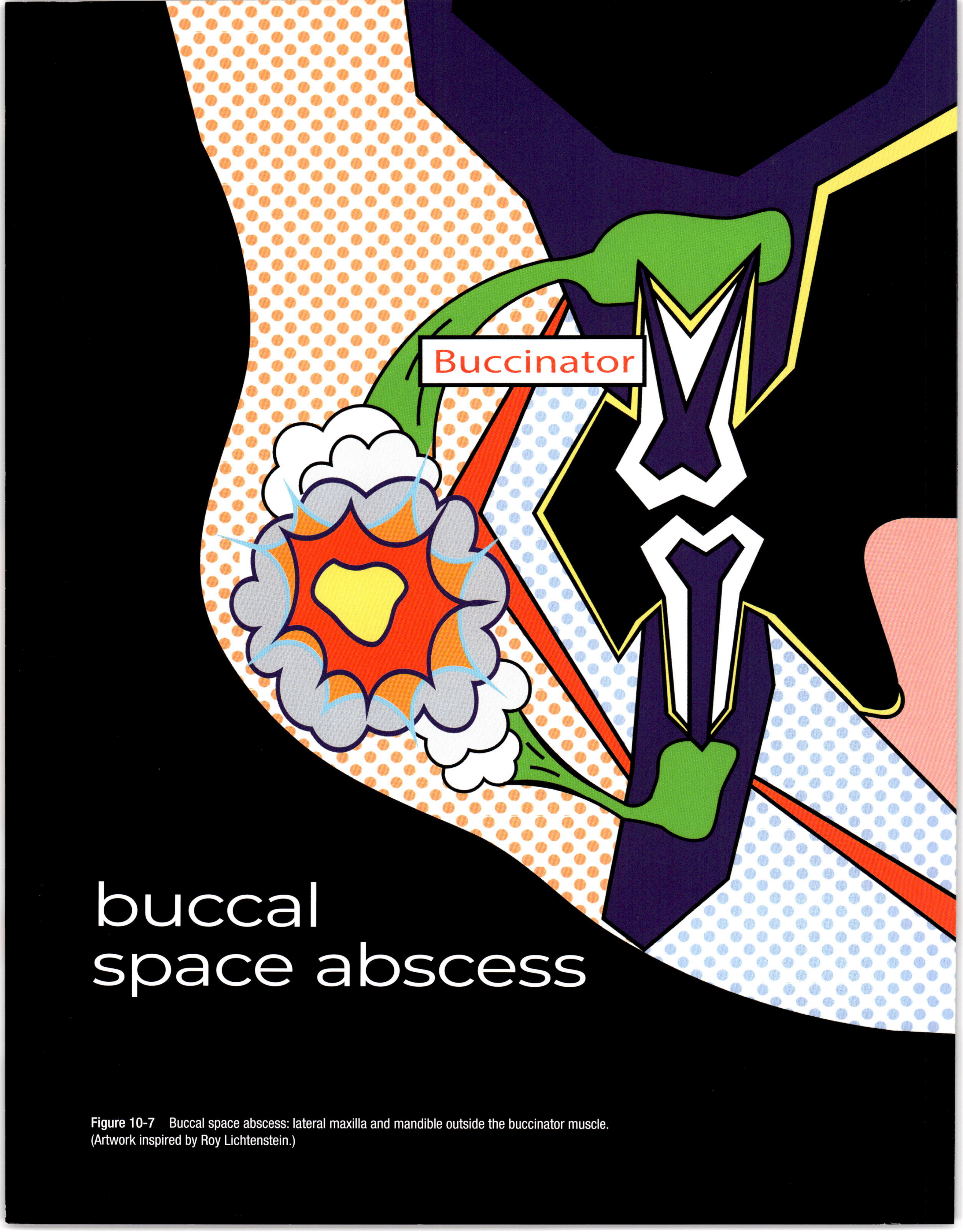

Figure 10-7 Buccal space abscess: lateral maxilla and mandible outside the buccinator muscle. (Artwork inspired by Roy Lichtenstein.)

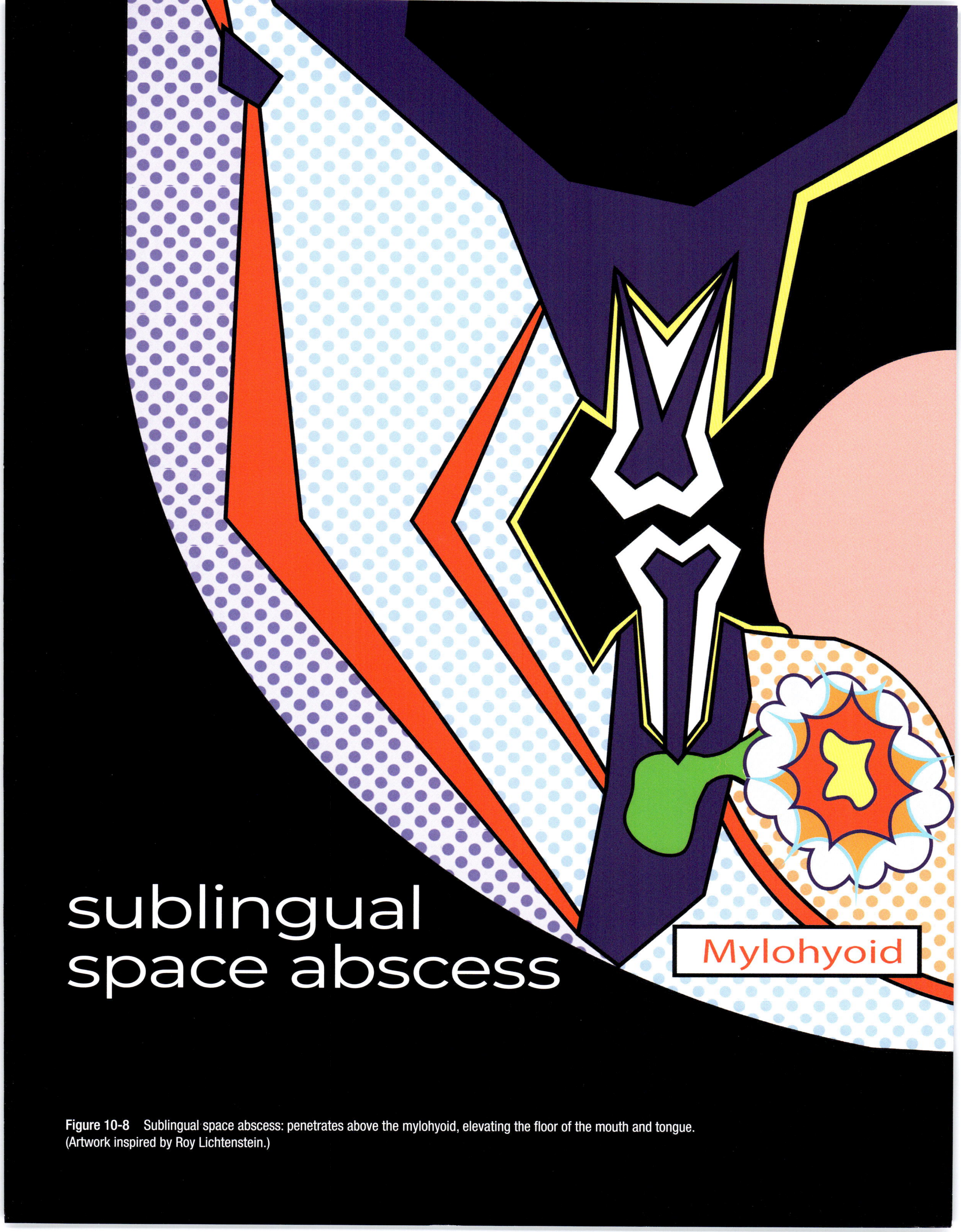

Figure 10-8 Sublingual space abscess: penetrates above the mylohyoid, elevating the floor of the mouth and tongue. (Artwork inspired by Roy Lichtenstein.)

Evaluation

You can learn a lot about an infection by listening to the patient's story. Without even looking at the patient, you can often determine the source, course, duration, onset and location. Did something cause it? Does it hurt? How and when did the pain start? Is there swelling? Could someone off the street see the swelling if they looked at you? Is it spreading? Is there any difficulty breathing or swallowing? Are you running a fever? While a conversation with the patient can't provide all the information necessary to manage an infection, it likely provides some of the most useful information.

Clinical evaluation

Pain, swelling and pus are three pertinent clinical findings. Ask patients to point with one finger to where the pain is the worst. This can guide you to the epicenter of the infection and the most likely place to find an abscess. If they use their whole hand instead of one finger, it may be in a cellulitic phase or may have progressed to involve multiple spaces.

The firmness of the tissue can provide insight on what is going on beneath the surface. I like to think of it this way: more firm means the tissue is more "cooked." Like a steak on the grill, it gets firmer as it gets more well done. When it is rare, it is quite soft and supple, like what you would find very early in the infection process. When the entire area is slightly firm, like medium-well, and a bit swollen, it is more likely cellulitis. If the tissue feels well-done or over-done, it may be cellulitis or may have developed into an abscess. It is usually much more painful when it gets to that point.

The shape of the swelling is also valuable. Cellulitis spreads out like a broad flood light within the tissue. It diffuses laterally over a much wider area. An abscess is more focal, like a spotlight. The challenge is, an abscess will typically be surrounded by cellulitic changes. It is like one of those flashlights that is super bright in the middle but also sheds light more broadly. When palpating, feel for the spotlight in the middle of the swelling. If the infection needs to be drained, that is where you look for pus.

I was taught to evaluate for fluctuance, that feeling of fluid collected beneath the surface. Does it wave or slosh when you push it from side to side? Patients hate this because it hurts, and it doesn't seem to guide my treatment very well. I find it difficult to feel the actual fluid collection. Just because you don't feel the fluid doesn't mean there isn't any.

Important questions

There are a few key clinical questions that provide insight on the severity of the infection:

1. How far does the tenderness to palpation extend down the neck? The farther it spreads, the worse it is. This is especially true if it extends beyond the inferior border of the mandible. And it is even more dangerous when it goes below the thyroid cartilage.
2. Is the floor of the mouth elevated? Is it tender? This can indicate sublingual space involvement. When the sublingual space is involved, it will elevate the tongue and floor of mouth. The tongue may feel bigger to patients, like it is taking up more space in their mouth.
3. Does it feel like it is hard to swallow, or does it just hurt to swallow? Differentiating between pain with swallowing and difficulty swallowing is important. If it feels like there is something blocking the movement of the swallowing (not just pain), it is

far more serious. This happens when the airway spaces are obstructed by swelling. If it just hurts to swallow, the muscles may be irritated, or the tissue inflamed. But tenderness with swallowing is a very different condition than inability to swallow. When a patient cannot manage their own secretions, that is a huge red flag. Take it very seriously.

4. Is the oropharyngeal airway deviated? "Open wide and say aah." When the pharyngeal drape is deviated, the lateral pharyngeal space is likely involved. From there, the infection can quickly spread around the airway, down the neck and into the lethal zones below.
5. Is it difficult to breathe? Does it feel like you are breathing through a small straw? If the answer is yes, secure that airway STAT! Get these patients to the emergency department. If they are already there, get them sedated and intubated. Patients in this state could be moments away from complete and fatal airway obstruction.

With potential for major complications, it is critical to clearly document pertinent positive and negative clinical findings of an infection. The clinical checklist below can help establish a diagnosis and plan. It can also bolster a legal defense if needed.

CLINICAL EXAMINATION CHECKLIST

When performing the clinical examination, it is important to evaluate and document at least these following points. Having this in the form of a checklist can be helpful.

Extraoral swelling:

- Location and extent:
- Firmness: (focal or diffuse)
- Inferior mandibular border: (palpable)
- Tenderness to palpation: (location and severity)

Intraoral swelling:

- Location and extent:
- Firmness: (focal or diffuse)
- Floor of mouth: (tender or elevated)
- Airway: (pharyngeal curtain deviation)
- Tenderness to palpation: (location and severity)

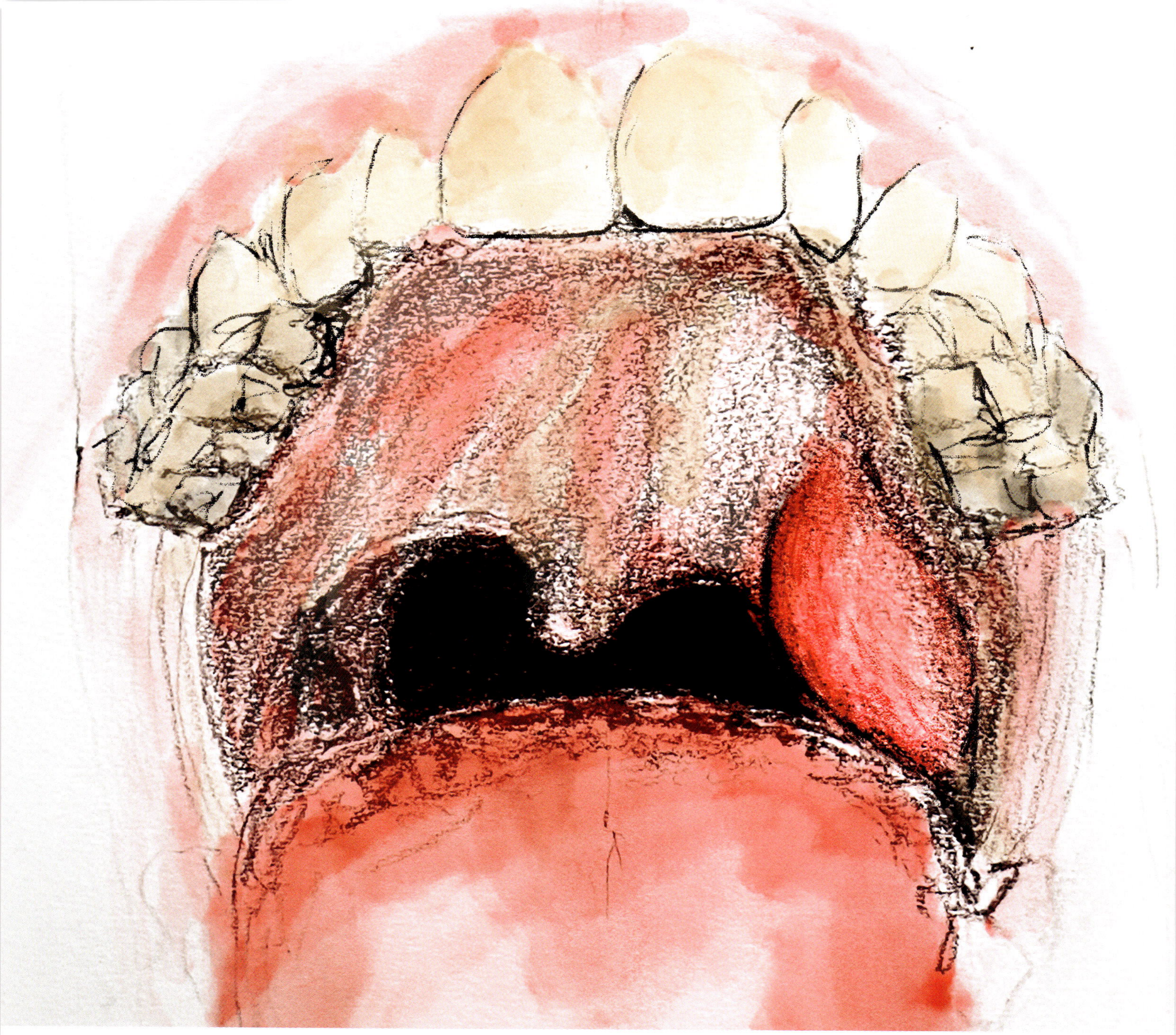

Figure 10-9 Deviated oropharyngeal airway with fullness in the left pharyngeal wall. This abscess is heading in a dangerous direction. Soon the airway could be compromised, and the abscess could spread down the parapharyngeal spaces.

Previous treatment

Previous treatment is an important piece of the puzzle. Have antibiotics previously failed? Or were they initially successful but there has been a resurgence of the infection? Has there been recent treatment at the site? Extraction? Endodontic therapy? Incision and drainage?

It should be an alert if an infection is progressing despite antibiotic treatment, or if the offending tooth was removed and the infection seems to continue to get worse. In these cases, consider more thorough evaluation and medical imaging. More aggressive treatment may be needed. The infection is declaring that it won't go down without a fight.

Evaluating the patient

Understanding the host is critically important in managing an infection. If a patient has little physiologic reserve and is not likely to do well with the stress of an infection, early and aggressive treatment is necessary. The physiologic reserve can be evaluated by the patient's diagnoses, medications, history, and sometimes just by eyeballing a patient.

Medications can compromise the immune system. Some immune-modulating medications hamper the immune system, giving the infection the advantage. These patients should be treated more aggressively and followed more closely. It will take more intervention on our part to get the immune system to successfully subdue the bacteria and restore balance. Steroids, chemotherapy and immunosuppressants are a few of the most common medications that weaken the immune system. It is important to keep up to date on current medications and classes of medications that compromise the immune system as they are always changing.

Alcohol consumption

Chronic alcohol consumption has a profound impact on almost all the cells and pathways of our immune system. It can negatively affect every organ system. This often goes unnoticed to a patient until it is exposed to the assault of an infection. Chronic alcohol users (whether they have been diagnosed with an alcohol use disorder) have impeded immune systems far less capable of fighting an infection. They also don't heal as well. Don't assume they will respond well to treatment. Treat them more aggressively and keep a close eye on them through their full recovery[5].

Past problems

History of recurrent or chronic infections could indicate higher likelihood of infection and potentially increased difficulty managing an infection. If patients have had a difficult time fighting infections in the past, their body and immune system will most likely have a difficult time again.

Diabetes

Poorly controlled diabetic patients are immunocompromised, especially regarding infections. Here are a few ways diabetes affects the ability to fight infection:

1. Macrovascular and microvascular damage impact the blood supply and resources available to fight an infection.
2. Suppressed cytokine production inhibits leukocyte recruitment.
3. Defects in phagocytosis lead to neutrophil and macrophage dysfunction.
4. Inhibition of antibody production reduces normal immune cell function that relies on direction from antibodies. Antibodies tell cells what to destroy.

With these and other physiologic limitations, diabetic patients are more likely to develop an infection. We need to do more of the work when fighting an infection in diabetics. We cannot rely as much on their bodies to effectively eradicate the infection. We may not need to kill every single organism in the infection, but we need to be prepared to do more of the work[6].

Another aspect of patient evaluation is the sixth sense. Sometimes you need to trust your gut. If a patient is infected and looks ill, be concerned. They may be decompensating or getting septic. Some patients look like they won't do well with the stress of an infection. Pay attention to these things. There is a lot to learn by looking at a patient as a whole.

Radiographic evaluation

Soft tissue computed tomography is a vital tool in diagnosing and treating infections. It provides information on the presence or absence of fluid collection. It identifies the location and spatial involvement of the cellulitis or abscess. It can also be vital in identifying potential airway compromise. When an infection is progressing rapidly or there are concerns of compromising the airway, consider obtaining a medical CT scan urgently. In hindsight, obtaining advanced imaging can almost never be criticized[7,8]. A medical grade CT scan can also reveal the extent of an abscess, identifying different loculations and providing a visual for the complex and often blind approach to the different spaces during incision and drainage. While this is not always necessary, it can be very beneficial in determining the extent of the infection as well as evaluating post-operative progression if it does not resolve.

Treatment

Surgery and antibiotics are our main weapons in the fight against infection. Not every patient needs both. Here are some things to consider when deciding whether to treat with antibiotics, surgery or both.

The case for antibiotic therapy without (or before) surgery

It can be exquisitely painful to drain an abscess or remove a tooth under local anesthetic in the presence of an acute infection. Profound anesthesia is thwarted in a couple of ways. An abscess decreases tissue pH due to the effects of inflammation. This reduces the effectiveness of local anesthetic, which requires a slightly higher pH to cross the nerve membrane. It is also more difficult to block the signal in a nerve that is hyperactivated from pain. If the acute infection can be resolved or even reduced with antibiotics, the procedure may then be possible with local anesthesia instead of general anesthesia. If you treat with antibiotics alone, you risk the infection progressing and causing more harm. In discussing this with patients, it is important they understand both the benefits and the risks of delaying surgery.

When an acute infection is associated with an implant, bone graft or a necrotic tooth that is planned to undergo endodontic therapy, surgery may not be indicated immediately. In these cases, treating with antibiotics without removing the source of infection may be indicated. (At least we hope they will resolve the infection without needing to remove the tooth, implant or graft.)

These cases present a unique challenge. For instance, when an implant site is showing signs of post-operative infection, it is possible it could resolve with antibiotics. The implant may have a statistically increased risk of failure, but there still may be reasonable potential for long term success. It can be challenging to determine when to remove an implant, especially when a patient pushes hard to keep it. I have come to favor removing the implant earlier and giving the site a fresh start after a few months of healing.

Antibiotic therapy before surgery may reduce pain associated with surgery, reduce cost by avoiding general anesthesia, and save an implant or bone graft from removal, but there is an increased risk of the infection progressing and possibly causing more harm. This may be the only option if the patient needs to be referred to a specialist for endodontic or surgical treatment.

The case for surgery without antibiotics

If there isn't an indication for prescribing an antibiotic, there is inherently a contraindication. Antibiotics kill beneficial, healthy bacteria. Let me say that again. Antibiotics are contraindicated in the absence of a good indication. Localized, non-aggressive infections with a reasonably competent host will not likely benefit from antibiotics. In these cases, the risks often outweigh the benefits. Discernment is the artform.

The most definitive treatment we can provide is surgery. That is what the body needs from us. It cannot intrinsically remove the offending tooth or drain the abscess. But it can kill bacteria and fight the infections. Antibiotics should be viewed as an adjunct to the definitive treatment, which is often surgical treatment.

The case for combined surgical and antibiotic therapy

Combined surgical and antibiotic therapy has the highest likelihood of resolving an infection. Studies have shown the particular antibiotic is irrelevant when combined with surgery, as long as it has appropriate coverage[9]. This dual mode therapy directly eliminates the infection source and helps wipe out the bacterial invasion. This is the treatment most often recommended, but it is not always feasible or necessary.

Surgical drainage

Principles of surgical drainage

Surgery is often the best thing we can do for an infection. It is the most definitive move we can make in the battle. In an instant, the number of organisms in the infectious army can be decreased by the millions. The pus that was shielding the bacteria from the immune system can be dramatically reduced just by poking into it and draining it. The pus would have eventually gone away, but surgical drainage is much more efficient at cleaning up the mess than the body's lymphatic system. It is reported that between 10% to 83% of deep neck space infections require surgical drainage for successful management[10]. This broad range underscores the nuances of infection management. It is as much art as it is science.

MAIN OBJECTIVES OF INCISION AND DRAINAGE

- Drain and flush the pus to reduce bacterial load and disrupt proliferation.
- Increase bacterial exposure to the host immune system and antibiotic therapy by eliminating the protection of the abscess.
- Alter the environment by irrigating the site and introducing oxygen, thus making it inhospitable for obligate anaerobic bacteria.

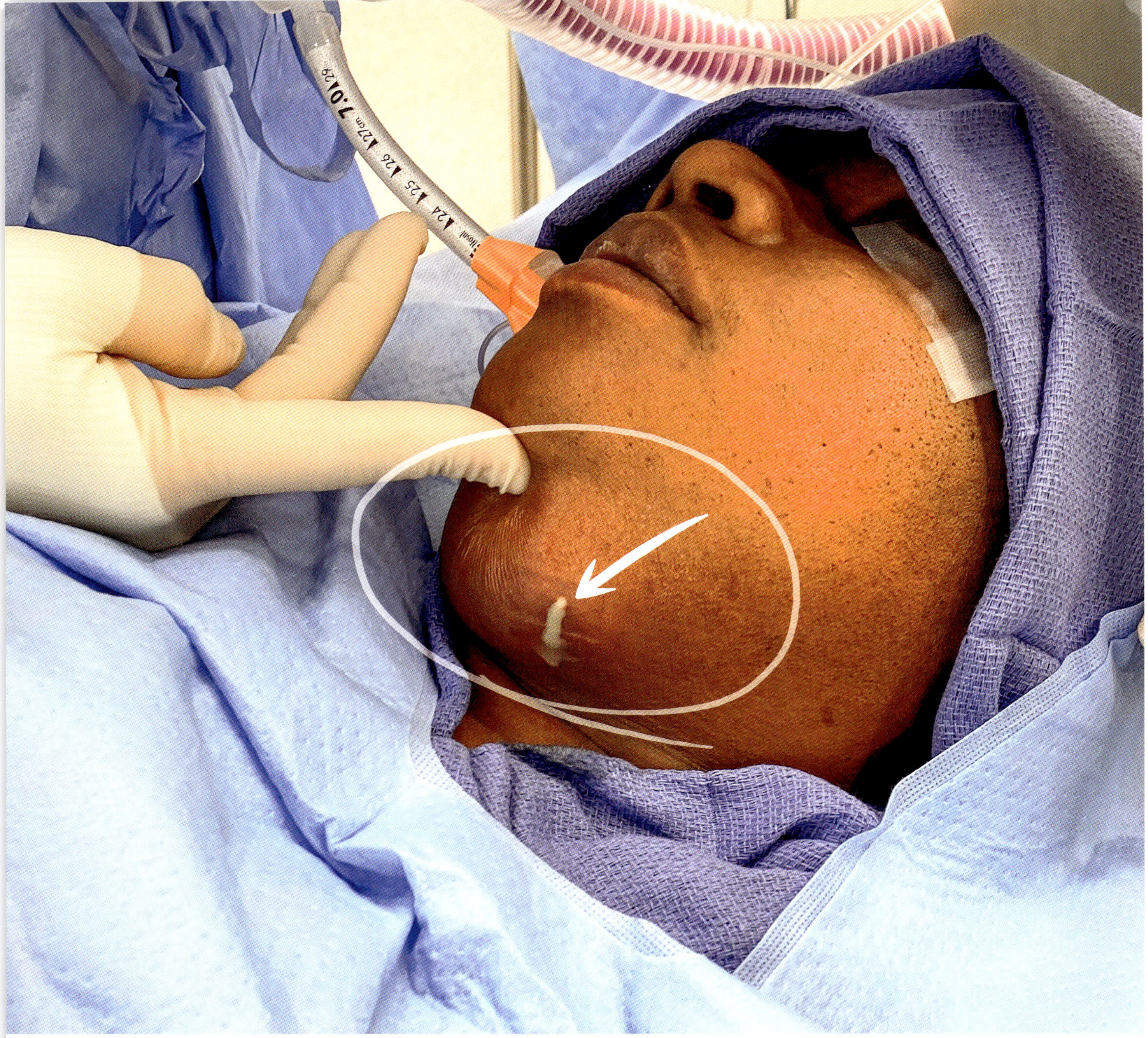

Figure 10-10 Surgical drainage under general anesthetic is sometimes necessary if the infection is not responding to treatment. In this case, the patient's airway was compromised when she presented to the hospital. The abscess was aspirated and cultured through sterile skin. It was explored and drained both intraorally and extraorally.

Strategy

Hit it where it counts. Generally, the most prominent area of swelling is the best point of entry for incision and drainage. There are two parts to this equation: knowledge of the anatomy and awareness of the current abscess location. The ideal approach is often in the vestibule, floor of mouth, submental or submandibular spaces. Ask the patient to point to where it feels the worst or most swollen. Palpate the tissue. Use your finger to point to where it feels the most tense and tender. That typically marks the spot. Make a stab incision through the epithelium. Advance closed hemostats into the wound and open wide to access the space. Remove the hemostat while it is still open. Never close hemostats within the wound. Blunt dissection is less likely to damage adjacent structures.

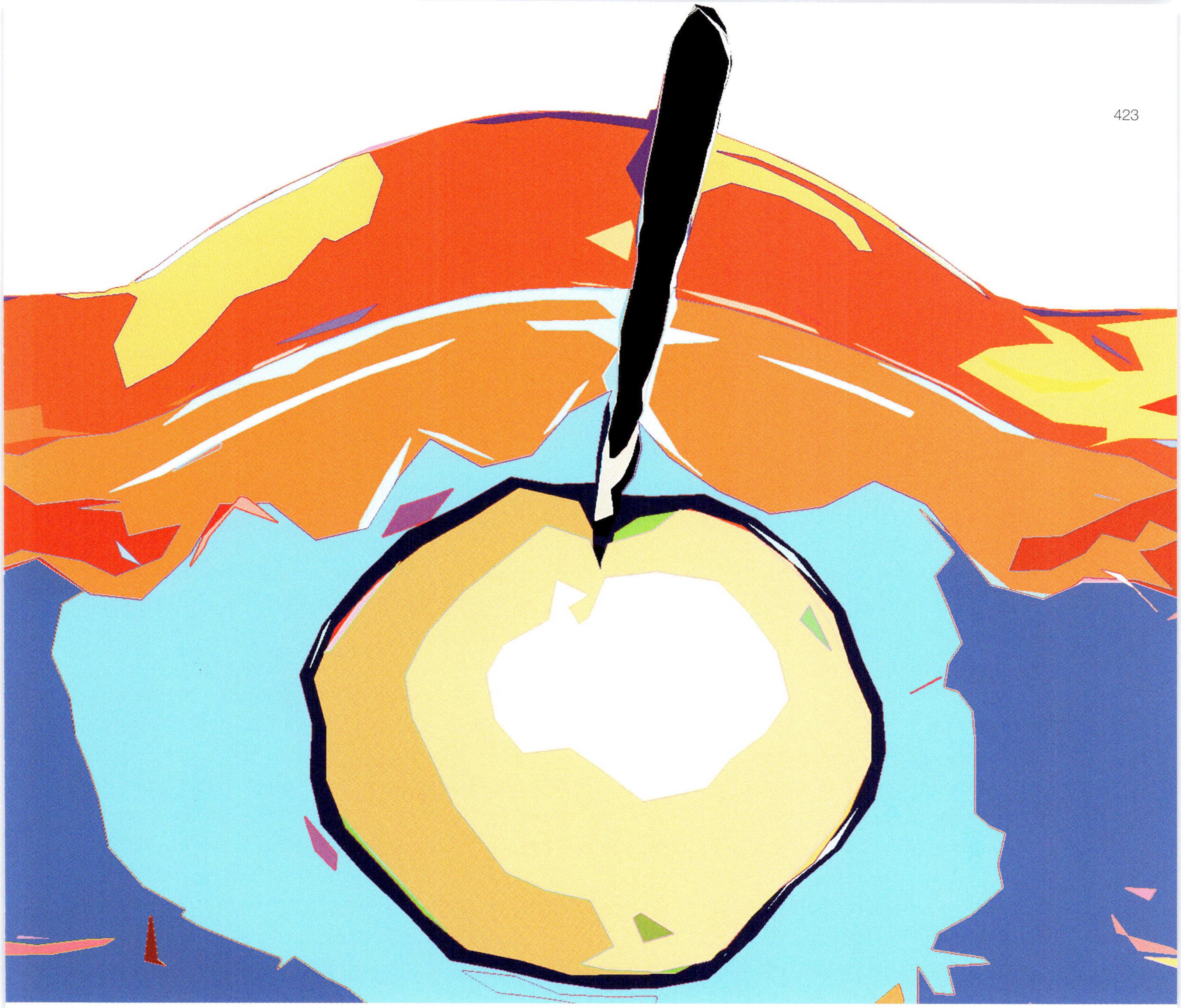

Figure 10-11 Abscesses often "point." The most prominent area of swelling is usually directly over the biggest collection of pus. That is usually the best spot to drain.

Primary space incision and drainage

Low risk

- **Vestibular space**: Stab incision with a #15 blade over the most prominent bulge of the abscess. This is usually in the vestibular mucosa. This space is fairly superficial and easy to access. At times, it is possible to access it through an extraction site. A curette can be passed subperiosteally down the lateral aspect of the mandible or through a cortical perforation. It may also be possible to flush the site through this access with a blunt tip syringe.
  - **Caution**: The mental nerve can be close to the surface. Use great care when making the incision to protect the nerve. Either access the site away from the nerve or be very careful with incision depth.

- **Buccal space**: Stab incision with a #15 blade at the height of contour in the buccal mucosa. The blade should pass through the mucosa and underlying connective tissue. Bluntly dissect toward the loculation with a closed hemostat. Upon entering the abscess, explore the margins of the space: up, down, front and back.
  - **Caution**: Branches of the facial artery run on the outside of the buccinator. Don't push the blade too deep. The artery should be safe with careful blunt dissection.
- **Infraorbital/canine space**: Intraoral access through the vestibule. Simple to approach and relatively easy to decompress through the vestibular mucosa, similar to the buccal space.

Moderate risk

- **Sublingual space**: Fairly superficial incision in the floor of the mouth, slightly lingual and parallel to the mandible.
  - **Caution**: Lingual nerve and submandibular ducts are in close proximity in this area. Delicate moves and cautious blunt dissection will help protect these critical structures. The blunt tips of closed hemostats will seldom cause any injury to these structures. A pinched hemostat or surgical blade can certainly cause harm.
- **Submandibular space**: Extraoral approach. Examine for a palpable inferior border. This helps differentiate buccal space from submandibular space. This is much more involved, similar to a secondary space infection.
- **Submental space**: Extraoral approach over the point or clinical height of the abscess. No significant anatomical structures to avoid. Just use good clinical judgment and you should be fine.

Secondary space incision and drainage

These are much higher risk sites for infection and surgical management. The same surgical principles apply when an infection progresses to the deeper spaces. We want to get rid of the pus, flush the site and change the environment. In these cases, the procedure's challenges and risk increase, as does the overall complexity and risk of complications to the patient. For further information on managing these more complex infections, consider reading[2,3,10-12]. This book doesn't have enough space to delve into these situations fully. But I do want to touch on one particular type of severe infection: Ludwig's Angina.

Ludwig's Angina is a very special infection. By definition, it is a severe, life-threatening cellulitis involving the five spaces of the upper neck: bilateral submandibular, bilateral sublingual and submental spaces. It spreads like wildfire through these spaces, causing a brawny or woody tension in the tissue. And it has a very high mortality rate. It demands emergency attention with airway stabilization, surgical exposure, and high-dose IV antibiotics. It is a truly impressive infection. It is important to understand the difference between Ludwig's Angina and any other routine deep neck space infection. The level of emergency and aggressive treatment can be completely different. In my career, I have often heard Ludwig's Angina applied by radiologists or emergency department staff when referring to any submandibular space swelling. The diagnosis of Ludwig's Angina should be reserved for rapidly progressing, brawny cellulitis impacting the multiple spaces of the upper neck.

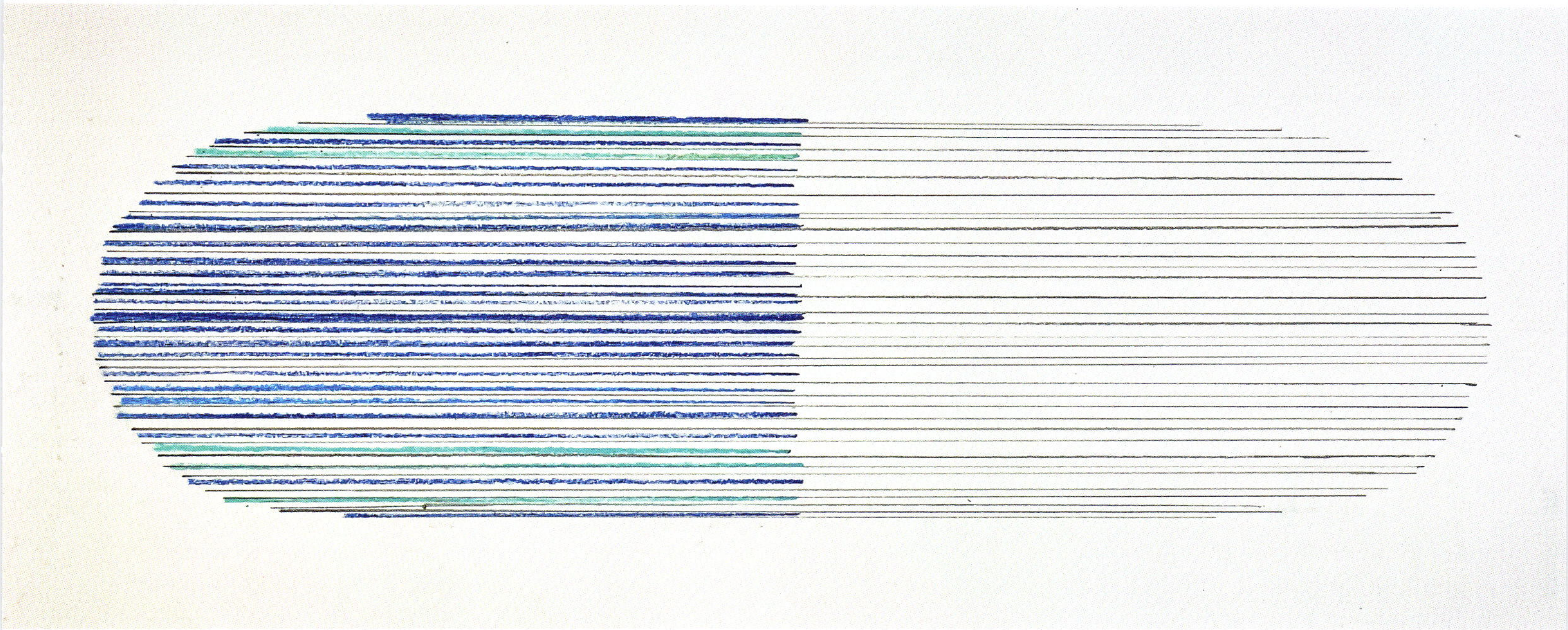

Figure 10-12 There is no perfect pill. No perfect antibiotic that only kills the bad bacteria. They all kill many innocent bystanders in the microbiological world. We need to be able to read between the lines. See beyond the obvious. (Artwork inspired by Agnes Martin.)

Antibiotics

Principles of antibiotic treatment

In a perfect world, antibiotic therapy would be directed by the individual strains of bacteria primarily responsible for causing the infection and its susceptibility to a particular antibiotic. In the real world, we treat empirically. We select the antibiotic that is most likely to kill the most commonly involved bacteria while not devastating other strains in the microbiome. This field is continually changing. Bacteria constantly evolve and new antibiotics are developed. Crucial research is continually being done on the microbiome and its tremendous impact on our overall health[13]. The art of antibiotic treatment is in the discerning application of the science. It is in knowing which therapies are most likely to succeed, when to administer them and when to withhold for the best possible outcome. Keeping up with current best practices is much easier with resources like Dr. Leslie S.T. Fang's "The Ultimate Cheat Sheets," which provides best practices and is frequently updated as the field changes.

To fight an infection, antibiotics can either kill the bacteria (bactericidal) or prevent them from reproducing (bacteriostatic). These are both very effective mechanisms. The lifespan of the average bacteria is short. In optimal conditions, *E. coli* doubles every 20 minutes[9]. Bacteria won't last long if we prevent their reproduction. And they certainly won't survive if we kill them.

Empiric treatment

Infections are polymicrobial, making them difficult to treat. Many different strains of bacteria are all competing against each other for resources. And the dominant strains typically evolve as the infection progresses. The initial environment of an odontogenic infection often favors more virulent, aerobic/facultative anaerobic organisms such as viridans streptococci. When oxygen is available, these bacteria use it to make ATP as their energy source through aerobic respiration. In the absence of oxygen, they produce ATP through fermentation. They can reproduce with or without oxygen. Early in an infection, these bacteria consume oxygen and deplete the local resources, putting pressure on themselves. The local environment in the infected tissue changes over the course of about 3 to 5 days. With less oxygen available, it becomes more favorable for anaerobic organisms, which often become the dominant strains as the infection progresses.

While the immune system fights an infection, antibiotics provide tremendous assistance. The immune system often benefits from the reinforcement of the antibiotics for a while, but not necessarily until every single bacterium in the infection is dead. As long as enough bacterial destruction has occurred and the milieu is shifted, the body can take over the rest. Identifying when to start and stop antibiotic therapy is part of the art of infection management.

Failed empiric treatment

When an infection persists, it may need surgical intervention or a change in antibiotic coverage. Most of the time, even severe infections resolve with adequate surgical care and proper antibiotic coverage[3,13]. Increasing antibiotic coverage can sometimes resolve an infection. But often, merely changing antibiotics is inadequate to successfully treat an infection when surgery is needed. When considering changing antibiotics for dental infections, increasing the gram-negative anaerobic coverage is usually most helpful, as they are most often the resistant organisms in dental infections. Obtaining a culture and sensitivity of the abscess ensures proper coverage in case the infection does not resolve.

Duration

Our prescribing practices are empirically driven, but we don't know if this patient with this infection will be adequately treated with a three, five or more than 10-day course of antibiotics. In the dance of infection management, the goal is to provide enough support so the body can wipe out the infection and reinstate an equilibrium within the microbiome. Longer exposure to antibiotics increases the pressure to select for resistant strains[14]. This seems to make sense logically, although clear evidence in the literature is lacking. It is our responsibility to be good stewards when prescribing antibiotics to patients, and it is their responsibility to follow our recommendations. As such, we must ensure we uphold our end of the bargain and prescribe the most judicious course of antibiotic treatment, tailored to the individual's needs. In short, if the infection is minimal and the patient is improving, consider discontinuing the antibiotic treatment before the prescribed course is complete. A patient need not complete the course, as if there is something magic about the number of days we chose to prescribe.

Bacteria

Bacteria reproduce. That sums up their mission statement. They are just single cell microorganisms doing everything they can to reproduce. Their mission objectives are vast and incredible. And in the process of their short life cycle, many of them contribute to critical tasks that help sustain their host and contribute to the broader ecosystem. We carry around more bacterial cells than human cells. In health, there are many beneficial byproducts of bacterial reproduction for digestion, immunity and synthesis of nutrients and vitamins to name a few. In the case of oral related infections, however, their reproduction can be quite harmful. As they reproduce, they apply physical and physiological pressure on surrounding tissue. They can produce toxins that break down tissue and cause tremendous destruction. They can advance and claim more territory from the host. It truly is a microscopic battle.

Classifying bacteria

Clinical signs and symptoms are the initial indication that a battle has begun, with pain, swelling, redness and pus among them. When they show up, we know an infection is brewing. Tremendous research has been and is currently being done in this field. We know the most common organisms involved in these infections. We empirically treat with a few specific antibiotics that are typically quite effective. The vast majority of infections we encounter in our field are successfully treated without ever identifying the specific organisms involved[3].

Culture and sensitivity

When an infection is more severe or the host is compromised, it can be extremely helpful to obtain a culture and sensitivity. Obtaining a clean culture is vital for valuable results. While a "clean culture" of pus may be an oxymoron, it is important to only provide the lab with bacteria from within the abscess. If the swab or needle accidentally contacts contaminated skin or oral mucosa, it will grow normal flora and be of little value.

Aspirating the abscess provides the most accurate results because it obtains a larger sample and, when performed properly, is less likely to be contaminated. The technique involves applying a sterile prep, such as Betadine, to the skin overlying the most prominent site of the abscess. Pass a sterile 18-20 gauge needle on a sterile syringe through the skin into the abscess, taking care to avoid vital structures such as the facial artery. To perform aspiration, draw back on the needle as it advances to the abscess site. As you explore the area, you may need to redirect the needle a few times. There will be times when you don't find any pus. If pus is encountered later after further draining and exploring the site surgically, sample it and send it to the lab.

Swab collection is more common because it is easier, but it is potentially less accurate. In this technique, the sterile swab included in the culture kit is carefully used to sample the pus or swab the infected tissue if no pus is encountered. If pus is encountered during exploration, it can be advanced through the incision into the abscess. It can also be used to swab pus if it exudes from an extraction site. Ideally, this is accomplished without the swab or pus contacting any exposed tissue.

The sample should be processed for both aerobic and anaerobic evaluation by using appropriate transport media. The containers should be individually labeled with instructions for proper handling. The sample must quickly be placed into the anaerobic container and delivered to the lab. The more exposure the specimen has to oxygen, the less likely it is to give accurate anaerobic results. While the systems have improved, anaerobic cultures are still thought to be less accurate in growing all the anaerobic organisms involved.

The first report available from the lab indicates a rough estimate of the number of microorganisms seen under the microscope, as well as their gram stain and shape. It will also include the number of white blood cells visualized, which indicates the specimen likely included pus from the site. If no white blood cells are visualized, it is possible the sample did not adequately retrieve pus.

Over the following days, the lab team grows bacteria from the specimen on multiple petri dishes in aerobic and anaerobic environments. They monitor and report on growth. They also expose separate petri dishes to different antibiotics and observe the impact on growth. This provides a good indication of which antibiotics will be successful against the specific organisms collected during surgery. Obtaining clean aerobic and anaerobic cultures is important. Check to make sure the lab order that accompanies the specimen indicates both aerobic and anaerobic culture. If the infection is not resolving as test results are reported, antibiotic treatment can be adjusted. Select an antibiotic with a high reported sensitivity to the organisms identified. If there are multiple organisms growing, consider the antibiotic with the best overall sensitivity.

Gram stain

Some bacteria (gram-positive) have a thick outer layer made up of long-chain polymers based on amino acids (peptido) and sugar (glycan) called peptidoglycan. This is reinforced by extensive protein crosslinking that links the chains together as a mesh. Other types of bacteria (gram-negative) have a thin outer layer of long-chain polymers composed of fat (lipo) and sugars (polysaccharide) called lipopolysaccharide or LPS. These also have a peptidoglycan layer, but it is inside the LPS membrane, and it is much thinner.

Gram staining involves applying a stain called crystal violet, which is retained in the outer peptidoglycan wall of gram-positive organisms and washes out of the outer LPS membrane of gram-negative organisms. This distinction is important because it helps broadly categorize bacteria based on their primary defense: the cell wall. Many other properties and characteristics follow the gram stain. For example, gram-positive bacteria secrete exotoxins that destroy surrounding cells, whereas gram-negative bacteria have endotoxins within their LPS cell wall that damage the host tissue after the cell dies and the inner portion of the cell wall is exposed to the tissue.

The value of gram staining is limited in clinical oral surgery. If the infection is bad enough that I am obtaining cultures and sensitivity, the patient should probably already be on a broader coverage antibiotic therapy. This empiric treatment is quite predictable regardless of the gram stain results. I have found infection severity and duration, as well as host immune status, directs treatment far more than gram stain results. Usually, if the infection is less severe and the patient is only on first line therapy, obtaining a culture and sensitivity is not indicated.

Bacteria shape

The primary bacteria encountered in oral infections are round clusters (cocci) or rods (bacilli). Like gram staining, this does not routinely direct antibiotic therapy in odontogenic infections. It can be extremely valuable in other specialties or in rare instances, but not so much for oral surgery.

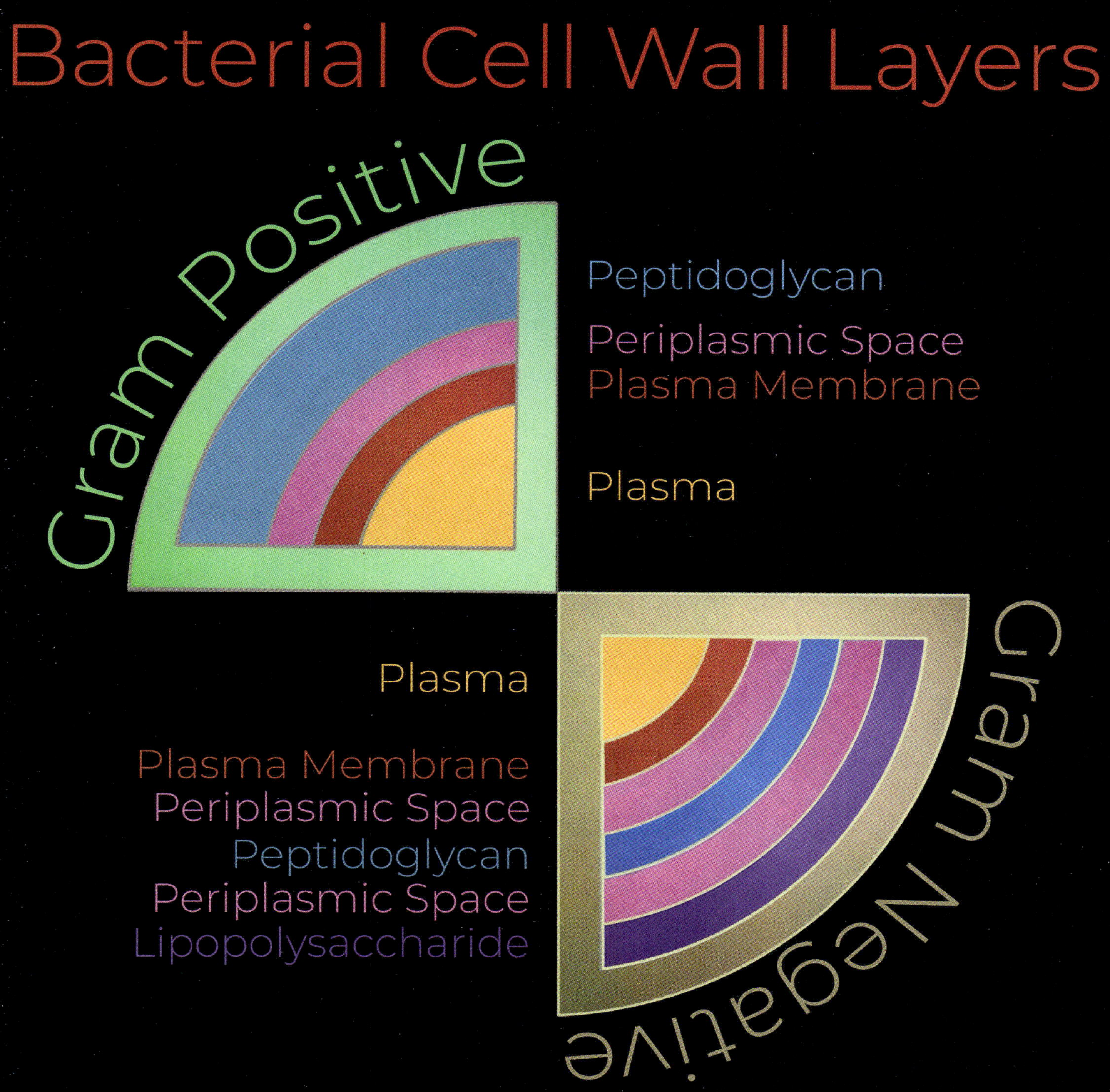

Figure 10-13 Gram-positive and gram-negative bacteria share multiple common layers. One of the biggest differences is in the outer layer. Gram-positive bacteria have a cross-linked peptidoglycan outer layer while gram-negative bacteria have a thick lipopolysaccharide (LPS) layer. (Artwork inspired by Frank Stella.)

Table 10-6 Most common bacterial species found in odontogenic infections

	Incidence	Impact
Gram-positive cocci	85%	Strep viridans (*S. milleri* or *S. anginosus.* Facultative anaerobic) *Peptostreptococcus* is noted but less common. Obligate anaerobes develop increasing resistance to drugs.
Gram-negative bacilli	50%	Bacteroides (fusobacteria and *Porphyromonas gingivalis*), *Prevotella, Pseudomonas aeruginosa. Eikenella* lower incidence, but are resistant to clindamycin.
Gram-positive bacilli	5%	*Staph aureus* (facultative aerobe). Little effect on treatment.
Gram-negative cocci	5%	Little effect on treatment

Common antibiotics of oral surgery

We attack bacteria with antibiotics. We learn from nature and figure out ways to dismantle them, disrupt their metabolism, and destroy their protection. Although they are single-cell organisms, these little buggers can be sneaky and develop antibiotic resistance. We develop different ways to modify the antibiotic or the environment and come back with a counterattack. And so it goes. Let's look at some of the most common antibiotics we use. This is not a comprehensive overview. I hope it can shed some new light on infections and give you a different perspective through which you can appreciate this microscopic universe.

ß-lactam antibiotics (Penicillins and cephalosporins)

The attack…antibiotic therapy

Amoxicillin, Augmentin, cephalexin.
Amoxicillin 500 mg TID (typically 5-7 days)
Augmentin 875/125 mg BID (typically 5-7 days)
Cephalexin 500 mg QID (typically 5-7 days)

The mechanism of the broad category of ß-lactam antibiotics makes bacterial cells burst. There is constant osmotic pressure within bacterial cells. The thick peptidoglycan cell wall of gram-positive bacteria maintains its shape and structural integrity of the cell under this constant pressure. The protein crosslinking reinforces the peptidoglycan chains. The ß-lactam ring prevents this crosslinking, causing the cell to explode. It does this by entering the cell, binding to and inhibiting the transpeptidase protein (also called the penicillin binding protein), which links the peptidoglycan layers together. It basically stops the cell from gluing the layers of its cell wall together. And it bursts under normal pressure.

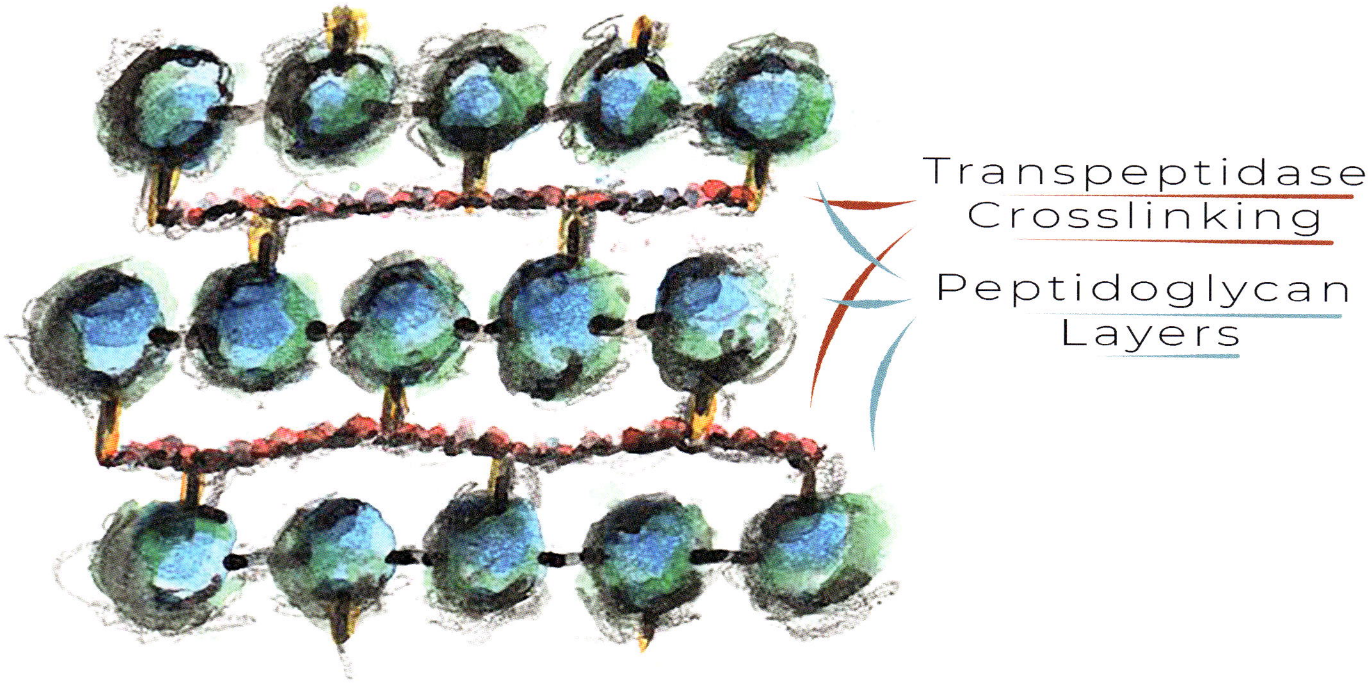

Figure 10-14 Transpeptidase crosslinking holds the cell wall's peptidoglycan layers together. When crosslinking is inhibited, the cell wall loses integrity and bursts under normal pressure, killing the bacterium.

ß-lactam antibiotics were initially most effective against gram-positive bacteria because of how well they destroy the thick outer peptidoglycan wall. They were commonly thought of as less effective against gram-negative bacteria. This seems to be due to the protective outer LPS membrane that prevents antibiotic penetration and their high incidence of ß-lactamase production. Broader spectrum ß-lactam development has increased penetration through the cell membrane, improving coverage for both gram-positive and gram-negative organisms. For example, gram-negative bacilli are often more sensitive to amoxicillin (third generation) than penicillin (first generation). Penicillin has generally fallen out of favor due to its mediocre, narrow coverage and decreased patient compliance. It must be taken four times per day on an empty stomach because gastric acid inactivates it and reduces its absorption to 30%[15]. Later generation cephalosporins also have very broad coverage and are less susceptible to ß-lactamase.

The resistance…Antibiotic resistance

Bacteria evolve to stay alive. In normal cellular function, ribosomes assemble proteins and enzymes with information from RNA one bond at a time. When the information in the delicate RNA changes even slightly, the ribosome will follow the altered instructions and build an altered protein. Sometimes, the altered protein is an enzyme. Enzymes are specialized proteins that actively change biochemistry by facilitating the formation or cleavage of a bond. The vast majority of the time, random mutations cause more harm than good to a cell, and they are not passed on. But sometimes, a mutant enzyme helps bacteria survive and reproduce. And bacteria evolve. For example, ß-lactamase enzymes that are produced by many bacteria break the lactam ring and protect the bacteria from its demise. It thus becomes resistant to ß-lactams. Because they reproduce so rapidly, they can undergo rapid genetic evolution[9].

This has been happening in nature long before the synthetic antimicrobial developments of the mid-20th century. The protective properties of various ß-lactamase enzymes are found in most bacterial species. Indeed, their prominence in gram-negative species further decreases the effect of ß-lactam antibiotics. While this type of enzyme is thought to be billions of years old, the numbers and variations have dramatically increased with the recent increased exposure to penicillins and cephalosporins, particularly in gram-negative bacteria.

The more pressure we put on bacteria with antibiotics, the more likely they are to adapt and become resistant. Afterall, the ß-lactamase enzyme is only beneficial for bacteria when they are threatened by the ß-lactam ring. They seem to have no other inherent benefit.

Bacteria have a few main ways to resist antibiotics. They can block the antibiotic from entering the cell by decreasing permeability. After it is inside, they can pump the antibiotic out with efflux pumps. They can physically inactivate the antibiotic or they can change the target site, making the antibiotic ineffective. The genetic coding for these various mechanisms is transferred to other bacteria in one of two main ways. It can go up the family tree when new bacteria are born through cell division (vertical) or out on the tree to bacteria that are already living (horizontal).

Transferring resistance: gene transfer

Vertical gene transfer is the easy way to think of genetics. We pass genes on to our babies. They pass them on to theirs and so on. In bacterial genetics, this can occur every 30 minutes resulting in a million bacteria babies in just 10 hours. Brand new mutations occur primarily through genetic alterations in this pathway. Thankfully, these novel mutations are extremely rare, especially compared to the transfer of existing resistance genes. Consider this: If a single bacterium has a resistance gene, such as a particular ß-lactamase, it can share that genetic material with the rest of the colony, effectively and rapidly spreading resistance to all the millions of bacteria. Next thing you know, the entire abscess is equipped to resist the antibiotic. It is a bit more complicated in reality, but hopefully this paints the picture for the purpose of this conversation.

Bacteria are always learning. Due to their elegant yet simplistic design, genetic material can pass through the cell wall and become incorporated directly into the DNA or it can be employed by ribosomes to produce proteins through RNA. There are three clever ways this can happen. Cells can hook up and share genetics, a bit like sex for an asexual species (conjugation). They can get infected with a virus called a bacteriophage that spreads the resistant genes instead of their own viral genetics (transduction). Everything inside a bacterium spills out when it dies. The naked DNA floating around can cross the cell membrane of surrounding bacteria and become integrated into their DNA (natural transformation).

The more pressure we put on bacteria with antibiotics, the more clever they become. And the more they share what they learn. We can't think of antibiotics as the ultimate weapon. They are a tool we can use to better equip the patient's own immune system to restore the proper balance of power. If we can shift the battle favorably for patients, their immune system can do the rest. If we rely on the antibiotic to kill every bug in the infection, that type of thinking will result in significant antibiotic overuse and, ultimately, further resistance.

The counterattack...

Antibiotic resistance is clearly a major problem. In the constant struggle for power between humans and microorganisms, we continue to develop strategies for the fight. When bacteria produce the ß-lactamase enzyme to break open the ß-lactam ring of amoxicillin, one of our counter attacks is a ß-lactamase inhibitor like clavulanic acid. Clavulanic acid is a "suicide enzyme" that attaches irreversibly to ß-lactamase and debilitates it. It is like sacrificial body armor that protects the ß-lactam ring as it effectively destroys the cell wall. Augmentin is the combination of amoxicillin and clavulanic acid. It broadens the coverage of amoxicillin against many ß-lactamase producing bacteria.

We discovered and employed ß-lactams. They evolved and produced ß-lactamases. We discovered and employed ß-lactamase inhibitors.

Clindamycin (Lincosamide)
Clindamycin 300 mg TID (typically 5-7 days)

Clindamycin effectively stops the protein synthesis assembly line in bacterial cells. It binds to and directly inhibits bacterial ribosomes from translating RNA and making proteins. By jamming up the protein-making machine, it prevents bacteria from doing much of anything. They get stopped in their tracks. They certainly cannot replicate without ribosome function. It is bacteriostatic. And it is quite effective in the realm of odontogenic infections.

Early and late odontogenic infections are often both susceptible to clindamycin. It is effective against the common early gram-positive aerobes as well as the later gram-negative anaerobes. It has similar effectiveness to amoxicillin in early pathogens but is much more effective against the later, abscess-related pathogens.

This antibiotic has particularly good bone penetration. It can be a good choice if there is concern for osteomyelitis, which is a beast all its own, but the culture and sensitivity of the particular infection is critical in determining optimal antibiotic treatment.

Resistance

Clindamycin is not as effective against gram-negative aerobes, such as pseudomonas. Their outer envelope prevents it from entering the cell. Thankfully these are not particularly common strains in odontogenic infections. Yet clindamycin may still be effective in managing infections where one species is clindamycin resistant. This is due to the interdependent polymicrobial nature of most infections. There are many different types of bacteria. Together they have created their environment. The bacteria become interdependent. If all the other bugs are wiped out, an antibiotic can still potentially eliminate the resistant bacteria because of the drastic change in the overall environment.

There has been some regional resistance to clindamycin reported in strep anginosus and prevotella (estimated at 20% to 30%). It would be worthwhile to reach out to your local infectious disease specialists to discuss local bacterial resistance. They are good people to have on your team, especially when encountering a particularly difficult infection.

Adverse effects: gastrointestinal complications

Clindamycin has earned a reputation for causing minor to severe GI complications, particularly pseudomembranous colitis. Many people get an upset stomach, nausea or diarrhea as a side effect. But it also has a significantly higher rate of causing *Clostridioides difficile* (*C. diff*) related pseudomembranous colitis. It is contraindicated in patients with a history of *C. diff* infection.

It is ineffective against *Eikenella*, which is commonly found in periodontal pockets. Consider adding metronidazole if gram-negative anaerobes are involved and infection is not responding to surgery and clindamycin.

Azithromycin. Z-Pak (macrolide)
Azithromycin 250 mg (Take two initially then one per day for 2 to 4 more days.)

Azithromycin has a very similar mechanism of action as clindamycin. It prevents bacteria from making the proteins necessary for survival and reproduction. It cuts off their protein manufacturing by binding to the 50S ribosomal subunit, which is specifically responsible for plugging the amino acids together to form proteins (in comparison with the 30S subunit that lines them up and prepares them for the 50S subunit). It is bacteriostatic in nature.

One main benefit of azithromycin is the long half-life. It has very high tissue uptake, slowing down its elimination, and increasing the maximum tissue concentration. This is favorable for single daily dosing, and it capitalizes on the fact it is concentration dependent. It also lingers in the tissue for up to 10 days after typical dosing. It can wreak havoc on the bacteria long after the last dose. The coverage is more limited than amoxicillin, making it a reasonable alternative if a patient doesn't tolerate penicillins.

Metronidazole (Flagyl)
Metronidazole 500 mg TID (typically 5-7 days. May consider loading dose. The package insert indicates 250 to 500 mg BID-TID for 8 days.)

Metronidazole is a fascinating little antibiotic. Its small size improves its ability to penetrate into bacterial cells and through tissue that is inaccessible to common larger antibiotics. Once inside, it actually hijacks the anaerobic portion of the Krebs cycle. It steals two electrons during fermentation and ultimately gives them to a couple of oxygen molecules. The pair of oxygen molecules, armed with a couple extra electrons, destroys the enemy's DNA. This triggers a self-destruct mechanism from within.

The mechanism of action for metronidazole, from uptake to the formation of the superoxide superhero, happens in the absence of oxygen. It only occurs in anaerobic conditions. Most severe oral infections that persist and spread transition to an anaerobic environment and can become more difficult to penetrate with other antibiotics. This is where metronidazole can save the day. If the initial report on a culture shows gram-negative rods, think about adding metronidazole. It won't do anything to the aerobic or facultative anaerobic bugs, so it works best in combination therapy with one of the other favorite drugs like Augmentin or clindamycin.

When antibiotic therapy disrupts the normal gut microbiome, the fastidious anaerobic organism *C. diff* flourishes. This overgrowth causes pseudomembranous colitis, which is inflammation and sloughing of the colon's lining. Many of our antibiotics of choice, like clindamycin, azithromycin and amoxicillin, are known to cause this devastating process. But metronidazole actually treats it. It can infiltrate the bacteria and destroy it. Consider including it when a patient with a history of *C. diff* needs antibiotics.

Mixing alcohol and metronidazole causes a severe hangover. It stops the body's process of ethanol metabolism at the worst possible step. Ethanol is initially converted by alcohol dehydrogenase into acetaldehyde, the toxic metabolite credited with causing many of the undesirable symptoms of a hangover like headache, flushing, dizziness and nausea. Apart from sobriety, aldehyde dehydrogenase is the ultimate hangover cure. It is the enzyme the body uses to break down the toxic acetaldehyde into acetic acid. It is speculated that metronidazole blocks aldehyde dehydrogenase, causing a huge buildup of acetaldehyde and its terrible sequelae. How much alcohol is safe while on or even for a few days after taking metronidazole? None. Absolutely none. Make sure patients know this so they can avoid turning a bit of wine into a raging hangover. Even the alcohol in mouth rinse can cause side effects.

Fluoroquinolones (moxifloxacin)

Moxifloxacin 400 mg QD (typically 5-10 days)

Bacterial cells have double stranded DNA that is duplicated before the cell splits into two. A replication fork unwinds and splits the DNA, which is followed by formation of matching strands by DNA transcriptase. As this goes, the coil gets tight in front of the fork. A protein called DNA gyrase helps keep it straight. The two new double DNA strands are untangled by a protein called Topoisomerase IV. The quinolone ring in fluoroquinolones binds to these proteins, destroying the DNA, triggering a self-destruct sequence of the cell. Fluoroquinolones are effective against both gram-positive and gram-negative organisms, although the mechanism is slightly different for each. It binds primarily to the DNA gyrase in gram-negative and primarily the topoisomerase IV in the gram-positive. Aren't the details fascinating?

This class of medications has its own Achilles heel. They cause a dangerous increase in an enzyme called matrix metalloproteinase (MMP). The expression of this type of enzyme is very tightly controlled. It is an important tool in tendon healing, breaking up the proteins holding the tendon together in a very calculated and strictly governed way. But the quinolones crank up MMP production, causing generalized tendon micro destruction. This increases the risk of tendon injury, ranging from an annoying tendonitis to a devastating rupture of the Achilles tendon. We must warn patients of this risk when we prescribe these antibiotics. They should be cautious when exercising and attentive to their body if they experience symptoms of tendonitis.

Concentration-dependent vs time-dependent killing

We want to prescribe the optimal dosage and antibiotic scheduling to quickly kill the most bacteria with the least side effects. The antibiotic's dynamic activity or effect on the bacteria is called pharmacodynamics. One key thing in pharmacodynamics is the minimum drug concentration needed in the tissue to inhibit bacteria growth. This is called the minimum inhibitory concentration, or MIC. We will come back to this in just a bit.

We also need to understand how much of the drug actually makes it to the site. This involves absorption in the GI tract, transportation through the blood, deposition in the site and metabolism. The kinetics or movement of the drug through the body or the system is called pharmacokinetics. When the patient takes the medication, how does it get to the site? And what is the concentration in that site over time after administration?

Pharmacodynamics: How the drug acts on the body. Study of drugs and what they change.
Pharmacokinetics: How the body acts on the drug. Study of drugs and their movement.

As clinicians, we rely on the dedicated scientists, doctors and companies studying these medications to help us optimize the pharmacodynamics and pharmacokinetics for our patients. There is a lot yet to learn in these areas, and there is some contradicting information. It seems to me that when good science is contradictory, there is something yet to be discovered that can resolve the inconsistency.

Some antibiotics exhibit concentration dependent killing, relying on a high concentration to be effective, while others are time dependent, keeping the concentration above the MIC during treatment.

Concentration-dependent: The heavy hitter. Hits them with a big slug of antibiotics less frequently. Does not need to maintain a high concentration throughout the treatment. Max concentration is what matters. This is the peak of the curve. When adequate peak level is achieved, the effects persist as the concentration decreases. Increasing administration frequency is not necessarily beneficial. (Azithromycin and metronidazole)

Time-dependent: The long squeeze. Maintaining adequate concentration above the MIC over time keeps the pressure on. Higher concentration has no real benefit. Higher doses are not better. (Amoxicillin, Augmentin, cephalexin)

Concentration and time dependent: Keep hitting them. Hitting harder is better. This is visualized by the area under the curve. It is most effective when the area is greatest. (Clindamycin)

The two main ways this applies to our daily practice are loading doses and missed doses.

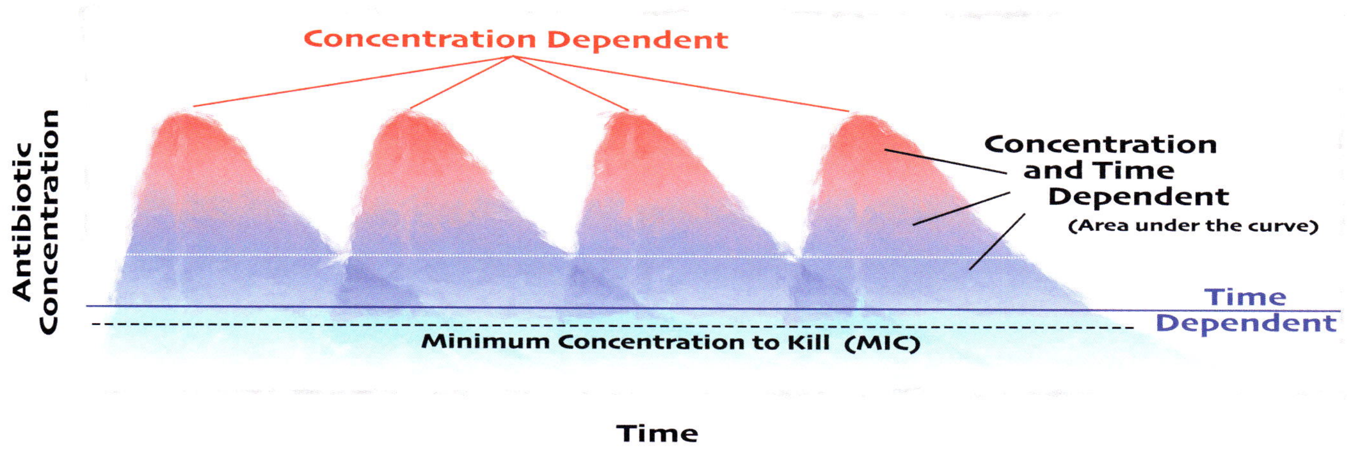

Figure 10-15 Antibiotics are classified as concentration dependent, time dependent, or concentration and time dependent. Concentration dependent antibiotics must reach adequate peak levels to be effective. Time dependent antibiotics must remain above a minimum concentration continually throughout treatment to be effective. Concentration and time dependent antibiotics benefit from both maximum concentration and consistent concentration above an effective amount. Notice the rough brush strokes on this graph. In practice, antibiotic dosing is not a perfect science. Rather, it is an art guided by these basic principles.

Loading dose

If an antibiotic is concentration dependent, a higher initial dose known as a loading dose may be beneficial. We see this in dosing azithromycin as a Z-Pak. The initial dose is 500 mg (two 250 mg tablets) followed by one tablet per day for three or five days. There is some potential benefit in a loading dose of clindamycin as it is both time and concentration dependent. A loading dose is much less beneficial for time dependent antibiotics such as amoxicillin.

Missed dose

When patients miss a dose of an antibiotic, what should they do? If it is time dependent, they should get the dose in as soon as possible to raise the concentration back above the MIC. Sometimes patients may decide to take a double dose to make up for the missed dose. This is not helpful in time dependent antibiotics, but it may be beneficial if the antibiotic is concentration dependent. This is a clinical decision that depends on the severity of the infection. Azithromycin's half life is so long patients may be fine just taking it as soon as possible and then continuing on that timeline.

Risks of antibiotic treatment

Allergy

Allergic reaction is the most common risk associated with antibiotic treatment. Proper evaluation and documenting previous antibiotic tolerance is important. If patients experience itchiness, rash, tongue, or throat swelling or difficulty breathing, they should be instructed to immediately take 50 mg of oral Benadryl, discontinue the antibiotic and go to the nearest emergency department if their symptoms become severe.

Many patients report allergies to medications that are not true allergies. They may have had previous untoward side effects or may have been told they had an allergy as a child that may not be clinically relevant as they age. It is advisable to avoid prescribing medications patients report on their allergy list. If a particular antibiotic on their list is strongly preferred and they didn't have true allergic symptoms, or if they report it only as a young child, consider referral for allergy testing.

At times, trying an antibiotic may be considered with sound clinical judgment and a well-documented conversation about the risks and benefits. In these cases, bear in mind the risk to the patient and potential medicolegal risk. The patient must have either had a very minimal reaction at a young age or clearly non-allergic reaction. And the potential antibiotic must clearly be the best choice for the situation. If this is the case, proceed with caution and document your discussion and decision-making process clearly and completely.

Diarrhea and *C. diff*

There is solid evidence showing risks of antibiotics increase with treatment duration. This is especially true regarding microbiome disruption and the potential risk of a *C. diff* infection[21]. Our first line antibiotics for odontogenic infections are quite effective because of their broad spectrum of coverage. They kill a lot of different bugs. But they don't often kill *C. diff*, a gram-positive anaerobic rod common in the normal gut flora. This particular bacterium has developed multiple mechanisms of resistance to many different antibiotics, including the common antibiotics we use for oral infections.

Table 10-7 Relationship between our most common antibiotics and *C. diff*

Highest risk	Lower risk	Treatment for *C. diff*
Clindamycin	Other penicillins (Penicillin, Augmentin)	Metronidazole
Amoxicillin	Macrolides (Azithromycin)	Vancomycin
Cephalosporins		
Fluoroquinolones (Moxifloxacin)		

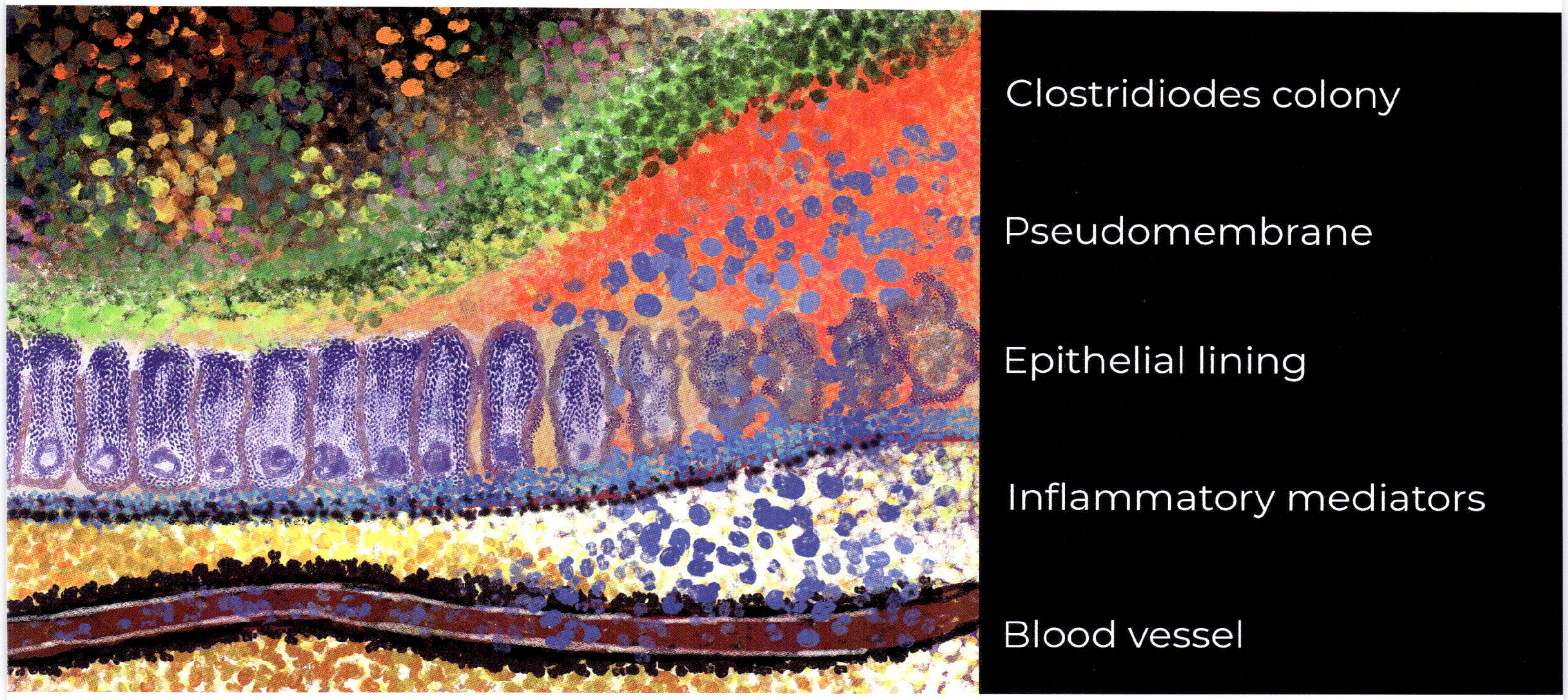

Figure 10-16 When clostridiodes difficile bacteria overwhelm the columnar lining of the colon, a tremendous increase in inflammatory mediators rushes to the area. The inflammation, in combination with toxins from the bacteria, cause significant destruction of the epithelial cells forming an inflamed pseudo membrane. This disrupts normal function, leading to debilitating diarrhea and devastating complications.

Administering these antibiotics wipes out the competition in the colon, clearing the way for *C. diff* overgrowth. The accompanying increase in exotoxin production by *C. diff* is the main issue. This bacterium excretes a few proteins that are extremely toxic to the cells lining the colon. They end up dying and sloughing off. Large portions of this sloughing debris look like white-yellow patches called pseudomembranes. This causes enormous, localized swelling in the colon referred to as colitis. The dysfunction and debilitation caused by pseudomembranous colitis ranges from severely disruptive to deadly, depending on the host and virulence of the infection.

Many antibiotics cause GI symptoms: nausea, vomiting and diarrhea. But if a patient has more than three watery stools in 24 hours during or shortly after antibiotic treatment, they must be evaluated and treated for a *C. diff* infection. In these cases, it would be wise to consider immediately referring to a primary care physician or GI specialist. Early and effective treatment can significantly improve the outcome of this potentially devastating illness. Two common antibiotic treatments are oral vancomycin (125-250 mg QID) or metronidazole (500 mg TID). *C. diff* infection and pseudomembranous colitis have been the cause for many lawsuits, so make sure documentation is clear regarding the reason for prescribing the antibiotic and for timely referral if patients are experiencing significant GI symptoms.

Yeast infection

Our microbiome includes yeast. When the normal flora is disrupted, an opportunistic Candidal overgrowth can occur. Oral thrush and yeast vaginitis occur commonly after antibiotic therapy. If a patient develops signs of oral thrush (creamy white areas covering areas of the oral cavity and/or oropharynx with or without pain or burning symptoms), consider a nystatin rinse or other topical treatment. Vaginal symptoms can be treated with topical OTC treatment, such as miconazole cream. Additionally, a single dose of oral fluconazole 150 mg is often effective. If the symptoms persist after 72 hours, another dose may be indicated. Patients may report a history of yeast infection. Consider prophylactic treatment or possibly providing a prescription in the event they develop symptoms.

Interesting aside. Dentures can harbor yeast and cause persistent candida infection if not cleaned properly. In addition to commercially available denture cleaners, one study showed the potential benefit of microwave disinfection[22].

Probiotics

There are hundreds of different species of bacteria in the gut, all playing their part in our health. And they rely on each other. Having lived my entire life with them, I find it difficult to truly grasp their expanse and impact on my life. When I write out 39 trillion (an estimated population of your microbiome at a recent census) it just doesn't really compute. There are a lot of zeroes. And they are all playing together in the symphony of our health. As you sit here reading this, your body is far more than just the cells present after generations of mitotic division and cell differentiation that began in utero. You are profoundly influenced by the bacterial colonists that join you on your journey through life.

The broad-spectrum antibiotics we often take for granted for preventing and treating oral infections ravage this delicate ecosystem. The colorful and diverse system can lose its balance—and that is a huge number of microorganisms to get back on track. One of the big frontiers in medicine transforming the way we think and work is the microbiome. We have learned a lot in the past 20 years. And we have a lot left to learn.

TREATMENT OPTIONS FOR ORAL CANDIDA INFECTION

Nystatin rinse, 400,000-600,000 units 4-6 mL. Swish and gargle for 30 seconds and swallow. Continue for 48 hours after resolution of symptoms.

Clotrimazole troche, 10 mg. Dissolve in mouth completely and slowly five times per day for 14 days.

Miconazole gel, QID. Apply after meals to affected areas for 10 days.

Oral fluconazole, 200 mg 1st day, then 100 mg daily for 14 days.

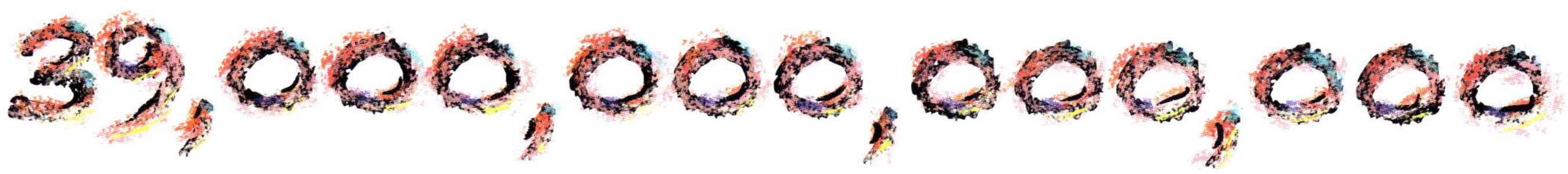

Figure 10-17 Average microbiome population.

I get the sense many people erroneously believe probiotics help restore the microbiome population in the wake of antibiotics. They have been shown to decrease the risk of antibiotic related diarrhea and the development of *C. diff* infections. They are protective indeed. But probiotics actually delay microbiome homeostasis[23]. Think about this: The microbiome is like a coral reef. The more diverse and colorful, the healthier. And each reef is unique. The balance of the fragile ecosystem is built on the interdependence of the various species on each other. Let's say a bunch of the Blue Tangs and Sergeant Majors were suddenly wiped out. Would it make sense to introduce 50 billion clownfish, expecting them to restore the reef to its original diversity? Repopulating or "proactively engineering" the microbiome through probiotics decreases the likelihood of a hostile takeover by such strains as *C. diff*, but reef dynamics take a long time to return to their baseline. Major research is going into identifying and studying microbiome genetics and compositions.

Coadministration of probiotics and antibiotics has been shown to reduce antibiotic associated diarrhea by 58% and *C. diff* infection by 66%[24]. Current supporting data appears to be of moderate quality. More studies are needed to increase the confidence and scientific support to further dial in treatment protocols. It seems like we are heading for a time when analyzing a fecal sample could direct precise therapies to control and optimize the microbiome. In the meantime, the best information I can find seems to promote taking Lactobacillus rhamnosus GG with a minimal daily dose of 2×10^9 CFU concurrently with antibiotics and for 7 to 14 days afterward. A multi-strain formulation of Lactobacillus rhamnosus GG, Lactobacillus acidophilus LA-5, Bifidobacterium lactis BB-12 has also been shown to be quite effective at preventing antibiotic associated diarrhea. A general rule of thumb is to get refrigerated probiotics. The bacteria are better preserved and more effective.

Fecal microbiota transplantation (FMT) is an astounding new territory. It has been shown to be effective as a treatment and even a cure for many different diseases and illnesses[25]. It impacts metabolism, energy level, mood, hormones—pretty much everything. Undoubtedly, significant progress is being made between when I am sitting here writing this and when you read it. Fecal transplants may be a key to health care in the future. (That is some good shit.)

Topical antibiotic and antiseptic therapy

Chlorhexidine

The chlorhexidine molecule has fantastic antimicrobial properties. It dissociates into a positively charged cation that binds to the negatively charged phospholipids found in bacterial cell walls. Depending on the concentration, this can disrupt or destroy the cell wall. It is bacteriostatic at lower concentrations and bactericidal at higher concentrations. By compromising the cell wall, it can pass into the cytoplasm, causing disruption from within the cell by its positive charge. The increased permeability also causes the smaller stuff in the cytoplasm to leak out, further compromising the microorganism's viability.

This broad-spectrum agent seems to bind a bit better to gram-positive cell walls, requiring slightly lower concentration for cell death than gram-negative bacteria. In adequate concentration, it is quite effective against most bacteria.

The positive charge of chlorhexidine gluconate binds to the surface proteins of skin and mucosa, causing it to hang around for a few hours. This further improves the effects as an oral rinse or topical antiseptic. Its positive charge can also bind to negatively charged components in the biofilm and even the surface of titanium. By killing plaque producing bacteria, it effectively reduces plaque accumulation[16].

Uses

Commercially available chlorhexidine gluconate 0.12% (Peridex) is commonly used perioperatively in oral surgery as well as in various periodontal treatment protocols. It is most commonly prescribed to swish for 30 seconds and spit. The 30 seconds is important as it allows adequate protein binding and exposure of the bacteria. Less time will decrease protein binding to both the bacterial cell wall (decreasing bactericidal effects) and the mucosal cells (decreasing duration of effect). As humans, we tend to underestimate time on things like this, so I recommend patients set a timer. Even if they don't set a timer, they may be more likely to rinse longer if they were instructed to time it.

The benefit of chlorhexidine application lasts longer than the 30 second rinse due to the protein binding. As such, it is important to instruct patients to avoid putting anything in their mouth for 30 minutes after rinsing. If possible, it should be the last thing they do before going to bed, after they brush and floss. It is also most beneficial if applied in the morning after routine hygiene and even after breakfast, if that is reasonably possible. Sometimes we need to find the line between ideal and practical.

There are three main perioperative timeframes when chlorhexidine is often used: days leading up to surgery, immediately before surgery and after surgery. When prescribed for the days leading up to surgery, it may decrease infection related post-operative complications by decreasing the bacterial load. Immediate pre-operative use also decreases the bacterial burden. It doesn't result in a sterile environment, but it certainly can make it cleaner. The standard operating procedure in my practice is for every surgical patient to rinse for 30 seconds prior to surgery.

Post-operative use also can be beneficial. I have found it is most valuable in more invasive cases or after grafting or implant placement. I also prescribe it after coronectomy procedures, which have a slightly higher potential for infection due to the retained tooth root. The risk of post-operative infection decreases after the initial healing when the epithelium has been restored. Treatment duration may be debated, but I typically recommend patients continue it for 7 to 10 days, longer if there is a concern with healing.

Chlorhexidine is a great option to treat symptomatic pericoronitis of a partially impacted third molar. Consider instructing the patient to irrigate under the inflamed tissue with a curved tip syringe and then rinse for 30 seconds to optimize the benefit. The ideal treatment would be removing the offending tooth, but when it cannot be immediately removed, this may be very helpful.

Side effects

The biggest complaint I encounter is the undesirable dark staining of the teeth and tongue. There are several potential causes for this, the most likely related to plaque and chromogenic or pigmented foods, such as coffee, tea and red wine. The more plaque, the more staining. Patients don't seem happy when they are told their coffee or wine is contributing to their unpleasant smile. There is some evidence a dental cleaning prior to starting the rinse can decrease staining. While chlorhexidine gluconate effectively decreases plaque accumulation, it somehow increases calculus formation. This also seems to be impacted by the presence of plaque prior to treatment.

Some patients don't tolerate the bitter taste very well. It often resolves in 30 minutes but can persist for hours. And some may report a generalized metallic taste during and after treatment. While this may be disturbing for patients, it is typically transient[16-18].

Homeopathic alternative

Other topical antibacterial products that show potential benefits over chlorhexidine are coming to the market. To date, the most promoted of these is VEGA gel (StellaLife). While it has been shown to have decreased but adequate overall antibacterial properties compared to chlorhexidine in lab studies, it has significantly better cellular compatibility[19]. This alternative has been shown to improve the overall outcome by reducing infection and optimizing tissue healing[20]. And it does this without the bitter taste and staining that accompanies chlorhexidine.

OraCare

Another fascinating topical antiseptic gaining popularity is chlorine dioxide (OraCare). When the two liquids containing HCl and $NaClO_2$ are combined, they form chlorine dioxide gas (ClO_2). The unique properties of the dissolved gas allow it to penetrate into areas inaccessible to traditional liquid agents. The oxidizing power of ClO_2 permeates farther into the deepest darkest areas harboring the most tenacious bacteria.

The unresolving infection and post-operative infection

Proceed with caution!

These can be the worst. As providers, we are less likely to provide an appropriate level of care if we have seen the patient multiple times as they progress, or if the infection is following our own treatment[26]. When patients come in seeking a second opinion, it is much more common for more appropriate or aggressive diagnostics and treatment to be rendered. It is in our psyche as highly trained and experienced providers to put on blinders and protect ourselves from our own internal critics. We are much less likely to catch a case of osteomyelitis if we have seen the patient multiple times in the weeks following a procedure. It seems we are much more likely to properly work up a patient and suspect and adequately treat it if we were not the initial provider. In an article by the Risk Assessment department of the Oral and Maxillofacial Surgeons National Insurance Company (OMSNIC), it was recommended that we implement a system for assessing patients if their problem doesn't resolve after the third post-operative visit[26].

Set up a system to protect the patients in your practice before the need arises. Systems make it easier to do the best thing. It would also be helpful to think through when patients might benefit from referral to another oral surgeon within a group practice or to an outside surgeon in a solo practice.

This system should include:

1. A radiograph of the affected area.
2. A review of the chart, including the temperature trend of the patient (taken on all post-operative visits).
3. Questioning the patient on his or her progress (whether there was improvement with antibiotic therapy or when dressings were changed and for how long).
4. An assessment of whether the symptoms and treatment rendered supported the post-operative diagnosis or whether there could be another diagnosis.

"Much of the trouble we face [medicolegally] stems from failure to diagnose a bigger underlying issue, failure to recruit the help of our surgical or infectious disease colleagues, failure to obtain adequate studies (CT scan, cultures, blood workup) and failure to recognize the progression of something that seemed minor but didn't resolve."[26]

Real World Challenge

Decision making is most challenging when there isn't an obvious indication or contraindication. The ends of the spectrum are obvious, but the art is in the shades of gray. And that is the real world we all live in every day.

When a patient is scheduled in three days for surgery and the tooth flares up, what do you do? It seems to be minor swelling and there is no sign of airway compromise.

You get a call on Saturday about some increasing swelling on post-op day 5 after uncomplicated removal of third molars.

These are the real dilemmas our patients rely on us to navigate with them. I have provided some navigational beacons and a compass of sorts, but the actual journey is the art of infection management. It isn't always pretty, but it is essential.

References

1. Deo PN, Deshmukh R. Oral microbiome: Unveiling the fundamentals. J Oral Maxillofac Pathol. 2019;23(1):122-128.
2. Vieira F, Allen SM, Stocks RMS, et al. Deep neck infection. Otolaryngol Clin North Am. 2008 Jun;41(3):459-483, vii.
3. Taub D, Yampolsky A, Diecidue R, Gold L. Controversies in the Management of Oral and Maxillofacial Infections. Oral Maxillofac Surg Clin North Am. 2017 Nov;29(4):465-473.
4. Aas JA, Paster BJ, Stokes LN, et al. Defining the normal bacterial flora of the oral cavity. J Clin Microbiol. 2005 Nov;43(11):5721-5732.
5. Szabo G, Saha B. Alcohol's Effect on Host Defense. Alcohol Res. 2015;37(2):159-170.
6. Berbudi A, Rahmadika N, Tjahjadi AI, et al. Type 2 Diabetes and its Impact on the Immune System. Curr Diabetes Rev. 2020 May;16(5):442-449.
7. Ogura I, Minami Y, Sugawara Y, et al. Odontogenic Infection Pathway to the Parapharyngeal Space: CT Imaging Assessment. J Maxillofac Oral Surg. 2022 Mar;21(1):235-239.
8. Kinzer S, Pfeiffer J, Becker S, et al. Severe deep neck space infections and mediastinitis of odontogenic origin: clinical relevance and implications for diagnosis and treatment. Acta Otolaryngol. 2009 Jan;129(1):62-70.
9. Allen RJ, Waclaw B. Bacterial growth: a statistical physicist's guide. Rep Prog Phys. 2019 Jan;82(1):016601.
10. Osborn TM, Assael LA, Bell RB. Deep space neck infection: principles of surgical management. Oral Maxillofac Surg Clin North Am. 2008 Aug;20(3):353-365.
11. Hupp JR, Tucker MR, Ellis E, editors. Contemporary oral and maxillofacial surgery. 7th ed. Philadelphia, PA: Elsevier; 2019.
12. Miloro M, Ghali GE, Larsen P, et al. Peterson's principles of oral and maxillofacial surgery. 3rd ed. Shelton: People's Medical Publishing House; 2012.
13. Caruso SR, Yamaguchi E, Portnof JE. Update on Antimicrobial Therapy in Management of Acute Odontogenic Infection in Oral and Maxillofacial Surgery. Oral Maxillofac Surg Clin North Am. 2022 Feb;34(1):169-177.
14. Costelloe C, Metcalfe C, Lovering A, et al. Effect of antibiotic prescribing in primary care on antimicrobial resistance in individual patients: systematic review and meta-analysis. BMJ. 2010 May 18;340:c2096.
15. Yip DW, Gerriets V. Penicillin. In: StatPearls [Internet]. Treasure Island (FL): StatPearls Publishing; 2022 [cited 2022 Dec 17]. Available from: http://www.ncbi.nlm.nih.gov/books/NBK554560/
16. Lim KS, Kam PCA. Chlorhexidine - Pharmacology and Clinical Applications. Anaesth Intensive Care. 2008 Jul;36(4):502-512.
17. Cheung HY, Wong MMK, Cheung SH, et al. Differential Actions of Chlorhexidine on the Cell Wall of Bacillus subtilis and Escherichia coli. PLoS One. 2012;7(5):e36659.
18. Zanatta FB, Antoniazzi RP, Rösing CK. Staining and calculus formation after 0.12% chlorhexidine rinses in plaque-free and plaque covered surfaces: a randomized trial. J Appl Oral Sci. 2010 Sep-Oct;18(5):515-521.
19. Fujioka-Kobayashi M, Schaller B, Pikos MA, et al. Cytotoxicity and Gene Expression Changes of a Novel Homeopathic Antiseptic Oral Rinse in Comparison to Chlorhexidine in Gingival Fibroblasts. Materials (Basel). 2020 Jul 17;13(14):3190.
20. Wyganowska-Swiatkowska M, Kotwicka M, Urbaniak P, et al. Clinical implications of the growth-suppressive effects of chlorhexidine at low and high concentrations on human gingival fibroblasts and changes in morphology. Int J Mol Med. 2016 Jun;37(6):1594-1600.
21. Zar FA, Bakkanagari SR, Moorthi KMLST, et al. A comparison of vancomycin and metronidazole for the treatment of Clostridium difficile-associated diarrhea, stratified by disease severity. Clin Infect Dis. 2007 Aug 1;45(3):302-307.
22. Klironomos T, Katsimpali A, Polyzois G. The Effect of Microwave Disinfection on Denture Base Polymers, Liners and Teeth: A Basic Overview. Acta Stomatol Croat. 2015 Sep;49(3):242-253.
23. Suez J, Zmora N, Zilberman-Schapira G, et al. Post-Antibiotic Gut Mucosal Microbiome Reconstitution Is Impaired by Probiotics and Improved by Autologous FMT. Cell. 2018 Sep 6;174(6):1406-1423.e16.
24. Goodman C, Keating G, Georgousopoulou E, et al. Probiotics for the prevention of antibiotic-associated diarrhoea: a systematic review and meta-analysis. BMJ Open. 2021 Aug 12;11(8):e043054.
25. Vindigni SM, Surawicz CM. Fecal Microbiota Transplantation. Gastroenterol Clin North Am. 2017 Mar;46(1):171-185.
26. Holmes SM, Udey DK. What are the lessons we can glean from a review of recent closed malpractice cases involving oral and maxillofacial infections? Oral Maxillofac Surg Clin North Am. 2011 Nov;23(4):601-607, vii.

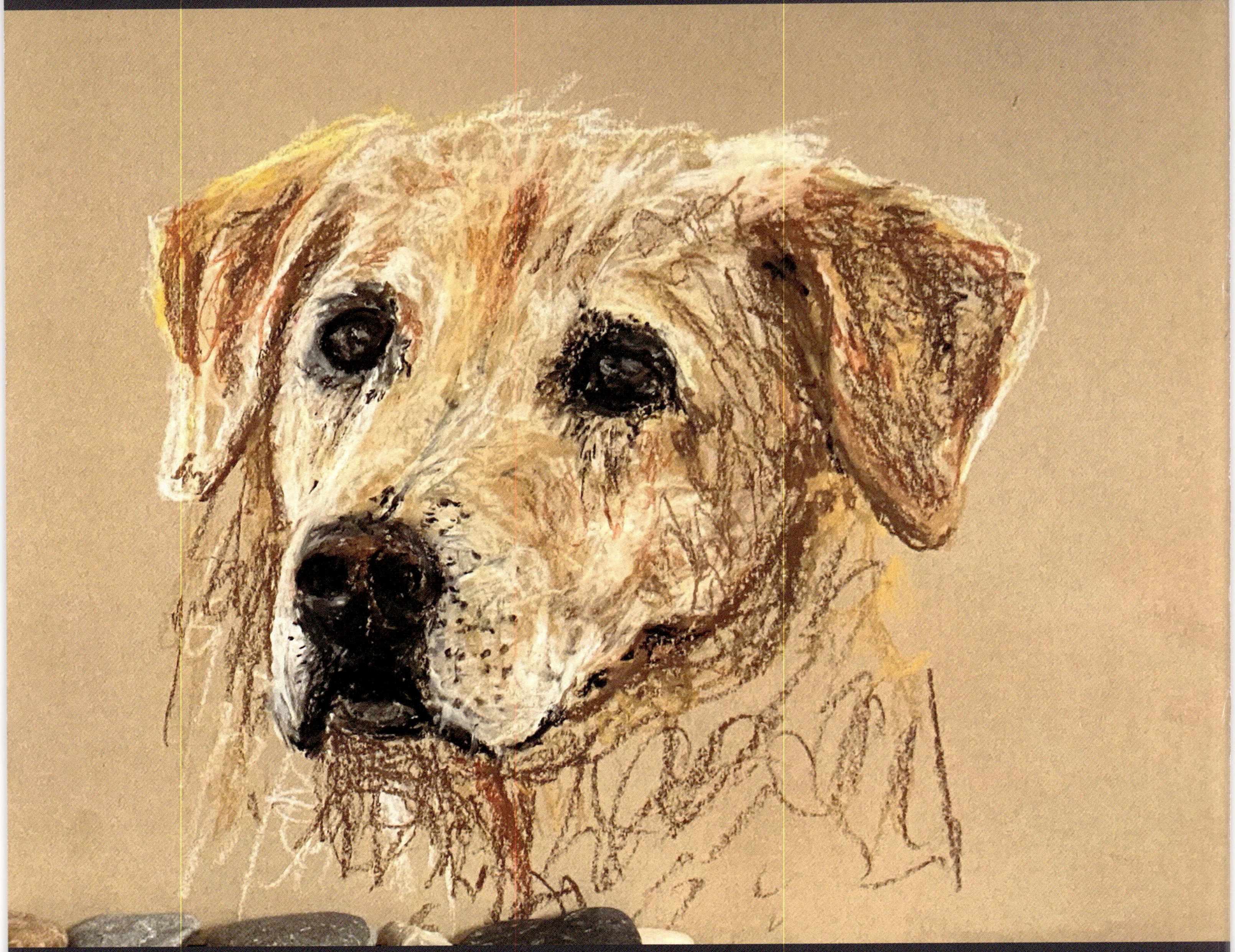

Jack and the Rocks. (Oil pastel accompanied by Lake Michigan rocks.)
Knowing eyes. Jack saw us through thick and thin for 14 years. He loved it when we would go to the beach to pick rocks. It was his favorite place.

ACKNOWLEDGMENTS

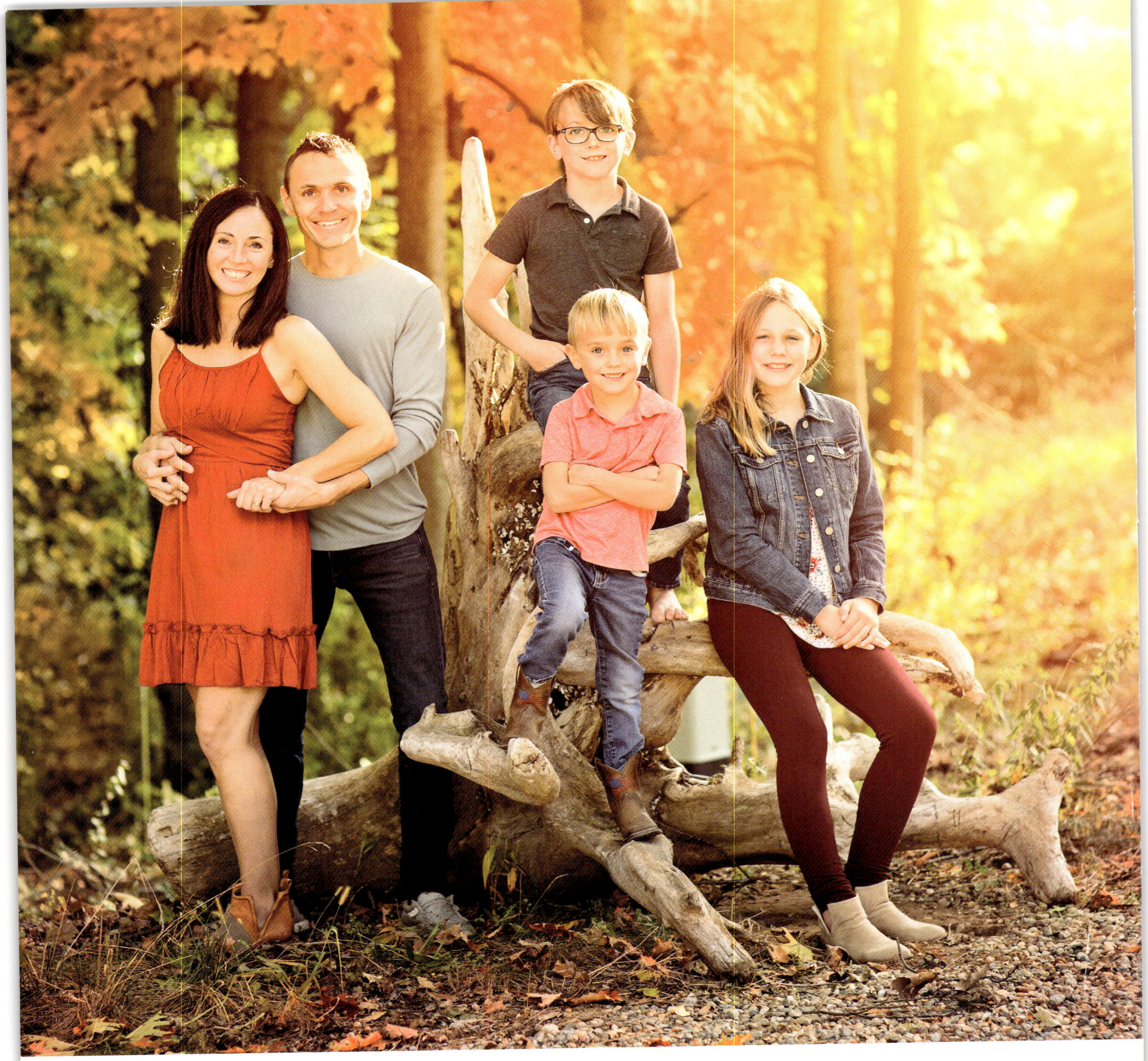

Anderson family photo courtesy of Christi and Corban Nelson Photography.

To Lindsey, the love of my life and my best friend.

To Ellyana, Silas and Micah. Pursue your dreams. Try the impossible. Stay curious and loving. Life is a whole lot bigger and more beautiful than we can even imagine.

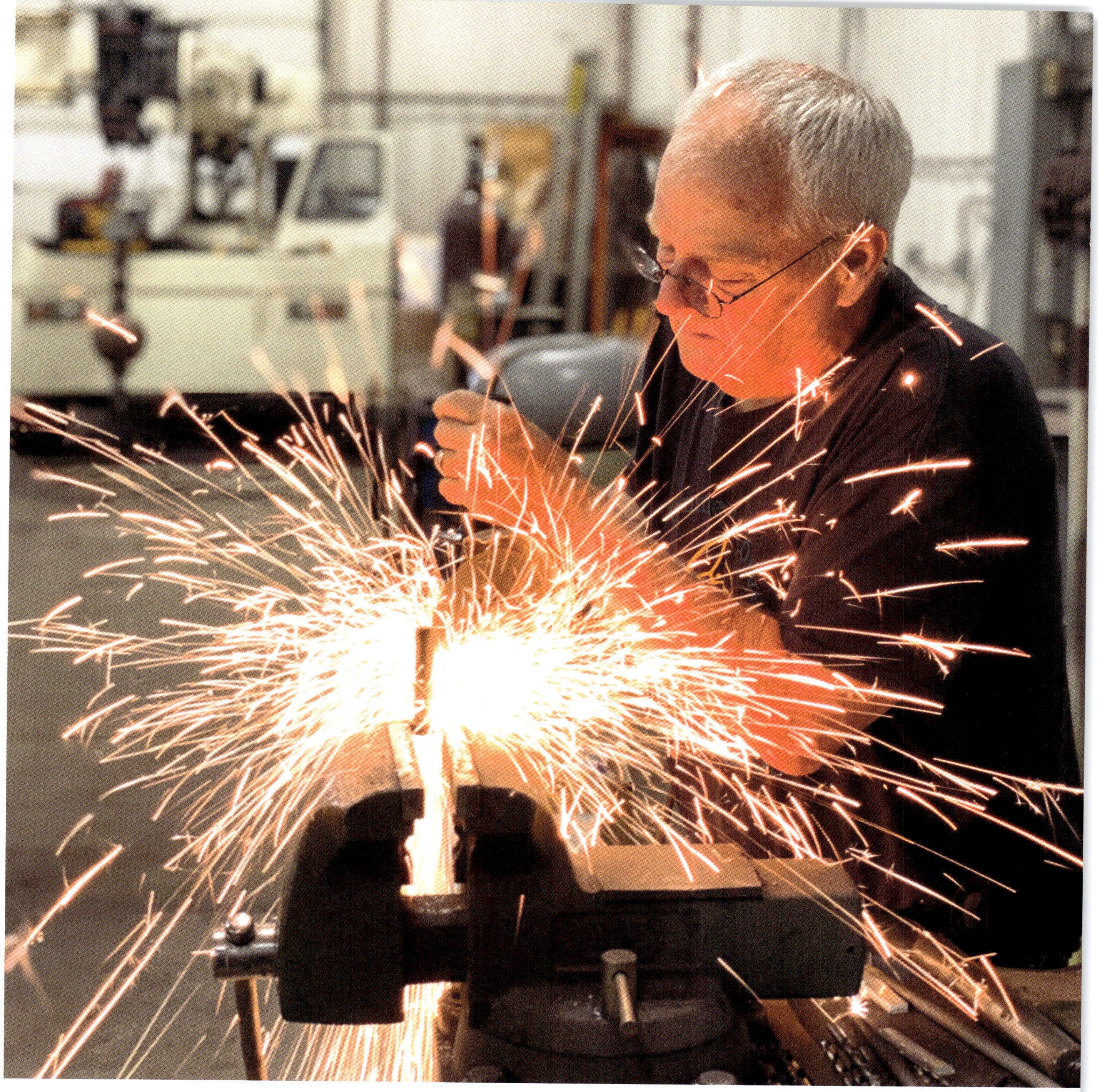

To Bill Carnes, your friendship meant the world to me.
Here's to overthinking every solution, and then welding them into existence in your shop. No matter what wild project we were working on, I could always just be me with you. I learned so much from you. Wish I could have shared this final project with you. My kids miss their grandpa. I miss you.

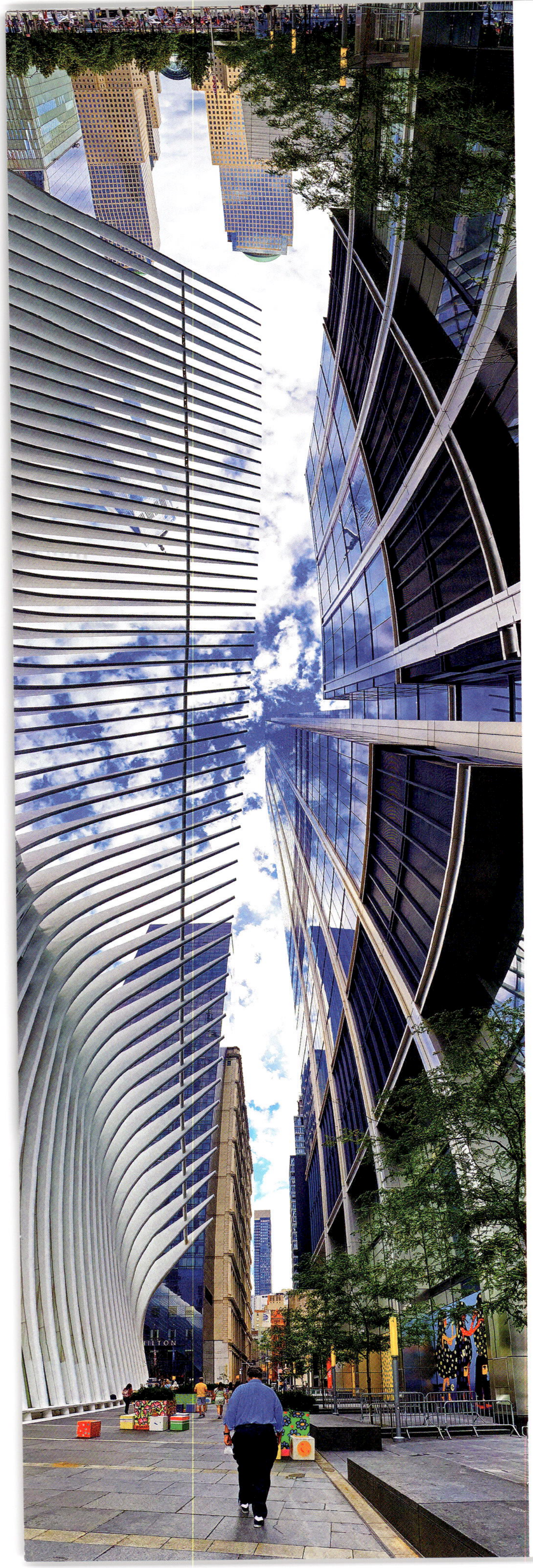

To Mark Ferber, for seeing more in me than I could have ever imagined was there and for gently helping me see it too. My deep appreciation for your guidance and mentorship are surpassed only by your friendship. Thank you for your gracious discernment as you worked so closely with me to bring this to life, not only for our own entertainment, but for the greater good. Thank you for believing in me.

To mom and dad, for all the talent and feedback you have given me on this project. For teaching me to question and lean in.

To my team, you believe in me and graciously trust me. Your endless patience created space for me to explore and develop *The Art of Oral Surgery*. Your gloved hands in the pictures throughout the pages of this book are proof of your support.

To my patients, who put up with me taking photos in some of the most awkward ways. Thank you for your patience as you allowed me to share this work with the world.

Catching and keeping the vision.
NYC 2021

To my family. Go out and be creative. As we grow up, it seems like some of us become scared of making our own art. It feels like our creative spirit gets shut down. I want to encourage every person reading this book to go out and try creating some art, just for the fun of it. Give yourself space to make something beautiful or awful. No judging. Anything you don't like, call it a study. Then when you make something that looks or feels beautiful to you, enjoy it. Maybe even share it.

Family Beach Sunset. Micah Anderson age 5. (Oil Pastel on paper.)

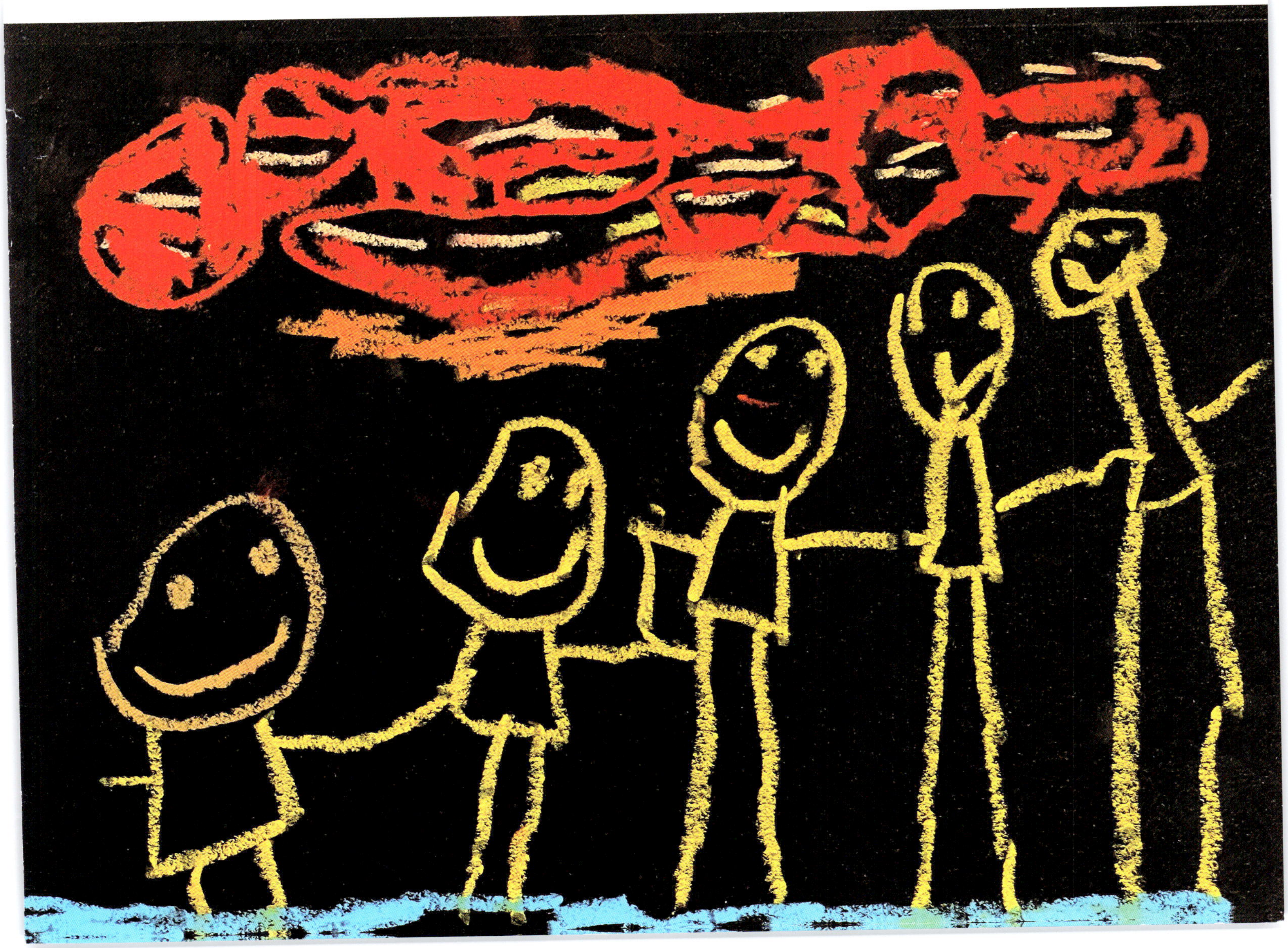